Pediatric Mental Health

A Compendium of AAP Clinical Practice Guidelines and Policies

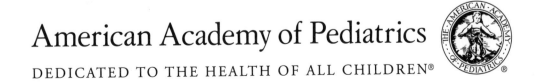

American Academy of Pediatrics

DEDICATED TO THE HEALTH OF ALL CHILDREN®

AMERICAN ACADEMY OF PEDIATRICS
PUBLISHING STAFF

Mary Lou White
Chief Product and Services Officer/SVP, Membership, Marketing, and Publishing

Mark Grimes
Vice President, Publishing

Jennifer McDonald
Senior Editor, Digital Publishing

Sean Rogers
Digital Content Specialist

Leesa Levin-Doroba
Production Manager, Practice Management

Linda Smessaert, MSIMC
Senior Marketing Manager, Professional Resources

Mary Louise Carr
Marketing Manager, Clinical Publications

Published by the American Academy of Pediatrics
345 Park Blvd
Itasca, IL 60143
Telephone: 630/626-6000
Facsimile: 847/434-8000
www.aap.org

The American Academy of Pediatrics is an organization of 67,000 primary care pediatricians, pediatric medical subspecialists, and pediatric surgical specialists dedicated to the health, safety, and well-being of infants, children, adolescents, and young adults.

The recommendations in this publication do not indicate an exclusive course of treatment or serve as a standard of medical care. Variations, taking into account individual circumstances, may be appropriate.

Products are mentioned for informational purposes only. Inclusion in this publication does not imply endorsement by the American Academy of Pediatrics.

Every effort has been made to ensure that the drug selection and dosage set forth in this publication are in accordance with the current recommendations and practice at the time of publication. It is the responsibility of the health care professional to check the package insert of each drug for any change in indications and dosage and for added warnings and precautions.

This publication has been developed by the American Academy of Pediatrics. The authors, editors, and contributors are expert authorities in the field of pediatrics. No commercial involvement of any kind has been solicited or accepted in the development of the content of this publication.

Special discounts are available for bulk purchases of this publication. Email Special Sales at aapsales@aap.org for more information.

Printed in the United States of America
9-429/0419   1 2 3 4 5 6 7 8 9 10
MA0943

ISBN: 978-1-61002-364-1
eBook ISBN: 978-1-61002-365-8
Library of Congress Control Number: 2019937940

INTRODUCTION

Clinical practice guidelines have long provided physicians with evidence-based decision-making tools for managing common pediatric conditions. Policy statements issued by the American Academy of Pediatrics (AAP) are developed to provide physicians with a quick reference guide to the AAP position on child health care issues. We have combined these 2 authoritative resources into 1 comprehensive manual to provide easy access to important clinical and policy information.

This manual contains an AAP clinical practice guideline, as well as AAP policy statements, clinical reports, and technical reports.

Additional information about AAP policy can be found in a variety of professional publications such as *Pediatric Clinical Practice Guidelines & Policies*, 19th Edition; *Red Book*®, 31st Edition; and *Red Book*® *Online* (http://redbook.solutions.aap.org).

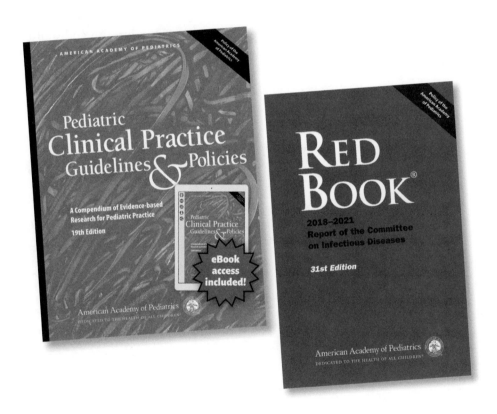

AMERICAN ACADEMY OF PEDIATRICS

The American Academy of Pediatrics (AAP) and its member pediatricians dedicate their efforts and resources to the health, safety, and well-being of infants, children, adolescents, and young adults. The AAP has approximately 67,000 members in the United States, Canada, and Latin America. Members include pediatricians, pediatric medical subspecialists, and pediatric surgical specialists.

Core Values. *We believe*

- In the inherent worth of all children; they are our most enduring and vulnerable legacy.
- Children deserve optimal health and the highest quality health care.
- Pediatricians, pediatric medical subspecialists, and pediatric surgical specialists are the best qualified to provide child health care.
- Multidisciplinary teams including patients and families are integral to delivering the highest quality health care.
- The AAP is the organization to advance child health and well-being and the profession of pediatrics.

Vision. Children have optimal health and well-being and are valued by society. American Academy of Pediatrics members practice the highest quality health care and experience professional satisfaction and personal well-being.

Mission. The mission of the AAP is to attain optimal, physical, mental, and social health and well-being for all infants, children, adolescents, and young adults. To accomplish this mission, the AAP shall support the professional needs of its members.

TABLE OF CONTENTS

FOREWORD

This is the first compendium of polices and clinical practice guidelines related to pediatric mental health from the American Academy of Pediatrics (AAP). It is timely. As highlighted in the final policy statement, "[t]he prevalence of mental health conditions in children and adolescents is increasing and, alarmingly, suicide rates are now the second leading cause of death in young people from 10 to 24 years of age." Pediatric clinicians practicing in both primary care and subspecialty settings have a unique advantage: longitudinal, trusting relationships with children, adolescents, and their families on which to build a therapeutic alliance. With frequent contact and this bond of trust, we can elicit our patients' and families' concerns, recognize risks and strengths in their social environment, partner with parents to build their children's resilience, and address emerging mental health symptoms. Our pediatric advantage positions us to provide help…and $H E L^2 P^3$ (described below).

Policies in the compendium provide clinical guidance aimed at all clinicians who provide care to children and adolescents with mental health needs—pediatricians, family physicians, emergency medicine physicians, nurse practitioners, and physician assistants. Topics run the gamut of acuity from preventive care to emergency care, with management of common conditions and care of special populations in between. Several policies include content on clinician self-care. Many go beyond the interface between clinician and patient to offer guidance on preparing the practice and organizing the health care team; collaborating with developmental and mental health specialists; engaging with other community providers of health and social services; and advocating for improvements in payment, access to care, and mental health systems of care. As such, the compendium is also a resource for child advocates and policy makers. The compendium concludes with a policy statement on the competencies—knowledge, skills, and attitudes—pediatricians need to provide mental health care to children and adolescents (including "common factors" communication techniques, abbreviated by the mnemonic $H E L^2 P^3$—an approach that is intuitive to experienced clinicians and proven effective across a wide range of mental health concerns). The statement also offers resources to assist in achieving the competencies.

The compendium is a publication of the AAP, whose mission is "to attain optimal physical, mental, and social health and well-being for all infants, children, adolescents, and young adults." Among the AAP strengths are a commitment to evidence-based medicine and hundreds of pediatric experts willing to share their expertise with others. Serving on leadership groups—committees, councils, and sections—these experts are charged with providing policies, educational programming, and resources for AAP members and the public. Given the crosscutting nature of mental health, policies in this compendium draw on the expertise of leaders across many of these leadership entities. Authors of policies do not prescribe an exclusive course of action or a standard of care. Rather, based on their review of all available data, they offer evidence-based recommendations when supported by data and consensus when data are lacking. American Academy of Pediatrics policies allow flexibility in individual situations and encourage sound clinical judgment.

I believe the guidance and resources in this compendium will motivate and help clinicians to improve the mental health of children and adolescents in their care and, as a result, enhance their patients' lifelong well-being. I also believe this compendium will assist child advocates and policy makers in creating a framework of payment, mental health consultation and specialty services, and public policy to support pediatric clinicians' critical role in providing mental health care.

Jane Meschan Foy, MD, FAAP
AAP Board of Directors, 2013–2019

SECTION 1
Attention-Deficit/ Hyperactivity Disorder

CLINICAL PRACTICE GUIDELINE

American Academy
of Pediatrics
DEDICATED TO THE HEALTH OF ALL CHILDREN™

Clinical Practice Guideline for the Diagnosis, Evaluation, and Treatment of Attention-Deficit/Hyperactivity Disorder in Children and Adolescents

Mark L. Wolraich, MD, FAAP,[a] Joseph F. Hagan, Jr, MD, FAAP,[b,c] Carla Allan, PhD,[d,e] Eugenia Chan, MD, MPH, FAAP,[f,g] Dale Davison, MSpEd, PCC,[h,i] Marian Earls, MD, MTS, FAAP,[j,k] Steven W. Evans, PhD,[l,m] Susan K. Flinn, MA,[n] Tanya Froehlich, MD, MS, FAAP,[o,p] Jennifer Frost, MD, FAAFP,[q,r] Joseph R. Holbrook, PhD, MPH,[s] Christoph Ulrich Lehmann, MD, FAAP,[t] Herschel Robert Lessin, MD, FAAP,[u] Kymika Okechukwu, MPA,[v] Karen L. Pierce, MD, DFAACAP,[w,x] Jonathan D. Winner, MD, FAAP,[y] William Zurhellen, MD, FAAP,[z] SUBCOMMITTEE ON CHILDREN AND ADOLESCENTS WITH ATTENTION-DEFICIT/HYPERACTIVE DISORDER

abstract

Attention-deficit/hyperactivity disorder (ADHD) is 1 of the most common neurobehavioral disorders of childhood and can profoundly affect children's academic achievement, well-being, and social interactions. The American Academy of Pediatrics first published clinical recommendations for evaluation and diagnosis of pediatric ADHD in 2000; recommendations for treatment followed in 2001. The guidelines were revised in 2011 and published with an accompanying process of care algorithm (PoCA) providing discrete and manageable steps by which clinicians could fulfill the clinical guideline's recommendations. Since the release of the 2011 guideline, the *Diagnostic and Statistical Manual of Mental Disorders* has been revised to the fifth edition, and new ADHD-related research has been published. These publications do not support dramatic changes to the previous recommendations. Therefore, only incremental updates have been made in this guideline revision, including the addition of a key action statement related to diagnosis and treatment of comorbid conditions in children and adolescents with ADHD. The accompanying process of care algorithm has also been updated to assist in implementing the guideline recommendations. Throughout the process of revising the guideline and algorithm, numerous systemic barriers were identified that restrict and/or hamper pediatric clinicians' ability to adopt their recommendations. Therefore, the subcommittee created a companion article (available in the Supplemental Information) on systemic barriers to the care of children and adolescents with ADHD, which identifies the major systemic-level barriers and presents recommendations to address those barriers; in this article, we support the recommendations of the clinical practice guideline and accompanying process of care algorithm.

[a]Section of Developmental and Behavioral Pediatrics, University of Oklahoma, Oklahoma City, Oklahoma; [b]Department of Pediatrics, The Robert Larner, MD, College of Medicine, The University of Vermont, Burlington, Vermont; [c]Hagan, Rinehart, and Connolly Pediatricians, PLLC, Burlington, Vermont; [d]Division of Developmental and Behavioral Health, Department of Pediatrics, Children's Mercy Kansas City, Kansas City, Missouri; [e]School of Medicine, University of Missouri-Kansas City, Kansas City, Missouri; [f]Division of Developmental Medicine, Boston Children's Hospital, Boston, Massachusetts; [g]Harvard Medical School, Harvard University, Boston, Massachusetts; [h]Children and Adults with Attention-Deficit/Hyperactivity Disorder, Lanham, Maryland; [i]Dale Davison, LLC, Skokie, Illinois; [j]Community Care of North Carolina, Raleigh, North Carolina; [k]School of Medicine, University of North Carolina, Chapel Hill, North Carolina; [l]Department of Psychology, Ohio University, Athens, Ohio; [m]Center for Intervention Research in Schools, Ohio University, Athens, Ohio; [n]American Academy of Pediatrics, Alexandria, Virginia; [o]Department of Pediatrics, University of Cincinnati, Cincinnati, Ohio; [p]Cincinnati Children's Hospital Medical Center, Cincinnati, Ohio; [q]Swope Health Services, Kansas City, Kansas; [r]American Academy of Family Physicians, Leawood, Kansas; [s]National Center on Birth Defects and Developmental Disabilities, Centers for Disease Control and Prevention, Atlanta, Georgia; [t]Departments of Biomedical Informatics and Pediatrics, Vanderbilt University, Nashville, Tennessee; [u]The Children's Medical Group, Poughkeepsie, New York;

To cite: Wolraich ML, Hagan JF, Allan C, et al. AAP SUBCOMMITTEE ON CHILDREN AND ADOLESCENTS WITH ATTENTION-DEFICIT/HYPERACTIVE DISORDER. Clinical Practice Guideline for the Diagnosis, Evaluation, and Treatment of Attention-Deficit/Hyperactivity Disorder in Children and Adolescents. *Pediatrics.* 2019;144(4):e20192528

FROM THE AMERICAN ACADEMY OF PEDIATRICS

INTRODUCTION

This article updates and replaces the 2011 clinical practice guideline revision published by the American Academy of Pediatrics (AAP), "Clinical Practice Guideline: Diagnosis and Evaluation of the Child with Attention-Deficit/Hyperactivity Disorder."[1] This guideline, like the previous document, addresses the evaluation, diagnosis, and treatment of attention-deficit/hyperactivity disorder (ADHD) in children from age 4 years to their 18th birthday, with special guidance provided for ADHD care for preschool-aged children and adolescents. (Note that for the purposes of this document, "preschool-aged" refers to children from age 4 years to the sixth birthday.) Pediatricians and other primary care clinicians (PCCs) may continue to provide care after 18 years of age, but care beyond this age was not studied for this guideline.

Since 2011, much research has occurred, and the *Diagnostic and Statistical Manual of Mental Disorders, Fifth Edition (DSM-5)*, has been released. The new research and *DSM-5* do not, however, support dramatic changes to the previous recommendations. Hence, this new guideline includes only incremental updates to the previous guideline. One such update is the addition of a key action statement (KAS) about the diagnosis and treatment of coexisting or comorbid conditions in children and adolescents with ADHD. The subcommittee uses the term "comorbid," to be consistent with the *DSM-5*.

Since 2011, the release of new research reflects an increased understanding and recognition of ADHD's prevalence and epidemiology; the challenges it raises for children and families; the need for a comprehensive clinical resource for the evaluation, diagnosis, and treatment of pediatric ADHD; and the barriers that impede the

implementation of such a resource. In response, this guideline is supported by 2 accompanying documents, available in the Supplemental Information: (1) a process of care algorithm (PoCA) for the diagnosis and treatment of children and adolescents with ADHD and (2) an article on systemic barriers to the care of children and adolescents with ADHD. These supplemental documents are designed to aid PCCs in implementing the formal recommendations for the evaluation, diagnosis, and treatment of children and adolescents with ADHD. Although this document is specific to children and adolescents in the United States in some of its recommendations, international stakeholders can modify specific content (ie, educational laws about accommodations, etc) as needed. (Prevention is addressed in the Mental Health Task Force recommendations.[2])

PoCA for the Diagnosis and Treatment of Children and Adolescents With ADHD

In this revised guideline and accompanying PoCA, we recognize that evaluation, diagnosis, and treatment are a continuous process. The PoCA provides recommendations for implementing the guideline steps, although there is less evidence for the PoCA than for the guidelines. The section on evaluating and treating comorbidities has also been expanded in the PoCA document.

Systems Barriers to the Care of Children and Adolescents With ADHD

There are many system-level barriers that hamper the adoption of the best-practice recommendations contained in the clinical practice guideline and the PoCA. The procedures recommended in this guideline necessitate spending more time with patients and their families, developing a care management system of contacts with school and other community stakeholders, and providing continuous, coordinated

care to the patient and his or her family. There is some evidence that African American and Latino children are less likely to have ADHD diagnosed and are less likely to be treated for ADHD. Special attention should be given to these populations when assessing comorbidities as they relate to ADHD and when treating for ADHD symptoms.[3] Given the nationwide problem of limited access to mental health clinicians,[4] pediatricians and other PCCs are increasingly called on to provide services to patients with ADHD and to their families. In addition, the AAP holds that primary care pediatricians should be prepared to diagnose and manage mild-to-moderate ADHD, anxiety, depression, and problematic substance use, as well as co-manage patients who have more severe conditions with mental health professionals. Unfortunately, third-party payers seldom pay appropriately for these time-consuming services.[5,6]

To assist pediatricians and other PCCs in overcoming such obstacles, the companion article on systemic barriers to the care of children and adolescents with ADHD reviews the barriers and makes recommendations to address them to enhance care for children and adolescents with ADHD.

ADHD EPIDEMIOLOGY AND SCOPE

Prevalence estimates of ADHD vary on the basis of differences in research methodologies, the various age groups being described, and changes in diagnostic criteria over time.[7] Authors of a recent meta-analysis calculated a pooled worldwide ADHD prevalence of 7.2% among children[8]; estimates from some community-based samples are somewhat higher, at 8.7% to 15.5%.[9,10] National survey data from 2016 indicate that 9.4% of children in the United States 2 to 17 years of age have ever had an ADHD diagnosis, including 2.4% of children 2 to 5 years of age.[11] In that national survey, 8.4% of children 2 to 17 years of age currently had ADHD, representing 5.4 million children.[11] Among children and adolescents with current ADHD, almost two-thirds were taking medication, and approximately half had received behavioral treatment of ADHD in the past year. Nearly one quarter had received neither type of treatment of ADHD.[11]

Symptoms of ADHD occur in childhood, and most children with ADHD will continue to have symptoms and impairment through adolescence and into adulthood. According to a 2014 national survey, the median age of diagnosis was 7 years; approximately one-third of children were diagnosed before 6 years of age.[12] More than half of these children were first diagnosed by a PCC, often a pediatrician.[12] As individuals with ADHD enter adolescence, their overt hyperactive and impulsive symptoms tend to decline, whereas their inattentive symptoms tend to persist.[13,14] Learning and language problems are common comorbid conditions with ADHD.[15]

Boys are more than twice as likely as girls to receive a diagnosis of ADHD,[9,11,16] possibly because hyperactive behaviors, which are easily observable and potentially disruptive, are seen more frequently in boys. The majority of both boys and girls with ADHD also meet diagnostic criteria for another mental disorder.[17,18] Boys are more likely to exhibit externalizing conditions like oppositional defiant disorder or conduct disorder.[17,19,20] Recent research has established that girls with ADHD are more likely than boys to have a comorbid internalizing condition like anxiety or depression.[21]

Although there is a greater risk of receiving a diagnosis of ADHD for children who are the youngest in their class (who are therefore less developmentally capable of compensating for their weaknesses), for most children, retention is not beneficial.[22]

METHODOLOGY

As with the original 2000 clinical practice guideline and the 2011 revision, the AAP collaborated with several organizations to form a subcommittee on ADHD (the subcommittee) under the oversight of the AAP Council on Quality Improvement and Patient Safety.

The subcommittee's membership included representation of a wide range of primary care and subspecialty groups, including primary care pediatricians, developmental-behavioral pediatricians, an epidemiologist from the Centers for Disease Control and Prevention; and representatives from the American Academy of Child and Adolescent Psychiatry, the Society for Pediatric Psychology, the National Association of School Psychologists, the Society for Developmental and Behavioral Pediatrics (SDBP), the American Academy of Family Physicians, and Children and Adults with Attention-Deficit/Hyperactivity Disorder (CHADD) to provide feedback on the patient/parent perspective.

This subcommittee met over a 3.5-year period from 2015 to 2018 to review practice changes and newly identified issues that have arisen since the publication of the 2011 guidelines. The subcommittee members' potential conflicts were identified and taken into consideration in the group's deliberations. No conflicts prevented subcommittee member participation on the guidelines.

Research Questions

The subcommittee developed a series of research questions to direct an evidence-based review sponsored by 1 of the Evidence-based Practice Centers of the US Agency for Healthcare Research and Quality (AHRQ).[23] These questions assessed 4 diagnostic areas and 3 treatment areas on the basis of research published in 2011 through 2016.

The AHRQ's framework was guided by key clinical questions addressing diagnosis as well as treatment interventions for children and adolescents 4 to 18 years of age.

The first clinical questions pertaining to ADHD diagnosis were as follows:

1. What is the comparative diagnostic accuracy of approaches that can be used in the primary care practice setting or by specialists to diagnose ADHD among children younger than 7 years of age?

2. What is the comparative diagnostic accuracy of EEG, imaging, or executive function approaches that can be used in the primary care practice setting or by specialists to diagnose ADHD among individuals aged 7 to their 18th birthday?

3. What are the adverse effects associated with being labeled correctly or incorrectly as having ADHD?

4. Are there more formal neuropsychological, imaging, or genetic tests that improve the diagnostic process?

The treatment questions were as follows:

1. What are the comparative safety and effectiveness of pharmacologic and/or nonpharmacologic treatments of ADHD in improving outcomes associated with ADHD?

2. What is the risk of diversion of pharmacologic treatment?

3. What are the comparative safety and effectiveness of different monitoring strategies to evaluate the effectiveness of treatment or changes in ADHD status (eg, worsening or resolving symptoms)?

In addition to this review of the research questions, the subcommittee considered information from a review of evidence-based psychosocial treatments for children and adolescents with ADHD[24] (which, in some cases, affected the evidence grade) as well as updated information on prevalence from the Centers for Disease Control and Prevention.

Evidence Review

This article followed the latest version of the evidence base update format used to develop the previous 3 clinical practice guidelines.[24–26] Under this format, studies were only included in the review when they met a variety of criteria designed to ensure the research was based on a strong methodology that yielded confidence in its conclusions.

The level of efficacy for each treatment was defined on the basis of child-focused outcomes related to both symptoms and impairment. Hence, improvements in behaviors on the part of parents or teachers, such as the use of communication or praise, were not considered in the review. Although these outcomes are important, they address how treatment reaches the child or adolescent with ADHD and are, therefore, secondary to changes in the child's behavior. Focusing on improvements in the child or adolescent's symptoms and impairment emphasizes the disorder's characteristics and manifestations that affect children and their families.

The treatment-related evidence relied on a recent review of literature from 2011 through 2016 by the AHRQ of citations from Medline, Embase, PsycINFO, and the Cochrane Database of Systematic Reviews.

The original methodology and report, including the evidence search and review, are available in their entirety and as an executive summary at https://effectivehealthcare.ahrq.gov/

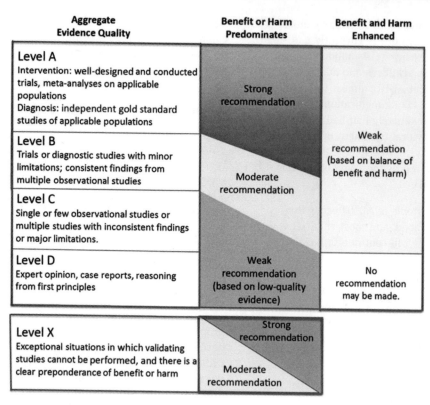

FIGURE 1
AAP rating of evidence and recommendations.

sites/default/files/pdf/cer-203-adhd-final_0.pdf.

The evidence is discussed in more detail in published reports and articles.[25]

Guideline Recommendations and Key Action Statements

The AAP policy statement, "Classifying Recommendations for Clinical Practice Guidelines," was followed in designating aggregate evidence quality levels for the available evidence (see Fig 1).[27] The AAP policy statement is consistent with the grading recommendations advanced by the University of Oxford Centre for Evidence Based Medicine.

The subcommittee reached consensus on the evidence, which was then used to develop the clinical practice guideline's KASs.

When the scientific evidence was at least "good" in quality and demonstrated a preponderance of benefits over harms, the KAS provides a "strong recommendation" or "recommendation."[27] Clinicians should follow a "strong recommendation" unless a clear and compelling rationale for an alternative approach is present; clinicians are prudent to follow a "recommendation" but are advised to remain alert to new information and be sensitive to patient preferences[27] (see Fig 1).

When the scientific evidence comprised lower-quality or limited data and expert consensus or high-quality evidence with a balance between benefits and harms, the KAS provides an "option" level of recommendation. Options are clinical interventions that a reasonable health care provider might or might not wish to implement in the practice.[27] Where the evidence was lacking, a combination of evidence and expert consensus would be used, although this did not occur in these guidelines, and all KASs achieved a "strong recommendation" level except for KAS 7, on comorbidities, which received a recommendation level (see Fig 1).

As shown in Fig 1, integrating evidence quality appraisal with an assessment of the anticipated balance between benefits and harms leads to a designation of a strong recommendation, recommendation, option, or no recommendation.

Once the evidence level was determined, an evidence grade was assigned. AAP policy stipulates that the evidence supporting each KAS be prospectively identified, appraised, and summarized, and an explicit link between quality levels and the grade of recommendation must be defined. Possible grades of recommendations range from "A" to "D," with "A" being the highest:

- grade A: consistent level A studies;
- grade B: consistent level B or extrapolations from level A studies;
- grade C: level C studies or extrapolations from level B or level C studies;
- grade D: level D evidence or troublingly inconsistent or inconclusive studies of any level; and
- level X: not an explicit level of evidence as outlined by the Centre for Evidence-Based Medicine. This level is reserved for interventions that are unethical or impossible to test in a controlled or scientific fashion and for which the preponderance of benefit or harm is overwhelming, precluding rigorous investigation.

Guided by the evidence quality and grade, the subcommittee developed 7 KASs for the evaluation, diagnosis, and treatment of ADHD in children and adolescents (see Table 1).

These KASs provide for consistent and high-quality care for children and adolescents who may have symptoms suggesting attention disorders or problems as well as for their families. In developing the 7 KASs, the subcommittee considered the requirements for establishing the diagnosis; the prevalence of ADHD; the effect of untreated ADHD; the efficacy and adverse effects of treatment; various long-term outcomes; the importance of coordination between pediatric and mental health service providers; the value of the medical home; and the common occurrence of comorbid conditions, the importance of addressing them, and the effects of not treating them.

The subcommittee members with the most epidemiological experience assessed the strength of each recommendation and the quality of evidence supporting each draft KAS.

Peer Review

The guidelines and PoCA underwent extensive peer review by more than 30 internal stakeholders (eg, AAP committees, sections, councils, and task forces) and external stakeholder groups identified by the subcommittee. The resulting comments were compiled and reviewed by the chair and vice chair; relevant changes were incorporated into the draft, which was then reviewed by the full subcommittee.

KASS FOR THE EVALUATION, DIAGNOSIS, TREATMENT, AND MONITORING OF CHILDREN AND ADOLESCENTS WITH ADHD

KAS 1

The pediatrician or other PCC should initiate an evaluation for ADHD for any child or adolescent age 4 years to the 18th birthday who presents with academic or behavioral problems and symptoms of inattention, hyperactivity, or impulsivity

(Table 2). (Grade B: strong recommendation.)

The basis for this recommendation is essentially unchanged from the previous guideline. As noted, ADHD is the most common neurobehavioral disorder of childhood, occurring in approximately 7% to 8% of children and youth.[8,18,28,29] Hence, the number of children with this condition is far greater than can be managed by the mental health system.[4] There is evidence that appropriate diagnosis can be accomplished in the primary care setting for children and adolescents.[30,31] Note that there is insufficient evidence to recommend diagnosis or treatment for children younger than 4 years (other than parent training in behavior management [PTBM], which does not require a diagnosis to be applied); in instances in which ADHD-like symptoms in children younger than 4 years bring substantial impairment, PCCs can consider making a referral for PTBM.

KAS 2

To make a diagnosis of ADHD, the PCC should determine that *DSM-5* criteria have been met, including documentation of symptoms and impairment in more than 1 major setting (ie, social, academic, or occupational), with information obtained primarily from reports from parents or guardians, teachers, other school personnel, and mental health clinicians who are involved in the child or adolescent's care. The PCC should also rule out any alternative cause (Table 3). (Grade B: strong recommendation.)

The American Psychiatric Association developed the *DSM-5* using expert consensus and an expanding research foundation.[32] The *DSM-5* system is used by professionals in psychiatry, psychology, health care systems, and primary care; it is also well established with third-party payers.

TABLE 1 Summary of KASs for Diagnosing, Evaluating, and Treating ADHD in Children and Adolescents

KASs	Evidence Quality, Strength of Recommendation
KAS 1: The pediatrician or other PCC should initiate an evaluation for ADHD for any child or adolescent age 4 years to the 18th birthday who presents with academic or behavioral problems and symptoms of inattention, hyperactivity, or impulsivity.	Grade B, strong recommendation
KAS 2: To make a diagnosis of ADHD, the PCC should determine that *DSM-5* criteria have been met, including documentation of symptoms and impairment in more than 1 major setting (ie, social, academic, or occupational), with information obtained primarily from reports from parents or guardians, teachers, other school personnel, and mental health clinicians who are involved in the child or adolescent's care. The PCC should also rule out any alternative cause.	Grade B, strong recommendation
KAS 3: In the evaluation of a child or adolescent for ADHD, the PCC should include a process to at least screen for comorbid conditions, including emotional or behavioral conditions (eg, anxiety, depression, oppositional defiant disorder, conduct disorders, substance use), developmental conditions (eg, learning and language disorders, autism spectrum disorders), and physical conditions (eg, tics, sleep apnea).	Grade B, strong recommendation
KAS 4: ADHD is a chronic condition; therefore, the PCC should manage children and adolescents with ADHD in the same manner that they would children and youth with special health care needs, following the principles of the chronic care model and the medical home.	Grade B, strong recommendation
KAS 5a: For preschool-aged children (age 4 years to the sixth birthday) with ADHD, the PCC should prescribe evidence-based PTBM and/or behavioral classroom interventions as the first line of treatment, if available.	Grade A, strong recommendation for PTBM
Methylphenidate may be considered if these behavioral interventions do not provide significant improvement and there is moderate-to-severe continued disturbance in the 4- through 5-year-old child's functioning. In areas in which evidence-based behavioral treatments are not available, the clinician needs to weigh the risks of starting medication before the age of 6 years against the harm of delaying treatment.	Grade B, strong recommendation for methylphenidate
KAS 5b. For elementary and middle school-aged children (age 6 years to the 12th birthday) with ADHD, the PCC should prescribe FDA-approved medications for ADHD, along with PTBM and/or behavioral classroom intervention (preferably both PTBM and behavioral classroom interventions). Educational interventions and individualized instructional supports, including school environment, class placement, instructional placement, and behavioral supports, are a necessary part of any treatment plan and often include an IEP or a rehabilitation plan (504 plan).	Grade A, strong recommendation for medications Grade A, strong recommendation for training and behavioral treatments for ADHD with family and school
KAS 5c. For adolescents (age 12 years to the 18th birthday) with ADHD, the PCC should prescribe FDA-approved medications for ADHD with the adolescent's assent. The PCC is encouraged to prescribe evidence-based training interventions and/or behavioral interventions as treatment of ADHD, if available. Educational interventions and individualized instructional supports, including school environment, class placement, instructional placement, and behavioral supports, are a necessary part of any treatment plan and often include an IEP or a rehabilitation plan (504 plan).	Grade A, strong recommendation for medications Grade A, strong recommendation for training and behavioral treatments for ADHD with the family and school
KAS 6. The PCC should titrate doses of medication for ADHD to achieve maximum benefit with tolerable side effects.	Grade B, strong recommendation
KAS 7. The PCC, if trained or experienced in diagnosing comorbid conditions, may initiate treatment of such conditions or make a referral to an appropriate subspecialist for treatment. After detecting possible comorbid conditions, if the PCC is not trained or experienced in making the diagnosis or initiating treatment, the patient should be referred to an appropriate subspecialist to make the diagnosis and initiate treatment.	Grade C, recommendation

The *DSM-5* criteria define 4 dimensions of ADHD:

1. attention-deficit/hyperactivity disorder primarily of the inattentive presentation (ADHD/I) (314.00 [F90.0]);

2. attention-deficit/hyperactivity disorder primarily of the hyperactive-impulsive presentation (ADHD/HI) (314.01 [F90.1]);

3. attention-deficit/hyperactivity disorder combined presentation (ADHD/C) (314.01 [F90.2]); and

4. ADHD other specified and unspecified ADHD (314.01 [F90.8]).

As with the previous guideline recommendations, the *DSM-5* classification criteria are based on the best available evidence for ADHD diagnosis and are the

standard most frequently used by clinicians and researchers to render the diagnosis and document its appropriateness for a given child. The use of neuropsychological testing has not been found to improve diagnostic accuracy in most cases, although it may have benefit in clarifying the child or adolescent's learning strengths and weaknesses. (See the

TABLE 2 KAS 1: The pediatrician or other PCC should initiate an evaluation for ADHD for any child or adolescent age 4 years to the 18th birthday who presents with academic or behavioral problems and symptoms of inattention, hyperactivity, or impulsivity. (Grade B: strong recommendation.)

Aggregate evidence quality	Grade B
Benefits	ADHD goes undiagnosed in a considerable number of children and adolescents. Primary care clinicians' more-rigorous identification of children with these problems is likely to decrease the rate of undiagnosed and untreated ADHD in children and adolescents.
Risks, harm, cost	Children and adolescents in whom ADHD is inappropriately diagnosed may be labeled inappropriately, or another condition may be missed, and they may receive treatments that will not benefit them.
Benefit-harm assessment	The high prevalence of ADHD and limited mental health resources require primary care pediatricians and other PCCs to play a significant role in the care of patients with ADHD and assist them to receive appropriate diagnosis and treatment. Treatments available have good evidence of efficacy, and a lack of treatment has the risk of impaired outcomes.
Intentional vagueness	There are limits between what a PCC can address and what should be referred to a subspecialist because of varying degrees of skills and comfort levels present among the former.
Role of patient preferences	Success with treatment is dependent on patient and family preference, which need to be taken into account.
Exclusions	None.
Strength	Strong recommendation.
Key references	Wolraich et al[31]; Visser et al[28]; Thomas et al[8]; Egger et al[30]

PoCA for more information on implementing this KAS.)

Special Circumstances: Preschool-Aged Children (Age 4 Years to the Sixth Birthday)

There is evidence that the diagnostic criteria for ADHD can be applied to preschool-aged children.[33–39] A review of the literature, including the multisite study of the efficacy of methylphenidate in preschool-aged children, found that the *DSM-5* criteria could appropriately identify children with ADHD.[25]

To make a diagnosis of ADHD in preschool-aged children, clinicians should conduct a clinical interview with parents, examine and observe the child, and obtain information from parents and teachers through *DSM*-based ADHD rating scales.[40] Normative data are available for the *DSM-5*–based rating scales for ages 5 years to the 18th birthday.[41] There are, however, minimal changes in the specific behaviors from the *DSM-IV*, on which all the other *DSM*-based ADHD rating scales obtained normative data. Both the ADHD Rating Scale-IV and the Conners Rating Scale have preschool-age normative data based on the *DSM-IV*. The specific behaviors in the *DSM-5* criteria for ADHD are the same for all

children younger than 18 years (ie, preschool-aged children, elementary and middle school–aged children, and adolescents) and are only minimally different from the *DSM-IV*. Hence, if clinicians do not have the ADHD Rating Scale-5 or the ADHD Rating Scale-IV Preschool Version,[42] any other *DSM*-based scale can be used to provide a systematic method for collecting information from parents and teachers, even in the absence of normative data.

Pediatricians and other PCCs should be aware that determining the presence of key symptoms in this age group has its challenges, such as

TABLE 3 KAS 2: To make a diagnosis of ADHD, the PCC should determine that *DSM-5* criteria have been met, including documentation of symptoms and impairment in more than 1 major setting (ie, social, academic, or occupational), with information obtained primarily from reports from parents or guardians, teachers, other school personnel, and mental health clinicians who are involved in the child or adolescent's care. The PCC should also rule out any alternative cause. (Grade B: strong recommendation.)

Aggregate evidence quality	Grade B
Benefits	Use of the *DSM-5* criteria has led to more uniform categorization of the condition across professional disciplines. The criteria are essentially unchanged from the *Diagnostic and Statistical Manual of Mental Disorders, Fourth Edition (DSM-IV)*, for children up to their 18th birthday, except that *DSM-IV* required onset prior to age 7 for a diagnosis, while *DSM-5* requires onset prior to age 12.
Risks, harm, cost	The *DSM-5* does not specifically state that symptoms must be beyond expected levels for developmental (rather than chronologic) age to qualify for an ADHD diagnosis, which may lead to some misdiagnoses in children with developmental disorders.
Benefit-harm assessment	The benefits far outweigh the harm.
Intentional vagueness	None.
Role of patient preferences	Although there is some stigma associated with mental disorder diagnoses, resulting in some families preferring other diagnoses, the need for better clarity in diagnoses outweighs this preference.
Exclusions	None.
Strength	Strong recommendation.
Key references	Evans et al[25]; McGoey et al[42]; Young[43]; Sibley et al[46]

observing symptoms across multiple settings as required by the *DSM-5*, particularly among children who do not attend a preschool or child care program. Here, too, focused checklists can be used to aid in the diagnostic evaluation.

PTBM is the recommended primary intervention for preschool-aged children with ADHD as well as children with ADHD-like behaviors whose diagnosis is not yet verified. This type of training helps parents learn age-appropriate developmental expectations, behaviors that strengthen the parent-child relationship, and specific management skills for problem behaviors. Clinicians do not need to have made an ADHD diagnosis before recommending PTBM because PTBM has documented effectiveness with a wide variety of problem behaviors, regardless of etiology. In addition, the intervention's results may inform the subsequent diagnostic evaluation. Clinicians are encouraged to recommend that parents complete PTBM, if available, before assigning an ADHD diagnosis.

After behavioral parent training is implemented, the clinician can obtain information from parents and teachers through *DSM-5*–based ADHD rating scales. The clinician may obtain reports about the parents' ability to manage their children and about the child's core symptoms and impairments. Referral to an early intervention program or enrolling in a PTBM program can help provide information about the child's behavior in other settings or with other observers. The evaluators for these programs and/or early childhood special education teachers may be useful observers, as well.

Special Circumstances: Adolescents (Age 12 Years to the 18th Birthday)

Obtaining teacher reports for adolescents is often more challenging than for younger children because many adolescents have multiple teachers. Likewise, an adolescent's parents may have less opportunity to observe their child's behaviors than they did when the child was younger. Furthermore, some problems experienced by children with ADHD are less obvious in adolescents than in younger children because adolescents are less likely to exhibit overt hyperactive behavior. Of note, adolescents' reports of their own behaviors often differ from other observers because they tend to minimize their own problematic behaviors.[43-45]

Despite these difficulties, clinicians need to try to obtain information from at least 2 teachers or other sources, such as coaches, school guidance counselors, or leaders of community activities in which the adolescent participates.[46] For the evaluation to be successful, it is essential that adolescents agree with and participate in the evaluation. Variability in ratings is to be expected because adolescents' behavior often varies between different classrooms and with different teachers. Identifying reasons for any variability can provide valuable clinical insight into the adolescent's problems.

Note that, unless they previously received a diagnosis, to meet *DSM-5* criteria for ADHD, adolescents must have some reported or documented manifestations of inattention or hyperactivity/impulsivity before age 12. Therefore, clinicians must establish that an adolescent had manifestations of ADHD before age 12 and strongly consider whether a mimicking or comorbid condition, such as substance use, depression, and/or anxiety, is present.[46]

In addition, the risks of mood and anxiety disorders and risky sexual behaviors increase during adolescence, as do the risks of intentional self-harm and suicidal behaviors.[31] Clinicians should also be aware that adolescents are at greater risk for substance use than are younger children.[44,45,47] Certain substances, such as marijuana, can have effects that mimic ADHD; adolescent patients may also attempt to obtain stimulant medication to enhance performance (ie, academic, athletic, etc) by feigning symptoms.[48]

Trauma experiences, posttraumatic stress disorder, and toxic stress are additional comorbidities and risk factors of concern.

Special Circumstances: Inattention or Hyperactivity/Impulsivity (Problem Level)

Teachers, parents, and child health professionals typically encounter children who demonstrate behaviors relating to activity level, impulsivity, and inattention but who do not fully meet *DSM-5* criteria. When assessing these children, diagnostic criteria should be closely reviewed, which may require obtaining more information from other settings and sources. Also consider that these symptoms may suggest other problems that mimic ADHD.

Behavioral interventions, such as PTBM, are often beneficial for children with hyperactive/impulsive behaviors who do not meet full diagnostic criteria for ADHD. As noted previously, these programs do not require a specific diagnosis to be beneficial to the family. The previous guideline discussed the diagnosis of problem-level concerns on the basis of the *Diagnostic and Statistical Manual for Primary Care (DSM-PC), Child and Adolescent Version*,[49] and made suggestions for treatment and care. The *DSM-PC* was published in 1995, however, and it has not been revised to be compatible with the *DSM-5*. Therefore, the *DSM-PC* cannot be used as a definitive source for diagnostic codes related to ADHD and comorbid conditions, although it can be used conceptually as a resource for enriching the understanding of problem-level manifestations.

KAS 3

In the evaluation of a child or adolescent for ADHD, the PCC should include a process to at least screen for comorbid conditions, including emotional or behavioral conditions (eg, anxiety, depression, oppositional defiant disorder, conduct disorders, substance use), developmental conditions (eg, learning and language disorders, autism spectrum disorders), and physical conditions (eg, tics, sleep apnea) (Table 4). (Grade B: strong recommendation.)

The majority of both boys and girls with ADHD also meet diagnostic criteria for another mental disorder.[17,18] A variety of other behavioral, developmental, and physical conditions can be comorbid in children and adolescents who are evaluated for ADHD, including emotional or behavioral conditions or a history of these problems. These include but are not limited to learning disabilities, language disorder, disruptive behavior, anxiety, mood disorders, tic disorders, seizures, autism spectrum disorder, developmental coordination disorder, and sleep disorders.[50–66] In some cases, the presence of a comorbid

condition will alter the treatment of ADHD.

The SDBP is developing a clinical practice guideline to support clinicians in the diagnosis of treatment of "complex ADHD," which includes ADHD with comorbid developmental and/or mental health conditions.[67]

Special Circumstances: Adolescents (Age 12 Years to the 18th Birthday)

At a minimum, clinicians should assess adolescent patients with newly diagnosed ADHD for symptoms and signs of substance use, anxiety, depression, and learning disabilities. As noted, all 4 are common comorbid conditions that affect the treatment approach. These comorbidities make it important for the clinician to consider sequencing psychosocial and medication treatments to maximize the impact on areas of greatest risk and impairment while monitoring for possible risks such as stimulant abuse or suicidal ideation.

KAS 4

ADHD is a chronic condition; therefore, the PCC should manage children and adolescents with ADHD in the same manner that they would children and youth with special health care needs, following the principles of the chronic care model

and the medical home (Table 5). (Grade B: strong recommendation.)

As in the 2 previous guidelines, this recommendation is based on the evidence that for many individuals, ADHD causes symptoms and dysfunction over long periods of time, even into adulthood. Available treatments address symptoms and function but are usually not curative. Although the chronic illness model has not been specifically studied in children and adolescents with ADHD, it has been effective for other chronic conditions, such as asthma.[68] In addition, the medical home model has been accepted as the preferred standard of care for children with chronic conditions.[69]

The medical home and chronic illness approach may be particularly beneficial for parents who also have ADHD themselves. These parents can benefit from extra support to help them follow a consistent schedule for medication and behavioral programs.

Authors of longitudinal studies have found that ADHD treatments are frequently not maintained over time[13] and impairments persist into adulthood.[70] It is indicated in prospective studies that patients with ADHD, whether treated or not, are at increased risk for early death, suicide, and increased psychiatric

---

TABLE 4 KAS 3: In the evaluation of a child or adolescent for ADHD, the PCC should include a process to at least screen for comorbid conditions, including emotional or behavioral conditions (eg, anxiety, depression, oppositional defiant disorder, conduct disorders, substance use), developmental conditions (eg, learning and language disorders, autism spectrum disorders), and physical conditions (eg, tics, sleep apnea). (Grade B: strong recommendation.)

Aggregate evidence quality	Grade B
Benefits	Identifying comorbid conditions is important in developing the most appropriate treatment plan for the child or adolescent with ADHD.
Risks, harm, cost	The major risk is misdiagnosing the comorbid condition(s) and providing inappropriate care.
Benefit-harm assessment	There is a preponderance of benefits over harm.
Intentional vagueness	None.
Role of patient preferences	None.
Exclusions	None.
Strength	Strong recommendation.
Key references	Cuffe et al[51]; Pastor and Reuben[52]; Bieiderman et al[53]; Bieiderman et al[54]; Bieiderman et al[72]; Crabtree et al[57]; LeBourgeois et al[58]; Chan[115]; Newcorn et al[60]; Sung et al[61]; Larson et al[66]; Mahajan et al[65]; Antshel et al[64]; Rothenberger and Roessner[63]; Froehlich et al[62]

TABLE 5 KAS 4: ADHD is a chronic condition; therefore, the PCC should manage children and adolescents with ADHD in the same manner that they would children and youth with special health care needs, following the principles of the chronic care model and the medical home. (Grade B: strong recommendation.)

Aggregate evidence quality	Grade B
Benefits	The recommendation describes the coordinated services that are most appropriate to manage the condition.
Risks, harm, cost	Providing these services may be more costly.
Benefit-harm assessment	There is a preponderance of benefits over harm.
Intentional vagueness	None.
Role of patient preferences	Family preference in how these services are provided is an important consideration, because it can increase adherence.
Exclusions	None
Strength	Strong recommendation.
Key references	Brito et al[69]; Biederman et al[72]; Scheffler et al[74]; Barbaresi et al[75]; Chang et al[71]; Chang et al[78]; Lichtenstein et al[77]; Harstad and Levy[80]

comorbidity, particularly substance use disorders.[71,72] They also have lower educational achievement than those without ADHD[73,74] and increased rates of incarceration.[75–77] Treatment discontinuation also places individuals with ADHD at higher risk for catastrophic outcomes, such as motor vehicle crashes[78,79]; criminality, including drug-related crimes[77] and violent reoffending[76]; depression[71]; interpersonal issues[80]; and other injuries.[81,82]

To continue providing the best care, it is important for a treating pediatrician or other PCC to engage in bidirectional communication with teachers and other school personnel as well as mental health clinicians involved in the child or adolescent's care. This communication can be difficult to achieve and is discussed in both the PoCA and the section on systemic barriers to the care of children and adolescents with ADHD in the Supplemental Information, as is the medical home model.[69]

Special Circumstances: Inattention or Hyperactivity/Impulsivity (Problem Level)

Children with inattention or hyperactivity/impulsivity at the problem level, as well as their families, may also benefit from the chronic illness and medical home principles.

Recommendations for the Treatment of Children and Adolescents With ADHD: KAS 5a, 5b, and 5c

Recommendations vary depending on the patient's age and are presented for the following age ranges:

a. preschool-aged children: age 4 years to the sixth birthday;

b. elementary and middle school–aged children: age 6 years to the 12th birthday; and

c. adolescents: age 12 years to the 18th birthday.

The KASs are presented, followed by information on medication, psychosocial treatments, and special circumstances.

KAS 5a

For preschool-aged children (age 4 years to the sixth birthday) with ADHD, the PCC should prescribe evidence-based behavioral PTBM and/or behavioral classroom interventions as the first line of treatment, if available (grade A: strong recommendation). Methylphenidate may be considered if these behavioral interventions do not provide significant improvement and there is moderate-to-severe continued disturbance in the 4- through 5-year-old child's functioning. In areas in which evidence-based behavioral treatments are not available, the clinician needs to weigh the risks of starting medication before the age of

6 years against the harm of delaying treatment (Table 6). (Grade B: strong recommendation.)

A number of special circumstances support the recommendation to initiate PTBM as the first treatment of preschool-aged children (age 4 years to the sixth birthday) with ADHD.[25,83] Although it was limited to children who had moderate-to-severe dysfunction, the largest multisite study of methylphenidate use in preschool-aged children revealed symptom improvements after PTBM alone.[83] The overall evidence for PTBM among preschoolers is strong.

PTBM programs for preschool-aged children are typically group programs and, although they are not always paid for by health insurance, they may be relatively low cost. One evidence-based PTBM, parent-child interaction therapy, is a dyadic therapy for parent and child. The PoCA contains criteria for the clinician's use to assess the quality of PTBM programs. If the child attends preschool, behavioral classroom interventions are also recommended. In addition, preschool programs (such as Head Start) and ADHD-focused organizations (such as CHADD[84]) can also provide behavioral supports. The issues related to referral, payment, and communication are discussed in the section on systemic barriers in the Supplemental Information.

TABLE 6 KAS 5a: For preschool-aged children (age 4 years to the sixth birthday) with ADHD, the PCC should prescribe evidence-based behavioral PTBM and/or behavioral classroom interventions as the first line of treatment, if available (grade A: strong recommendation). Methylphenidate may be considered if these behavioral interventions do not provide significant improvement and there is moderate-to-severe continued disturbance in the 4- through 5-year-old child's functioning. In areas in which evidence-based behavioral treatments are not available, the clinician needs to weigh the risks of starting medication before the age of 6 years against the harm of delaying treatment (grade B: strong recommendation).

Aggregate evidence quality	Grade A for PTBM; Grade B for methylphenidate
Benefits	Given the risks of untreated ADHD, the benefits outweigh the risks.
Risks, harm, cost	Both therapies increase the cost of care; PTBM requires a high level of family involvement, whereas methylphenidate has some potential adverse effects.
Benefit-harm assessment	Both PTBM and methylphenidate have relatively low risks; initiating treatment at an early age, before children experience repeated failure, has additional benefits. Thus, the benefits outweigh the risks.
Intentional vagueness	None.
Role of patient preferences	Family preference is essential in determining the treatment plan.
Exclusions	None.
Strength	Strong recommendation.
Key references	Greenhill et al[83]; Evans et al[25]

In areas in which evidence-based behavioral treatments are not available, the clinician needs to weigh the risks of starting methylphenidate before the age of 6 years against the harm of delaying diagnosis and treatment. Other stimulant or nonstimulant medications have not been adequately studied in children in this age group with ADHD.

KAS 5b

For elementary and middle school–aged children (age 6 years to the 12th birthday) with ADHD, the PCC should prescribe US Food and Drug Administration (FDA)–approved medications for ADHD, along with PTBM and/or behavioral classroom intervention (preferably both PTBM and behavioral classroom interventions). Educational interventions and individualized instructional supports, including school environment, class placement, instructional placement, and behavioral supports, are a necessary part of any treatment plan and often include an Individualized Education Program (IEP) or a rehabilitation plan (504 plan) (Table 7). (Grade A: strong recommendation for medications; grade A: strong recommendation for PTBM training and behavioral treatments for ADHD implemented with the family and school.)

The evidence is particularly strong for stimulant medications; it is sufficient, but not as strong, for atomoxetine, extended-release guanfacine, and extended-release clonidine, in that order (see the Treatment section, and see the PoCA for more information on implementation).

KAS 5c

For adolescents (age 12 years to the 18th birthday) with ADHD, the PCC should prescribe FDA-approved medications for ADHD with the adolescent's assent (grade A: strong recommendation). The PCC is encouraged to prescribe evidence-based training interventions and/or behavioral interventions as treatment of ADHD, if available. Educational interventions and individualized instructional supports, including school environment, class placement, instructional placement, and behavioral supports, are a necessary part of any treatment plan and often include an IEP or a rehabilitation plan (504 plan) (Table 8). (Grade A: strong recommendation.)

Transition to adult care is an important component of the chronic care model for ADHD. Planning for the transition to adult care is an ongoing process that may culminate after high school or, perhaps, after college. To foster a smooth transition,

it is best to introduce components at the start of high school, at about 14 years of age, and specifically focus during the 2 years preceding high school completion.

Psychosocial Treatments

Some psychosocial treatments for children and adolescents with ADHD have been demonstrated to be effective for the treatment of ADHD, including behavioral therapy and training interventions.[24–26,85] The diversity of interventions and outcome measures makes it challenging to assess a meta-analysis of psychosocial treatment's effects alone or in association with medication treatment. As with medication treatment, the long-term positive effects of psychosocial treatments have yet to be determined. Nonetheless, ongoing adherence to psychosocial treatment is a key contributor to its beneficial effects, making implementation of a chronic care model for child health important to ensure sustained adherence.[86]

Behavioral therapy involves training adults to influence the contingencies in an environment to improve the behavior of a child or adolescent in that setting. It can help parents and school personnel learn how to effectively prevent and respond to adolescent behaviors such as

TABLE 7 KAS 5b: For elementary and middle school–aged children (age 6 years to the 12th birthday) with ADHD, the PCC should prescribe US Food and Drug Administration (FDA)–approved medications for ADHD, along with PTBM and/or behavioral classroom intervention (preferably both PTBM and behavioral classroom interventions). Educational interventions and individualized instructional supports, including school environment, class placement, instructional placement, and behavioral supports, are a necessary part of any treatment plan and often include an Individualized Education Program (IEP) or a rehabilitation plan (504 plan). (Grade A: strong recommendation for medications; grade A: strong recommendation for PTBM training and behavioral treatments for ADHD implemented with the family and school.)

Aggregate evidence quality	Grade A for Treatment with FDA-Approved Medications; Grade A for Training and Behavioral Treatments for ADHD With the Family and School.
Benefits	Both behavioral therapy and FDA-approved medications have been shown to reduce behaviors associated with ADHD and to improve function.
Risks, harm, cost	Both therapies increase the cost of care. Psychosocial therapy requires a high level of family and/or school involvement and may lead to increased family conflict, especially if treatment is not successfully completed. FDA-approved medications may have some adverse effects and discontinuation of medication is common among adolescents.
Benefit-harm assessment	Given the risks of untreated ADHD, the benefits outweigh the risks.
Intentional vagueness	None.
Role of patient preferences	Family preference, including patient preference, is essential in determining the treatment plan and enhancing adherence.
Exclusions	None.
Strength	Strong recommendation.
Key references	Evans et al[25]; Barbaresi et al[73]; Jain et al[103]; Brown and Bishop[104]; Kambeitz et al[105]; Bruxel et al[106]; Kieling et al[107]; Froehlich et al[108]; Joensen et al[109]

interrupting, aggression, not completing tasks, and not complying with requests. Behavioral parent and classroom training are well-established treatments with preadolescent children.[25,87,88] Most studies comparing behavior therapy to stimulants indicate that stimulants have a stronger immediate effect on the 18 core symptoms of ADHD. Parents, however, were more satisfied with the effect of behavioral therapy, which addresses symptoms and functions in addition to ADHD's core symptoms. The positive effects of behavioral therapies tend to persist, but the positive effects of medication cease when medication stops. Optimal care is likely to occur when both therapies are used, but the decision about therapies is heavily dependent on acceptability by, and feasibility for, the family.

Training interventions target skill development and involve repeated practice with performance feedback over time, rather than modifying behavioral contingencies in a specific setting. Less research has been conducted on training interventions compared to behavioral treatments; nonetheless, training interventions are well-established treatments to target disorganization of materials and time that are exhibited by most youth with ADHD; it is likely that they will benefit younger children, as well.[25,89] Some training interventions, including social skills training, have not been shown to be effective for children with ADHD.[25]

TABLE 8 KAS 5c: For adolescents (age 12 years to the 18th birthday) with ADHD, the PCC should prescribe FDA-approved medications for ADHD with the adolescent's assent (grade A: strong recommendation). The PCC is encouraged to prescribe evidence-based training interventions and/or behavioral interventions as treatment of ADHD, if available. Educational interventions and individualized instructional supports, including school environment, class placement, instructional placement, and behavioral supports, are a necessary part of any treatment plan and often include an IEP or a rehabilitation plan (504 plan). (Grade A: strong recommendation.)

Aggregate evidence quality	Grade A for Medications; Grade A for Training and Behavioral Therapy
Benefits	Training interventions, behavioral therapy, and FDA-approved medications have been demonstrated to reduce behaviors associated with ADHD and to improve function.
Risks, harm, cost	Both therapies increase the cost of care. Psychosocial therapy requires a high level of family and/or school involvement and may lead to unintended increased family conflict, especially if treatment is not successfully completed. FDA-approved medications may have some adverse effects, and discontinuation of medication is common among adolescents.
Benefit-harm assessment	Given the risks of untreated ADHD, the benefits outweigh the risks.
Intentional vagueness	None.
Role of patient preferences	Family preference, including patient preference, is likely to predict engagement and persistence with a treatment.
Exclusions	None.
Strength	Strong recommendation.
Key references	Evans et al[25]; Webster-Stratton et al[87]; Evans et al[95]; Fabiano et al[93]; Sibley and Graziano et al[94]; Langberg et al[96]; Schultz et al[97]; Brown and Bishop[104]; Kambeitz et al[105]; Bruxel et al[106]; Froehlich et al[108]; Joensen et al[109]

Some nonmedication treatments for ADHD-related problems have either too little evidence to recommend them or have been found to have little or no benefit. These include mindfulness, cognitive training, diet modification, EEG biofeedback, and supportive counseling. The suggestion that cannabidiol oil has any effect on ADHD is anecdotal and has not been subjected to rigorous study. Although it is FDA approved, the efficacy for external trigeminal nerve stimulation (eTNS) is documented by one 5-week randomized controlled trial with just 30 participants receiving eTNS.[90] To date, there is no long-term safety and efficacy evidence for eTNS. Overall, the current evidence supporting treatment of ADHD with eTNS is sparse and in no way approaches the robust strength of evidence documented for established medication and behavioral treatments for ADHD; therefore, it cannot be recommended as a treatment of ADHD without considerably more extensive study on its efficacy and safety.

Special Circumstances: Adolescents

Much less research has been published on psychosocial treatments with adolescents than with younger children. PTBM has been modified to include the parents and adolescents in sessions together to develop a behavioral contract and improve parent-adolescent communication and problem-solving (see above).[91] Some training programs also include motivational interviewing approaches. The evidence for this behavioral family approach is mixed and less strong than PTBM with pre-adolescent children.[92–94] Adolescents' responses to behavioral contingencies are more varied than those of younger children because they can often effectively obstruct behavioral contracts, increasing parent-adolescent conflict.

Training approaches that are focused on school functioning skills have consistently revealed benefits for adolescents.[95–97] The greatest benefits from training interventions occur when treatment is continued over an extended period of time, performance feedback is constructive and frequent, and the target behaviors are directly applicable to the adolescent's daily functioning.

Overall, behavioral family approaches may be helpful to some adolescents and their families, and school-based training interventions are well established.[25,94] Meaningful improvements in functioning have not been reported from cognitive behavioral approaches.

Medication for ADHD

Preschool-aged children may experience increased mood lability and dysphoria with stimulant medications.[83] None of the nonstimulants have FDA approval for use in preschool-aged children. For elementary school–aged students, the evidence is particularly strong for stimulant medications and is sufficient, but less strong, for atomoxetine, extended-release guanfacine, and extended-release clonidine (in that order). The effect size for stimulants is 1.0 and for nonstimulants is 0.7. An individual's response to methylphenidate verses amphetamine is idiosyncratic, with approximately 40% responding to both and about 40% responding to only 1. The subtype of ADHD does not appear to be a predictor of response to a specific agent. For most adolescents, stimulant medications are highly effective in reducing ADHD's core symptoms.[73]

Stimulant medications have an effect size of around 1.0 (effect size = [treatment M − control M)/control SD]) for the treatment of ADHD.[98] Among nonstimulant medications, 1 selective norepinephrine reuptake inhibitor, atomoxetine,[99,100] and 2 selective α-2 adrenergic agonists, extended-release guanfacine[101,102] and extended-release clonidine,[103] have also demonstrated efficacy in reducing core symptoms among school-aged children and adolescents, although their effect sizes, —around 0.7 for all 3, are less robust than that of stimulant medications. Norepinephrine reuptake inhibitors and α-2 adrenergic agonists are newer medications, so, in general, the evidence base supporting them is considerably less than that for stimulants, although it was adequate for FDA approval.

A free list of the currently available, FDA-approved medications for ADHD is available online at www. ADHDMedicationGuide.com. Each medication's characteristics are provided to help guide the clinician's prescription choice. With the expanded list of medications, it is less likely that PCCs need to consider the off-label use of other medications. The section on systemic barriers in the Supplemental Information provides suggestions for fostering more realistic and effective payment and communication systems.

Because of the large variability in patients' response to ADHD medication, there is great interest in pharmacogenetic tools that can help clinicians predict the best medication and dose for each child or adolescent. At this time, however, the available scientific literature does not provide sufficient evidence to support their clinical utility given that the genetic variants assayed by these tools have generally not been fully studied with respect to medication effects on ADHD-related symptoms and/or impairment, study findings are inconsistent, or effect sizes are not of sufficient size to ensure clinical utility.[104–109] For that reason, these pharmacogenetics tools are not recommended. In addition, these tests may cost thousands of dollars and are typically not covered by insurance. For a pharmacogenetics tool to be recommended for clinical use, studies would need to reveal (1) the genetic variants assayed have consistent, replicated associations with medication response; (2) knowledge about a patient's genetic profile would change clinical decision-making, improve outcomes and/or reduce costs or burden; and (3) the acceptability of the test's operating characteristics has been demonstrated (eg, sensitivity, specificity, and reliability).

Side Effects

Stimulants' most common short-term adverse effects are appetite loss, abdominal pain, headaches, and sleep disturbance. The Multimodal Treatment of Attention Deficit Hyperactivity Disorder (MTA) study results identified stimulants as having a more persistent effect on decreasing growth velocity compared to most previous studies.[110] Diminished growth was in the range of 1 to 2 cm from predicted adult height. The results of the MTA study were particularly noted among children who were on higher and more consistently administered doses of stimulants.[110] The effects diminished by the third year of treatment, but no compensatory rebound growth was observed.[110] An uncommon significant adverse effect of stimulants is the occurrence of hallucinations and other psychotic symptoms.[111]

Stimulant medications, on average, increase patient heart rate (HR) and blood pressure (BP) to a mild and clinically insignificant degree (average increases: 1–2 beats per minute for HR and 1–4 mm Hg for systolic and diastolic BP).[112] However, because stimulants have been linked to more substantial increases in HR and BP in a subset of individuals (5%–15%), clinicians are encouraged to monitor these vital signs in patients receiving stimulant treatment.[112] Although concerns have been raised about sudden cardiac death among children and adolescents using stimulant and medications,[113] it is an extremely rare occurrence. In fact, stimulant medications have not been shown to increase the risk of sudden death

beyond that observed in children who are not receiving stimulants.[114–118] Nevertheless, before initiating therapy with stimulant medications, it is important to obtain the child or adolescent's history of specific cardiac symptoms in addition to the family history of sudden death, cardiovascular symptoms, Wolff-Parkinson-White syndrome, hypertrophic cardiomyopathy, and long QT syndrome. If any of these risk factors are present, clinicians should obtain additional evaluation to ascertain and address potential safety concerns of stimulant medication use by the child or adolescent.[112,114]

Among nonstimulants, the risk of serious cardiovascular events is extremely low, as it is for stimulants. The 3 nonstimulant medications that are FDA approved to treat ADHD (ie, atomoxetine, guanfacine, and clonidine) may be associated with changes in cardiovascular parameters or other serious cardiovascular events. These events could include increased HR and BP for atomoxetine and decreased HR and BP for guanfacine and clonidine. Clinicians are recommended to not only obtain the personal and family cardiac history, as detailed above, but also to perform additional evaluation if risk factors are present before starting nonstimulant medications (ie, perform an electrocardiogram [ECG] and possibly refer to a pediatric cardiologist if the ECG is not normal).[112]

Additional adverse effects of atomoxetine include initial somnolence and gastrointestinal tract symptoms, particularly if the dosage is increased too rapidly, and decreased appetite.[119–122] Less commonly, an increase in suicidal thoughts has been found; this is noted by an FDA black box warning. Extremely rarely, hepatitis has been associated with atomoxetine. Atomoxetine has also been linked to growth delays compared to expected trajectories in the first 1 to 2 years of treatment, with a return to expected measurements

after 2 to 3 years of treatment, on average. Decreases were observed among those who were taller or heavier than average before treatment.[123]

For extended-release guanfacine and extended-release clonidine, adverse effects include somnolence, dry mouth, dizziness, irritability, headache, bradycardia, hypotension, and abdominal pain.[30,124,125] Because rebound hypertension after abrupt guanfacine and clonidine discontinuation has been observed,[126] these medications should be tapered off rather than suddenly discontinued.

Adjunctive Therapy

Adjunctive therapies may be considered if stimulant therapy is not fully effective or limited by side effects. Only extended-release guanfacine and extended-release clonidine have evidence supporting their use as adjunctive therapy with stimulant medications sufficient to have achieved FDA approval.[127] Other medications have been used in combination on an off-label basis, with some limited evidence available to support the efficacy and safety of using atomoxetine in combination with stimulant medications to augment treatment of ADHD.[128]

Special Circumstances: Preschool-Aged Children (Age 4 Years to the Sixth Birthday)

If children do not experience adequate symptom improvement with PTBM, medication can be prescribed for those with moderate-to-severe ADHD. Many young children with ADHD may require medication to achieve maximum improvement; methylphenidate is the recommended first-line pharmacologic treatment of preschool children because of the lack of sufficient rigorous study in the preschool-aged population for nonstimulant ADHD medications and dextroamphetamine. Although amphetamine is the only medication with FDA approval for use in children younger than 6 years, this authorization was issued at a time when approval criteria were less stringent than current requirements. Hence, the available evidence regarding dextroampheta- mine's use in preschool-aged children with ADHD is not adequate to recommend it as an initial ADHD medication treatment at this time.[80]

No nonstimulant medication has received sufficient rigorous study in the preschool-aged population to be recommended for treatment of ADHD of children 4 through 5 years of age.

Although methylphenidate is the ADHD medication with the strongest evidence for safety and efficacy in preschool-aged children, it should be noted that the evidence has not yet met the level needed for FDA approval. Evidence for the use of methylphenidate consists of 1 multisite study of 165 children[83] and 10 other smaller, single-site studies ranging from 11 to 59 children, for a total of 269 children.[129] Seven of the 10 single-site studies revealed efficacy for methylphenidate in preschoolers. Therefore, although there is moderate evidence that methylphenidate is safe and effective in preschool-aged children, its use in this age group remains on an "off-label" basis.

With these caveats in mind, before initiating treatment with medication, the clinician should assess the severity of the child's ADHD. Given current data, only preschool-aged children with ADHD and moderate-to-severe dysfunction should be considered for medication. Severity criteria are symptoms that have persisted for at least 9 months; dysfunction that is manifested in both home and other settings, such as preschool or child care; and dysfunction that has not responded adequately to PTBM.[83]

The decision to consider initiating medication at this age depends, in part, on the clinician's assessment of the estimated developmental impairment, safety risks, and potential

consequences if medications are not initiated. Other considerations affecting the treatment of preschool-aged children with stimulant medications include the lack of information and experience about their longer-term effects on growth and brain development, as well as the potential for other adverse effects in this population. It may be helpful to obtain consultation from a mental health specialist with specific experience with preschool-aged children, if possible.

Evidence suggests that the rate of metabolizing methylphenidate is slower in children 4 through 5 years of age, so they should be given a low dose to start; the dose can be increased in smaller increments. Maximum doses have not been adequately studied in preschool-aged children.[83]

Special Circumstances: Adolescents (Age 12 Years to the 18th Birthday)

As noted, before beginning medication treatment of adolescents with newly diagnosed ADHD, clinicians should assess the patient for symptoms of substance use. If active substance use is identified, the clinician should refer the patient to a subspecialist for consultative support and guidance.[2,130–134]

In addition, diversion of ADHD medication (ie, its use for something other than its intended medical purposes) is a special concern among adolescents.[135] Clinicians should monitor the adolescent's symptoms and prescription refill requests for signs of misuse or diversion of ADHD medication, including by parents, classmates, or other acquaintances of the adolescent. The majority of states now require prescriber participation in prescription drug monitoring programs, which can be helpful in identifying and preventing diversion activities. They may consider prescribing nonstimulant medications that minimize abuse potential, such as atomoxetine and extended-release guanfacine or extended-release clonidine.

Given the risks of driving for adolescents with ADHD, including crashes and motor vehicle violations, special concern should be taken to provide medication coverage for symptom control while driving.[79,136,137] Longer-acting or late-afternoon, short-acting medications may be helpful in this regard.[138]

Special Circumstances: Inattention or Hyperactivity/Impulsivity (Problem Level)

Medication is not appropriate for children whose symptoms do not meet *DSM-5* criteria for ADHD. Psychosocial treatments may be appropriate for these children and adolescents. As noted, psychosocial treatments do not require a specific diagnosis of ADHD, and many of the studies on the efficacy of PTBM included children who did not have a specific psychiatric or ADHD diagnosis.

Combination Treatments

Studies indicate that behavioral therapy has positive effects when it is combined with medication for pre-adolescent children.[139] (The combined effects of training interventions and medication have not been studied.)

In the MTA study, researchers found that although the combination of behavioral therapy and stimulant medication was not significantly more effective than treatment with medication alone for ADHD's core symptoms, after correcting for multiple tests in the primary analysis,[139] a secondary analysis of a combined measure of parent and teacher ratings of ADHD symptoms did find a significant advantage for the combination, with a small effect of $d = 0.28$.[140] The combined treatment also offered greater improvements on academic and conduct measures, compared to medication alone, when the ADHD was comorbid with anxiety and the child or adolescent lived in a lower socioeconomic environment.

In addition, parents and teachers of children who received combined therapy reported that they were significantly more satisfied with the treatment plan. Finally, the combination of medication management and behavioral therapy allowed for the use of lower stimulant dosages, possibly reducing the risk of adverse effects.[141]

School Programming and Supports

Encouraging strong family-school partnerships helps the ADHD management process.[142] Psychosocial treatments that include coordinating efforts at school and home may enhance the effects.

Children and adolescents with ADHD may be eligible for services as part of a 504 Rehabilitation Act Plan (504 plan) or special education IEP under the "other health impairment" designation in the Individuals with Disability Education Act (IDEA).[143] (ADHD qualifies as a disability under a 504 plan. It does not qualify under an IEP unless its severity impairs the child's ability to learn. See the PoCA for more details.) It is helpful for clinicians to be aware of the eligibility criteria in their states and school districts to advise families of their options. Eligibility decisions can vary considerably between school districts, and school professionals' independent determinations might not agree with the recommendations of outside clinicians.

There are essentially 2 categories of school-based services for students with ADHD. The first category includes interventions that are intended to help the student independently meet age-appropriate academic and behavioral expectations. Examples of these interventions include daily report cards, training interventions, point systems, and academic remediation of skills. If successful, the student's impairment will resolve, and the student will no longer need services.

The second category is intended to provide changes in the student's program so his or her ADHD-related problems no longer result in failure and cause distress to parents, teachers, and the student.[144] These services are referred to as "accommodations" and include extended time to complete tests and assignments, reduced homework demands, the ability to keep study materials in class, and provision of the teacher's notes to the student. These services are intended to allow the student to accomplish his work successfully and communicate that the student's impairment is acceptable. Accommodations make the student's impairment acceptable and are separate from interventions aimed at improving the students' skills or behaviors. In the absence of such interventions, long-term accommodations may lead to reduced expectations and can lead to the need for accommodations to be maintained throughout the student's education.

Encouraging strong family-school partnerships helps the ADHD management process, and addressing social determinants of health is essential to these partnerships.[145,146] Psychosocial treatments that include coordinating efforts at school and home may enhance the effects.

KAS 6

The PCC should titrate doses of medication for ADHD to achieve maximum benefit with tolerable side effects (Table 9). (Grade B: strong recommendation.)

The MTA study is the landmark study comparing effects of methylphenidate and behavioral treatments in children with ADHD. Investigators compared treatment effects in 4 groups of children who received optimal medication management, optimal behavioral management, combined medication and behavioral management, or community treatment. Children in the optimal medication management and combined medication and behavioral management groups underwent a systematic trial with 4 different doses of methylphenidate, with results suggesting that when this full range of doses is administered, more than 70% of children and adolescents with ADHD are methylphenidate responders.[140]

Authors of other reports suggest that more than 90% of patients will have a beneficial response to 1 of the psychostimulants if a range of medications from both the methylphenidate and amphetamine and/or dextroamphetamine classes

TABLE 9 KAS 6: The PCC should titrate doses of medication for ADHD to achieve maximum benefit with tolerable side effects. (Grade B: strong recommendation.)

Aggregate evidence quality	Grade B
Benefits	The optimal dose of medication is required to reduce core symptoms to, or close to, the levels of children without ADHD.
Risks, harm, cost	Higher levels of medication increase the chances of side effects.
Benefit-harm assessment	The importance of adequately treating ADHD outweighs the risk of adverse effects.
Intentional vagueness	None.
Role of patient preferences	The families' preferences and comfort need to be taken into consideration in developing a titration plan, as they are likely to predict engagement and persistence with a treatment.
Exclusions	None
Strength	Strong recommendation
Key references	Jensen et al[140]; Solanto[147]; Brinkman et al[149]

are tried.[147] Of note, children in the MTA study who received care in the community as usual, either from a clinician they chose or to whom their family had access, showed less beneficial results compared with children who received optimal medication management. The explanation offered by the study investigators was that the community treatment group received lower medication doses and less frequent monitoring than the optimal medication management group.

A child's response to stimulants is variable and unpredictable. For this reason, it is recommended to titrate from a low dose to one that achieves a maximum, optimal effect in controlling symptoms without adverse effects. Calculating the dose on the basis of milligrams per kilogram has not usually been helpful because variations in dose have not been found to be related to height or weight. In addition, because stimulant medication effects are seen rapidly, titration can be accomplished in a relatively short time period. Stimulant medications can be effectively titrated on a 7-day basis, but in urgent situations, they may be effectively titrated in as few as 3 days.[140]

Parent and child and adolescent education is an important component in the chronic illness model to ensure cooperation in efforts to achieve appropriate titration, remembering that the parents themselves may be significantly challenged by ADHD.[148,149] The PCC should alert parents and children that changing medication dose and occasionally changing a medication may be necessary for optimal medication management, may require a few months to achieve optimal success, and that medication efficacy should be monitored at regular intervals.

By the 3-year (ie, 36-month) follow-up to the MTA interventions, there were no differences among the 4 groups (ie, optimal medications management, optimal behavioral management,

a combination of medication and behavioral management, and community treatment). This equivalence in poststudy outcomes may, however, have been attributable to convergence in ongoing treatments received for the 4 groups. After the initial 14-month intervention, the children no longer received the careful monthly monitoring provided by the study and went back to receiving care from their community providers; therefore, they all effectively received a level of ongoing care consistent with the "community treatment" study arm of the study. After leaving the MTA trial, medications and doses varied for the children who had been in the optimal medication management or combined medication and behavioral management groups, and a number stopped taking ADHD medication. On the other hand, some children who had been in the optimal behavioral management group started taking medication after leaving the trial. The results further emphasize the need to treat ADHD as a chronic illness and provide continuity of care and, where possible, provide a medical home.[140]

See the PoCA for more on implementation of this KAS.

KAS 7

The PCC, if trained or experienced in diagnosing comorbid conditions, may initiate treatment of such conditions or make a referral to an appropriate subspecialist for treatment. After detecting possible comorbid conditions, if the PCC is not trained or experienced in making the diagnosis or initiating treatment, the patient should be referred to an appropriate subspecialist to make the diagnosis and initiate treatment (Table 10). (Grade C: recommendation.)

The effect of comorbid conditions on ADHD treatment is variable. In some cases, treatment of the ADHD may resolve the comorbid condition. For example, treatment of ADHD may lead to improvement in coexisting aggression and/or oppositional

defiant, depressive, or anxiety symptoms.[150,151]

Sometimes, however, the comorbid condition may require treatment in addition to the ADHD treatment. If the PCC is confident of his or her ability to diagnose and treat certain comorbid conditions, the PCC may do so. The PCC may benefit from additional consultative support and guidance from a mental health subspecialist or may need to refer a child with ADHD and comorbid conditions, such as severe mood or anxiety disorders, to subspecialists for assessment and management. The subspecialists could include child and adolescent psychiatrists, clinical child psychologists, developmental-behavioral pediatricians, neurodevelopmental disability physicians, child neurologists, or child- or school-based evaluation teams.

IMPLEMENTATION: PREPARING THE PRACTICE

It is generally the role of the primary care pediatrician to manage mild-to-moderate ADHD, anxiety, depression, and substance use. The AAP statement "The Future of Pediatrics: Mental Health Competencies for Pediatric Primary Care" describes the competencies needed in both pediatric primary and specialty care to address the social-emotional and mental health needs of children and families.[152] Broadly, these include incorporating mental health content and tools into health promotion, prevention, and primary care intervention, becoming knowledgeable about use of evidence-based treatments, and participating as a team member and comanaging with pediatric and mental health specialists.

The recommendations made in this guideline are intended to be integrated with the broader mental health algorithm developed as part of the AAP Mental Health Initiatives.[2,133,153] Pediatricians have unique opportunities

TABLE 10 KAS 7: The PCC, if trained or experienced in diagnosing comorbid conditions, may initiate treatment of such conditions or make a referral to an appropriate subspecialist for treatment. After detecting possible comorbid conditions, if the PCC is not trained or experienced in making the diagnosis or initiating treatment, the patient should be referred to an appropriate subspecialist to make the diagnosis and initiate treatment. (Grade C: recommendation.)

Aggregate evidence quality	Grade C
Benefits	Clinicians are most effective when they know the limits of their practice to diagnose comorbid conditions and are aware of resources in their community.
Risks, harm, cost	Under-identification or inappropriate identification of comorbidities can lead to inadequate or inappropriate treatments.
Benefit-harm assessment	The importance of adequately identifying and addressing comorbidities outweighs the risk of inappropriate referrals or treatments.
Intentional vagueness	None.
Role of patient preferences	The families' preferences and comfort need to be taken into consideration in identifying and treating or referring their patients with comorbidities, as they are likely to predict engagement and persistence with a treatment.
Exclusions	None.
Strength	Recommendation.
Key references	Pliszka et al[150]; Pringsheim et al[151]

to identify conditions, including ADHD, intervene early, and partner with both families and specialists for the benefit of children's health. A wealth of useful information is available at the AAP Mental Health Initiatives Web site (https://www.aap.org/en-us/advocacy-and-policy/aap-health-initiatives/Mental-Health/Pages/Tips-For-Pediatricians.aspx).

It is also important for PCCs to be aware of health disparities and social determinants that may impact patient outcomes and strive to provide culturally appropriate care to all children and adolescents in their practice.[145,146,154,155]

The accompanying PoCA provides supplemental information to support PCCs as they implement this guideline's recommendations. In particular, the PoCA describes steps for preparing the practice that provide useful recommendations to clinicians. For example, the PoCA includes information about using standardized rating scales to diagnose ADHD, assessing for comorbid conditions, documenting all aspects of the diagnostic and treatment procedures in the patient's records, monitoring the patient's treatment and outcomes, and providing families with written management plans.

The AAP acknowledges that some PCCs may not have the training,

experience, or resources to diagnose and treat children and adolescents with ADHD, especially if severity or comorbid conditions make these patients complex to manage. In these situations, comanagement with specialty clinicians is recommended. The SDBP is developing a guideline to address such complex cases and aid pediatricians and other PCCs to manage these cases; the SDBP currently expects to publish this document in 2019.[67]

AREAS FOR FUTURE RESEARCH

There is a need to conduct research on topics pertinent to the diagnosis and treatment of ADHD, developmental variations, and problems in children and adolescents in primary care. These research opportunities include the following:

- assessment of ADHD and its common comorbidities: anxiety, depression, learning disabilities, and autism spectrum disorder;
- identification and/or development of reliable instruments suitable for use in primary care to assess the nature or degree of functional impairment in children and adolescents with ADHD and to monitor improvement over time;
- refinement of developmentally informed assessment procedures

for evaluating ADHD in preschoolers;

- study of medications and other therapies used clinically but not FDA approved for ADHD;
- determination of the optimal schedule for monitoring children and adolescents with ADHD, including factors for adjusting that schedule according to age, symptom severity, and progress reports;
- evaluation of the effectiveness and adverse effects of medications used in combination, such as a stimulant with an α-adrenergic agent, selective serotonin reuptake inhibitor, or atomoxetine;
- evaluation of processes of care to assist PCCs to identify and treat comorbid conditions;
- evaluation of the effectiveness of various school-based interventions;
- comparisons of medication use and effectiveness in different ages, including both harms and benefits;
- development of methods to involve parents, children, and adolescents in their own care and improve adherence to both psychosocial and medication treatments;
- conducting research into psychosocial treatments, such as cognitive behavioral therapy and cognitive training, among others;

- development of standardized and documented tools to help primary care providers identify comorbid conditions;
- development of effective electronic and Web-based systems to help gather information to diagnose and monitor children and adolescents with ADHD;
- improvements to systems for communicating with schools, mental health professionals, and other community agencies to provide effective collaborative care;
- development of more objective measures of performance to more objectively monitor aspects of severity, disability, or impairment;
- assessment of long-term outcomes for children in whom ADHD was first diagnosed at preschool ages; and
- identification and implementation of ideas to address the barriers that hamper the implementation of these guidelines and the PoCA.

CONCLUSIONS

Evidence is clear with regard to the legitimacy of the diagnosis of ADHD and the appropriate diagnostic criteria and procedures required to establish a diagnosis, identify comorbid conditions, and effectively treat with both psychosocial and pharmacologic interventions. The steps required to sustain appropriate treatments and achieve successful long-term outcomes remain challenging, however.

As noted, this clinical practice guideline is supported by 2 accompanying documents available in the Supplemental Information: the PoCA and the article on systemic barriers to the car of children and adolescents with ADHD. Full implementation of the guideline's KASs, the PoCA, and the recommendations to address barriers to care may require changes in office procedures and the identification of community resources. Fully addressing systemic barriers requires identifying local, state, and national entities with which to partner to advance solutions and manifest change.[156]

SUBCOMMITTEE ON CHILDREN AND ADOLESCENTS WITH ADHD (OVERSIGHT BY THE COUNCIL ON QUALITY IMPROVEMENT AND PATIENT SAFETY)

Mark L. Wolraich, MD, FAAP, Chairperson, Section on Developmental Behavioral Pediatrics

Joseph F. Hagan Jr, MD, FAAP, Vice Chairperson, Section on Developmental Behavioral Pediatrics
Carla Allan, PhD, Society of Pediatric Psychology
Eugenia Chan, MD, MPH, FAAP, Implementation Scientist
Dale Davison, MSpEd, PCC, Parent Advocate, Children and Adolescents with Attention-Deficit/Hyperactivity Disorder
Marian Earls, MD, MTS, FAAP, Mental Health Leadership Work Group
Steven W. Evans, PhD, Clinical Psychologist
Tanya Froehlich, MD, FAAP, Section on Developmental Behavioral Pediatrics/Society for Developmental and Behavioral Pediatrics
Jennifer Frost, MD, FAAFP, American Academy of Family Physicians
Joseph R. Holbrook, PhD, MPH, Epidemiologist, Centers for Disease Control and Prevention
Herschel Robert Lessin, MD, FAAP, Section on Administration and Practice Management
Karen L. Pierce, MD, DFAACAP, American Academy of Child and Adolescent Psychiatry
Christoph Ulrich Lehmann, MD, FAAP, Partnership for Policy Implementation
Jonathan D. Winner, MD, FAAP, Committee on Practice and Ambulatory Medicine
William Zurhellen, MD, FAAP, Section on Administration and Practice Management

STAFF

Kymika Okechukwu, MPA, Senior Manager, Evidence-Based Medicine Initiatives
Jeremiah Salmon, MPH, Program Manager, Policy Dissemination and Implementation

CONSULTANT

Susan K. Flinn, MA, Medical Editor

ABBREVIATIONS

AAP: American Academy of Pediatrics
ADHD: attention-deficit/hyperactivity disorder
ADHD/C: attention-deficit/hyperactivity disorder combined presentation
ADHD/HI: attention-deficit/hyperactivity disorder primarily of the hyperactive-impulsive presentation
ADHD/I: attention-deficit/hyperactivity disorder primarily of the inattentive presentation

AHRQ: Agency for Healthcare Research and Quality
BP: blood pressure
CHADD: Children and Adults with Attention-Deficit/Hyperactivity Disorder
DSM-5: *Diagnostic and Statistical Manual of Mental Disorders, Fifth Edition* DSM-IV: *Diagnostic and Statistical Manual of Mental Disorders Fourth Edition*
DSM-PC: *Diagnostic and Statistical Manual for Primary Care*
ECG: electrocardiogram
eTNS: external trigeminal nerve stimulation

FDA: US Food and Drug Administration
HR: heart rate
IDEA: Individuals with Disability Education Act
IEP: Individualized Education Program
KAS: key action statement
MTA: The Multimodal Treatment of Attention Deficit Hyperactivity Disorder
PCC: primary care clinician
PoCA: process of care algorithm
PTBM: parent training in behavior management
SDBP: Society for Developmental and Behavioral Pediatrics

ᵛAmerican Academy of Pediatrics, Itasca, Illinois; ʷAmerican Academy of Child and Adolescent Psychiatry, Washington, District of Columbia; ˣFeinberg School of Medicine, Northwestern University, Chicago, Illinois; ʸAtlanta, Georgia; and ᶻHolderness, New Hampshire

The guidance in this report does not indicate an exclusive course of treatment or serve as a standard of medical care. Variations, taking into account individual circumstances, may be appropriate.

All clinical practice guidelines from the American Academy of Pediatrics automatically expire 5 years after publication unless reaffirmed, revised, or retired at or before that time.

The findings and conclusions in this report are those of the authors and do not necessarily represent the official position of the Centers for Disease Control and Prevention. Dr Holbrook was not an author of the accompanying supplemental section on barriers to care.

This document is copyrighted and is property of the American Academy of Pediatrics and its Board of Directors. All authors have filed conflict of interest statements with the American Academy of Pediatrics. Any conflicts have been resolved through a process approved by the Board of Directors. The American Academy of Pediatrics has neither solicited nor accepted any commercial involvement in the development of the content of this publication.

DOI: https://doi.org/10.1542/peds.2019-2528

Address correspondence to Mark L. Wolraich, MD, FAAP. Email: mark-wolraich@ouhsc.edu

PEDIATRICS (ISSN Numbers: Print, 0031-4005; Online, 1098-4275).

FINANCIAL DISCLOSURE: The authors have indicated they have no financial relationships relevant to this article to disclose.

FUNDING: No external funding.

POTENTIAL CONFLICT OF INTEREST: All authors have filed conflict of interest statements with the American Academy of Pediatrics. Any conflicts have been resolved through a process approved by the American Academy of Pediatrics board of directors. Dr Allan reports a relationship with ADDitude Magazine; Dr Chan reports relationships with TriVox Health and Wolters Kluwer; Dr Lehmann reports relationships with International Medical Informatics Association, Springer Publishing, and Thieme Publishing Group; Dr Wolraich reports a Continuing Medical Education trainings relationship with the Resource for Advancing Children's Health Institute; the other authors have indicated they have no potential conflicts of interest to disclose.

REFERENCES

1. American Academy of Pediatrics. Subcommittee on Attention-Deficit/Hyperactivity Disorder, Steering Committee on Quality Improvement and Management. ADHD: Clinical guideline for the diagnosis, evaluation, and treatment of attention-deficit/hyperactivity disorder in children and adolescents. *Pediatrics.* 2011;128(5):1007–1022

2. American Academy of Pediatrics Task Force on Mental Health. *Addressing Mental Health Concerns in Primary Care: A Clinician's Toolkit [CD-ROM].* Elk Grove Village, IL: American Academy of Pediatrics; 2010

3. Pastor PN, Reuben CA. Racial and ethnic differences in ADHD and LD in young school-age children: parental reports in the National Health Interview Survey. *Public Health Rep.* 2005;120(4):383–392

4. US Department of Health and Human Services; Health Resources and Services Administration. Designated health professional shortage areas statistics: designated HPSA quarterly summary. Rockville, MD: Health Resources and Services Administration; 2018

5. Pelech D, Hayford T. Medicare advantage and commercial prices for mental health services. *Health Aff (Millwood).* 2019;38(2):262–267

6. Melek SP, Perlman D, Davenport S. *Differential Reimbursement of Psychiatric Services by Psychiatrists and Other Medical Providers.* Seattle, WA: Milliman;2017

7. Holbrook JR, Bitsko RH, Danielson ML, Visser SN. Interpreting the prevalence of mental disorders in children: tribulation and triangulation. *Health Promot Pract.* 2017;18(1):5–7

8. Thomas R, Sanders S, Doust J, Beller E, Glasziou P. Prevalence of attention-deficit/hyperactivity disorder: a systematic review and meta-analysis. *Pediatrics.* 2015;135(4). Available at: www.pediatrics.org/cgi/content/full/135/4/e994

9. Wolraich ML, McKeown RE, Visser SN, et al. The prevalence of ADHD: its diagnosis and treatment in four school districts across two states. *J Atten Disord.* 2014;18(7):563–575

10. Rowland AS, Skipper BJ, Umbach DM, et al. The prevalence of ADHD in a population-based sample. *J Atten Disord.* 2015;19(9):741–754

11. Danielson ML, Bitsko RH, Ghandour RM, Holbrook JR, Kogan MD, Blumberg SJ. Prevalence of parent-reported ADHD diagnosis and associated treatment among U.S. children and adolescents, 2016. *J Clin Child Adolesc Psychol.* 2018; 47(2):199–212

12. Visser SN, Zablotsky B, Holbrook JR, et al. *National Health Statistics Reports, No 81: Diagnostic Experiences of Children with Attention-Deficit/Hyperactivity Disorder.* Hyattsville, MD: National Center for Health Statistics; 2015

13. Molina BS, Hinshaw SP, Swanson JM, et al; MTA Cooperative Group. The MTA at 8 years: prospective follow-up of children treated for combined-type ADHD in a multisite study. *J Am Acad Child Adolesc Psychiatry.* 2009;48(5):484–500

14. Holbrook JR, Cuffe SP, Cai B, et al. Persistence of parent-reported ADHD symptoms from childhood through adolescence in a community sample. *J Atten Disord.* 2016;20(1):11–20

15. Mueller KL, Tomblin JB. Examining the comorbidity of language disorders and ADHD. *Top Lang Disord*. 2012;32(3): 228–246

16. Pastor PN, Reuben CA, Duran CR, Hawkins LD. *Association Between Diagnosed ADHD and Selected Characteristics Among Children Aged 4–17 Years: United States, 2011–2013*. NCHS Data Brief, No. 201. Hyattsville, MD: National Center for Health Statistics; 2015

17. Elia J, Ambrosini P, Berrettini W. ADHD characteristics: I. Concurrent co-morbidity patterns in children & adolescents. *Child Adolesc Psychiatry Ment Health*. 2008;2(1):15

18. Centers for Disease Control and Prevention (CDC). Mental health in the United States. Prevalence of diagnosis and medication treatment for attention-deficit/hyperactivity disorder--United States, 2003. *MMWR Morb Mortal Wkly Rep*. 2005;54(34):842–847

19. Cuffe SP, Visser SN, Holbrook JR, et al. ADHD and psychiatric comorbidity: functional outcomes in a school-based sample of children [published online ahead of print November 25, 2015]. *J Atten Disord*. doi:10.1177/1087054715613437

20. Gaub M, Carlson CL. Gender differences in ADHD: a meta-analysis and critical review. *J Am Acad Child Adolesc Psychiatry*. 1997;36(8):1036–1045

21. Tung I, Li JJ, Meza JI, et al. Patterns of comorbidity among girls with ADHD: a meta-analysis. *Pediatrics*. 2016;138(4): e20160430

22. Layton TJ, Barnett ML, Hicks TR, Jena AB. Attention deficit-hyperactivity disorder and month of school enrollment. *N Engl J Med*. 2018;379(22): 2122–2130

23. Kemper AR, Maslow GR, Hill S, et al. *Attention Deficit Hyperactivity Disorder: Diagnosis and Treatment in Children and Adolescents. Comparative Effectiveness Reviews, No. 203*. Rockville, MD: Agency for Healthcare Research and Quality; 2018

24. Pelham WE Jr, Wheeler T, Chronis A. Empirically supported psychosocial treatments for attention deficit hyperactivity disorder. *J Clin Child Psychol*. 1998;27(2):190–205

25. Evans SW, Owens JS, Wymbs BT, Ray AR. Evidence-based psychosocial treatments for children and adolescents with attention deficit/hyperactivity disorder. *J Clin Child Adolesc Psychol*. 2018;47(2):157–198

26. Pelham WE Jr, Fabiano GA. Evidence-based psychosocial treatments for attention-deficit/hyperactivity disorder. *J Clin Child Adolesc Psychol*. 2008;37(1): 184–214

27. American Academy of Pediatrics Steering Committee on Quality Improvement and Management. Classifying recommendations for clinical practice guidelines. *Pediatrics*. 2004;114(3):874–877

28. Visser SN, Lesesne CA, Perou R. National estimates and factors associated with medication treatment for childhood attention-deficit/hyperactivity disorder. *Pediatrics*. 2007;119(suppl 1):S99–S106

29. Centers for Disease Control and Prevention (CDC). Increasing prevalence of parent-reported attention-deficit/hyperactivity disorder among children—United States, 2003 and 2007. *MMWR Morb Mortal Wkly Rep*. 2010;59(44):1439–1443

30. Egger HL, Kondo D, Angold A. The epidemiology and diagnostic issues in preschool attention-deficit/hyperactivity disorder: a review. *Infants Young Child*. 2006;19(2):109–122

31. Wolraich ML, Wibbelsman CJ, Brown TE, et al. Attention-deficit/hyperactivity disorder among adolescents: a review of the diagnosis, treatment, and clinical implications. *Pediatrics*. 2005;115(6): 1734–1746

32. American Psychiatric Association. *Diagnostic and Statistical Manual of Mental Disorders (DSM-5)*. 5th ed. Arlington, VA: American Psychiatric Association; 2013

33. Lahey BB, Pelham WE, Stein MA, et al. Validity of DSM-IV attention-deficit/hyperactivity disorder for younger children. *J Am Acad Child Adolesc Psychiatry*. 1998;37(7):695–702

34. Pavuluri MN, Luk SL, McGee R. Parent reported preschool attention deficit hyperactivity: measurement and validity. *Eur Child Adolesc Psychiatry*. 1999;8(2):126–133

35. Harvey EA, Youngwirth SD, Thakar DA, Errazuriz PA. Predicting attention-deficit/hyperactivity disorder and oppositional defiant disorder from preschool diagnostic assessments. *J Consult Clin Psychol*. 2009;77(2): 349–354

36. Keenan K, Wakschlag LS. More than the terrible twos: the nature and severity of behavior problems in clinic-referred preschool children. *J Abnorm Child Psychol*. 2000;28(1):33–46

37. Gadow KD, Nolan EE, Litcher L, et al. Comparison of attention-deficit/hyperactivity disorder symptom subtypes in Ukrainian schoolchildren. *J Am Acad Child Adolesc Psychiatry*. 2000;39(12):1520–1527

38. Sprafkin J, Volpe RJ, Gadow KD, Nolan EE, Kelly K. A DSM-IV-referenced screening instrument for preschool children: the Early Childhood Inventory-4. *J Am Acad Child Adolesc Psychiatry*. 2002;41(5):604–612

39. Poblano A, Romero E. ECI-4 screening of attention deficit-hyperactivity disorder and co-morbidity in Mexican preschool children: preliminary results. *Arq Neuropsiquiatr*. 2006;64(4):932–936

40. American Academy of Pediatrics. *Mental Health Screening and Assessment Tools for Primary Care*. Elk Grove Village, IL: American Academy of Pediatrics; 2012. Available at: https://www.aap.org/en-us/advocacy-and-policy/aap-health-initiatives/Mental-Health/Documents/MH_ScreeningChart.pdf. Accessed September 8, 2019

41. DuPaul GJ, Power TJ, Anastopoulos AD, Reid R. *ADHD Rating Scale – 5 for Children and Adolescents: Checklists, Norms, and Clinical Interpretation*. 2nd ed. New York, NY: Guilford Press; 2016

42. McGoey KE, DuPaul GJ, Haley E, Shelton TL. Parent and teacher ratings of attention-deficit/hyperactivity disorder in preschool: the ADHD rating scale-IV preschool version. *J Psychopathol Behav Assess*. 2007;29(4):269–276

43. Young J. Common comorbidities seen in adolescents with attention-deficit/hyperactivity disorder. *Adolesc Med State Art Rev*. 2008;19(2):216–228, vii

44. Freeman RD; Tourette Syndrome International Database Consortium. Tic disorders and ADHD: answers from

a world-wide clinical dataset on Tourette syndrome. *Eur Child Adolesc Psychiatry.* 2007;16(suppl 1):15–23

45. Riggs PD. Clinical approach to treatment of ADHD in adolescents with substance use disorders and conduct disorder. *J Am Acad Child Adolesc Psychiatry.* 1998;37(3):331–332

46. Sibley MH, Pelham WE, Molina BSG, et al. Diagnosing ADHD in adolescence. *J Consult Clin Psychol.* 2012;80(1): 139–150

47. Kratochvil CJ, Vaughan BS, Stoner JA, et al. A double-blind, placebo-controlled study of atomoxetine in young children with ADHD. *Pediatrics.* 2011;127(4). Available at: www.pediatrics.org/cgi/content/full/127/4/e862

48. Harrison AG, Edwards MJ, Parker KC. Identifying students faking ADHD: preliminary findings and strategies for detection. *Arch Clin Neuropsychol.* 2007; 22(5):577–588

49. Wolraich ML, Felice ME, Drotar DD. *The Classification of Child and Adolescent Mental Conditions in Primary Care: Diagnostic and Statistical Manual for Primary Care (DSM-PC), Child and Adolescent Version.* Elk Grove Village, IL: American Academy of Pediatrics; 1996

50. Rowland AS, Lesesne CA, Abramowitz AJ. The epidemiology of attention-deficit/hyperactivity disorder (ADHD): a public health view. *Ment Retard Dev Disabil Res Rev.* 2002;8(3):162–170

51. Cuffe SP, Moore CG, McKeown RE. Prevalence and correlates of ADHD symptoms in the national health interview survey. *J Atten Disord.* 2005; 9(2):392–401

52. Pastor PN, Reuben CA. Diagnosed attention deficit hyperactivity disorder and learning disability: United States, 2004-2006. *Vital Health Stat 10.* 2008; 10(237):1–14

53. Biederman J, Faraone SV, Wozniak J, Mick E, Kwon A, Aleardi M. Further evidence of unique developmental phenotypic correlates of pediatric bipolar disorder: findings from a large sample of clinically referred preadolescent children assessed over the last 7 years. *J Affect Disord.* 2004; 82(suppl 1):S45–S58

54. Biederman J, Kwon A, Aleardi M, et al. Absence of gender effects on attention deficit hyperactivity disorder: findings in nonreferred subjects. *Am J Psychiatry.* 2005;162(6):1083–1089

55. Biederman J, Ball SW, Monuteaux MC, et al. New insights into the comorbidity between ADHD and major depression in adolescent and young adult females. *J Am Acad Child Adolesc Psychiatry.* 2008;47(4):426–434

56. Biederman J, Melmed RD, Patel A, McBurnett K, Donahue J, Lyne A. Long-term, open-label extension study of guanfacine extended release in children and adolescents with ADHD. *CNS Spectr.* 2008;13(12):1047–1055

57. Crabtree VM, Ivanenko A, Gozal D. Clinical and parental assessment of sleep in children with attention-deficit/hyperactivity disorder referred to a pediatric sleep medicine center. *Clin Pediatr (Phila).* 2003;42(9):807–813

58. LeBourgeois MK, Avis K, Mixon M, Olmi J, Harsh J. Snoring, sleep quality, and sleepiness across attention-deficit/hyperactivity disorder subtypes. *Sleep.* 2004;27(3):520–525

59. Chan E, Zhan C, Homer CJ. Health care use and costs for children with attention-deficit/hyperactivity disorder: national estimates from the Medical Expenditure Panel Survey. *Arch Pediatr Adolesc Med.* 2002;156(5):504–511

60. Newcorn JH, Miller SR, Ivanova I, et al. Adolescent outcome of ADHD: impact of childhood conduct and anxiety disorders. *CNS Spectr.* 2004;9(9): 668–678

61. Sung V, Hiscock H, Sciberras E, Efron D. Sleep problems in children with attention-deficit/hyperactivity disorder: prevalence and the effect on the child and family. *Arch Pediatr Adolesc Med.* 2008;162(4):336–342

62. Froehlich TE, Fogler J, Barbaresi WJ, Elsayed NA, Evans SW, Chan E. Using ADHD medications to treat coexisting ADHD and reading disorders: a systematic review. *Clin Pharmacol Ther.* 2018;104(4):619–637

63. Rothenberger A, Roessner V. The phenomenology of attention-deficit/hyperactivity disorder in tourette syndrome. In: Martino D, Leckman JF, eds. *Tourette Syndrome.* New York, NY: Oxford University Press; 2013:26–49

64. Antshel KM, Zhang-James Y, Faraone SV. The comorbidity of ADHD and autism spectrum disorder. *Expert Rev Neurother.* 2013;13(10):1117–1128

65. Mahajan R, Bernal MP, Panzer R, et al; Autism Speaks Autism Treatment Network Psychopharmacology Committee. Clinical practice pathways for evaluation and medication choice for attention-deficit/hyperactivity disorder symptoms in autism spectrum disorders. *Pediatrics.* 2012;130(suppl 2):S125–S138

66. Larson K, Russ SA, Kahn RS, Halfon N. Patterns of comorbidity, functioning, and service use for US children with ADHD, 2007. *Pediatrics.* 2011;127(3): 462–470

67. Society for Developmental and Behavioral Pediatrics. ADHD special interest group. Available at: www.sdbp.org/committees/sig-adhd.cfm. Accessed September 8, 2019

68. Medical Home Initiatives for Children With Special Needs Project Advisory Committee. American Academy of Pediatrics. The medical home. *Pediatrics.* 2002;110(1 pt 1):184–186

69. Brito A, Grant R, Overholt S, et al. The enhanced medical home: the pediatric standard of care for medically underserved children. *Adv Pediatr.* 2008;55:9–28

70. Sibley MH, Swanson JM, Arnold LE, et al; MTA Cooperative Group. Defining ADHD symptom persistence in adulthood: optimizing sensitivity and specificity. *J Child Psychol Psychiatry.* 2017;58(6): 655–662

71. Chang Z, D'Onofrio BM, Quinn PD, Lichtenstein P, Larsson H. Medication for attention-deficit/hyperactivity disorder and risk for depression: a nationwide longitudinal cohort study. *Biol Psychiatry.* 2016;80(12):916–922

72. Biederman J, Monuteaux MC, Spencer T, Wilens TE, Faraone SV. Do stimulants protect against psychiatric disorders in youth with ADHD? A 10-year follow-up study. *Pediatrics.* 2009;124(1):71–78

73. Barbaresi WJ, Katusic SK, Colligan RC, Weaver AL, Jacobsen SJ. Modifiers of long-term school outcomes for children with attention-deficit/hyperactivity disorder: does treatment with

stimulant medication make a difference? Results from a population-based study. *J Dev Behav Pediatr.* 2007; 28(4):274–287

74. Scheffler RM, Brown TT, Fulton BD, Hinshaw SP, Levine P, Stone S. Positive association between attention-deficit/ hyperactivity disorder medication use and academic achievement during elementary school. *Pediatrics.* 2009; 123(5):1273–1279

75. Barbaresi WJ, Colligan RC, Weaver AL, Voigt RG, Killian JM, Katusic SK. Mortality, ADHD, and psychosocial adversity in adults with childhood ADHD: a prospective study. *Pediatrics.* 2013;131(4):637–644

76. Chang Z, Lichtenstein P, Långström N, Larsson H, Fazel S. Association between prescription of major psychotropic medications and violent reoffending after prison release. *JAMA.* 2016; 316(17):1798–1807

77. Lichtenstein P, Halldner L, Zetterqvist J, et al. Medication for attention deficit-hyperactivity disorder and criminality. *N Engl J Med.* 2012;367(21):2006–2014

78. Chang Z, Quinn PD, Hur K, et al. Association between medication use for attention-deficit/hyperactivity disorder and risk of motor vehicle crashes. *JAMA Psychiatry.* 2017;74(6):597–603

79. Chang Z, Lichtenstein P, D'Onofrio BM, Sjölander A, Larsson H. Serious transport accidents in adults with attention-deficit/hyperactivity disorder and the effect of medication: a population-based study. *JAMA Psychiatry.* 2014;71(3):319–325

80. Harstad E, Levy S; Committee on Substance Abuse. Attention-deficit/ hyperactivity disorder and substance abuse. *Pediatrics.* 2014;134(1). Available at: www.pediatrics.org/cgi/content/ full/134/1/e293

81. Dalsgaard S, Leckman JF, Mortensen PB, Nielsen HS, Simonsen M. Effect of drugs on the risk of injuries in children with attention deficit hyperactivity disorder: a prospective cohort study. *Lancet Psychiatry.* 2015;2(8):702–709

82. Raman SR, Marshall SW, Haynes K, Gaynes BN, Naftel AJ, Stürmer T. Stimulant treatment and injury among children with attention deficit hyperactivity disorder: an application of

the self-controlled case series study design. *Inj Prev.* 2013;19(3):164–170

83. Greenhill L, Kollins S, Abikoff H, et al. Efficacy and safety of immediate-release methylphenidate treatment for preschoolers with ADHD. *J Am Acad Child Adolesc Psychiatry.* 2006;45(11): 1284–1293

84. Children and Adults with Attention-Deficit/Hyperactivity Disorder. CHADD. Available at: www.chadd.org. Accessed September 8, 2019

85. Sonuga-Barke EJ, Daley D, Thompson M, Laver-Bradbury C, Weeks A. Parent-based therapies for preschool attention-deficit/hyperactivity disorder: a randomized, controlled trial with a community sample. *J Am Acad Child Adolesc Psychiatry.* 2001;40(4):402–408

86. Van Cleave J, Leslie LK. Approaching ADHD as a chronic condition: implications for long-term adherence. *J Psychosoc Nurs Ment Health Serv.* 2008;46(8):28–37

87. Webster-Stratton CH, Reid MJ, Beauchaine T. Combining parent and child training for young children with ADHD. *J Clin Child Adolesc Psychol.* 2011;40(2):191–203

88. Shepard SA, Dickstein S. Preventive intervention for early childhood behavioral problems: an ecological perspective. *Child Adolesc Psychiatr Clin N Am.* 2009;18(3):687–706

89. Evans SW, Langberg JM, Egan T, Molitor SJ. Middle school-based and high school-based interventions for adolescents with ADHD. *Child Adolesc Psychiatr Clin N Am.* 2014;23(4):699–715

90. McGough JJ, Sturm A, Cowen J, et al. Double-blind, sham-controlled, pilot study of trigeminal nerve stimulation for attention-deficit/hyperactivity disorder. *J Am Acad Child Adolesc Psychiatry.* 2019;58(4):403–411.e3

91. Robin AL, Foster SL. *The Guilford Family Therapy Series. Negotiating Parent–Adolescent Conflict: A Behavioral–Family Systems Approach.* New York, NY: Guilford Press; 1989

92. Barkley RA, Guevremont DC, Anastopoulos AD, Fletcher KE. A comparison of three family therapy programs for treating family conflicts in adolescents with attention-deficit

hyperactivity disorder. *J Consult Clin Psychol.* 1992;60(3):450–462

93. Fabiano GA, Schatz NK, Morris KL, et al. Efficacy of a family-focused intervention for young drivers with attention-deficit hyperactivity disorder. *J Consult Clin Psychol.* 2016;84(12):1078–1093

94. Sibley MH, Graziano PA, Kuriyan AB, et al. Parent-teen behavior therapy + motivational interviewing for adolescents with ADHD. *J Consult Clin Psychol.* 2016;84(8):699–712

95. Evans SW, Langberg JM, Schultz BK, et al. Evaluation of a school-based treatment program for young adolescents with ADHD. *J Consult Clin Psychol.* 2016;84(1):15–30

96. Langberg JM, Dvorsky MR, Molitor SJ, et al. Overcoming the research-to-practice gap: a randomized trial with two brief homework and organization interventions for students with ADHD as implemented by school mental health providers. *J Consult Clin Psychol.* 2018; 86(1):39–55

97. Schultz BK, Evans SW, Langberg JM, Schoemann AM. Outcomes for adolescents who comply with long-term psychosocial treatment for ADHD. *J Consult Clin Psychol.* 2017;85(3): 250–261

98. Newcorn JH, Kratochvil CJ, Allen AJ, et al; Atomoxetine/Methylphenidate Comparative Study Group. Atomoxetine and osmotically released methylphenidate for the treatment of attention deficit hyperactivity disorder: acute comparison and differential response. *Am J Psychiatry.* 2008;165(6): 721–730

99. Cheng JY, Chen RY, Ko JS, Ng EM. Efficacy and safety of atomoxetine for attention-deficit/hyperactivity disorder in children and adolescents-meta-analysis and meta-regression analysis. *Psychopharmacology (Berl).* 2007; 194(2):197–209

100. Michelson D, Allen AJ, Busner J, et al. Once-daily atomoxetine treatment for children and adolescents with attention deficit hyperactivity disorder: a randomized, placebo-controlled study. *Am J Psychiatry.* 2002;159(11): 1896–1901

101. Biederman J, Melmed RD, Patel A, et al; SPD503 Study Group. A randomized,

double-blind, placebo-controlled study of guanfacine extended release in children and adolescents with attention-deficit/hyperactivity disorder. *Pediatrics*. 2008;121(1). Available at: www.pediatrics.org/cgi/content/full/121/1/e73

102. Sallee FR, Lyne A, Wigal T, McGough JJ. Long-term safety and efficacy of guanfacine extended release in children and adolescents with attention-deficit/hyperactivity disorder. *J Child Adolesc Psychopharmacol*. 2009; 19(3):215–226

103. Jain R, Segal S, Kollins SH, Khayrallah M. Clonidine extended-release tablets for pediatric patients with attention-deficit/hyperactivity disorder. *J Am Acad Child Adolesc Psychiatry*. 2011; 50(2):171–179

104. Brown JT, Bishop JR. Atomoxetine pharmacogenetics: associations with pharmacokinetics, treatment response and tolerability. *Pharmacogenomics*. 2015;16(13):1513–1520

105. Kambeitz J, Romanos M, Ettinger U. Meta-analysis of the association between dopamine transporter genotype and response to methylphenidate treatment in ADHD. *Pharmacogenomics J*. 2014;14(1):77–84

106. Bruxel EM, Akutagava-Martins GC, Salatino-Oliveira A, et al. ADHD pharmacogenetics across the life cycle: new findings and perspectives. *Am J Med Genet B Neuropsychiatr Genet*. 2014;165B(4):263–282

107. Kieling C, Genro JP, Hutz MH, Rohde LA. A current update on ADHD pharmacogenomics. *Pharmacogenomics*. 2010;11(3): 407–419

108. Froehlich TE, McGough JJ, Stein MA. Progress and promise of attention-deficit hyperactivity disorder pharmacogenetics. *CNS Drugs*. 2010; 24(2):99–117

109. Joensen B, Meyer M, Aagaard L. Specific genes associated with adverse events of methylphenidate use in the pediatric population: a systematic literature review. *J Res Pharm Pract*. 2017;6(2): 65–72

110. Swanson JM, Elliott GR, Greenhill LL, et al. Effects of stimulant medication on growth rates across 3 years in the MTA follow-up. *J Am Acad Child Adolesc Psychiatry*. 2007;46(8):1015–1027

111. Mosholder AD, Gelperin K, Hammad TA, Phelan K, Johann-Liang R. Hallucinations and other psychotic symptoms associated with the use of attention-deficit/hyperactivity disorder drugs in children. *Pediatrics*. 2009; 123(2):611–616

112. Cortese S, Holtmann M, Banaschewski T, et al; European ADHD Guidelines Group. Practitioner review: current best practice in the management of adverse events during treatment with ADHD medications in children and adolescents. *J Child Psychol Psychiatry*. 2013;54(3):227–246

113. Avigan M. *Review of AERS Data From Marketed Safety Experience During Stimulant Therapy: Death, Sudden Death, Cardiovascular SAEs (Including Stroke). Report No. D030403*. Silver Spring, MD: Food and Drug Administration, Center for Drug Evaluation and Research; 2004

114. Perrin JM, Friedman RA, Knilans TK; Black Box Working Group; Section on Cardiology and Cardiac Surgery. Cardiovascular monitoring and stimulant drugs for attention-deficit/hyperactivity disorder. *Pediatrics*. 2008; 122(2):451–453

115. McCarthy S, Cranswick N, Potts L, Taylor E, Wong IC. Mortality associated with attention-deficit hyperactivity disorder (ADHD) drug treatment: a retrospective cohort study of children, adolescents and young adults using the general practice research database. *Drug Saf*. 2009;32(11):1089–1096

116. Gould MS, Walsh BT, Munfakh JL, et al. Sudden death and use of stimulant medications in youths. *Am J Psychiatry*. 2009;166(9):992–1001

117. Cooper WO, Habel LA, Sox CM, et al. ADHD drugs and serious cardiovascular events in children and young adults. *N Engl J Med*. 2011;365(20):1896–1904

118. Schelleman H, Bilker WB, Strom BL, et al. Cardiovascular events and death in children exposed and unexposed to ADHD agents. *Pediatrics*. 2011;127(6): 1102–1110

119. Garnock-Jones KP, Keating GM. Atomoxetine: a review of its use in attention-deficit hyperactivity disorder in children and adolescents. *Paediatr Drugs*. 2009;11(3):203–226

120. Reed VA, Buitelaar JK, Anand E, et al. The safety of atomoxetine for the treatment of children and adolescents with attention-deficit/hyperactivity disorder: a comprehensive review of over a decade of research. *CNS Drugs*. 2016;30(7):603–628

121. Bangs ME, Tauscher-Wisniewski S, Polzer J, et al. Meta-analysis of suicide-related behavior events in patients treated with atomoxetine. *J Am Acad Child Adolesc Psychiatry*. 2008;47(2): 209–218

122. Bangs ME, Jin L, Zhang S, et al. Hepatic events associated with atomoxetine treatment for attention-deficit hyperactivity disorder. *Drug Saf*. 2008; 31(4):345–354

123. Spencer TJ, Kratochvil CJ, Sangal RB, et al. Effects of atomoxetine on growth in children with attention-deficit/hyperactivity disorder following up to five years of treatment. *J Child Adolesc Psychopharmacol*. 2007;17(5):689–700

124. Elbe D, Reddy D. Focus on guanfacine extended-release: a review of its use in child and adolescent psychiatry. *J Can Acad Child Adolesc Psychiatry*. 2014; 23(1):48–60

125. Croxtall JD. Clonidine extended-release: in attention-deficit hyperactivity disorder. *Paediatr Drugs*. 2011;13(5): 329–336

126. Vaughan B, Kratochvil CJ. Pharmacotherapy of pediatric attention-deficit/hyperactivity disorder. *Child Adolesc Psychiatr Clin N Am*. 2012; 21(4):941–955

127. Hirota T, Schwartz S, Correll CU. Alpha-2 agonists for attention-deficit/hyperactivity disorder in youth: a systematic review and meta-analysis of monotherapy and add-on trials to stimulant therapy. *J Am Acad Child Adolesc Psychiatry*. 2014;53(2):153–173

128. Treuer T, Gau SS, Méndez L, et al. A systematic review of combination therapy with stimulants and atomoxetine for attention-deficit/hyperactivity disorder, including patient characteristics, treatment strategies, effectiveness, and tolerability. *J Child Adolesc Psychopharmacol*. 2013;23(3): 179–193

129. Greenhill LL, Posner K, Vaughan BS, Kratochvil CJ. Attention deficit hyperactivity disorder in preschool children. *Child Adolesc Psychiatr Clin N Am.* 2008;17(2):347–366, ix

130. Wilens TE, Spencer TJ. Understanding attention-deficit/hyperactivity disorder from childhood to adulthood. *Postgrad Med.* 2010;122(5):97–109

131. Foy JM, ed. Psychotropic medications in primary care. In: *Mental Health Care of Children and Adolescents: A Guide for Primary Care Clinicians.* Itasca, IL: American Academy of Pediatrics; 2018: 315–374

132. Wilens TE, Adler LA, Adams J, et al. Misuse and diversion of stimulants prescribed for ADHD: a systematic review of the literature. *J Am Acad Child Adolesc Psychiatry.* 2008;47(1): 21–31

133. American Academy of Pediatrics. Mental health initiatives. Available at: https://www.aap.org/en-us/advocacy-and-policy/aap-health-initiatives/Mental-Health/Pages/default.aspx. Accessed September 8, 2019

134. Levy S, Campbell MD, Shea CL, DuPont R. Trends in abstaining from substance use in adolescents: 1975-2014. *Pediatrics.* 2018;142(2):e20173498

135. Graff Low K, Gendaszek AE. Illicit use of psychostimulants among college students: a preliminary study. *Psychol Health Med.* 2002;7(3):283–287

136. Barkley RA, Cox D. A review of driving risks and impairments associated with attention-deficit/hyperactivity disorder and the effects of stimulant medication on driving performance. *J Safety Res.* 2007;38(1):113–128

137. Jerome L, Habinski L, Segal A. Attention-deficit/hyperactivity disorder (ADHD) and driving risk: a review of the literature and a methodological critique. *Curr Psychiatry Rep.* 2006;8(5): 416–426

138. Cox DJ, Merkel RL, Moore M, Thorndike F, Muller C, Kovatchev B. Relative benefits of stimulant therapy with OROS methylphenidate versus mixed amphetamine salts extended release in improving the driving performance of adolescent drivers with attention-deficit/hyperactivity disorder. *Pediatrics.* 2006;118(3). Available at: www.pediatrics.org/cgi/content/full/118/3/e704

139. The MTA Cooperative Group; Multimodal Treatment Study of Children with ADHD. A 14-month randomized clinical trial of treatment strategies for attention-deficit/hyperactivity disorder. *Arch Gen Psychiatry.* 1999;56(12):1073–1086

140. Jensen PS, Hinshaw SP, Swanson JM, et al. Findings from the NIMH Multimodal Treatment Study of ADHD (MTA): implications and applications for primary care providers. *J Dev Behav Pediatr.* 2001;22(1):60–73

141. Pelham WE Jr, Gnagy EM. Psychosocial and combined treatments for ADHD. *Ment Retard Dev Disabil Res Rev.* 1999; 5(3):225–236

142. Homer CJ, Klatka K, Romm D, et al. A review of the evidence for the medical home for children with special health care needs. *Pediatrics.* 2008;122(4). Available at: www.pediatrics.org/cgi/content/full/122/4/e922

143. Davila RR, Williams ML, MacDonald JT. Memorandum on clarification of policy to address the needs of children with attention deficit disorders within general and/or special education. In: Parker HC, ed. *The ADD Hyperactivity Handbook for Schools.* Plantation, FL: Impact Publications Inc; 1991:261–268

144. Harrison JR, Bunford N, Evans SW, Owens JS. Educational accommodations for students with behavioral challenges: a systematic review of the literature. *Rev Educ Res.* 2013;83(4): 551–597

145. Committee on Pediatric Workforce. Enhancing pediatric workforce diversity and providing culturally effective pediatric care: implications for practice, education, and policy making. *Pediatrics.* 2013;132(4). Available at: www.pediatrics.org/cgi/content/full/132/4/e1105

146. Berman RS, Patel MR, Belamarich PF, Gross RS. Screening for poverty and poverty-related social determinants of health. *Pediatr Rev.* 2018;39(5):235–246

147. Solanto MV. Neuropsychopharmacological mechanisms of stimulant drug action in attention-deficit hyperactivity disorder: a review and integration. *Behav Brain Res.* 1998;94(1):127–152

148. Wagner E. Chronic disease management: what will it take to improve care for chronic illness? *Effect Clin Pract.* 1998;1(1):2–4

149. Brinkman WB, Sucharew H, Majcher JH, Epstein JN. Predictors of medication continuity in children with ADHD. *Pediatrics.* 2018;141(6):e20172580

150. Pliszka SR, Crismon ML, Hughes CW, et al; Texas Consensus Conference Panel on Pharmacotherapy of Childhood Attention Deficit Hyperactivity Disorder. The Texas Children's Medication Algorithm Project: revision of the algorithm for pharmacotherapy of attention-deficit/hyperactivity disorder. *J Am Acad Child Adolesc Psychiatry.* 2006;45(6):642–657

151. Pringsheim T, Hirsch L, Gardner D, Gorman DA. The pharmacological management of oppositional behaviour, conduct problems, and aggression in children and adolescents with attention-deficit hyperactivity disorder, oppositional defiant disorder, and conduct disorder: a systematic review and meta-analysis. Part 1: psychostimulants, alpha-2 agonists, and atomoxetine. *Can J Psychiatry.* 2015; 60(2):42–51

152. Committee on Psychosocial Aspects of Child and Family Health and Task Force on Mental Health. Policy statement--The future of pediatrics: mental health competencies for pediatric primary care. *Pediatrics.* 2009;124(1):410–421

153. Foy JM, ed. Algorithm: a process for integrating mental health care into pediatric practice. In: *Mental Health Care of Children and Adolescents: A Guide for Primary Care Clinicians.* Itasca, IL: American Academy of Pediatrics; 2018:815

154. Cheng TL, Emmanuel MA, Levy DJ, Jenkins RR. Child health disparities: what can a clinician do? *Pediatrics.* 2015;136(5):961–968

155. Stein F, Remley K, Laraque-Arena D, Pursley DM. New resources and strategies to advance the AAP's values of diversity, inclusion, and health equity. *Pediatrics.* 2018;141(4):e20180177

156. American Academy of Pediatrics, Committee on Child Health Financing. Scope of health care benefits for children from birth through age 26. *Pediatrics.* 2012;129(1):185–189

Supplemental Information

IMPLEMENTING THE KEY ACTION STATEMENTS OF THE AAP ADHD CLINICAL PRACTICE GUIDELINES: AN ALGORITHM AND EXPLANATION FOR PROCESS OF CARE FOR THE EVALUATION, DIAGNOSIS, TREATMENT, AND MONITORING OF ADHD IN CHILDREN AND ADOLESCENTS

I. INTRODUCTION

Practice guidelines provide a broad outline of the requirements for high-quality, evidence-based care. The AAP "Clinical Practice Guideline: Diagnosis and Evaluation of the Child With Attention-Deficit/Hyperactivity Disorder" provides the evidence-based processes for caring for children and adolescents with ADHD symptoms or diagnosis. This document supplements that guideline. It provides a PoCA that details processes to implement the guidelines; describes procedures for the evaluation, treatment, and monitoring of children and adolescents with ADHD; and addresses practical issues related to the provision of ADHD-related care within a typical, busy pediatric practice. The algorithm is entirely congruent with the guidelines and is based on the practical experience and expert advice of clinicians who are experienced in the diagnosis and management of children and adolescents with ADHD. Unlike the guidelines, this algorithm is based primarily on expert opinion and has a less robust evidence base because of the lack of clinical studies specifically addressing this approach. Understanding that providing appropriate care to children with

ADHD in a primary care setting faces a number of challenges and barriers, the subcommittee has also provided an additional article describing needed changes to address barriers to care (found in the Supplemental Information).

In this algorithm, we describe a continuous process; as such, its constituent steps are not intended to be completed in a single office visit or in a specific number of visits. Evaluation, treatment, and monitoring are ongoing processes to be addressed throughout the child's and adolescent's care within the practice and in transition planning as the adolescent moves into the adult care system. Many factors will influence the pace of the process, including the experience of the PCC, the practice's volume, the longevity of the relationship between the PCC and family, the severity of concerns, the availability of academic records and school input, the family's schedule, and the payment structure.

An awareness of the AAP "Primary Care Approach to Mental Health Care Algorithm," which is available on the AAP Mental Health Initiatives Web site, will enhance the integration of the procedures described in this document (http://www.aap.org/mentalhealth). That algorithm describes the process to integrate an initial psychosocial assessment at well visits and a brief mental health update at acute and chronic care visits. Mental health concerns, including symptoms of

inattention and impulsivity, may present when (1) elicited during the initial psychosocial assessment at a routine well visit, (2) elicited during a brief mental health update at an acute or chronic visit, or (3) presented during a visit triggered by a family or school concern.

When concerns are identified, the algorithm describes the process of conducting a brief primary care intervention, secondary screening, diagnostic assessment, treatment, and follow-up. Like this document, the mental health algorithm is intended to present a process that may involve more than 1 visit and may be completed over time.

This algorithm assumes that the primary care practice has adopted the initial psychosocial assessment and mental health update, as described by the AAP Mental Health Initiatives.[153] It begins with steps paralleling the secondary assessment of the general mental health algorithm. Both algorithms focus on the care team and include the family as a part of that team.

In light of the prevalence of ADHD, the severe consequences of untreated ADHD, and the availability of effective ADHD treatments, the AAP recommends that every child and adolescent identified with signs or symptoms suggestive of ADHD be evaluated for ADHD or other conditions that may share its symptomatology. Documenting all aspects of the diagnostic and treatment procedures in the patient's records will improve the ability of the

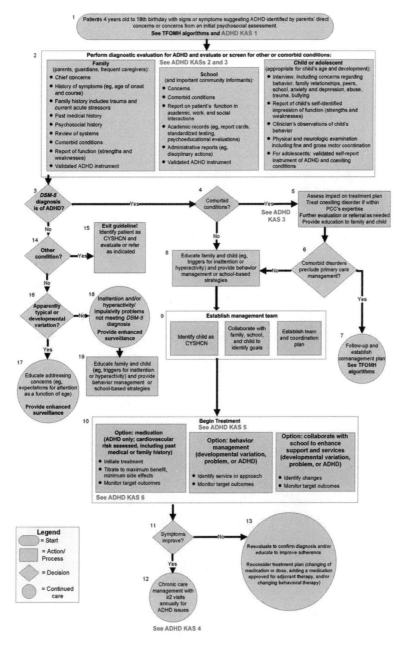

SUPPLEMENTAL FIGURE 2
ADHD care algorithm. CYSHCN, children and youth with special health care needs; TFOMH, Task Force on Mental Health.

pediatrician to best treat children with ADHD.

II. EVALUATION FOR ADHD

II a. A Child or Adolescent Presents With Signs and Symptoms Suggesting ADHD

The algorithm's steps can be implemented when a child or adolescent presents to a PCC for an assessment for ADHD. This may occur in a variety of ways.

Pediatricians and other PCCs traditionally have long-standing relationships with the child and family, which foster the opportunity to identify concerns early on. The young child may have a history of known ADHD risks, such as having parents who have been diagnosed with ADHD or having extremely low birth weight.

In those instances, the PCC would monitor for emerging issues.

Many parents bring their child or adolescent to the PCC with specific concerns about the child's or adolescent's ability to sustain attention, curb activity levels, and/or inhibit impulsivity at home, school, or in the community. In many instances, the parents may express concerns about behaviors and characteristics

1 Patients 4 years old to 18th birthday with signs or symptoms suggesting ADHD identified by parents' direct
concerns or concerns from an initial psychosocial assessment.
See TFOMH algorithms and ADHD KAS 1

SUPPLEMENTAL FIGURE 3
Evaluate for ADHD. TFOMH, Task Force on Mental Health.

that are associated with ADHD but may not mention the core ADHD symptoms. For example, parents may report that their child is getting poor grades, does not perform well in team sports (despite being athletic), has few friends, or is moody and quick to anger. These children and adolescents may have difficulty remaining organized; planning activities; or inhibiting their initial thoughts, actions, or emotions, which are behaviors that fall under the umbrella of executive functioning (ie, planning, prioritizing, and producing) or cognitive control. Problems with executive functions may be correlated with ADHD and are common among children and adolescents with ADHD. As recommended by Bright Futures (a national health promotion and prevention initiative led by the AAP[157]), routine psychosocial screening at preventive visits may identify concerns on the part of parent or another clinician (see below for more information on co-occurring conditions.)

Finally, parents may bring a child to a PCC for ADHD evaluation on the basis of the recommendation of a teacher, tutor, coach, etc.

(See the ADHD guideline's KAS 1.)

II b. Perform a Diagnostic Evaluation for ADHD and Evaluate or Screen for Comorbid Disorders

When a child or adolescent presents with concerns about ADHD, as described above, the clinician should initiate an evaluation for ADHD. (See the ADHD guideline's KASs 2 and 3.)

II c. Gather Information From the Family

As noted previously, the recommendations in the accompanying guideline are intended to be integrated with the broader mental health algorithm developed as part of the AAP Mental Health Initiatives.[2,133,153] It is also important for pediatricians and other PCCs to be aware of health disparities and social determinants that may affect patient outcomes and to provide culturally appropriate care to all children and adolescents in their practice, including during the initial evaluation

and assessment of the patient's condition.[145,146,154,155,158]

Ideally, the PCC's office staff obtains information from the family about the visit's purpose at scheduling so that an extended visit or multiple visits can be made available for the initial ADHD evaluation. This also increases the efficiency of an initial evaluation. Data on the child's or adolescent's symptoms and functioning can be gathered from parents, school personnel, and other sources before the visit. Parents can be given rating scales that are to be completed before the visit by teachers, coaches, and others who interact with the child. This strategy allows the PCC to focus on the most pertinent issues for that child or adolescent and family at the time of the visit. (See later discussion for more information on rating scales.) Note that schools will not release data to pediatric providers without written parental consent.

During the office evaluation session, the PCC reviews the patient's medical, family, and psychosocial history. Developmental history is presumed to be part of the patient's medical

2

Perform diagnostic evaluation for ADHD and evaluate or screen for other or comorbid conditions:
See ADHD KASs 2 and 3

Family (parents, guardians, frequent caregivers):	**School** (and important community informants):	**Child or adolescent** (appropriate for child's age and development):
• Chief concerns	• Concerns	• Interview, including concerns regarding behavior, family relationships, peers, school, anxiety and depression, abuse, trauma, bullying
• History of symptoms (eg, age of onset and course)	• Comorbid conditions	• Report of child's self-identified impression of function (strengths and weaknesses)
• Family history includes trauma and current acute stressors	• Report on patient's function in academic, work, and social interactions	• Clinician's observations of child's behavior
• Past medical history	• Academic records (eg, report cards, standardized testing, psychoeducational evaluations)	• Physical and neurologic examination includes fine and gross motor coordination
• Psychosocial history	• Administrative reports (eg, disciplinary actions)	• For adolescents: validated self-report instrument of ADHD and coexisting conditions
• Review of systems	• Validated ADHD instrument	
• Comorbid conditions		
• Report of function (strengths and weaknesses)		
• Validated ADHD instrument		

SUPPLEMENTAL FIGURE 4
Perform a diagnostic evaluation for ADHD and evaluate or screen for comorbid disorders

history. Family members (including parents, guardians, and other frequent caregivers) are asked to identify their chief concerns and provide a history of the onset, frequency, and duration of problem behaviors, situations that increase or decrease the problems, previous treatments and their results, and the caregivers' understanding of the issues. It is important to assess behaviors and conditions that are frequent side effects of stimulant medication (ie, sleep difficulties, tics, nail-biting, skin-picking, headaches, stomachaches, or afternoon irritability) and preexisting conditions, so they are not confused with the frequent side effects of stimulants. This enables the PCC to compare changes if medication is initiated later.

A sound assessment of symptoms and functioning in major areas can be used to construct an educational and behavioral profile that includes the child's strengths and talents. Many children with ADHD exhibit enthusiasm, exuberance, creativity, flexibility, the ability to detect and quickly respond to subtle changes in the environment, a sense of humor, a desire to please, etc. The most common areas of functioning affected by ADHD include academic achievement; relationships with peers, parents, siblings, and adult authority figures; participation in recreational activities, such as sports; and behavior and emotional regulation, including risky behavior.

The child's and family's histories can provide information about the status of symptoms and functioning and help determine age of onset and other factors that may be associated with the presenting problems. It also identifies any potential traumatic events that the child may have experienced, such as a family death, separation from the family, or physical or mental abuse.

The child or adolescent's medical history can help identify factors associated with ADHD, such as

prenatal and perinatal complications and exposures (eg, preterm delivery, maternal hypertension, prenatal alcohol exposure), childhood exposures, and head trauma.

The family history includes any medical syndromes, developmental delays, cognitive limitations, learning disabilities, trauma or toxic stress, or mental illness in the patient and family members, including ADHD, mood, anxiety, and bipolar disorders. Ask what the family has already tried, what works, and what does not work to avoid wasting time on interventions that have already been attempted unsuccessfully. Parental tobacco and substance use, including their use prenatally, are relevant risk factors for, and correlate with, ADHD.[159] ADHD is highly heritable and is often seen in other family members who may or may not have been formally diagnosed with ADHD. For this reason, asking about family members' school experience, including time and task management, grades, and highest grade level achieved, can aid in treatment decisions.

The psychosocial history is important in any ADHD evaluation and usually includes queries about environmental factors, such as family stress and problematic relationships, which sometime contribute to the child or adolescent's overall functioning. The caregivers' current and past approaches to parenting and the child's misbehavior can provide important information that may explain discrepancies between reporters. For example, parents may reduce their expectations for their child with ADHD as a means to relieve parenting stress. When these expectations are reduced (eg, eliminating chores, not monitoring homework completion, etc), parents may experience far fewer problems with the child than do teachers who may have maintained expectations for the child to complete tasks and follow rules. Knowing the parents' approach

to parenting may help the PCC understand differences in ratings completed by parents versus teachers.

Further evidence for an ADHD diagnosis includes an inability to independently complete daily routines in an age-appropriate manner as well as multiple and short-lasting friendships, trouble keeping and/or making friends, staying up late to complete assignments, and late, incomplete, and/or lost assignments. Somatic symptoms and school avoidance are more common among girls and may mask an ADHD diagnosis. With information obtained from the parents and school personnel, the PCC can make a clinical judgment about the effect of the core and associated ADHD symptoms on academic achievement, classroom performance, family and social relationships, independent functioning, and safety and/or unintentional injuries.

If other issues exist, such as self-injuries, comorbid mental health issues also need to be evaluated. Possible areas of functional impairment that require evaluation include domains such as self-perception, leisure activities, and self-care (ie, bathing, toileting, dressing, and eating). Additional guidance regarding functional assessment is available through the AAP ADHD Toolkit[2] and the AAP Mental Health Initiatives.[133,160] The ADHD Toolkit[2] is being revised concurrently with the development of these updated guidelines. After publication, the toolkit may be accessed at https://www.aap.org/en-us/professional-resources/quality-improvement/Pages/Quality-Improvement-Implementation-Guide.aspx. Additionally, a new Education in Quality Improvement for Pediatric Practice Module was developed on the basis of the new clinical recommendations and can also be accessed by using the same link above.

The patient needs to be screened for hearing and/or visual problems because these can mimic inattention. A full review of systems may reveal other symptoms or disorders, such as sleep disturbances, absence seizures, or tic disorders, which may assist in formulating a differential diagnosis and/or developing management plans. Internal feelings such as anxiety and depression can occur but may not be noticeable to parents and teachers, so it is important to elicit feedback about them from the patient as well.

The information gathered from this diagnostic interview, combined with the data from the rating scales (see below), provides an excellent foundation for determining the presence of symptoms and impairment criteria needed to diagnose ADHD.

II d. Use Parent Rating Scales and Other Tools

Rating scales that use the *DSM-5* criteria for ADHD can help obtain the information that will contribute to making a diagnosis. Rating scales for parents that use *DSM-5* criteria for ADHD are helpful in obtaining the core symptoms required to make a diagnosis on the basis of the *DSM-5*.[161] Because changes in the 18 core symptoms are essentially unchanged from *DSM-IV* criteria, *DSM-IV*–based rating scales can be used if *DSM-5* rating scales are not readily available. Some of these symptom rating scales include symptoms of commonly comorbid conditions and measures of impairment in a variety of domains that are also required for a diagnosis.[41,162] Some available measures are limited because they provide only a global rating.[163,164]

Caregiver and teacher endorsement of the requisite number of ADHD symptoms on the rating scales is not sufficient for diagnosis. A rating scale documents the presence of inattention, hyperactivity, and impulsivity symptoms but not whether these symptoms are actually attributable to ADHD versus a mimicking condition. Caregivers may misread or misunderstand some of the behaviors. Furthermore, rating scales do not inform the PCC about contextual influences that may account for the symptoms and impairment. Likewise, broadband rating scales that assess general mental health functioning do not provide reliable and valid indications of ADHD diagnoses, although they can help to screen for concurrent behavioral conditions.[165]

Nevertheless, parent ratings provide valuable information on their perspective of the child's symptoms and impairment and add information about normative levels of the parents' perspectives, which help the PCC determine the degree with which the problems are or are not in the typical range for the child's age and sex. Finally, broad rating scales that assess general mental health functioning do not provide sufficient information about all the ADHD core symptoms but may help screen for the concurrent behavioral conditions.[165]

To address the rating scales' limitations, pediatricians and other PCCs need to interview parents and may need to review documents such as report cards and standardized test results and historical records of detentions, suspensions, and/or expulsions from school, which can serve as evidence of functional impairment. Further evidence may include difficulty developing and maintaining lasting friendships. This information is discussed below.

II e. Gather Information From School and Community Informants

Information from parents is not the only source that informs diagnostic decisions for children and adolescents because a key criterion for an ADHD diagnosis is the display of symptoms and impairments in multiple settings. Gathering data from other adults who regularly interact with the child or adolescent being evaluated provides rich additional information for the evaluation.

The information from various sources may be inconsistent because parents and teachers observe the children at different times and under different circumstances, as described previously.[166] Disagreement may result from differences in students' behavior and performance in different classrooms, their relationship with the teachers, or variations in teachers' expectations, as well as training in or experience with behavior management. Classes with high homework demands or classes with less structure are often the most problematic for students with ADHD. Investigating these inconsistencies can lead to hypotheses about the child that help inform the eventual clinical diagnoses and treatment decisions.[167]

Teachers and Other School Personnel

Teachers and other school personnel can provide critically important information because they develop a rich sense of the typical range of behaviors within a specific age group over time. School and classrooms settings provide the greatest social and performance expectations that potentially tax children and adolescents with ADHD. Parents and older children may be the best sources for identifying the school personnel who can best complete rating scales for an ADHD evaluation.

The value of school ratings increases as children age because parents often have less detailed information about their child's behavior and performance at school as the student moves into the higher grades. With elementary and middle school children, the classroom teacher is usually the best source; he or she may be the only source necessary. Other school staff, such as a special education teacher or school counselor, may be valuable sources of information. Direct communication with a school psychologist and/or school counselor may provide additional information on the child's functioning within the context of the classroom and school.

In secondary schools, students interact with many teachers who often instruct >100 students daily. As a result, high school teachers may not know the students as well as elementary and middle school teachers do. Parents and students may be encouraged to choose the 2 or 3 teachers who they believe know the student best and solicit their input (eg, math and English teachers or, for children or adolescents with learning disabilities, a teacher in an area of strong function and a teacher in an area of weak function). Regardless of the presence of a learning disability, it is helpful to obtain feedback from the teacher of the class in which the child or adolescent is having the most difficulty. The ADHD Toolkit provides materials relevant to school data collection.

Teachers may communicate their major concerns using questionnaires or verbally in person, via secure e-mail (if available), or over the telephone. It is important to ask an appropriate school representative to complete a validated ADHD instrument or behavior scale based on the *DSM-5* criteria for ADHD. A school representative's report might include information about any comorbid or alternative conditions, including disruptive behavior disorders, depression and anxiety disorders, tics, or learning disabilities. As noted, some parent rating scales have a version for teachers and assess symptoms and impairment in multiple domains.[41] Teacher rating scales exist that specifically target behavior and performance at school,[168] which provide a comprehensive and detailed description of a student's school functioning relative to normative data.

In addition to the academic information, it is important to request information characterizing the child or adolescent's level of functioning with regard to peer, teacher, and other authority figure relationships, ability to follow directions, organizational skills, history of classroom disruption, and assignment completion.

Academic Records

In addition to ratings from teachers and other school staff, academic records are sometimes available to inform a PCC's evaluation. These records include report cards; results from reading, math, and written expression standardized tests; and other assessments of academic competencies. If a child were referred for an evaluation for special education services, his or her file is likely to contain a report on the evaluation, which can be useful during an ADHD evaluation. School records pertaining to office discipline referrals, suspensions, absences, and detentions can provide valuable information about social function and behavioral regulation. Parents often keep report cards from early grades, which can provide valuable information about age of onset for children older than 12 years. Teachers in primary grades often provide information pertaining to important information about the history of the presenting problems.

Other Community Sources

It can be helpful to obtain information not only from school professionals but also from additional sources, such as grandparents, faith-based organization group leaders, scouting leaders, sports coaches, and others. Depending on the areas in which the child or adolescent exhibits impairment, these adults may be able to provide a valuable perspective on the nature of the presenting problems, although the accuracy of their reporting has not been studied.

II f. Gather Information From the Child or Adolescent

Another source of information is from the child or adolescent. This information is often collected but carries less weight than information from other sources because of children's and adolescents' limited ability to accurately report their strengths and weaknesses, including those associated with ADHD.[169] As a result, information gathered from the child about specific ADHD behaviors may do little to inform the presence or absence of symptoms and impairments because evidence suggests that children tend to minimize their problems and blame others for concerns.[170]

Nevertheless, self-report may provide other values. First, self-report is the primary means by which one can screen for internalizing conditions such as depression and anxiety. The AAP Mental Health Initiatives[133] and the *Guidelines for Adolescent Depression in Primary Care*[171-173] recommend the use of validated diagnostic rating scales for adolescent mood and anxiety disorders for clinicians who wish to use this format.[174-178] As measures of internal mental disorders, these data are likely to be more valid than the reports of adults about their children's behaviors.

Second, youth with ADHD are prone to talk impulsively and excessively when adults show an interest in them. They may share useful information about the home or classroom that parents and teachers do not know or impart. In addition, many share their experience with risky and dangerous behaviors that may be unknown to the adults in their lives. This information can be critical in both determining a diagnosis and designing treatment.

Third, even if little information of value is obtained, the fact that the PCC takes the time to meet alone and ask questions of the child or adolescents demonstrates respect and lays the foundation for collaboration in the decision-making and treatment process to follow. This relationship building is particularly important for adolescents.

Fourth, by gaining an understanding of the child's perspective, the PCC can anticipate the likely acceptance or resistance to treatment.

Interviewing the child or adolescent provides many important benefits beyond the possibility of informing the diagnosis and warrants its inclusion in the evaluation. For example, part of this interview includes asking the child or adolescent to identify personal goals (eg, What do you want to be when you grow up? What do you think that requires? How can we help you get there?). It is helpful when children perceive the pediatrician and other PCCs as seeking to help them achieve their goals rather than arbitrarily labeling them as deficient, defective, or needing to be fixed in some way.

II g. Clinical Observations and Physical Examination of the Child or Adolescent

The physical and neurologic examination needs to be comprehensive to determine if further medical or developmental assessments are indicated. Baseline height, weight, BP, and pulse measurements are required to be recorded in the medical record. It is important to look for behaviors that are consistent with ADHD's symptoms, including the child's level of attention, activity, and impulsivity during the encounter. Yet, ADHD is context dependent, and for this reason, behaviors and core symptoms that are seen in other settings are often not observed during an office visit.[179] Although the presence of hyperactivity and inattention during an office visit may provide supporting evidence of ADHD symptoms, their absence is not considered evidence that the child does not have ADHD.

Observations of a broad range of behaviors can be important for

considering their contribution to the presenting problems and the potential diagnosis of other conditions. Careful attention to these various behaviors can provide useful information when beginning the next step involving making diagnostic decisions. For example, hearing and visual acuity problems can often lead to inattention and overactivity at school. Attending to concerns about anxiety is also important given that young children may become overactive when they are in anxiety-provoking situations like a clinic visit.

In addition, observing the child's language skills is important because difficulties with language can be a symptom of a language disorder and predictor of subsequent reading problems. This observation is particularly important with young children given that language disorders may present as problems with sustaining attention and impulsivity. A language disorder may also involve pragmatic usage or the social use of language, which can contribute to social impairment. If the PCC, family, and/or school have concerns about receptive, expressive, or pragmatic language, it is important to make a referral for a formal speech and language evaluation. Dysmorphic features also need to be noted because symptoms of ADHD are similar to characteristics of children with some prenatal exposures and genetic syndromes (eg, fetal alcohol exposure,[180,181] fragile X syndrome).

Many children with ADHD have poor coordination, which may be severe enough to warrant a diagnosis of developmental coordination disorder and referral to occupational and/or physical therapy. Findings of poor coordination can affect how well the child performs in competitive sports, a frequent source of social interactions for children, and can adversely affect the child's writing skills. Detecting any motor or verbal tics is important as well, particularly because the use of stimulant

medications may cause or exacerbate tics.

Finally, it is important to evaluate the child's cardiovascular status because cardiovascular health must be considered if ADHD medication becomes an option. Cardiac illness is rare, and more evidence is required to determine if children or adolescents with ADHD are at increased risk when taking ADHD medications. Nevertheless, before initiating therapy with stimulant medications, it is important to obtain the child or adolescent's history of specific cardiac symptoms, as well as the family history of sudden death, cardiovascular symptoms, Wolff-Parkinson-White syndrome, hypertrophic cardiomyopathy, and long QT syndrome. If any of these risk factors are present, clinicians should obtain additional evaluation with an ECG and possibly consult with a pediatric cardiologist.

II h. Gather Information About Conditions That Mimic or Are Comorbid With ADHD

It is important for the PCC to obtain information about the status and history of conditions that may mimic or are comorbid with ADHD, such as depression, anxiety disorders, and posttraumatic stress disorder. Several validated rating scales are within the public domain and can help identify comorbid conditions. Examples include the Pediatric Symptom Checklist-17 as a screen for depression and anxiety[182]; the Screen for Child Anxiety Related Emotional Disorders, more specifically for anxiety disorders[176]; the Patient Health Questionnaire modified for adolescents; the Screening to Brief Intervention tool[183,184]; and the Child and Adolescent Trauma Screen for exposure to trauma.[185] All include questionnaire forms for both parents and patients.[2] The results help the PCC assess the extent to which reported impairment and/or distress are associated with ADHD versus comorbid conditions. These conditions are described in greater detail later.

Safety and Serious Mental Illness Concerns

PCCs may be asked to complete mental health or safety assessments, particularly for adolescents. Assessment requests may come from schools or other settings after a behavioral crisis, aggressive behavior, or destructive behaviors have occurred. With patient or guardian consent, information may be shared regarding diagnosis and current treatment strategies. Pediatricians and other PCCs are encouraged to exercise caution when asked to predict the likelihood of future behaviors in the absence of detailed understanding of the environment in which the behaviors occurred. Self-injurious behaviors or threats of self-harm are serious concerns that, when possible, should immediately be referred to community mental health crisis services or experienced child mental health professionals. PCCs are encouraged to provide further monitoring of the child or adolescent with these comorbidities.

III. MAKING DIAGNOSTIC DECISIONS

After gathering all of the relevant available information, the PCC will consider an ADHD diagnosis as well as a diagnosis of other related and/or comorbid disorders. The primary

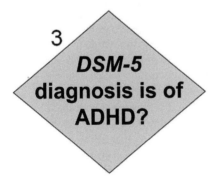

SUPPLEMENTAL FIGURE 5
Making diagnostic decisions.

decision-making process involves comparing the information obtained to the *DSM-5* criteria for ADHD. Although this assessment is straightforward, there are some issues the PCC needs to consider, including development, sex, and other disorders that may fit the presenting problems better than ADHD (see below for more on these issues).

III a. DSM-5 Criteria for ADHD

The *DSM-5* criteria define 4 dimensions of ADHD:

1. ADHD/I (314.00 [F90.0]);
2. ADHD/HI (314.01 [F90.1]);
3. ADHD/C (314.01 [F90.2]); and
4. ADHD other specified and unspecified ADHD (314.01 [F90.8]).

To make a diagnosis of ADHD, the PCC needs to establish that 6 or more (5 or more if the adolescent is 17 years or older) core symptoms are present in either or both of the inattention dimension and/or the hyperactivity-impulsivity dimension and occur inappropriately often. The core symptoms and dimensions are presented in Supplemental Table 2.

- ADHD/I: having at least 6 of 9 inattention behaviors and less than 6 hyperactive-impulsive behaviors;
- ADHD/HI: having at least 6 of 9 hyperactive-impulsive behaviors and less than 6 inattention behaviors;
- ADHD/C: having at least 6 of 9 behaviors in both the inattention and hyperactive-impulsive dimensions; and
- ADHD other specified and unspecified ADHD: These categories are meant for children who meet many of the criteria for ADHD, but not the full criteria, and who have significant impairment. "ADHD other specified" is used if the PCC specifies those criteria that have not been met; "unspecified ADHD" is used if the PCC does not specify these criteria.

In school-aged children and adolescents, diagnostic criteria for ADHD include documentation of the following criteria:

- At least 6 of the 9 behaviors described in the inattentive domain occur often, and to a degree, that is inconsistent with the child's developmental age. (For adolescents 17 years and older, documentation of at least 5 of the 9 behaviors is required.)
- At least 6 of the 9 behaviors described in the hyperactive-impulsive domain occur often, and to a degree, that is inconsistent with the child's developmental age. (For adolescents 17 years and older, documentation of at least 5 of the 9 behaviors is required.)
- Several inattentive or hyperactive-impulsive symptoms were present before age 12 years.
- There is clear evidence that the child's symptoms interfere with or reduce the quality of his or her social, academic, and/or occupational functioning.
- The symptoms have persisted for at least 6 months.
- The symptoms are not attributable to another physical, situational, or mental health condition.

Clear evidence exists that these criteria are appropriate for preschool-aged children (ie, age 4 years to the sixth birthday), elementary and middle school-aged children (ie, age 6 years to the 12th birthday), and adolescents (ie, age 12 years to the 18th birthday).[30,31] *DSM-5* criteria have also been updated to better describe how inattentive and hyperactive-impulsive symptoms present in older adolescents and adults.

DSM-5 criteria require evidence of symptoms before age 12 years. In some cases, however, parents and teachers may not recognize ADHD symptoms until the child is older than 12 years, when school tasks and responsibilities become more challenging and exceed the child's ability to perform effectively in school. For these children, history can often identify an earlier age of onset of some ADHD symptoms. Delayed recognition may also be seen more often in ADHD/I, which is more commonly diagnosed in girls.

If symptoms arise suddenly without previous history, the PCC needs to consider other conditions, including mood or anxiety disorders, substance use, head trauma, physical or sexual abuse, neurodegenerative disorders, sleep disorders (including sleep apnea), or a major psychological stress in the family or school (such as bullying). In adolescents and young adults, PCCs are encouraged to consider the potential for false reporting and misrepresentation of symptoms to obtain medications for other than appropriate medicinal use (ie, diversion, secondary gain). The majority of states now require prescriber participation in prescription drug monitoring programs, which can be helpful in identifying and preventing diversion activities. Pediatricians and other PCCs may consider prescribing nonstimulant medications that minimize abuse potential, such as atomoxetine and extended-release guanfacine or extended-release clonidine.

In the absence of other concerns and findings on prenatal or medical history, further diagnostic testing will not help to reach an ADHD diagnosis. Compared to clinical interviews, standardized psychological tests, such as computerized attention tests, have not been found to reliably differentiate between youth with and without ADHD.[187,188] Appropriate further assessment is indicated if an underlying etiology is suspected. Imaging studies or screening for high lead levels and abnormal thyroid hormone levels can be pursued if they are suggested by other historic or physical information, such as history or symptoms of a tumor or significant

brain injury. When children experience trauma, their evaluation needs to include the consideration of both the trauma and ADHD because they can co-occur and can exacerbate ADHD symptoms. Toxic stress has shown to be associated with the incidence of pediatric ADHD, but the conclusion that ADHD is a manifestation of this stress has not been demonstrated.[188]

Patients with ADHD commonly have comorbid conditions, such as oppositional defiant disorder, anxiety, depression, and language and learning disabilities. These conditions may present with ADHD symptoms and need evaluation because their treatment may relieve symptoms. Additionally, some conditions may present with ADHD symptoms and respond to treatment of the primary condition, such as sleep disorders, absence seizures, and hyperthyroidism. (Comorbid conditions are discussed later in this document.)

In addition, the behavioral characteristics specified in the *DSM-5* remain subjective and may be interpreted differently by various observers. Rates of ADHD and its treatment have been found to be different for different racial and/or ethnic groups.[50,189] Cultural norms and the expectations of parents or teachers may influence reporting of symptoms. Hence, the clinician benefits from being sensitive to cultural differences about the appropriateness of behaviors and perceptions of mental health conditions.[145,155]

After the diagnostic evaluation, a PCC will be able to answer the following questions:

- How many inattentive and hyperactive/impulsive behavior criteria for ADHD does the child or adolescent manifest across major settings of his or her life?
- Have these criteria been present for 6 months or longer?

- Was the onset of these or similar behaviors present before the child's 12th birthday?
- What functional impairments are caused by these behaviors?
- Could any other condition be a better explanation for the behaviors?
- Is there evidence of comorbid problems or disorders?

On the basis of this information, the clinician is usually able to arrive at a preliminary diagnosis of whether the child or adolescents has ADHD or not. (For children and adolescents who do not receive an ADHD diagnosis, see below.)

III b. Developmental Considerations

Considerations About the Child or Adolescent's Age

Although the diagnostic criteria for ADHD are the same for children up to age 17 years, developmental considerations affect the interpretation of whether a symptom is present. Before school age, the primary set of distinguishing symptoms involve hyperactivity, although this can be difficult to identify as outside of the normal range given the large variability in this young age group. Similarly, difficulties sustaining attention are difficult to determine with young children because of considerable variability in presentation and the limited demands for children in this age group to sustain attention over time. (See below for more information on developmental delays.)

Some children demonstrate hyperactivity and inattention that are clearly beyond the normal range. They may experience substantial impairment to an extent that baby-sitters or child care agencies refuse to care for them, parents are unable to take them shopping or to restaurants, or they routinely engage in dangerous or risky behaviors. In these extreme cases, the PCC may be able to make the decision for an ADHD diagnosis more quickly than other scenarios that require a thorough assessment. For other young children, the diagnosis will be less obvious, and developmental and environmental issues may lead the PCC to be cautious in making an ADHD diagnosis. In these situations, monitoring for the emergence or clarification of ADHD symptoms and/or providing a diagnosis of other specified *ADHD* or unspecified *ADHD* are appropriate options.

Adolescence is another developmental period when developmental considerations are warranted. Beginning at age 17 years, there are only 5 symptoms of inattention and/or 5 symptoms of hyperactivity/impulsivity required for an ADHD diagnosis. Hyperactivity typically diminishes for most children during adolescence, but problems associated with impulsivity can be dangerous and can include impaired driving, substance use, risky sexual behavior, and suicide. Disorganization of time and resources can be associated with substantial academic problems at school. Parent-child conflict and disengagement from school can provide a context that contributes toward poor long-term outcomes. Comorbid depression and conduct disorder are common but do not negate the importance of diagnosing ADHD when the developmental path warrants it and the ADHD symptoms exacerbate problems associated with the comorbid conditions.

Adolescence is the first developmental period for which age of onset of symptoms must be documented before 12 years. School records and parent reports are often the richest source for making this determination. It is important to try to identify adolescents (or their parents) who are pursuing a diagnosis of ADHD for secondary gains such as school accommodations, standardized testing

accommodations, and/or stimulant prescriptions. In addition, impairment sometimes emerges when expectations for the adolescent markedly increase or when accommodations are removed. The teenager's level of functioning may stay the same, but when faced with the expectations of advanced placement courses or a part-time job, failure to keep pace with increasing expectations may lead to concerns that warrant an evaluation for ADHD. These examples emphasize the importance of determining an early age of onset.

Considerations About the Child or Adolescent's Sex

ADHD is diagnosed in boys about twice as often as it is diagnosed in girls. There are many hypotheses about reasons for this difference; the primary reason appears to simply be that the disorder is more common in boys than girls. Some have raised concerns that the difference may be attributable to variances in society's expectations for boys versus girls or underdiagnosis in girls, but these reasons are unlikely to account for the large difference in diagnoses. Hence, no adjustment is needed in terms of the standards for girls to meet the criteria for an ADHD diagnosis compared with boys.

Girls are less likely to exhibit hyperactivity symptoms, which are the most easily observable of all ADHD symptoms, particularly in younger patients. This fact may account for a portion of the difference in diagnosis between girls and boys. As a result, it is important to fully consider a diagnosis of ADHD, predominantly inattentive presentation, when evaluating girls.

Symptoms of inattention alone can complicate the diagnosis because inattention is 1 of the most common symptoms across all disorders in the *DSM-5*. After puberty, it is more common for depression and anxiety to be diagnosed in girls than in boys,

and symptoms of inattention may be a result of these disorders as well as ADHD. Examining the age of onset and considering other distinguishing features, such as avoidance and anhedonia, can help the PCC clarify this challenging differential when evaluating girls for ADHD. For example, does the inattention occur primarily in anxiety-provoking situations or when the child or adolescent is experiencing periods of low mood and then remit when the anxiety or mood improves?

III c. Consideration of Comorbid Conditions

If other disorders are suspected or detected during the diagnostic evaluation, an assessment of the urgency of these conditions and their impact on the ADHD treatment plan should be made. Comorbid conditions provide unique challenges for treatment planning. Urgent conditions need to be addressed immediately with services capable of handling crisis situations. These conditions include suicidal thoughts or acts and other behaviors with the potential to severely injure the child, adolescent, and/or other people, including severe temper outbursts or child abuse. Note that adolescents are potentially more likely to provide honest answers if the PCC asks sensitive questions in the absence of the parents and may respond more readily to rating scales that assess mood or anxiety. In addition, substance use disorders require immediate attention and may precede or coincide with beginning treatment of ADHD. Additional information is available in the complex ADHD guideline published by the SDBP.[67]

Evidence shows that comorbid conditions may improve with treatment of ADHD, including oppositional behaviors and anxiety.[140] For example, children with ADHD and comorbid anxiety disorders may find that addressing the ADHD symptoms with

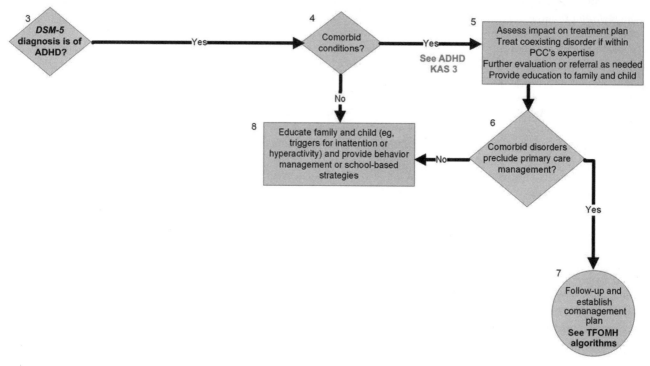

SUPPLEMENTAL FIGURE 6
Consideration of comorbid conditions. TFOMH, Task Force on Mental Health.

medications also decreases anxiety or mood symptoms. Other children may require additional therapeutic treatments to treat the ADHD adequately and treat comorbid conditions, including cognitive behavioral therapy (CBT), academic interventions, or different and/or additional medications.

The PCC may evaluate and treat the comorbid disorder if it is within his or her training and expertise. In addition, the PCC can provide education to the family and child or adolescent about triggers for inattention and/or hyperactivity. If the PCC requires the advice of a subspecialist, the clinician is encouraged to consider carefully when to initiate treatment of ADHD. In some cases, it may be advisable to delay the start of medication until the role of each member of the treatment team is established (see below). Integrated care models can be helpful (see www.integratedcareforkids.org).

The following are brief discussions of sleep disorders, psychiatric disorders,

emotion dysregulation, exposure to trauma, and learning disabilities, all of which can manifest in manners similar to ADHD and can complicate making a diagnosis.

(See the ADHD guideline's KAS 3.)

Sleep Disorders

Sleepiness impairs most people's ability to sustain attention and often leads to caffeine consumption to counter these effects. In the same way, sleep disturbance can lead to symptoms and impairment that mimic or exacerbate ADHD symptoms. A child with ADHD may have difficulty falling asleep because of the busy thoughts caused by ADHD. Some sleep disorders are frequently associated with ADHD or present as symptoms of inattention, hyperactivity, and impulsivity, such as obstructive sleep apnea syndrome and restless legs syndrome and/or periodic limb movement disorder (RLS/PLMD).[190–193]

The differential diagnosis of insomnia in children and adolescents with ADHD includes the following:

- inadequate sleep hygiene (eg, inconsistent bedtimes and wake times, absence of a bedtime routine, electronics in the bedroom, caffeine use)[194];

- ADHD medication (stimulant and nonstimulant) effects:

  o direct effects on sleep architecture: prolonged sleep onset, latency, and decreased sleep duration, increased night wakings[195–197]; and

  o indirect effects: inadequate control of ADHD symptoms in the evening and medication withdrawal or rebound symptoms[198,199];

- sleep problems associated with comorbid psychiatric conditions (eg, anxiety and mood disorders, disruptive behavior disorders)[200];

- circadian-based phase delay in sleep-wake patterns, which have been shown to occur in some children with ADHD, resulting in both prolonged sleep onset and difficulty waking in the morning[201]; and

- intrinsic deficit associated with ADHD. Authors of numerous studies have reported that nonmedicated children with ADHD without comorbid mood or anxiety disorders have significantly greater bedtime resistance, more sleep onset difficulties, and more frequent night awakenings when compared with typically developing children in control groups.[202] In addition, some children with ADHD appear to have evidence of increased daytime sleepiness, even in the absence of a primary sleep disorder.[202–204]

For this reason, all children and adolescents who are evaluated for ADHD need to be systematically screened for symptoms of primary sleep disorders, such as frequent snoring, observed breathing pauses, restless sleep, urge to move one's legs at night, and excessive daytime sleepiness. (Issues of access to these services are discussed in the accompanying section, Systemic Barriers to the Care of Children and Adolescents with ADHD.) In addition, screenings generally include primary sleep disorders' risk factors, such as adenotonsillar hypertrophy, asthma and allergies, obesity, a family history of RLS/PLMD, and iron deficiency.[199] Sleep assessment measures that have been shown to be useful in the pediatric primary care practice setting include brief screening tools[205] and parent-report surveys.[206,207] Overnight polysomnography is generally required for children who have symptoms suggestive of and/or risk factors for obstructive sleep apnea syndrome and RLS/PLMD.[208,209]

If the results suggest the presence of a sleep disorder, the PCC needs to obtain a comprehensive sleep history, including assessment of the environment in which the child sleeps; the cohabitants in the room; the bedtime routine, including its initiation, how long it takes for the child fall asleep, sleep duration, and

any night-time awakenings; and what time the child wakes up in the morning and his or her state when awakening. It is important to determine sleep interventions attempted and their results. Even when no primary sleep disorders occur, modest reductions in sleep duration or increases in sleep disruption may be associated with increased, detectable problems with attention in children and adolescents with ADHD.[210] Although fully disentangling sleep disruption from ADHD may not be possible because significant sleep problems and their associated impairment are often comorbid with ADHD, sleep disruptions often warrant consideration as an additional target for treatment. In addition, some children with ADHD appear to show evidence of increased daytime sleepiness, even in the absence of a primary sleep disorder.[203,204] Significant sleep problems and their associated impairment are often comorbid with ADHD and, for many children, are considered as an additional target for treatment.

A variety of issues need to be considered when determining if sleep problems constitute an additional diagnosis of insomnia disorder or are linked to ADHD-related treatment issues. First, a child's sleep can be affected if he or she is already taking stimulant medication or regularly consuming caffeine. The dosage and timing of this consumption needs to be tracked and manipulated to examine its effects; simple modifications of timing and dosage of stimulant consumption can improve sleep onset, duration, and quality. Second, sleep problems can occur from inadequate sleep health and/or hygiene[194] or from other disorders, such as anxiety and mood disorders, when the rumination and worry associated with them impairs or disrupts the child's sleep. Restructuring behavior preceding and at bedtime can dramatically improve

sleep and diminish associated impairments. These potential causes of sleep disturbance and the related impairments that mimic or exacerbate ADHD symptoms need to be considered before diagnosing ADHD, related problems, or insomnia disorder.

Trauma

Children with ADHD are at higher-than-normal risk of experiencing some forms of trauma, including corporal punishment and accidents (often because of their risk-taking behaviors). In addition, posttraumatic stress disorder may manifest some similar symptoms. Depending on the child, the trauma may have been a one-time event or one to which they are consistently exposed. Exposure to trauma may exacerbate or lead to symptoms shared by trauma disorders and ADHD (eg, inattention). As a result, when evaluating a child for ADHD, obtaining a brief trauma history and screening for indicators of impairing responses to trauma can be helpful. Although a trauma history does not inform the diagnosis of ADHD, it may identify an alternative diagnosis and inform treatment and other interventions, including referral for trauma-focused therapy and reporting suspected abuse.

Mental Health Conditions

In children or adolescents who have coexisting mild depression, anxiety, or obsessive-compulsive disorder, the PCC may undertake the treatment of all disorders if doing so is within his or her abilities. Another option is to collaborate with a mental health clinician to treat the coexisting condition while the PCC oversees the ADHD treatment. As a third option, the consulting specialists may advise about the treatment of the coexisting condition to the extent that the PCC is comfortable treating both ADHD and the coexisting problems. With some coexisting psychiatric disorders, such as severe anxiety, depression, autism, schizophrenia, obsessive-compulsive disorder, oppositional defiant disorder, conduct disorder, and bipolar disorder, a comanaging developmental-behavioral pediatrician or child and adolescent psychiatrist might take responsibility for treatment of both ADHD and the coexisting illness.

Many children with ADHD exhibit emotion dysregulation, which is considered to be a common feature of the disorder and one that is potentially related to other executive functioning deficits.[211] A child exhibiting emotion dysregulation with either or both positive (eg, exuberance) or negative (eg, anger) emotions along with symptoms of ADHD can be considered as a good candidate for an ADHD diagnosis. Sometimes behavior related to emotion dysregulation can lead the PCC to consider other diagnoses such as disruptive mood dysregulation disorder, intermittent explosive disorder, and bipolar disorder. All 3 may be diagnosed with ADHD. Intermittent explosive disorder and bipolar disorder are rare in children, and data are currently inadequate to know the prevalence of disruptive mood dysregulation disorder. Given the base rates, these other diagnoses are unlikely, although they do occur in childhood. If the PCC has any uncertainty about making these distinctions, referring the child to a clinical child psychologist or child mental health professionals may be warranted.

Learning Disabilities

Learning disabilities frequently co-occur with ADHD and can lead to symptoms and impairment that are similar to those in children with ADHD. As a result, screening for learning disabilities' presence, such as via the Vanderbilt ADHD Rating Scale,[212] is important given that treatment of ADHD and learning disabilities differ markedly.

Learning disabilities involve impairment related to learning specific academic content, usually reading or math, although there is increased awareness about disorders of written expression. The impairment is not attributable to difficulties with sustaining attention; however, some children with learning disabilities have trouble sustaining attention in class because they cannot keep up and then disengage. A careful evaluation for learning disabilities includes achievement testing, cognitive ability testing, and measures of the child's learning in response to evidence-based instruction. Such thorough evaluations are typically not available in a PCC practice. If screening suggests the possibility of learning disabilities, the PCC can help advise parents on how to obtain school psychoeducational evaluations or refer the child to a psychologist or other specialist trained in conducting these evaluations.

The PCC's attention is directed to language skills in preschool-aged and young school-aged children because difficulties in language skills can be a symptom of a language disorder and predictor of subsequent reading problems. Language disorders may present as problems with attention and impulsivity. Likewise, social interactions need to be noted during the examination because they may be impaired when the child or adolescent's language skills are delayed or disordered.

Children who have intellectual or other developmental disabilities may have ADHD, but assessment of these patients is more difficult because a diagnosis of ADHD would only be appropriate if the child or adolescent's level of inattention or hyperactivity/impulsivity is disproportionate to his or her developmental rather than chronological age. Therefore, assessment of ADHD in individuals with intellectual disabilities requires input from the child or adolescent's education specialists, school psychologists, and/or independent psychologists. Although it is important to attempt to differentiate whether the presenting problems are associated with learning disabilities, ADHD, or something else, it is important to consider the possibility that a child has multiple disorders. Pediatricians and other PCCs who are involved in assessing ADHD in children with intellectual disabilities will need to collaborate closely with school or independent psychologists.

Summary

Overall, there are many factors that influence a diagnostic decision. Frequently, these decisions must be made without the benefit of all of the relevant information described. Family and cultural issues that affect parents' expectations for their child and perceptions about mental health can further complicate this process. Poverty, family history, access to care, and many other factors that a PCC will probably not know when making the diagnosis can also be formative in the child's presenting problems.[145,146,154,155,158] The PCC will wisely remain sensitive to individual variations in parents' beliefs, values, and perception of their culture and community when completing the assessment and determining a diagnosis. These factors add complexities to the assessment and diagnostic process and make a good evaluation and diagnosis a function of clinical experience, judgment, and a foundation in science.

IV. TREATMENT

If the child meets the *DSM-5* criteria for ADHD, including commensurate functional disabilities, progress through the PoCA.

(See the AHDH guideline's KASs 5 and 6.)

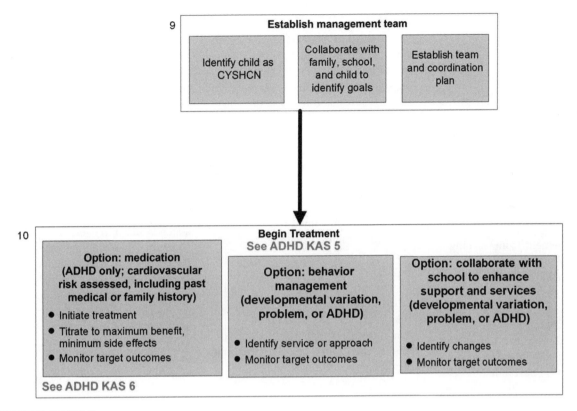

SUPPLEMENTAL FIGURE 7
Treatment. CYSHCN, children and youth with special health care needs.

IV a. Establish Management Team: Identify the Patient as a Child With Special Health Care Needs

Any child who meets the criteria for ADHD is considered a "child or youth with special health care needs"; these children are best managed in a medical home.[213–217] In addition, the AAP encourages clinicians to develop systems to allow the medical home to meet all needs of children with chronic illnesses. These needs and strategies for meeting them are discussed in further detail in AAP resources such as the Building Your Medical Home toolkit and Addressing Concerns in Primary Care: A Clinician's Toolkit. Care in the medical home is reviewed in the AAP publication *Bright Futures: Guidelines for Health Supervision of Infants, Children, and Adolescents, Fourth Edition*. Pediatricians and other PCCs who provide effective

medical homes identify family strengths and recognize the importance of parents in the care team.[218–221] The PCC may provide education about the disorder and treatment options, medication, and/or psychosocial treatment and monitor response to treatments over time as well as the child's development.

IV b. Establish Management Team: Collaborate With Family, School, and Child to Identify Target Goals

ADHD is a chronic illness; hence, education for both the child or adolescent and other family members is a critical element in the care plan. Family education involves all members of the family, including the provision of developmentally age-appropriate information for the affected child or adolescent and any siblings. Topics may include the disorder's potential causes and typical symptoms, the assessment

process; common coexisting disorders; ADHD's effect on school performance and social participation; long-term sequelae; and treatment options and their potential benefits, adverse effects, and long-term outcomes. It is important to address the patient's self-concept and clarify that having ADHD does not mean that the child is less smart than others. At every stage, education must continue in a manner consistent with the child or adolescent's level of understanding.

The emphasis for parental education is on helping parents understand the disorder, how to obtain additional accurate information about ADHD and treatments, and how to effectively advocate for their child. This may include addressing parental concerns about labeling the child or adolescent with a disorder by providing information on the benefits of diagnosis and treatment.

Some guidance about effective parenting strategies may be helpful, but PTBM is likely to be most beneficial for most parents (see the section on Psychosocial Treatments). Pediatricians and other PCCs are encouraged to be cognizant of the challenges families may face to attend such training, including taking time off from work and covering the costs associated with the intervention.

Parents may benefit from learning about optimal ways to partner with schools, particularly their child's teachers, and become part of the educational and intervention teams. Educating parents about special education and other services can be helpful, but school interventions and advocacy may be best aided by partnering closely with an advocate or clinician experienced in working with schools (see the Psychosocial Treatment section). With the parent's permission, the clinician may provide educators at the school with information from the evaluation that will help the school determine eligibility for special education services or accommodations and/or develop appropriate services.

In addition, it is helpful to provide assistance to the parent or other caregiver in understanding and using any relevant electronic health record (EHR) system. Sometimes, the health literacy gap around EHRs can lead to confusion and frustration on the family's side. Also, providing information on community resources, such as other health care providers or specialists, can be beneficial in addressing fragmentation and communication barriers.

Family education continues throughout the course of treatment and includes anticipatory guidance in areas such as transitions (eg, from elementary to middle school, middle to high school, and high school to college or employment); working with schools; and developmental challenges that may be affected by ADHD, including driving, sexual activity, and substance use and abuse. For parents who are interested in understanding the developmental aspects of children's understanding about ADHD (ie, causes, manifestations, treatments), several AAP publications may be useful.[222-224]

Although having a child diagnosed with ADHD can sometimes provide relief for families, it is important to check on the parents' well-being. Having a disruptive child who has trouble interacting with others can be stressful for parents, and learning that their child has a disorder sometimes gives them something to blame other than themselves. Helping families cope with parenting challenges or making referrals for services to address their stress or depression can be an important part of care. These concerns are particularly relevant when a parent has ADHD or associated conditions. Parents may require support balancing the needs of their child with ADHD and their other children's needs. Advocacy and support groups such as the National Resource on ADHD (a program of CHADD: https://chadd.org/about/about-nrc/) and the Attention Deficit Disorder Association (www.add.org) can provide information and support for families. There also may be local support organizations. The ADHD Toolkit provides lists of educational resources including Internet-based resources, organizations, and books that may be useful to parents and children.

IV c. Establish Management Team: Establish Team and Coordination Plan

Treatment Team

The optimal treatment team includes everyone involved in the care of the child: the child, parents, teachers, PCC, therapists, subspecialists, and other adults (such as coaches or faith leaders) who will be actively engaged in supporting and monitoring the treatment of ADHD.[218-221] It is helpful for the PCC or another assigned care coordinator to make each team member aware of his or her role, the process and timing of routine and as-needed communication strategies, and expectations for reports (ie, frequency, scope). Collaboration with school personnel goes beyond the initial report of diagnosis and is best facilitated by agreement on a standardized, reliable communication system. Although there are obstacles to achieving this level of coordination, if successful, it enhances care and improves outcomes for the child. (See Systemic Barriers to the Care of Children and Adolescents With ADHD section in the Supplemental Information for a discussion of systemic challenges.)

Treatment Goals

Management plans include the establishment of treatment goals for the areas of concern, such as those most commonly affected by ADHD: academic performance; relationships with peers, parents, and siblings; and safety. It is not necessary to develop goals in every area at once. Families might be encouraged to identify up to 3 of the most impairing areas to address initially. Parents and the child or adolescent can add other targets as indicated by their relative importance. Other goals may be identified using the International Classification of Function, Disability, and Health analysis conducted in the diagnostic phase of the clinical pathway. This process increases the understanding of ADHD's effects on each family member and may lead to improved collaboration in developing a few specific and measurable outcomes. It is helpful to incorporate a child's strengths and resilience when considering target goals and generating the treatment plan. Academic or school goals require the input of teachers and other personnel for both identification and measurement.

Establishing measurable goals in interpersonal domains and improving behavior in unstructured settings may be particularly important. Wherever possible, progress should be quantifiable to monitor the frequency of behaviors. The number of achieved and missed goals per day can be recorded by the parent, child, and/or teacher. Charts may be suggested as strategies to record events so that parents, teachers, children, and PCCs can agree on how much progress has been made building success in a systematic and measurable way. Keeping the focus on progress toward the identified goals can keep all family members engaged, provide a rubric for measuring response to various treatments, and offer a vehicle for rewarding success. Such strategies can help a family accurately assess and see progress of behavior changes. A single-page daily report card can be used to identify and monitor 4 or 5 behaviors that affect function at school and the card can be shared with parents. Other strategies and tools are available to clinicians in the AAP *ADHD Provider Toolkit, Third Edition*,[225] and for parents, *ADHD: What Every Parent Needs to Know.*[226]

As treatment proceeds, in addition to using a *DSM-5*–based ADHD rating scale to monitor core symptom changes, formal and informal queries can be made in the areas affected by ADHD. At every visit, it is helpful for the PCC to gradually further empower children and adolescents so they are able to be full partners in the treatment plan by adolescence. Data from school are helpful at these visits, including rating scales completed by the child or adolescent's teacher, grades, daily behavior ratings (when available), and formal test results.

Management Plan

In addition to educating the family, the PCC can consider developing a management plan that, over time, addresses the following questions:

- Does the family need further assistance in understanding the core symptoms of ADHD and the child or adolescent's target symptoms and coexisting conditions?
- Does the family need support in learning how to establish, measure, and monitor target goals?
- Have the family's goals been identified and addressed in the care plan?
- Does the family have an understanding of effective behavior management techniques for responding to tantrums, oppositional behavior, and/or poor compliance with requests or commands?
- Does the family need help on normalizing peer and family relationships?
- Does the child need help in academic areas? If so, has a formal evaluation been performed and reviewed to distinguish work production problems secondary to ADHD or attributable to coexisting learning or language disabilities?
- Does the child or adolescent need assistance in achieving independence in self-help or schoolwork?
- Does the child or adolescent or family require help with optimizing, organizing, planning, or managing schoolwork?
- Does the family need help in recognizing, understanding, or managing coexisting conditions?
- Does the family have a plan to educate the child or adolescent systematically about ADHD and its treatment, as well as the child's own strengths and weaknesses?
- Does the family have a plan to empower the child or adolescent with the knowledge and understanding that will increase their adherence to treatments? Has

that plan been initiated, and is it pitched at the child or adolescent's developmental level?

- Does the family have a copy of a care plan that summarizes the evaluation findings and treatment recommendations?
- Does the follow-up plan provide comprehensive, coordinated, family-centered, and culturally competent ongoing care?
- Does the family have any needed referrals to specialists to provide additional evaluations, treatments, and support?
- Does the family have a plan for the transition from pediatric to adult care that provides the transitioning youth with the necessary ADHD self-management skills, understanding of health care and educational privacy laws, identified adult clinician to continue his or her ADHD care, and health insurance coverage?

IV d. Treatment: Medication, Psychosocial Treatment, and Collaboration With the School to Enhance Support Services

The decision about the most acceptable treatment of the child rests with the family and its decisions about treatment. The PCC needs to encourage that this decision is based on accurate and adequate information, which often involves correcting misinformation or unwarranted concerns about medication. If the family still declines medication treatment, the PCC can encourage all other types of effective treatment and provide appropriate monitoring (families who decline medication are discussed in more detail below).

Pediatricians and other PCCs need to educate families about the benefits and characteristics of evidence-based ADHD psychosocial treatment and explicitly communicate that play therapy and sensory-related therapies have not been demonstrated to be effective. Likewise, for children younger than 7 years, individual CBT lacks demonstrated effectiveness; CBT has some, but not strong, evidence for children 7 to 17 years of age. Families should be made aware that for psychosocial treatments to be effective, the therapist needs to work with the family (not just the child or adolescent) on setting and maintaining routines, discipline and reward-related procedures, training programs, and creating a home environment that will bring out the best in the child and minimize ADHD-related dysfunction.

(See the ADHD guideline KASs 5 and 6.)

Treatment: Medication

This treatment option is restricted to children and adolescents who meet diagnostic criteria for ADHD.

The FDA has approved stimulant medications (ie, methylphenidate and amphetamines) and several nonstimulant medications for the treatment of ADHD in children and adolescents. New brands of methylphenidate and amphetamines continue to be introduced, including longer-acting products, various isomeric products, and delayed-release products. Hence, it is increasingly unlikely that pediatricians and other PCCs need to consider the off-label use of other medications. A free and continually updated list of medications is available at www. adhdmedicationguide.com. (See the ADHD guideline for information on off-label use.)

With the expanded choices and considerations of the clinical effects comes the reality that clinical choices are often heavily restricted by insurance coverage. Some, but not all, of the problems include changes in insurance and formulary that preclude the use of certain medications or force a stable patient

to change medications, step therapy requirements that may delay effective treatment, and financial barriers that preclude a patient's use of newer drugs or those not preferred by the payer. (See Systemic Barriers to the Care of Children and Adolescents with ADHD section in the Supplemental Information for a discussion of this issue.)

The choice of stimulant medication formulation depends on such factors as the efficacy of each agent for a given child, the preferred length of coverage, whether a child can swallow pills or capsules, and out-of-pocket costs. The extended-release formulations are generally more expensive than the immediate-release formulations. Families and children may prefer them, however, because of the benefits of consistent and sustained coverage with fewer daily administrations. Long-acting formulations usually avoid the need for school-based administration of ADHD medication. Better coverage with fewer daily administrations leads to greater convenience to the family and is linked with increased adherence to the medication management plan.[227]

Some patients, particularly adolescents, may require more than 12 hours of coverage daily to ensure adequate focus and concentration during the evening, when they are more likely to be studying and/or driving. In these cases, a nonstimulant medication or short-acting preparation of stimulant medication may be used in the evening in addition to a long-acting preparation in the morning. Of note, stimulant medication treatment of individuals with ADHD has been linked to better driving performance and a significant reduced risk of motor vehicle crashes.[78]

The ease with which preparations can be administered and the minimization of adverse effects are key quality-of-life factors and are

important concerns for children, adolescents, and their parents. When making medication recommendations, PCCs have to consider the time of day when the targeted symptoms occur, when homework is usually done, whether medication remains active when teenagers are driving, whether medication alters sleep initiation, and risk status for substance use or stimulant misuse or diversion.

All FDA-approved stimulant medications are methylphenidate or amphetamine compounds and have similar desired and adverse effects. Given the extensive evidence of efficacy and safety, these drugs remain the first choice in medication treatment. The decision about what compound a PCC prescribes first should be made on the basis of individual clinician and family preferences and the child's age. Some children will respond better to, or experience more adverse effects with, 1 of the 2 stimulants groups (ie, methylphenidate or amphetamine) over another. Because this cannot be determined in advance, medication trials are appropriate. If a trial with 1 group is unsuccessful because of poor efficacy or significant adverse effects, a medication trial with medication from the other group should be undertaken. At least half of children who fail to respond to 1 stimulant medication have a positive response to the alternative medication.[228]

Of note, recent meta-analyses have documented some subtle group-level differences in amphetamine and/or dextroamphetamine and methylphenidate response. Authors of 1 such analysis found that, on average, youth with ADHD who were treated with either amphetamine- or methylphenidate-based medications showed improvement in ADHD symptoms.[229] There was a marginally larger improvement in clinicians' ADHD symptom ratings for amphetamine-based versus methylphenidate-based preparations.[229] This meta-analysis indicated that overall adverse effects (including sleep problems and emotional side effects) were more prominent among those using amphetamine-based preparations. The findings were corroborated by a 2018 meta-analysis in which authors found that amphetamine and/or dextroamphetamine worsened emotional lability compared to the premedication baseline. Authors of the meta-analysis found there was a tendency for methylphenidate to reduce irritability and anxiety compared to the patients' premedication ratings.[230] Among individual patients, medication's efficacy and adverse effects can vary from these averages.

Families who are concerned about the use of stimulants or the potential for their abuse and/or diversion may choose to start with atomoxetine, extended-release guanfacine, or extended-release clonidine. In addition, those not responding to either stimulant group may still respond to atomoxetine, extended-release guanfacine, or extended-release clonidine.

There is a black box warning on atomoxetine about the possibility of suicidal ideation when initiating medication management. Early symptoms of suicidal ideation may include thinking about self-harm and increasing agitation. If there are any concerns about suicidal ideation in children prescribed atomoxetine, further evaluation (ie, using the Patient Health Questionnaire-9 rating scale, asking about suicidal ideation, reviewing presence of firearms in the home, determining if there is good communication between the patient and parents or trusted adults, etc), reconsideration about the use of atomoxetine, and more frequent monitoring should be considered; referral to a mental health clinician may be necessary.

Atomoxetine is a selective norepinephrine reuptake inhibitor

that may demonstrate maximum response after approximately 4 to 6 weeks of use, although some patients experience modest benefits after 1 week of atomoxetine treatment. Extended-release guanfacine and extended-release clonidine are α-2A adrenergic agonists that may demonstrate maximum response in about 2 to 4 weeks. It is worth making families aware that symptom change is more gradual with atomoxetine and α-2A adrenergic agonists than the rapid effect seen with stimulant medications. Atomoxetine may cause gastrointestinal tract symptoms and sedation early on, so it is recommended to prescribe half the treatment dose (0.5 mg/kg) for the first week. Appetite suppression can also occur. Both α-2A agonists can cause the adverse effect of somnolence. It is recommended that α-2A agonists be tapered when discontinued to prevent possible rebound hypertension.

In patients who only respond partially to stimulant medications, it is possible to combine stimulant and nonstimulant α-2 agonist medications to obtain better efficacy (see Medication for ADHD section in the clinical practice guideline). It is helpful to ask the family if they have any previous experience with any of the medications because a previous good or bad experience in other family members may indicate a willingness or reluctance to use 1 type or a specific stimulant medication. When there is concern about possible use or diversion of the medication or a strong family preference against stimulant medication, an FDA-approved nonstimulant medication may be considered as the first choice of medication.

Medications that use a microbead technology can be opened and sprinkled on food and are, therefore, suitable for children who have difficulty swallowing tablets or

capsules. For patients who are unable to swallow pills, alternative options include immediate- and extended-release methylphenidate and amphetamine in a liquid and chewable form, a methylphenidate transdermal patch, and an orally disintegrating tablet.

It is often helpful to inform families that the initial medication titration process may take several weeks to complete, medication changes can be made on a weekly basis, and subsequent changes in medication may be necessary. Completion of ADHD rating scales before dose adjustment helps promote measurement-based treatment. The usual procedure is to begin with a low dose of medication and titrate to the dose that provides maximum benefit and minimal adverse effects. Core symptom reduction can be seen immediately with stimulant medication initiation, but improvements in function require more time to manifest. Stimulant medications can be effectively titrated with changes occurring in a 3- to 7-day period. During the first month of treatment, the medication dose may be titrated with a weekly or biweekly follow-up. The increasing doses can be provided either by prescriptions that allow dose adjustments upward or, for some of medications, by 1 prescription of tablets or capsules of the same strength with instructions to administer progressively higher amounts by doubling or tripling the initial dose.

Another approach, similar to the one used in the MTA study,[228] is for parents to be directed to administer different doses of the same preparation, each for 1 week at a time (eg, Saturday through Friday). At the end of each week, feedback from parents and teachers and/or *DSM-5*–based ADHD rating scales can be obtained through a phone interview, fax, or a secure electronic system. In addition to the ADHD rating scale, parents and teachers can be asked to review adverse effects and progress on target goals.

Follow-up Visits

A face-to face follow-up visit is recommended at about the fourth week after starting the medication. At this visit, the PCC reviews the child or adolescent's responses to the varying doses and monitors adverse effects, pulse, BP, and weight. To promote progress in controlling symptoms is maintained, PCCs will continue to monitor levels of core symptoms and improvement in specified target goals. ADHD rating scales should be completed at each visit, particularly before any changes in medication and/or dose.

In the first year of treatment, face-to-face visits to the PCC are recommended to occur on a monthly basis until consistent and optimal response has been achieved, then they should occur every 3 months. Subsequent face-to-face visits will be dependent on the response; they typically occur quarterly but need to occur at least twice annually until it is clear that target goals are progressing and that symptoms have stabilized. Thereafter, visits occur periodically as determined by the family and the PCC. After several years, if the child or adolescent is doing well and wants to attempt a trial off of the medication, this can be initiated.

Results from the MTA study suggest that there are some children who, after 3 years of medication treatment, continue to improve even if the medication is discontinued.[13] These findings suggest that children who are stable in their improvement of ADHD symptoms may be given a trial off medication after extended periods of use to determine if medication is still needed. This process is best undertaken with close monitoring of the child's core symptoms and function at home, in school, and in the community. If pharmacologic interventions do not improve the child or adolescent's symptoms, the

diagnosis needs to be reassessed (see Treatment Failure section).

Whenever possible, improvements in core symptoms and target goals should be monitored in an objective way (eg, an increase from 40% goal attainment to 80% per week; see the ADHD Toolkit for more information). Core symptoms can be monitored with 1 of the *DSM-5*–based ADHD rating scales.

Pediatricians and other PCCs are encouraged to educate parents that although medications can be effective in facilitating schoolwork, they have not been shown to be effective in addressing learning disabilities or a child's level of motivation. A child or adolescent who continues to experience academic underachievement after attaining some control of his or her ADHD behavioral symptoms needs to be assessed for a coexisting condition. Such coexisting conditions include learning and language disabilities, other mental health disorders, and other psychosocial stressors. This assessment is part of the initial assessment in children who present with difficulties in keeping up with their schoolwork and grades and who are rated as having problems in the 3 academic areas (ie, reading, writing, and math).

Treatment: Psychosocial Treatment

Two types of psychosocial treatments are well established for children and adolescents with ADHD, including some behavioral treatments and training.[25]

Behavioral Treatments

There is a great deal of evidence supporting the use of behavioral treatments for preschool-aged and elementary and middle school–aged children, including several types of PTBM and classroom interventions (see the clinical practice guideline for more information). There are multiple PTBM programs available,

which are reviewed in the ADHD Toolkit.[225]

Evidence-based PTBM training typically begins with 7 to 12 weekly group or individual sessions with a trained or certified therapist. Although PTBM treatments differ, the primary focus is on helping parents improve the methods they use to reward and motivate their child to reduce the behavioral difficulties posed by ADHD and improve their child's behavior. Therapists help parents establish consistent relationships or contingencies between the child's specific behaviors and the parents' use of rewards or logical consequences for misbehavior. These treatments typically use specific directed praise, point systems, time-outs, and privileges to shape behavior. Parents learn how to effectively communicate expectations and responses to desirable and undesirable behaviors.

PTBM programs offer specific techniques for reinforcing adaptive and positive behaviors and decreasing or eliminating inappropriate behaviors, which alter the motivation of the child or adolescent to control attention, activity, and impulsivity. These programs emphasize establishing positive interactions between parents and children, shaping children's behaviors through praising and strengths spotting, giving successful commands, and reinforcing positive behaviors. They help parents to extinguish inappropriate behaviors through ignoring, to identify behaviors that are most appropriately handled through natural consequences, and to use natural consequences in in a responsible way.

These programs all emphasize teaching self-control and building positive family relationships. If parents strongly disagree about behavior management or have contentious relationships, parenting programs will likely be unsuccessful.

Depending on the severity of the child or adolescent's behaviors and the capabilities of the parents, group or individual training programs will be required. Programs may also include support for maintenance and relapse prevention.

Although all effective parenting uses behavioral techniques, applying these strategies to children or adolescents with ADHD requires additional rigor, adherence, and persistence, compared with children without the disorder. Some PTBM programs include additional components such as education about ADHD, development and other related issues, motivational interviewing, and support for parents coping with a child with ADHD.

PTBM training has been modified for use with adolescents to incorporate a family therapy approach that includes communication, problem-solving, and negotiation. Initially developed for adolescents with a wide range of problems,[94,231] this approach has been modified for adolescents with ADHD.[94,233] The approach's effects are not as large as with PTBM training with children, but clear benefits have been reported; this is a feasible clinic-based approach that warrants a referral, if available.

Although PTBM training is typically effective, such programs may not be available in many areas (see Systemic Barriers to the Care of Children and Adolescents with ADHD section in the Supplemental Information for further discussion of this issue[153]). Factors that may diminish PTBM's effects and/or render them ineffective include the time commitment required to attend sessions and practice the recommendations at home, particularly given other competing demands for the family's time. Parental disagreements about implementing the PTBM program, conflicts between parents, and separated parents who share

caretaking responsibilities can adversely affect the results. Careful monitoring of progress and follow-up by the therapist or PCC can reduce the likelihood of these risks. PTBM training may not be covered by health insurance (insurance issues are discussed in the Systemic Barriers to the Care of Children and Adolescents With ADHD section).

Training Interventions

Training interventions are likely to be effective with children and adolescents with ADHD. These interventions involve targeting specific deficiencies in skills such as study, organization, and interpersonal skills. Effective training approaches involve targeting a set of behaviors that are useful to the child in daily life and providing extensive training, practice, and coaching over an extended period of time. For some children, the combination of behavioral treatments and training may be most effective. Psychosocial treatments are applicable for children who have problems with inattentive or hyperactive/impulsive behaviors but do not meet the *DSM-5* criteria for a diagnosis of ADHD.

Many of the behavioral and training treatments described above can be provided at school. Coaching, which has emerged as a treatment modality over the last decade, can be a useful alternative to clinic- or school-based treatments. There has yet to be rigorous studies to support its benefits, although it has good face validity. Currently, there is no standardized training or certification for coaches.

Other Considerations

PCCs can make recommendations about treatments that are most likely to help a child or adolescent with ADHD and discourage the use of nonmedication treatments that are unlikely to be effective. Pediatricians and other PCCs are encouraged to discuss what parents have tried in the

past and what has been beneficial for the child and his or her family.

Treatments for which there is insufficient evidence include large doses of vitamins and other dietary alterations, vision and/or visual training, chelation, EEG biofeedback, and working memory (ie, cognitive training) programs.[25] To date, there is insufficient evidence to determine that these therapies lead to changes in ADHD's core symptoms or functioning. There is a lack of information about the safety of many of these alternative therapies. Although there is some minimal information that significant doses of essential fatty acids may help with ADHD symptoms, further study on effectiveness, negative impacts, and adverse effects is needed before it can be considered a recommended treatment.[233]

As noted, some therapies that are effective for other disorders are not supported for use with children or adolescents with ADHD. These include CBT (which has documented effectiveness for the treatment of anxiety and depressive disorders), play therapy, social skills training, and interpersonal talk therapy. Although it is possible that these treatments may improve ADHD symptoms in a specific child or adolescent, they are less likely to do so compared to evidence-based treatments. As a result, the PCC should discourage use of these approaches. If these ineffective treatments are attempted before evidence-based modalities, parents may erroneously conclude that all mental health treatments are ineffective. For example, if CBT or play therapy does not help their child's ADHD, parents may dismiss other treatments, like PTBM, which could be helpful. Parents also may discount CBT if it subsequently is recommended for an emerging anxiety disorder.

Pediatricians and other PCCs are unlikely to be effective in providing psychosocial treatment unless they are specifically trained, have trained staff, are colocated with a therapist, or dedicate multiple visits to providing this treatment. Clinicians may have difficulty determining if the therapists listed in the patient's health insurance plan have the requisite skills to provide evidence-based, psychosocial ADHD-related treatment. This determination is important because many therapists focus on a play therapy or interpersonal talk therapy, which have not been shown to be effective in treating the impairments associated with ADHD.

Pediatricians and other PCCs may want to develop a resource list of local therapists, agencies, and other mental health clinicians who can treat these impairments. Clinicians might request references from other parents of children with ADHD, professional organizations (eg, the Association for Behavioral and Cognitive Therapies), and ADHD advocacy organizations (eg, CHADD). Parents who have read authoritatively written books about psychosocial treatment may be in a better position to know what they are looking for in a therapist. Some of these resources are available in the ADHD Toolkit[225] and in *ADHD: What Every Parent Needs to Know*[226] as well as other online sources.[226,234–236] Unfortunately, lack of insurance coverage, availability, and accessibility of effective services may limit the implementation of this process (see Systemic Barriers to the Care of Children and Adolescents with ADHD section in the Supplemental Information for further discussion).

Treatment: Collaborate With School to Enhance Support and Services

School-based approaches have demonstrated both short- and long-term benefits for at least 1 year beyond treatment.[95,97] Schools can implement behavioral or training interventions that directly target ADHD symptoms and interventions to

enhance academic and social functioning. Schools may use strategies to enhance communication with families, such as daily behavior report cards. All schools should have specialists (eg, school psychologists, counselors, special educators) who can observe the child or adolescent, identify triggers and reinforcers, and support teachers in improving the classroom environment. School specialists can recommend accommodations to address ADHD symptoms, such as untimed testing, testing in less distracting environments, and routine reminders. As children and adolescents get older, their executive functioning skills continue developing. Thus, their delays may decrease, and they may no longer need the accommodations. Alternatively, further intervention may be indicated to facilitate the development of these independent skills.

It is helpful for PCCs to be aware of the eligibility criteria for 504 Rehabilitation Act and the IDEA support in their state and local school districts.[143] It is helpful to understand the process for referral and the specific individuals to contact about these issues. Providing this information to parents will support their efforts to secure classroom adaptations for their child or adolescent, including the use of empirically supported academic interventions to address the achievement difficulties that are often associated with ADHD symptoms.

Educate Parents About School Services

School is often the place where many problems of a child or adolescent with ADHD occur. Although services are available through special education, IDEA, and Section 504 plans, classroom teachers can help students with ADHD. Students with ADHD are most likely to succeed in effectively managed classrooms in which teachers provide engaging

instruction, support their students, and implement rules consistently. School staff can sometimes consult with classroom teachers to help them improve their skills in these areas. In many schools, parents can ask the principal for a specific teacher for their child the following academic year.

In some schools, teachers may implement activities to help a student before he or she is considered for special services, including a daily report card, organization interventions, behavioral point systems, and coordinating with the parents, such as using Web sites or portal systems for communication. Individualized behavioral interventions, if implemented well and consistently, are some of the most effective interventions for children with ADHD. In addition to individualized interventions, encouraging parents to increase communication with the teacher can help parents reinforce desirable behavior at school.

If these approaches are not adequate or teachers are unwilling to provide them, parents can be encouraged to write to the principal or the director of special education requesting an evaluation for special education services. An evaluation from a PCC can help this evaluation process but is unlikely to replace it. A child who has an ADHD diagnosis may be eligible for special education services in the category of "other health impaired." Depending on the specific nature of a child's impairment at school, he or she may be eligible for the categories of "emotional and behavioral disorders" or "specific learning disability." The category of eligibility does not affect the services available to the child but usually reflect the nature of the problems that resulted in his or her eligibility for special education services.

Although a PCC may recommend that a child is eligible for special education and specific services, these are only recommendations, as specific evaluation procedures and criteria for eligibility are determined by each school district within federal guidelines. If the ADHD is severe and interfering with school performance, services are usually provided under the other health impaired category. It is important for PCCs to avoid using language in the report that could alienate people in the school or create conflict between the parents and school staff. After school staff complete the evaluation, a meeting will be held to review the results of all evaluation information (including the PCC report) and determine the student's eligibility for an IEP or a 504 plan. If they wish, the parents may invite others to attend the meeting. Some communities have individuals who are trained to help parents effectively advocate for services; being aware of existing resources, if they exist, can help the PCC refer parents to them. Additional details about eligibility are usually available on the Web sites of the school district and the state department of education.

A PCC can help educate the parents about the types of services they can request at the meeting. There are generally 2 categories of services. Some of the most common services are often referred to as accommodations, including extending time on tests, reducing homework, or providing a child with class notes from the teacher or a peer. These services reduce the expectations for a child and can quickly eliminate school problems. For example, if a child is failing classes because he or she is not completing homework and the teacher stops assigning the child homework, then the child's grade in the class is likely to improve quickly. Similarly, parent-child conflict regarding homework will quickly cease. Although these outcomes are desirable, if discontinuing the expectation for completing homework results does not help improve the student's ability to independently complete tasks outside school, which is an important life skill, it may not be beneficial. Although appealing, these services may not improve and in some cases may decrease the child's long-term competencies. They need to be considered with this in mind.

The second set of services consists of interventions that enhance the student's competencies. These take much more work to implement than the services described above and do not solve the problem nearly as quickly. Although appealing, these services may decrease the child's long-term competencies if they are not combined with interventions that are aimed at improving the student's skills and behaviors. Accommodations need to be considered with this broader context in mind. The advantage of interventions is that many students improve their competencies and become able to independently meet age-appropriate expectations over time (for more information on this approach, see information on the Life Course Model[237]).[238] Interventions include organization interventions, daily report cards, and training study skills. The following school-based interventions have been found to be effective in improving academic and interpersonal skills for students with ADHD: Challenging Horizons Program,[95] Child Life and Attention Skills Program,[239] and Homework and Organization Planning Skills.[96] If these are available in area schools, it is important to encourage their use.

V. AGE-RELATED ISSUES

V a. Preschool-Aged Children (Age 4 Years to the Sixth Birthday)

Clinicians can initiate treatment of preschool-aged children with ADHD (ie, children age 4 years to the sixth birthday) with PTBM training and assess for other developmental problems, especially with language. If children continue to have moderate-to-severe dysfunction, the PCC needs to reevaluate the extent to which the parents can implement the therapy; the PCC can also consider prescribing methylphenidate, as described previously. Titration should start with a small dose of immediate-release methylphenidate because preschool-aged children metabolize medication at a slower rate. They have shown lower optimal milligrams-per-kilogram daily doses than older children and may be more sensitive to emotional side effects such as irritability and crying.[83,98]

Currently, dextroamphetamine is the only FDA-approved ADHD medication to treat preschool-aged children. However, when dextroamphetamine received FDA approval, the criteria were less stringent than they are now, so there is only sparse evidence to support its safety and efficacy in this age group. There is more abundant evidence that methylphenidate is safe and efficacious for preschool-aged children with ADHD. For this reason, methylphenidate is the first-line recommended ADHD medication treatment of this age group despite not having FDA approval.[28]

The Preschool ADHD Treatment Study,[83] the landmark trial documenting methylphenidate's safety and efficacy in this age group, included children with moderate-to-severe dysfunction. Therefore, the recommendation for methylphenidate treatment is reserved for children with significant, rather than mild, ADHD-related impairment. In the Preschool ADHD Treatment Study trial, moderate-to-severe impairment was defined as having symptoms present for at least 9 months and clear impairment in both the home and child care and/or preschool settings that did not respond to an appropriate intervention.

There is limited published evidence of the safety and efficacy for the preschool-aged group of atomoxetine, extended-release guanfacine, or extended-release clonidine. None of these nonstimulant medications have FDA approval for this age group.[47]

V b. Adolescents (Age 12 Years to the 18th Birthday)

Pediatricians and other PCCs may increase medication adherence and engagement in the treatment process by closely involving adolescents (age 12 years to the 18th birthday) in medication treatment decisions. Collaborating with the adolescent to determine if the medication is beneficial can help align outcome measures with the adolescent's own goals. Special attention ought to be paid to provide medication coverage at times when the adolescent may exhibit risky behaviors, such as when he or she is driving or spending unsupervised time with friends. Longer-acting or late-afternoon administration of nonstimulant medications or short-acting medications may be helpful.

If pediatricians and other PCCs begin transitioning children to be increasingly responsible for treatment decisions during early adolescence, then transitioning to a primary care physician who specializes in care for adults will be a natural continuation of that process when the adolescent reaches the highest grades in high school. Preparation for the transition to adulthood is an important step that includes planning for transferring care, adapting treatment to new activities and schedules, and educating the patient about effective ways to obtain insurance and engage in services.

Counseling for adolescents around medication issues needs to include dealing with resistance to treatment and empowering the patient to take charge of and own his or her medication management as much as possible. Techniques of motivational interviewing may be useful in improving adherence.[240]

In addition to the numerous developmental changes encountered

when working with adolescents, PCCs should assess adolescent patients with ADHD for symptoms of substance use or abuse before beginning medication treatment. If substance use is revealed, the patient should stop the use. Referral for treatment of substance use must be provided before beginning treatment of ADHD (see the clinical practice guideline). Pediatricians and other PCCs should pay careful attention to potential substance use and misuse and diversion of medications. Screening for signs of substance use is important in the care of all adolescents and, depending on the amount of use, may lead a PCC to recommend treatment of substance use. Extensive use or abuse may result in concerns about continuing medication treatment of ADHD until the abuse is resolved. Similar concerns and consideration of discontinuing medication treatment of ADHD could emerge if there is evidence that the adolescent is misusing or diverting medications for other than its intended medical purposes. Pediatricians and other PCCs are encouraged to monitor symptoms and prescription refills for signs of misuse or diversion of ADHD medication. Diversion of ADHD medication is a special concern among adolescents.[132]

When misuse or diversion is a concern, the PCC might consider prescribing nonstimulant medications with much less abuse potential, such as atomoxetine, extended-release guanfacine, or extended-release clonidine. It is more difficult but not impossible to extract the methylphenidate or amphetamine for abuse from the stimulant medications lisdexamfetamine, dermal methylphenidate, and osmotic-release oral system methylphenidate, although these preparations still have some potential for abuse or misuse.

PCCs should be aware that short-acting, mixed amphetamine salts are the most commonly misused or

diverted ADHD medication. It is important to note that diversion and misuse of ADHD medications may be committed by individuals who have close contact with or live in the same house as the adolescent, not necessarily by the adolescent him- or herself; this is especially true for college-aged adolescents. Pediatricians and other PCCs are encouraged to discuss safe storage practices, such as lockboxes for controlled substances, when used by college-aged adolescents.

VI. MONITORING

Pediatricians and other PCCs should regularly monitor all aspects of ADHD treatment, including the following:

- systematic reassessment of core symptoms and function;
- regular reassessment of target goals;
- family satisfaction with the care it is receiving from other clinicians and therapists, if applicable;
- provision of anticipatory guidance, further child or adolescent and family education, and transition planning as needed and appropriate;
- occurrence and quality of care coordination to meet the needs of the child or adolescent and family;
- confirmation of adherence to any prescribed medication regimen, with adjustments made as needed;
- HR, BP, height, and weight monitoring; and
- furthering the therapeutic relationship with the child or adolescent and empowering families and children or adolescents to be strong, informed advocates.

Some treatment monitoring can occur during general health care visits if the PCC inquires about the child or adolescent's progress toward target goals, adherence to medication and behavior therapy, concerns, and

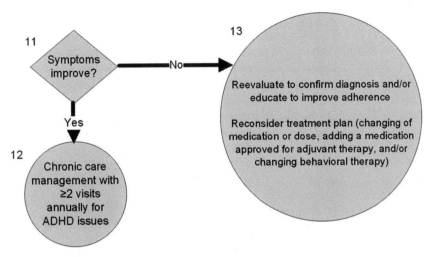

SUPPLEMENTAL FIGURE 8
Monitoring.

changes. This extra time and evaluation effort may generate an evaluate and management (E/M) code along with the well-child care code and may result in an additional cost to the family (see the section on barriers, specifically the compensation section[153]). Monitoring of a child or adolescent with inattention or hyperactivity/impulsivity problems can help to ensure prompt treatment should symptoms worsen to the extent that a diagnosis of ADHD is warranted.

As treatment proceeds, in addition to using a *DSM-5*–based ADHD rating scale to monitor core symptom changes, the PCC can make formal and informal queries in the areas of function most commonly affected by ADHD: academic achievement; peer, parent, or sibling relationships; and risk-taking behavior. Progress can be measured by monitoring the target goals established in collaboration with the child and family. Checklists completed by the school can facilitate medication monitoring. Data from the school, including ADHD symptom ratings completed by the teacher as well as grades and any other formal testing, are helpful at these visits. Screening for substance use and sleep problems is best continued throughout treatment because these

problems can emerge at any time. At every visit, it is helpful to gradually further empower children to become full partners in their treatment plan by adolescence.

In the early stages of treatment, after a successful titration period, the frequency of follow-up visits will depend on adherence, coexisting conditions, family willingness, and persistence of symptoms. As noted, a general guide for visits to the PCC is for these visits to occur initially on a monthly basis, then at least quarterly for the first year of treatment. More frequent visits may be necessary if comorbid conditions are present. Visits then need be held preferably quarterly but at least twice each year, with additional phone contact monitoring at the time of medication refill requests. Ongoing communication with the school regarding medication and services is needed.

There is little evidence establishing the optimal, practical follow-up regimen. It is likely that the regimen will need to be tailored to the individual child or adolescent and family needs on the basis of clinical judgment. Follow-up may incorporate electronic collection of rating scales, telehealth, or use of remote monitoring of symptoms and impairment. The time-intensive

nature of this process, insurance restrictions, and lack of payment may be significant barriers to adoption (see Systemic Barriers to the Care of Children and Adolescents with ADHD section in the Supplemental Information for more information on this issue).

(See the ADHD guideline's KAS 4.)

VI A. TREATMENT FAILURE

ADHD treatment failure may be a sign of inadequate dosing, lack of patient or family information or compliance, and/or incorrect or incomplete diagnosis. Family conflict and parental psychopathology can also contribute to treatment failure.

In the event of treatment failure, the PCC is advised to repeat the full diagnostic evaluation with increased attention to the possibility of another condition or comorbid conditions that mimic or are associated with ADHD, such as sleep disorders, autism spectrum disorders, or epilepsy (eg, absence epilepsy or partial seizures). Treatment failure may also arise from a new acute stressor or from an unrecognized or underappreciated traumatic event. A coexisting learning disability may cause an apparent treatment failure. In the case of a child or adolescent previously diagnosed with problem-level inattention or hyperactivity, repeating the diagnostic evaluation may result in a diagnosis of ADHD, which would allow for increased school support and the inclusion of medication in the treatment plan. A forthcoming complex ADHD guideline from the SDBP will provide additional information on diagnostic evaluation and treatment of children and adolescents with ADHD treatment failure and/or ADHD that is complicated by coexisting developmental or mental health conditions.

Treatment failure could result from poor adherence to the treatment plan. Increased monitoring and education, especially by including the patient, may increase adherence. It is helpful to try to identify the issues restricting adherence, including lack of information about or understanding of the treatment plan. It is also important to recognize that cultural factors may impact the patient's treatment and outcomes.

If the child continues to struggle despite the school's interventions and treatment of ADHD, further psychoeducational, neuropsychological, and/or language assessments are necessary to evaluate for a learning, language, or processing disorder. The clinician may recommend evaluation by an independent psychologist or neuropsychologist.

VII. CHILDREN AND ADOLESCENTS FOR WHOM AN ADHD DIAGNOSIS IS NOT MADE

If the evaluation identifies or suggests another disorder is the cause of the concerning signs and symptoms, it is appropriate to exit this algorithm.

VII a. Other Condition

The subsequent approach is dictated by the evaluation's results. If the PCC has the expertise and ability to evaluate and treat the other or

comorbid condition, he or she may do so. Many collaborative care models exist to help facilitate a pediatrician's comfort with comorbidity, as well as programs that teach pediatricians to manage comorbidities. It is important for the PCC to frame the referral questions clearly if a referral is made. A comanagement plan must be established that addresses the family's and child or adolescent's ongoing needs for education and general and specialty health care. Resources from the AAP Mental Health Initiatives and the forthcoming complex ADHD clinical practice guideline from the SDBP may be helpful.[67,133,241]

VII b. Apparently Typical or Developmental Variation

Evaluation may reveal that the child or adolescent's inattention, activity level, and impulsivity are within the typical range of development, mildly or inconsistently elevated in comparison with his or her peers, or is not associated with any functional impairment in behavior, academics, social skills, or other domains. The clinician can probe further to determine if the parents' concerns are attributable to other issues in the family, such as parental tension or drug use by a family member; whether they are caused by other issues in school, such as social pressures or bullying; or whether they are within the spectrum of typical development.

In talking with parents, it may help to explain that ADHD differs from a condition like pregnancy, which is a "yes" or "no" condition. With ADHD, behaviors follow a spectrum from variations on typical behavior, to atypical behaviors that cause problems but are not severe enough to be considered a disorder, to consistent behaviors that are severe enough to be considered a disorder. With problematic behaviors, it is helpful for the PCC to provide education about both the range of

typical development and strategies to improve the child or adolescent's behaviors. A schedule of enhanced surveillance absolves the family of the need to reinitiate contact if the situation deteriorates. If a recommendation for continued routine systematic surveillance is made by the PCC, it is important to provide reassurance that ongoing concerns can be revisited at future primary care visits.

VII c. Children and Adolescents With Inattention or Hyperactivity/Impulsivity (Problem Level)

Children and adolescents whose symptoms do not meet the criteria for diagnosis of ADHD may still encounter some difficulties or mild impairment in some settings, as described in the *DSM-PC, Child and Adolescent Version*.[49] For these patients, enhanced surveillance is recommended. PCCs are encouraged to provide education for both the patient and his or her family, specifically about triggers for inattention and/or hyperactivity as well as behavior management strategies.

Medication is not appropriate for children and adolescents whose symptoms do not meet *DSM-5* criteria for diagnosis of ADHD, but PTBM does not require a diagnosis of ADHD to be recommended.

VIII. COMPLEMENTARY AND ALTERNATIVE THERAPIES AND/OR INTEGRATIVE MEDICINE

Families of children and adolescents with ADHD increasingly ask their pediatrician and other PCCs about complementary and alternative therapies. These include megavitamins and other dietary alterations, vision and/or visual training, chelation, EEG biofeedback, and working memory (eg, cognitive training) programs.[242] As noted, there is insufficient evidence to suggest that these therapies lead to changes in ADHD's core symptoms or function.

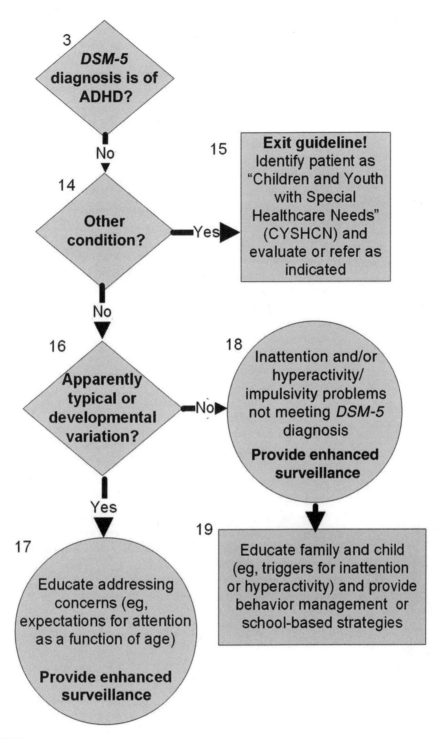

SUPPLEMENTAL FIGURE 9
Children and adolescents for whom an ADHD diagnosis is not made. CYSHCN, children and youth with special health care needs.

For many complementary and alternative therapies, limited information is available about their safety. Both chelation and megavitamins have been proven to cause adverse effects and are contraindicated.[243,244] For these reasons, complementary and alternative therapies are not recommended.

Pediatricians and other PCCs can play a constructive role in helping families make thoughtful treatment choices by reviewing the goals and/or effects claimed for a given treatment, the state of evidence to support or discourage use of the treatment, and known or potential adverse effects. If families are interested in trying complementary and alternative treatments, it is helpful to have them define specific measurable goals to monitor the treatment's impact. Families also need to be strongly encouraged to use evidence-based interventions while they explore complementary and alternative treatments. PCCs have to respect families' interests and preferences while they address and answer questions about complementary and alternative therapies.

Pediatricians and other PCCs should ask about additional therapies that families may be administering to adequately monitor for drug interactions. Parents and children or adolescents who do not feel that their choices in health care are respected by their PCCs may be less likely to communicate about complementary or alternative therapies and/or integrative medicine.

IX. IMPLEMENTATION ISSUES: PREPARING THE PRACTICE

Implementation of the process described in this algorithm can be enhanced with preparation of the practice to meet the needs of children and adolescents with ADHD. This preparation includes both internal practice characteristics and relationships within the community. (More detail can be found in the AAP Mental Health Initiatives' resources.[133,245])

The following office procedures and resources will help practices facilitate the steps in this algorithm:

- developing a packet of ADHD questionnaires and rating scales for parents and teachers to complete before a scheduled visit;
- allotting adequate time for ADHD-related visits;
- determining billing and documentation procedures and monitoring insurance payments to appropriately capture the services rendered to the extent possible;

- implementing methods to track and follow patients (see Systemic Barriers to the Care of Children and Adolescents with ADHD section in the Supplemental Information for more information on this issue);
- asking questions during all clinical encounters and promoting patient education materials (ie, brochures and posters) that alert parents and patients that appropriate issues to discuss with the PCC include problem behaviors, school problems, and concerns about attention and hyperactivity;
- developing an office system for monitoring and titrating medication, including communication with parents and teachers. For stimulant medications, which are controlled substances requiring new, monthly prescriptions, it is necessary to develop a monitoring and refill process including periodic review of the state's database of controlled substance prescriptions (any such system is based on the PCC's assessment of family organization, phone access, and parent-teacher communication effectiveness); and
- using the ADHD Toolkit resources.

Establishing relations with schools and other agencies can facilitate communication and establish clear expectations when collaborating on care for a child. A community-level system that reflects consensus among district school staff and local PCCs for key elements of diagnosis, interventions, and ongoing communication can help to provide consistent, well-coordinated, and cost-effective care. A community-based system with schools relieves the individual PCC from negotiating with each school about care and communication regarding each patient. Offices that have incorporated medical home principles are ideal for establishing this kind of community-level system. Although achieving the level of coordination described below

is ideal and takes consistent effort over the years, especially in areas with multiple separate school systems, some aspects may be achieved relatively quickly and will enhance services for children.

The key elements for a community-based collaborative system include consensus on the following:

- a clear and organized process by which an evaluation can be initiated when concerns are identified either by parents or school personnel;
- a packet of information completed by parents and teachers about each child and/or adolescent referred to the PCC;
- a contact person at the practice to receive information from parents and teachers at the time of evaluation and during follow-up;
- an assessment process to investigate coexisting conditions;
- a directory of evidence-based interventions available in the community;
- an ongoing process for follow-up visits, phone calls, teacher reports, and medication refills;
- availability of forms for collecting and exchanging information;
- a plan for keeping school staff and PCCs up to date on the process; and
- awareness of the network of mental health providers in your area and establishments of collaborative relationships with them.

The PCC may face challenges to developing such a collaborative process. For example, a PCC is typically caring for children from more than 1 school system, a school system may be large and not easily accessed, schools may have limited staff and resources to complete assessments, or scheduling may make it difficult for the PCC to communicate with school personnel. Further complicating these efforts is the fact that many providers encounter a lack of recognition and payment for the time involved in coordinating care. These barriers may hamper efforts to provide the internal resources within a practice and coordination across schools and other providers that are described above; nevertheless, some pediatricians and other PCCs have found ways to lessen some of these obstacles (see Systemic Barriers to the Care of Children and Adolescents with ADHD section in the Supplemental Information for more information on overcoming challenges).

In the case of multiple or large school systems in a community, the PCC may want to begin with 1 school psychologist or principal, or several practices can initiate contact collectively with a community school system. Agreement among the clinicians on the components of a good evaluation process facilitates cooperation and communication with the school toward common goals. Agreement on behavior rating scales used can facilitate completion by school personnel. Standard communication forms that monitor progress and specific interventions can

be exchanged among the school and the pediatric office to share information. Collaborative systems can extend to other providers who may comanage care with a PCC. Such providers may include a mental health professional who sees the child or adolescent for psychosocial interventions or a specialist to address difficult cases, such as a developmental-behavioral pediatrician, child and adolescent psychiatrist, child neurologist, neurodevelopmental disability physician, or psychologist. The AAP Mental Health Initiatives provide a full discussion of collaborative relationships with mental health professionals, including colocation and integrated models, in its Chapter Action Kit and PediaLink Module.[133,241]

Achieving this infrastructure in the practice and the coordination across schools and other providers will enhance the PCC's ability to implement the treatment guidelines and this algorithm. Achieving these ideals is not necessary for providing care consistent with these practices, however.

X. CONCLUSIONS

ADHD is the most common neurobiological disorder of children and adolescents. Untreated or undertreated ADHD can have far-reaching and serious consequences for the child or adolescent's health and well-being. Fortunately, effective treatments are available, as are methods for assessing and diagnosing ADHD in children and adolescents. The AAP is committed to supporting primary care physicians in providing quality care to children and adolescents with ADHD and their families. This algorithm represents a portion of that commitment and an effort to assist pediatricians and other PCCs to deliver care that meets the quality goals of the practice guideline. This PoCA, in combination with the guideline and Systemic Barriers to the Care of Children and Adolescents With ADHD section below, is intended to provide support and guidance in what is currently the best evidence-based care for their patients with ADHD. Additional support and guidance can be obtained through the work and publications of the AAP Mental Health Initiatives.[133,241]

SYSTEMIC BARRIERS TO THE CARE OF CHILDREN AND ADOLESCENTS WITH ADHD

INTRODUCTION

The AAP strives to improve the quality of care provided by PCCs through quality improvement initiatives including developing, promulgating, and regularly revising evidence-based clinical practice guidelines. The AAP has published a revision to its 2011 guideline on evaluating, diagnosing, and treating ADHD on the basis of the latest scientific evidence (see main article). This latest revision of the clinical practice guideline is accompanied by a PoCA (also found in the Supplemental Information), which outlines the applicable diagnostic and treatment processes needed to implement the guidelines. This section, which is a companion to the clinical guideline and PoCA, outlines common barriers that impede ADHD care and provides suggested strategies for clinicians seeking to improve care for children and adolescents with ADHD and work with other concerned public and private organizations, health care payers, government entities, state insurance regulators, and other stakeholders.

ADHD is the most common childhood neurobehavioral disorder in the United States and the second most commonly diagnosed childhood condition after asthma.[246] The *DSM-5* criteria define 4 dimensions of ADHD:

1. ADHD/I (314.00 [F90.0]);

2. ADHD/HI (314.01 [F90.1]);

3. ADHD/C (314.01 [F90.2]); and

4. ADHD other specified and unspecified ADHD (314.01 [F90.8]).

National survey data from 2016 reveal that 9.4% of 2- to 17-year-old US children received an ADHD diagnosis during childhood, and 8.4% currently have ADHD.[247] Prevalence estimates from community-based samples are somewhat higher, ranging from 8.7% to 15.5%.[9,10] Most children with ADHD (67%) had at least 1 other comorbidity, and 18% had 3 or more comorbidities, such as mental health disorders and/or learning disorders. These comorbidities increase the complexity of the diagnostic and treatment processes.[66]

The majority of care for children and adolescents with ADHD is provided by the child's PCC, particularly when the ADHD is uncomplicated in nature. In addition, families typically have a high degree of confidence and trust in pediatricians' ability to provide this professional care. Because of the high prevalence of ADHD in children and adolescents, it is essential that PCCs, particularly pediatricians, be able to diagnose, treat, and coordinate this care or identify an appropriate clinician who can provide this needed care. Despite having a higher prevalence than other conditions that PCCs see and manage, such as urinary tract infections and sports injuries, ADHD is often viewed as different from other pediatric conditions and beyond the purview of primary care. In addition, several barriers to care hamper effective and timely diagnosis and treatment of these children and adolescents and must be addressed and corrected to achieve optimum outcomes for these children.[153] These barriers include the following:

1. limited access to care because of inadequate developmental-behavioral and mental health care training during residencies and other clinical training and shortages of consultant specialists and referral resources;

2. inadequate payment for needed services and payer coverage limitations for needed medications;

3. challenges in practice organization and staffing; and

4. fragmentation of care and resulting communication barriers.

Addressing these barriers from a clinical and policy standpoint will enhance clinicians' ability to provide high-quality care for children and adolescents who are being evaluated and/or treated for ADHD. Strategies for improvement in the delivery of care to patients with ADHD and their families are offered for consideration for practice and for advocacy.

BARRIERS TO HIGH-QUALITY CARE FOR CHILDREN AND ADOLESCENTS WITH ADHD

Multiple barriers exist in the primary medical care of children and adolescents that are impediments to excellent ADHD care.

Limited Access to Care Because of Inadequate Developmental-Behavioral and Mental Health Care Training During Pediatric Residency and Other Clinical Training Programs and Shortages of Consultant Specialists and Referral Resources

There is an overall lack of adequate pediatric residency and other training programs for pediatric clinicians on developmental-behavioral and mental health conditions, including ADHD. The current curriculum and the nature of pediatric training still focus on the diagnosis and treatment of inpatient and intensive care conditions despite the fact that many primary care pediatricians spend less and less time providing these services, which are increasingly managed by pediatric hospitalists and intensive care specialists. Pediatric and family medicine residents do not receive sufficient training in the diagnosis and treatment of developmental-behavioral and mental health conditions, including ADHD, despite the high frequency in which they will encounter these conditions in their practices.[152,248]

SUPPLEMENTAL TABLE 2 Core Symptoms of ADHD From the *DSM-5*

Inattention Dimension	Hyperactivity-Impulsivity Dimension	
	Hyperactivity	Impulsivity
Careless mistakes	Fidgeting	Blurting answers before questions completed
Difficulty sustaining attention	Unable to stay seated	Difficulty awaiting turn
Seems not to listen	Moving excessively (restless)	Interrupting and/or intruding on others
Fails to finish tasks	Difficulty engaging in leisure activities quietly	—
Difficulty organizing	"On the go"	—
Avoids tasks requiring sustained attention	Talking excessively	—
Loses things	—	—
Easily distracted	—	—
Forgetful	—	—

Adapted from American Psychiatric Association. *Diagnostic and Statistical Manual of Mental Disorders.* 5th ed. Washington, DC: American Psychiatric Association; 2000:59–60. —, not applicable.

In addition, many experienced pediatric clinicians believe that general pediatric and family medicine residencies do not fully ensure that clinicians who enter primary care practice have the organizational tools to develop, join, or function in medical home settings and address chronic developmental and behavioral conditions like ADHD.[152] The current funding of residency and other training programs for pediatric clinicians and the needs of hospitals tend to limit those aspects of training. The training challenges are subsequently not sufficiently addressed by practicing pediatric and family medicine practitioners, in part because of the limited number and varying quality of continuing medical education (CME) opportunities and quality improvement projects focused on medical home models and/or the chronic care of developmental and behavioral pediatric and mental health conditions.

The lack of training is compounded by the national shortage of child and adolescent psychiatrists and developmental-behavioral pediatricians: the United States has only 8300 child psychiatrists[249] and 662 developmental-behavioral pediatricians.[250] The additional training required for child psychiatry and developmental-behavioral pediatrics certification increases education time and costs yet results

in little or no return on this investment in terms of increased compensation for these specialists.[249] Given the high cost of medical school and the increasing educational debt incurred by graduating medical students, physicians lack a financial incentive to add the extra years of training required for these specialties.[251] As a result, there are insufficient numbers of mental health professionals, including child psychiatrists and developmental-behavioral pediatricians, to serve as subspecialty referral options and/or provide PCCs with consultative support to comanage their patients effectively.

The specialist shortage is exacerbated by the geographically skewed distribution of extant child psychiatrists and developmental-behavioral pediatricians who are concentrated in academic medical centers and urban environments. Almost three quarters (74%) of US counties have no child and adolescent psychiatrists; almost half (44%) do not even have any pediatricians.[252] As a result, many PCCs lack an adequate pool of pediatric behavioral and mental health specialists who can accept referrals to treat complicated pediatric ADHD patients and an adequate pool of behavioral therapists to provide evidence-based behavioral interventions. The result is that patients must often travel untenable distances and endure long

waits to obtain these specialty services.

Suggested Strategies for Change to Address Limited Access to Care: Policy-Oriented Strategies for Change

- Promote changes in pediatric and family medicine residency curricula to devote more time to developmental, behavioral, learning, and mental health issues with a focus on prevention, early detection, assessment, diagnosis, and treatment. Changes in the national and individual training program requirements and in funding of training should foster practitioners' understanding of the family perspective; promote communication skills, including motivational interviewing; and bolster understanding and readiness in the use of behavioral interventions and medication as treatment options for ADHD.

- Emphasize teaching and practice activities within general pediatric residencies and other clinical training, so pediatricians and other PCCs gain the skills and ability they need to function within a medical home setting.

- Support pediatric primary care mental health specialist certification for advanced practice registered nurses through the

Pediatric Nursing Certification Board to provide advanced practice care to help meet evidence-based needs of children or adolescents with ADHD.

- Encourage the development and maintenance of affordable programs to provide CME and other alternative posttraining learning opportunities on behavioral and developmental health, including ADHD. These opportunities will help stakeholders, including PCCs, mental health clinicians, and educators, become more comfortable in providing such services within the medical home and/or educational settings.

- Develop, implement, and support collaborative care models that facilitate PCCs' rapid access to behavioral and mental health expertise and consultation. Examples include integration (such as collaborative care or colocation), on-call consultation, and support teams such as the Massachusetts Child Psychiatry Access Program,[253] the "Project Teach Initiative" of the New York State Department of Mental Health,[254] and Project Extension for Community Healthcare Outcomes, a collaborative model of medical education and care management that can be targeted to pediatric mental health.[255] In addition, federal funding had provided grants to18 states to develop Child Psychiatry Access Programs through Health Resources and Services Administration's Pediatric Mental Health Care Access Program.[256,257] Promote incentives such as loan forgiveness to encourage medical students to enter the fields of child and adolescent psychiatry and developmental and behavioral pediatrics, particularly for those who are willing to practice in underserved communities.

- Expand posttraining opportunities to include postpediatric portal programs, which provide alternative ways to increase number of child and adolescent psychiatrists.

Inadequate Payment for Needed Services and Payer Coverage Limitations for Needed Medications

Although proper diagnostic and procedure codes currently exist for ADHD care in pediatrics, effective and adequate third-party payment is not guaranteed for any covered services.[258] In addition, many payment mechanisms impede the delivery of comprehensive ADHD care. These impediments include restrictions to medication treatment choices such as step therapy, previous approval, narrow formularies, and frequent formulary changes. Some payers define ADHD as a "mental health problem" and implement a "carve-out" health insurance benefit that bars PCCs from participation.[259] This designation results in denial of coverage for primary care ADHD services. Some payers have restrictive service and/or medication approval practices that prevent patients from receiving or continuing needed care and treatment. Examples include approval of only a limited number of specialist visits, limited ADHD medication options, mandatory step therapy, frequent formulary changes resulting in clinical destabilization, and disproportionally high out-of-pocket copays for mental health care or psychotropic medications.

Payments for mental health and cognitive services are frequently lower than equivalents (by relative value unit measurement) paid for physical health care services, particularly those entailing specific procedures.[258] Longer and more frequent visits are often necessary to successfully address ADHD, yet time-based billing yields lower payment compared to multiple shorter visits. These difficulties financially limit a practice's ability to provide these needed services. Payments for E/M codes for chronic care are often insufficient to cover the staff and clinician time needed to provide adequate care. Furthermore, many payers deny payment for the use of rating scales, which are the currently recommended method for monitoring ADHD patients. The use of rating scales takes both the PCC's time and the practice's organizational resources. Arbitrary denial of payment is a disincentive to the provisions of this essential and appropriate service.

Finally, payers commonly decline to pay or provide inadequate payment for care coordination services. Yet, office staff and clinicians are asked to spend large amounts of uncompensated time on these activities, including communicating with parents, teachers, and other stakeholders. Proposed new practice structures such as accountable care organizations (ACOs) are predicated on value-based services and may provide new financial mechanisms to support expanded care coordination services. Originally implemented for Medicare, all-payer ACO models are under development in many states. To date, however, the specifics of these ACO models have not been delineated, and their effectiveness has not yet been documented.[260]

The seemingly arbitrary and ever-changing standards for approval of services; the time-consuming nature of previous approval procedures; and restrictive, opaque pharmacy rules combine to create substantial barriers that result in many PCCs declining to care for children and adolescents with ADHD.[252] According to a recent AAP Periodic Survey of Fellows, 41% of pediatricians reported that "inadequate reimbursement is a major barrier to providing mental health counseling."[258] Of note, 46% reported that they would be interested in hiring mental health clinicians in their practice "if payment and financial resources were not an issue."[258]

Payers' practices regarding medication approval also create challenges for treating pediatric ADHD. In conflict with best-practice or evidence-based guidelines, payers commonly favor 1 ADHD medication and refuse to approve others, even when the latter may be more appropriate for a specific patient. Decisions seem to be made on cost, which at times can be variable. Certain drugs may be allowed only after review processes; others are refused for poorly delineated reasons. Reviewers of insurance denial appeals often lack pediatric experience and are unfamiliar with the effect of the patient's coexisting condition(s) or developmental stage on the medication choice. Step therapy protocols that require specific medications at treatment initiation may require patients to undergo time-consuming treatment failures before an effective therapy can be started. Changes to formularies may force medication changes on patients whose ADHD had been well-controlled, leading to morbidity or delays in finding alternative covered medications that might be equally effective in restoring clinical control.

Similarly, payers may inappropriately insist that a newer replacement drug be used in a patient whose ADHD has been well-controlled by another drug of the same or similar class. The assumption that generic psychoactive preparations are equal to brand-name compounds in efficacy and duration of action is not always accurate.[261] Although generic substitution is generally appropriate, a change in a patient's response may necessitate return to the nongeneric formulation. In addition,

because of the variation in covered medications across insurance companies, when a family changes health plans, clinicians have to spend more time to clarify treatments and reduce family stress and their economic burden.

Suggested Strategies for Change to Address Inadequate Payment and Payer Coverage Limitations: Policy-Oriented Strategies

- Revise payment systems to reflect the time and cognitive effort required by primary care, developmental-behavioral, and mental health clinicians to diagnose, treat, and manage pediatric ADHD and compensate these services at levels that incentivize and support their use.

- Support innovative partnerships between payers and clinicians to facilitate high-quality ADHD care. As new payment models are proposed, include input from practicing clinicians to inform insurance plans' understanding of the resources needed to provide comprehensive ADHD care.

- Require that payers' medical directors who review pediatric ADHD protocols and medication formularies either have pediatric expertise or seek such expertise before making decisions that affect the management of pediatric patients with ADHD.

- Advocate that health care payers' rules for approval of developmental-behavioral and mental health care services and medications are consistent with best-practice recommendations based on scientific evidence such as the AAP ADHD guideline. Payers should not use arbitrary step-based medication approval practices or force changes to a patient's stable and effective medication plans

because of cost-based formulary changes.

- Advocate for better monitoring by the FDA of ADHD medication generic formulations to verify their equivalency to brand-name preparations in terms of potency and delivery.

- Partner with CHADD and other parent support groups to help advocate for positive changes in payers' rules; these organizations provide a strong voice from families who face the challenges on a day-to-day basis.

Challenges in Practice Organization

ADHD is a chronic condition. Comprehensive ADHD care requires additional clinician time for complex visits, consultation and communication with care team members, and extended staff time to coordinate delivery of chronic care. Children and adolescents with ADHD have a special health care condition and should be cared for in a manner similar to that of other children and youth with special health care needs.[262] Such care is ideally delivered by practices that are established as patient- and family-centered medical homes. Yet, the number of patient- and family-centered medical homes is insufficient to meet the needs of many children with ADHD and their families. Pediatricians and other PCCs who have not adopted a patient- and family-centered medical home model may benefit from the use of similar systems to facilitate ADHD management. For more information, see the recommendations and descriptions from the AAP and the American Academy of Family Medicine regarding medical homes.[262]

Caring for children and adolescents with ADHD requires practices to modify office systems to address their patients' mental health care needs. Specifically, practices need to be familiar with local area mental health referral options, where available, and communicate these options to families. Once a referral has been made, the office flow needs to support communication with other ADHD care team members.[263] Other team members, especially those in mental health, need to formally communicate with the referring clinician in a bidirectional process.

Making a referral does not always mean that the patient is able to access care, however. Practices need to consider that many families face difficulties in following through with referrals for ADHD diagnosis and treatment. These difficulties may arise for a variety of reasons, including lack of insurance coverage, lengthy wait lists for mental health providers, transportation difficulties, reluctance to engage with an unfamiliar care system, cultural factors, and/or the perceived stigma of receiving mental health–specific services.[145,146,155,158]

Many of these barriers can be addressed by the integration of mental health services within primary care practices and other innovative collaborative care models. These models can help increase the opportunities for families to receive care in a familiar and accessible location and provide a "warm hand off" of the patient into the mental health arena. The implementation of these models can be hindered by cost; collaboration with mental health agencies may be fruitful.

Another challenge is the difficulty in determining which mental health subspecialists use evidence-based treatments for ADHD. Pediatricians and other PCCs can increase the likelihood that families receive evidence-based services by establishing a referral network of clinicians who are known to use evidence-based practices and educating parents about effective

psychosocial treatments for children and adolescents to help them be wise consumers. It is also important to be cognizant of the fact that for some families, accessing these services may present challenges, such as the need to take time off from work or cover any program costs.

Finding professionals who use evidence-based treatments is of the utmost importance, because exposure to non–evidence-based treatments has the potential to harm patients in several ways. First, the treatment is less likely to be effective and may be harmful (eg, adverse events can and do occur in psychosocial treatments).[264] Second, the effort and money spent on ineffective treatment interferes with the ability to meaningfully engage in evidence-based treatments. Finally, when a treatment does not yield benefits, families are likely to become disillusioned with psychosocial treatments generally, even those that are evidence-based, decreasing the likelihood of future engagement. Each of these harms may place the child at greater risk of problematic outcomes over time.

Suggested Strategies to Address Challenges in Practice Organization

Clinician-Focused Implementation Strategies

- Develop ADHD-specific office workflows, as detailed in the Preparing the Practice section of the PoCA (see Supplemental Information).

- Ensure that the practice is welcoming and inclusive to patients and families of all backgrounds and cultures.

- Enable office systems to support communication with parents, education professionals, and mental health specialists, possibly through electronic communication systems (discussed below).

- Consider office certification as a patient- and family-centered medical home.

- If certification as a patient- and family-centered medical home is not feasible, implement medical home policies and procedures, including care conferences and management. Explore care management opportunities, including adequate resourcing and payment, with third-party payers.

- Identify and establish relationships with mental health consultation and referral sources in the community and within region, if available, and investigate integration of services as well as the resources to support them.

- Promote communication between ADHD care team members by integrating health and mental health services and using collaborative care model treatments when possible.

- Be aware of the community mental health crisis providers' referral processes and be prepared to educate families about evidence-based psychosocial treatments for ADHD across the life span.

Policy-Oriented Suggested Strategies

- Encourage efforts to support the development and maintenance of patient- and family-centered medical homes or related systems to enable patients with chronic complex disorders to receive comprehensive care.

- Support streamlined, coordinated ADHD care across systems by providing incentives for the integration of health and mental health services and collaborative care models.

Fragmentation of Care and Resulting Communication Barriers

Multiple team members provide care for children and adolescents with ADHD, including those in the fields of physical health, mental health, and education. Each of these systems has its own professional standards and terminologies, environments, and hierarchical systems. Moreover, they protect communication via different privacy rules: the Health Insurance Portability and Accountability Act (HIPAA)[265] for the physical and mental health systems and the Family Educational Rights and Privacy Act (FERPA)[266] for the education system. These factors complicate communication not only within but also across these fields. The lack of communication interferes with clinicians' abilities to make accurate diagnoses of ADHD and co-occurring conditions, monitor progress in symptom reduction when providing treatment, identify patient resources, and coordinate the most effective services for children and adolescents with ADHD.

Electronic systems can help address these communication barriers by facilitating asynchronous communication among stakeholders. This is particularly useful for disparate stakeholders, such as parents, teachers, and clinicians, who often cannot all be available simultaneously for a telephone or in-person conference. Electronic systems can also facilitate the timely completion and submission of standardized ADHD rating scales, which are the best tools to assess and treat the condition.[267] Because implementation of electronic systems lies partially within the PCC's control, additional information is provided below on the strengths and weaknesses of a variety of such systems, including telemedicine.

Stand-alone Software Platforms and EHRs

Stand-alone software platforms and EHRs have the potential to improve communication and care coordination among ADHD care team members. Commercially available stand-alone software platforms typically use electronic survey interfaces (either Web or mobile) to collect rating data from parents and teachers, use algorithms to score the data, and display the results cross-sectionally or longitudinally for the clinician's review. Advantages of stand-alone platforms include the fact that they are designed specifically for ADHD care and can be accessed via the Internet through computers and mobile devices. Once implemented, these user-friendly systems allow parents, teachers, and practitioners from multiple disciplines or practices to conveniently complete rating scales remotely. Stand-alone platforms also offer the ability to customize rating scales and their frequency of use for individual patients. Submitted data are stored automatically in a database, mitigating the transcription errors that are often associated with manual data entry. Data are available for clinical care, quality improvement, or research, including quality metrics.

A substantial downside to stand-alone ADHD care systems is the lack of data integration into EHRs. Practitioners must log in to disparate systems for different facets of patient care: the stand-alone system to track ADHD symptoms and the EHR to track medications records, visit notes, and patient or family phone calls. To achieve data accuracy in the 2 different systems, the practitioner must copy medication information from the EHR into the stand-alone system and ADHD symptom and adverse effect ratings from the stand-alone system into the EHR. In addition, stand-alone systems require clinicians to log in before each visit to review the relevant ADHD care data. Patients may use a variety of ADHD stand-alone tracking systems, requiring the PCC to remember several accounts and passwords in addition to his or her own office and hospital EHR systems, creating an added burden that may reduce enthusiasm for such platforms. Finally, stand-alone systems typically charge fees to support the maintenance of servers, cybersecurity, and technical and customer support functionalities.

An issue over which the PCC has little control is the fact that other stakeholders may use stand-alone systems inconsistently. Parents (who may themselves have ADHD) must log in to the platform and complete the requisite ADHD rating scales. Teachers may be required to log in and complete the evaluation process, often for several students, on top of their other obligations. The fact that different pediatricians may use different systems, each with their own log-in and interface, adds to the activity's complexity, particularly for teachers who need to report on multiple students to a variety of PCCs.

EHRs for ADHD Management

EHRs can be adapted to improve the timely collection of parent and teacher ratings of ADHD symptoms, impairment, and medication adverse effects. Some EHRs use an electronic survey functionality or patient portal, similar to that provided by ADHD care stand-alone systems, to allow parents' access to online rating scales. A clear advantage of these EHR systems is that they increase the ability to access documentation about an individual patient's past treatment modalities and medications in the same place as information about his or her ADHD symptoms. The functionality of these EHRs may facilitate other care-related activities, including evidence-based decision support, quality improvement efforts, and outcomes reporting.[268]

Despite these benefits, there are numerous limitations to managing ADHD care with EHRs. First, health care systems' confidentiality barriers often prevent teachers from entering ratings directly into the child's medical record. The large number and heterogeneity of EHR systems and their lack of interoperability are additional barriers to their use for ADHD care.[269] Even when institutions use the same vendor's EHR, exchanging respective ADHD documentation among a variety of clinicians and therapists is frequently impossible.[270] The inability to share information and the lack of interoperability often results in incomplete information in the EHR about a given patient's interventions, symptoms, impairments, and adverse effects over time. Systems for tracking and comparing these aspects of a patient's care are not standard for most EHR packages. The ability to construct templates that are congruent with a clinician's workflow may be limited by the EHR itself. ADHD functionality must often be custom-built for each organization, a cumbersome, expensive, and lengthy process, resulting in lost productivity, clinical effectiveness, and revenue.

General Issues With ADHD Electronic Tracking Systems

EHRs have been linked to increased clinician stress. For this reason, it is important to consider the potential for added burden when either stand-alone or EHR-embedded systems are used to facilitate ADHD care.[271] Although the use of electronic ADHD systems to monitor patients remotely may be advantageous, clinicians and practices may not be equipped or staffed to manage the burden of additional clinical information

arriving between visits (ie, intervisit data).

Clinicians must also consider the liability associated with potentially actionable information that families may report electronically without realizing the information might not be reviewed in real time. Examples of such liabilities include a severe medication adverse effect, free-text report of suicidal ideation, and sudden deterioration in ADHD symptoms and/or functioning. In addition, parents and teachers may receive numerous requests to complete rating scales, leading them to experience "survey fatigue" and ignore the requests to complete these scales. Conversely, they may forget how to use the system if they engage with it on an infrequent basis. Some parents or teachers may be uncomfortable using electronic systems and within the medical home might prefer paper rating scales, and others may not have ready access to electronic systems or the Internet.

Telemedicine for ADHD Management

Telemedicine is a new and rapidly growing technology that has the potential, when properly implemented within the medical home, to expand access to care and to improve clinicians' ability to communicate with schools, consultants, care management team members, and especially patients and parents.[213,272,273] Well-run telemedicine programs offer some promise as a way to deliver evidence-based psychosocial treatments, although few evidence-based programs have been tested via telemental health trials.[274,275] Telemedicine is one of the foundations of the new advanced medical home and offers advantages as follows:

- offering communication opportunities (either face-to-face and synchronous as a conversation or asynchronous as messaging),

which can be prescheduled to minimize interruption of office flow;

- enabling communication on a one-on-one basis or one-to-many basis (for conference situations);

- replacing repeated office visits for patient follow-up and monitoring, which reduces time and the need for patients to travel to the PCC's office;

- facilitating digital storage of the telemedicine episode and its incorporation into multiple EHR systems as part of the patient record; and

- enhancing cooperation among all parties in the evaluation and treatment processes.

Telemedicine has great potential but needs to be properly implemented and integrated into the practice workflow to achieve maximum effectiveness and flexibility. Although some new state insurance regulations mandate payment for telemedicine services, such mandates have not yet been implemented in all states, limiting telemedicine's utility. Finally, payment for services needs to include the added cost of equipment and staff to provide them.

Suggested Strategies to Address Fragmentation of Care and Resulting Communication Barriers

Clinician-Focused Implementation Strategies

- Ensure the practice is aware of, and in compliance with, HIPAA and FERPA policies, as well as confidentiality laws and cybersecurity safeguards that impact EHRs' communication with school personnel and parents.[276]

- Maintain open lines of communication with all team members involved in the patient's ADHD care within the practical limits of existing systems, time, and economic constraints. As noted, team members include teachers, other school personnel, clinicians, and mental health practitioners. This activity involves a team-based approach and agreeing on a communication method and process to track ADHD interventions, symptoms, impairments, and adverse effects over time. Communication can be accomplished through a variety of means, including electronic systems, face-to-face meetings, conference calls, emails, and/or faxes.

- Consider using electronic communication via stand-alone ADHD management systems and electronic portals, after evaluating EHR interoperability and other administrative considerations.

- Integrate electronic ADHD systems into the practice's clinical workflow: decide who will review the data and when, how actionable information will be flagged and triaged, how information and related decision-making will be documented in the medical record, etc.

- Set and clarify caregivers' expectations about the practice's review of information provided electronically versus actionable information that should be communicated directly by phone.

- Promote the implementation of telemedicine for ADHD management in states where payment for such services is established; ensure the telemedicine system chosen is patient centered, HIPAA and FERPA compliant, and practice enhancing.

Policy-Oriented Suggested Strategies

- Promote the development of mechanisms for online communication to enhance ADHD

care collaboration, including electronic portals and stand-alone ADHD software systems, to serve as communication platforms for families, health professionals, mental health professionals, and educators. Ideally, these portals would be integrated with the most commonly used EHR systems.

- Advocate for regulations that mandate a common standard of interoperability for certified EHR systems. Interoperability facilitates the use of EHRs as a common repository of ADHD care information and communication platform for ADHD care team members.[276]

- Advocate for exceptions to HIPAA and FERPA regulations to allow more communication between education and health and mental health practitioners while maintaining privacy protections.

- Ensure that billing, coding, and payment systems provide adequate resources and time for clinicians to communicate with teachers and mental health clinicians, as discussed previously.

- Provide incentives for integration of health and mental health services, collaborative care models, and telemedicine to facilitate communication among ADHD care team members, including telemedicine services that cross state lines.

- Fund research in telehealth to learn more about who responds well to these approaches and whether telehealth is feasible for underserved populations.

CONCLUSIONS

Appropriate and comprehensive ADHD care requires a well-trained and adequately resourced multidisciplinary workforce, with office workflows that are organized to

provide collaborative services that are consistent with a chronic care model and to promote communication among treatment team members.[277–280] Many barriers in the current health care system must be addressed to support this care.

First and foremost, the shortage of clinicians, such as child and adolescent psychiatrists and developmental-behavioral pediatricians who provide consultation and referral ADHD care, must also be addressed. The shortages are driven by the lack of residency and other training programs for pediatric clinicians in the management of ADHD and other behavioral health issues, the lack of return on investment in the additional training and debt required to specialize in this area, and inadequate resourcing at all levels of ADHD care. The shortage is exacerbated by geographic maldistribution of practitioners and lack of adequate mental health training as a whole during residency and in CME projects. These challenges must be addressed on a system-wide level.

A significant review and change in the ADHD care payment for cognitive services is required to ensure that practitioners are backed by appropriate resources that support the provision of high-quality ADHD care. The lack of adequate compensation for ADHD care is a major challenge to reaching children and adolescents with the care they need. Improved payment is a major need to encourage primary care clinicians to train in ADHD subspecialty care and incentivize child and adolescent psychiatry and developmental-behavioral pediatrics practitioners to provide ADHD care in the primary care setting, so the provision of such care does not result in financial hardship for the families or the practice. Improvement should also include changes to payer policies to improve compensation for care coordination services and mental health care.

Because the pediatrician is often the first contact for a parent seeking help for a child with symptoms that may be caused by ADHD, barriers to payment need to be addressed before providing these time-consuming services. Some insurance plans direct all claims with a diagnosis reported by *International Classification of Diseases, 10th Revision, Clinical Modification* codes F01–F99 to their mental and behavioral health benefits system. Because pediatricians are generally not included in networks for mental and behavioral health plans, this can create delays or denials of payment. This is not always the case, though, and with a little preventive footwork, practices can identify policy guidelines for plans that are commonly seen in the practice patient population.

The first step in identifying coverage for services to diagnose or treat ADHD is to determine what payment guidelines have been published by plans that contract with your practice. Many health plans post their payment guidelines on their Web sites, but even when publicly available, the documents do not always clearly address whether payment for primary care diagnosis and management of ADHD are covered. It may be necessary to send a written inquiry to provider relations and the medical director of a plan seeking clarification of what diagnoses and procedure codes should pass through the health benefit plan's adjudication system without denial or crossover to a mental health benefit plan. It is important to recognize that even with documentation that the plan covers primary care services related to ADHD, claims adjudication is an automated process that may erroneously cause denials. Billing and payment reconciliation staff should always refer such denials for appeal.

Once plans that do and do not provide medical benefits for the diagnosis and treatment of ADHD have been identified, advocacy to the medical directors of those plans that do not recognize the role of the medical home in mental health care can be initiated. The AAP template letter, Increasing Access to Mental Health Care, is a resource for this purpose. Practices should also be prepared to offer advance notice to parents when their plan is likely to deny or pay out of network for services. A list of referral sources for mental and behavioral health is also helpful for parents whose financial limitations may require alternative choices and for patients who may require referral for additional evaluation.

For services rendered, identify the codes that represent covered diagnoses and services and be sure that these codes are appropriately linked and reported on claims.

When ADHD is suspected but not yet diagnosed, symptoms such as attention and concentration deficit (R41.840) should be reported. Screening for ADHD in the absence of signs or symptoms may be reported with code Z13.4, encounter for screening for certain developmental disorders in childhood. *Current Procedural Terminology* codes 96110 and 96112 to 96113 should be reported for developmental screening and testing services.

Services related to diagnosis and management of ADHD are more likely to be paid under the patient's medical benefits when codes reported are not those for psychiatric or behavioral health services. Reporting of E/M service codes based on face-to-face time of the visit when more than 50% of that time was spent in counseling or coordination of care will likely be more effective than use of codes such as 90791, psychiatric diagnostic evaluation. *Current Procedural Terminology* E/M service

guidelines define counseling as a discussion with a patient or family concerning 1 or more of the following areas:

- diagnostic results, impressions, or recommended diagnostic studies;
- prognosis;
- risks and benefits of management (treatment) options;
- instructions for management (treatment) or follow-up;
- importance of compliance with chosen management (treatment) options;
- risk factor reduction; and
- patient and family education.

Finally, staff should track claim payment trends for services related to ADHD, including the number of claims requiring appeal and status of appeal determinations to inform future advocacy efforts and practice policy.

Many AAP chapters have developed pediatric councils that meet with payers on pediatric coding issues. Sharing your experiences with your chapter pediatric council will assist in its advocacy efforts. AAP members can also report carrier issues on the AAP Hassle Factor Form.

These system-wide barriers are challenging, if not impossible, for individual practitioners to address on their own. Practice organization and communication changes can be made, however, that have the potential to improve access to ADHD care. Clinicians and other practitioners can implement the office work-flow recommendations made in the Preparing the Practice section of the updated PoCA (see Supplemental Information). Implementing a patient- and family-centered medical home model, colocating health and mental health services, and adopting collaborative care models can also help overcome communication barriers and minimize fragmentation of care. It is noted that these models must be adequately resourced to be effective.

Finally, practitioners can implement innovative communication and record-keeping solutions to overcome barriers to ADHD care. Potential solutions could include the use of EHRs, other electronic systems, and high-quality telemedicine to support enhanced communication and record-keeping on the part of myriad ADHD care team members. These solutions can also aid with monitoring treatment responses on the part of the child or adolescent with ADHD. Telemedicine also has the distinct benefit of compensating for the maldistribution of specialists and other clinicians who can treat pediatric ADHD.

Many stakeholders have a role in addressing the barriers that prevent children and adolescents from receiving needed evidenced-based treatment of ADHD. Pediatric councils, the national AAP, and state and local AAP chapters must be advocates for broad changes in training, CME, and payment policies to overcome the systemic challenges that hamper access to care. On an individual level, practitioners can effect change in their own practice systems and professional approaches and implement systems that address fragmentation of care and communication. Practitioners are important agents for change in ADHD care. The day-to-day interactions that practitioners have with patients, families, educators, payers, state insurance regulators, and others can foster comprehensive, contemporary, and effective care that becomes a pillar of advocacy and change.

SUBCOMMITTEE ON CHILDREN AND ADOLESCENTS WITH ATTENTION-DEFICIT/HYPERACTIVITY DISORDER

The Council on Quality Improvement and Patient Safety oversees the Subcommittee

Mark L. Wolraich, MD, FAAP (Chairperson: Section on

Developmental Behavioral Pediatrics).

Joseph F. Hagan, Jr, MD, FAAP (Vice Chairperson: Section on Developmental Behavioral Pediatrics).

Carla Allan, PhD (Society of Pediatric Psychology).

Eugenia Chan, MD, MPH, FAAP (Implementation Scientist).

Dale Davison, MSpEd, PCC (Parent Advocate, Children and Adults with ADHD).

Marian Earls, MD, MTS, FAAP (Mental Health Leadership Work Group).

Steven W. Evans, PhD (Clinical Psychologist).

Tanya Froehlich, MD, FAAP (Section on Developmental Behavioral Pediatrics/Society for Developmental and Behavioral Pediatrics).

Jennifer L. Frost, MD, FAAFP (American Academy of Family Physicians).

Herschel R. Lessin, MD, FAAP, Section on Administration and Practice Management).

Karen L. Pierce, MD, DFAACAP (American Academy of Child and Adolescent Psychiatry).

Christoph Ulrich Lehmann, MD, FAAP (Partnership for Policy Implementation).

Jonathan D. Winner, MD, FAAP (Committee on Practice and Ambulatory Medicine).

William Zurhellen, MD, FAAP (Section on Administration and Practice Management).

STAFF

Kymika Okechukwu, MPA, Senior Manager, Evidence-Based Medicine Initiatives

Jeremiah Salmon, MPH, Program Manager, Policy Dissemination and Implementation

CONSULTANT

Susan K. Flinn, MA, Medical Editor

SUPPLEMENTAL REFERENCES

157. Bright Futures Available at: https://brightfutures.aap.org. Accessed September 8, 2019

158. American Academy of Pediatrics. AAP Diversity and Inclusion Statement. *Pediatrics.* 2018;141(4): e20180193

159. Chronis AM, Lahey BB, Pelham WE Jr, Kipp HL, Baumann BL, Lee SS. Psychopathology and substance abuse in parents of young children with attention-deficit/hyperactivity disorder. *J Am Acad Child Adolesc Psychiatry.* 2003;42(12):1424–1432

160. Foy JM, ed. Iterative Mental Health Assessement, Appendix 2: Mental Health Tools for Pediatrics. In: *Mental Health Care of Children and Adolescents: A Guide for Primary Care Clinicians.* Itasca, IL: American Academy of Pediatrics; 2018:817–868

161. Wolraich ML, Bard DE, Neas B, Doffing M, Beck L. The psychometric properties of the Vanderbilt attention-deficit hyperactivity disorder diagnostic teacher rating scale in a community population. *J Dev Behav Pediatr.* 2013;34(2):83–93

162. Bard DE, Wolraich ML, Neas B, Doffing M, Beck L. The psychometric properties of the Vanderbilt attention-deficit hyperactivity disorder diagnostic parent rating scale in a community population. *J Dev Behav Pediatr.* 2013;34(2):72–82

163. Goodman R. The extended version of the Strengths and Difficulties Questionnaire as a guide to child psychiatric caseness and consequent burden. *J Child Psychol Psychiatry.* 1999;40(5):791–799

164. Shaffer D, Gould MS, Brasic J, et al. A children's global assessment scale (CGAS). *Arch Gen Psychiatry.* 1983; 40(11):1228–1231

165. Brown RT, Freeman WS, Perrin JM, et al. Prevalence and assessment of attention-deficit/hyperactivity disorder in primary care settings. *Pediatrics.* 2001;107(3). Available at:

www.pediatrics.org/cgi/content/full/
107/3/E43

166. Evans SW, Allen J, Moore S, Strauss V. Measuring symptoms and functioning of youth with ADHD in middle schools. *J Abnorm Child Psychol.* 2005;33(6): 695–706

167. Wolraich ML, Lambert EW, Bickman L, Simmons T, Doffing MA, Worley KA. Assessing the impact of parent and teacher agreement on diagnosing attention-deficit hyperactivity disorder. *J Dev Behav Pediatr.* 2004;25(1):41–47

168. DiPerna JC, Elliott SN. *Academic Competence Evaluation Scales (ACES).* San Antonio, TX: The Psychological Corporation; 2000

169. Smith BH, Pelham WE, Gnagy E, Molina B, Evans S. The reliability, validity, and unique contributions of self-report by adolescents receiving treatment for attention-deficit/hyperactivity disorder. *J Consult Clin Psychol.* 2000; 68(3):489–499

170. Hoza B, Pelham WE Jr, Dobbs J, Owens JS, Pillow DR. Do boys with attention-deficit/hyperactivity disorder have positive illusory self-concepts? *J Abnorm Psychol.* 2002;111(2): 268–278

171. Zuckerbrot RA, Cheung AH, Jensen PS, Stein RE, Laraque D; GLAD-PC Steering Group. Guidelines for adolescent depression in primary care (GLAD-PC): I. Identification, assessment, and initial management. *Pediatrics.* 2007;120(5). Available at: www.pediatrics.org/cgi/content/full/120/5/e1299

172. Cheung AH, Zuckerbrot RA, Jensen PS, Ghalib K, Laraque D, Stein RE; GLAD-PC Steering Group. Guidelines for adolescent depression in primary care (GLAD-PC): II. Treatment and ongoing management. *Pediatrics.* 2007;120(5). Available at: www.pediatrics.org/cgi/content/full/120/5/e1313

173. Foy JM, ed. Low Mood, Appendix 2: Mental Health Tools for Pediatrics. In: *Mental Health Care of Children and Adolescents: A Guide for Primary Care Clinicians.* Itasca, IL: American Academy of Pediatrics; 2018:817–868

174. The Center for Adolescent Substance Use Research, Children's Hospital Boston. *CRAFFT: Screening Adolescents for Alcohol and Drugs.* Boston, MA:

Children's Hospital Boston; 2001. Available at: http://www.childrenshospital.org/~/media/microsites/ceasar/2016-2sided-crafft-card_clinician-interview.ashx?la=en. Accessed September 8, 2019

175. Levy S, Weiss R, Sherritt L, et al. An electronic screen for triaging adolescent substance use by risk levels. *JAMA Pediatr.* 2014;168(9): 822–828

176. University of Pittsburgh Child and Adolescent Bipolar Spectrum Services. Instruments: Screen for Child Anxiety Related Emotional Disorders (SCARED). Available at: https://www.pediatricbipolar.pitt.edu/resources/instruments. Accessed September 8, 2019

177. Kovacs M. *CDI 2: Children's Depression Inventory.* 2nd ed. North Tonawanda, NY: Multi-Health Systems Assessments; 2018. Available at: https://www.mhs.com/MHS-Assessment?prodname=cdi2. Accessed September 8, 2019

178. Richardson LP, McCauley E, Grossman DC, et al. Evaluation of the Patient Health Questionnaire-9 Item for detecting major depression among adolescents. *Pediatrics.* 2010;126(6): 1117–1123

179. Sleator EK, Ullmann RK. Can the physician diagnose hyperactivity in the office? *Pediatrics.* 1981;67(1):13–17

180. American Academy of Pediatrics. Fetal alcohol spectrum disorders program: toolkit. Available at: https://www.aap.org/en-us/advocacy-and-policy/aap-health-initiatives/fetal-alcohol-spectrum-disorders-toolkit/Pages/default.aspx. Accessed September 8, 2019

181. Hagan JF Jr, Balachova T, Bertrand J, et al; Neurobehavioral Disorder Associated With Prenatal Alcohol Exposure Workgroup; American Academy of Pediatrics. Neurobehavioral disorder associated with prenatal alcohol exposure. *Pediatrics.* 2016;138(4):e20151553

182. Gardner W, Murphy M, Childs G, et al. The PSC-17: a brief pediatric symptom checklist including psychosocial problem subscales: a report from PROS and ASPN. *Ambul Child Health.* 1999;5:225–236

183. National Institutes of Health. *Screening to Brief Intervention (S2BI).*

Bethesda, MD: National Institute on Drug Abuse. Available at: https://www.drugabuse.gov/ast/s2bi/#/. Accessed September 8, 2019

184. Levy SJ, Williams JF; Committee on Substance Use and Prevention. Substance use screening, brief intervention, and referral to treatment. *Pediatrics.* 2016;138(1): e20161211

185. University of Washington Harborview Center for Sexual Assault and Traumatic Stress. Standardized measures. Available at: https://depts.washington.edu/hcsats/PDF/TF-%20CBT/pages/assessment.html. Accessed September 8, 2019

186. Gordon M, Barkley RA, Lovett B. Tests and observational measures. In: Barkley RA, ed. *Attention-Deficit Hyperactivity Disorder Third Edition: A Handbook for Diagnosis and Treatment.* 3rd ed. New York, NY: Guilford Press; 2005:369–388

187. Edwards MC, Gardner ES, Chelonis JJ, Schulz EG, Flake RA, Diaz PF. Estimates of the validity and utility of the Conners' Continuous Performance Test in the assessment of inattentive and/or hyperactive-impulsive behaviors in children. *J Abnorm Child Psychol.* 2007;35(3):393–404

188. Li J, Olsen J, Vestergaard M, Obel C. Attention-deficit/hyperactivity disorder in the offspring following prenatal maternal bereavement: a nationwide follow-up study in Denmark. *Eur Child Adolesc Psychiatry.* 2010;19(10): 747–753

189. Angold A, Erkanli A, Egger HL, Costello EJ. Stimulant treatment for children: a community perspective. *J Am Acad Child Adolesc Psychiatry.* 2000;39(8): 975–984; discussion 984–994

190. Konofal E, Lecendreux M, Cortese S. Sleep and ADHD. *Sleep Med.* 2010; 11(7):652–658

191. Gozal D, Kheirandish-Gozal L. Neurocognitive and behavioral morbidity in children with sleep disorders. *Curr Opin Pulm Med.* 2007; 13(6):505–509

192. Capdevila OS, Kheirandish-Gozal L, Dayyat E, Gozal D. Pediatric obstructive sleep apnea: complications, management, and long-term

outcomes. *Proc Am Thorac Soc.* 2008; 5(2):274–282

193. Cortese S, Konofal E, Lecendreux M, et al. Restless legs syndrome and attention-deficit/hyperactivity disorder: a review of the literature. *Sleep.* 2005;28(8):1007–1013

194. Weiss MD, Wasdell MB, Bomben MM, Rea KJ, Freeman RD. Sleep hygiene and melatonin treatment for children and adolescents with ADHD and initial insomnia. *J Am Acad Child Adolesc Psychiatry.* 2006;45(5):512–519

195. Stein MA, Sarampote CS, Waldman ID, et al. A dose-response study of OROS methylphenidate in children and adolescents with attention-deficit/ hyperactivity disorder. *Pediatrics.* 2003;112(5). Available at: www.pediatrics. org/cgi/content/full/112/5/e404

196. Corkum P, Panton R, Ironside S, Macpherson M, Williams T. Acute impact of immediate release methylphenidate administered three times a day on sleep in children with attention-deficit/hyperactivity disorder. *J Pediatr Psychol.* 2008;33(4): 368–379

197. O'Brien LM, Ivanenko A, Crabtree VM, et al. The effect of stimulants on sleep characteristics in children with attention deficit/hyperactivity disorder. *Sleep Med.* 2003;4(4): 309–316

198. Owens J, Sangal RB, Sutton VK, Bakken R, Allen AJ, Kelsey D. Subjective and objective measures of sleep in children with attention-deficit/ hyperactivity disorder. *Sleep Med.* 2009;10(4):446–456

199. Owens JA. A clinical overview of sleep and attention-deficit/hyperactivity disorder in children and adolescents. *J Can Acad Child Adolesc Psychiatry.* 2009;18(2):92–102

200. Mick E, Biederman J, Jetton J, Faraone SV. Sleep disturbances associated with attention deficit hyperactivity disorder: the impact of psychiatric comorbidity and pharmacotherapy. *J Child Adolesc Psychopharmacol.* 2000;10(3):223–231

201. van der Heijden KB, Smits MG, van Someren EJ, Boudewijn Gunning W. Prediction of melatonin efficacy by pretreatment dim light melatonin

onset in children with idiopathic chronic sleep onset insomnia. *J Sleep Res.* 2005;14(2):187–194

202. Cortese S, Faraone SV, Konofal E, Lecendreux M. Sleep in children with attention-deficit/hyperactivity disorder: meta-analysis of subjective and objective studies. *J Am Acad Child Adolesc Psychiatry.* 2009;48(9):894–908

203. Golan N, Shahar E, Ravid S, Pillar G. Sleep disorders and daytime sleepiness in children with attention-deficit/hyperactive disorder. *Sleep.* 2004;27(2):261–266

204. Lecendreux M, Konofal E, Bouvard M, Falissard B, Mouren-Siméoni MC. Sleep and alertness in children with ADHD. *J Child Psychol Psychiatry.* 2000;41(6): 803–812

205. Owens JA, Dalzell V. Use of the 'BEARS' sleep screening tool in a pediatric residents' continuity clinic: a pilot study. *Sleep Med.* 2005;6(1):63–69

206. Chervin RD, Hedger K, Dillon JE, Pituch KJ. Pediatric sleep questionnaire (PSQ): validity and reliability of scales for sleep-disordered breathing, snoring, sleepiness, and behavioral problems. *Sleep Med.* 2000;1(1):21–32

207. Owens JA, Spirito A, McGuinn M. The Children's Sleep Habits Questionnaire (CSHQ): psychometric properties of a survey instrument for school-aged children. *Sleep.* 2000;23(8):1043–1051

208. Aurora RN, Zak RS, Karippot A, et al; American Academy of Sleep Medicine. Practice parameters for the respiratory indications for polysomnography in children. *Sleep (Basel).* 2011;34(3):379–388

209. Aurora RN, Lamm CI, Zak RS, et al. Practice parameters for the non-respiratory indications for polysomnography and multiple sleep latency testing for children. *Sleep (Basel).* 2012;35(11):1467–1473

210. Gruber R, Wiebe S, Montecalvo L, Brunetti B, Amsel R, Carrier J. Impact of sleep restriction on neurobehavioral functioning of children with attention deficit hyperactivity disorder. *Sleep (Basel).* 2011;34(3):315–323

211. Bunford N, Evans SW, Wymbs F. ADHD and emotion dysregulation among

children and adolescents. *Clin Child Fam Psychol Rev.* 2015;18(3):185–217

212. Langberg JM, Vaughn AJ, Brinkman WB, Froehlich T, Epstein JN. Clinical utility of the Vanderbilt ADHD Rating Scale for ruling out comorbid learning disorders. *Pediatrics.* 2010;126(5). Available at: www.pediatrics.org/cgi/ content/full/126/5/e1033

213. Kressly SJ. Extending the medical home to meet your patients' mental health needs: is telehealth the answer? *Pediatrics.* 2019;143(3): e20183765

214. Dudek E, Henschen E, Finkle E, Vyas S, Fiszbein D, Shukla A. Improving continuity in a patient centered medical home. *Pediatrics.* 2018;142(1): 366

215. Dessie AS, Hirway P, Gjelsvik A. Children with developmental, behavioral, or emotional problems are less likely to have a medical home. *Pediatrics.* 2018;141(1):23

216. Foy JM. The medical home and integrated behavioral health. *Pediatrics.* 2015;135(5):930–931

217. Ader J, Stille CJ, Keller D, Miller BF, Barr MS, Perrin JM. The medical home and integrated behavioral health: advancing the policy agenda. *Pediatrics.* 2015;135(5):909–917

218. American Academy of Pediatrics. Collaboration in practice: implementing team-based care. *Pediatrics.* 2016;138(2):e20161486

219. Kressley SJ. Team-based care for children: who should be included and who should lead? *AAP News.* July 24, 2017. Available at: https://www. aappublications.org/news/2017/07/ 24/TeamBased072417. Accessed September 8, 2019

220. Katkin JP, Kressly SJ, Edwards AR, et al; Task Force on Pediatric Practice Change. Guiding principles for team-based pediatric care. *Pediatrics.* 2017; 140(2):e20171489

221. Godoy L, Hodgkinson S, Robertson HA, et al. Increasing mental health engagement from primary care: the potential role of family navigation. *Pediatrics.* 2019;143(4):e20182418

222. Wolraich ML, Hagan JF Jr. *ADHD: What Every Parent Needs to Know.* 3rd ed.

Itasca, IL: American Academy of Pediatrics; 2019. Available at: https://shop.aap.org/adhd-paperback/. Accessed September 8, 2019

223. American Academy of Pediatrics. *Understanding ADHD*. Itasca, IL: American Academy of Pediatrics; 2017. Available at: https://shop.aap.org/understanding-adhd-brochure-50pk-brochure/. Accessed September 8, 2019

224. HealthyChildren.org. ADHD. 2018. Available at: https://www.healthychildren.org/English/health-issues/conditions/adhd/Pages/default.aspx. Accessed September 8, 2019

225. American Academy of Pediatrics. *ADHD Provider Toolkit*. 3rd ed. In production

226. Reiff MI. *ADHD: What Every Parent Needs to Know*. 2nd ed. Elk Grove Village, IL: American Academy of Pediatrics; 2011

227. Charach A, Fernandez R. Enhancing ADHD medication adherence: challenges and opportunities. *Curr Psychiatry Rep*. 2013;15(7):371

228. Greenhill LL, Abikoff HB, Arnold LE, et al. Medication treatment strategies in the MTA Study: relevance to clinicians and researchers. *J Am Acad Child Adolesc Psychiatry*. 1996;35(10):1304–1313

229. Cortese S, Adamo N, Del Giovane C, et al. Comparative efficacy and tolerability of medications for attention-deficit hyperactivity disorder in children, adolescents, and adults: a systematic review and network meta-analysis. *Lancet Psychiatry*. 2018;5(9):727–738

230. Pozzi M, Carnovale C, Peeters GGAM, et al. Adverse drug events related to mood and emotion in paediatric patients treated for ADHD: a meta-analysis. *J Affect Disord*. 2018;238:161–178

231. Robin AL, Foster SL. *Negotiating Parent Adolescent Conflict: A Behavioral-Family Systems Approach*. New York, NY: Guilford Press; 1989

232. Barkley RA, Edwards G, Laneri M, Fletcher K, Metevia L. The efficacy of problem-solving communication training alone, behavior management training alone, and their combination for parent-adolescent conflict in teenagers with ADHD and ODD. *J Consult Clin Psychol*. 2001;69(6):926–941

233. Bloch MH, Qawasmi A. Omega-3 fatty acid supplementation for the treatment of children with attention-deficit/hyperactivity disorder symptomatology: systematic review and meta-analysis. *J Am Acad Child Adolesc Psychiatry*. 2011;50(10):991–1000

234. Understood.org. Get personalized recommendations for you and your child. Available at: https://www.understood.org/en/learning-attention-issues/treatments-approaches/working-with-clinicians. Accessed September 8, 2019

235. ImpactADHD. Free resources for parents. Available at: https://impactadhd.com/resources/free-impactadhd-resources-for-parents/. Accessed September 8, 2019

236. ImpactADHD. ImpactADHD. Available at: https://www.youtube.com/user/ImpactADHD. Accessed September 8, 2019

237. Halfon N, Forrest CB, Lerner RM, Faustman EM. *Handbook of Life Course Health Development*. Cham, Switzerland: Springer; 2018

238. Evans SW, Owens JS, Mautone JA, DuPaul GJ, Power TJ. Toward a comprehensive, Life Course Model of care for youth with ADHD. In: Weist M, Lever N, Bradshaw C, Owens J, eds. *Handbook of School Mental Health*. 2nd ed. New York, NY: Springer; 2014:413–426

239. Pfiffner LJ, Hinshaw SP, Owens E, et al. A two-site randomized clinical trial of integrated psychosocial treatment for ADHD-inattentive type. *J Consult Clin Psychol*. 2014;82(6):1115–1127

240. Charach A, Volpe T, Boydell KM, Gearing RE. A theoretical approach to medication adherence for children and youth with psychiatric disorders. *Harv Rev Psychiatry*. 2008;16(2):126–135

241. Foy JM, ed. *Mental Health Care of Children and Adolescents: A Guide for Primary Care Clinicians*. Itasca, IL: American Academy of Pediatrics; 2018

242. Chan E. Complementary and alternative medicine in developmental-behavioral pediatrics. In: Wolraich ML, Drotar DD, Dworkin PH, Perrin EC, eds. *Developmental-Behavioral Pediatrics: Evidence and Practice*. Philadelphia, PA: Mosby Elsevier; 2008:259–280

243. Chan E. The role of complementary and alternative medicine in attention-deficit hyperactivity disorder. *J Dev Behav Pediatr*. 2002;23(suppl 1):S37–S45

244. James S, Stevenson SW, Silove N, Williams K. Chelation for autism spectrum disorder (ASD). *Cochrane Database Syst Rev*. 2015;(5):CD010766

245. Foy JM, ed. Office and network systems to support mental health care. In: *Mental Health Care of Children and Adolescents: A Guide for Primary Care Clinicians*. Itasca, IL: American Academy of Pediatrics; 2018:73–126

246. kidsdata.org. *Children With Special Health Care Needs, by Condition (California & U.S. Only)*. Palo Alto, CA: Lucille Packard Foundation for Children's Health; 2010. Available at: https://www.kidsdata.org/topic/486/special-needs-condition/table#fmt=640&loc=1,2&tf=74&ch=152,1039,854,154,845,1040,1041,858,157,158,1042,1043,160,161,861,1044,1045,1046,165,166. Accessed September 8, 2019

247. Danielson ML, Visser SN, Gleason MM, Peacock G, Claussen AH, Blumberg SJ. A national profile of attention-deficit hyperactivity disorder diagnosis and treatment among US children aged 2 to 5 years. *J Dev Behav Pediatr*. 2017;38(7):455–464

248. American Academy of Pediatrics. Mental health initiatives: residency curriculum. Available at: https://www.aap.org/en-us/advocacy-and-policy/aap-health-initiatives/Mental-Health/Pages/Residency-Curriculum.aspx. Accessed September 8, 2019

249. American Academy of Child & Adolescent Psychiatry. *Workforce Issues*. Washington, DC: American Academy of Child & Adolescent Psychiatry; 2016. Available at: https://www.aacap.org/aacap/Resources_for_Primary_Care/Workforce_Issues.aspx. Accessed September 8, 2019

250. Thomas CR, Holzer CE III. The continuing shortage of child and adolescent psychiatrists. *J Am Acad Child Adolesc Psychiatry.* 2006;45(9): 1023–1031

251. Rohlfing J, Navarro R, Maniya OZ, Hughes BD, Rogalsky DK. Medical student debt and major life choices other than specialty. *Med Educ Online.* 2014;19:25603

252. Centers for Disease Control and Prevention. *ADHD: Behavioral Health Services – Where They Are and Who Provides Them.* Atlanta, GA: Centers for Disease Control and Prevention; 2018. Available at: https://www.cdc.gov/ncbddd/adhd/stateprofiles-providers/index.html. Accessed September 8, 2019

253. Massachusetts Child Psychiatry Access Program. MCPAP: connecting primary care with child psychiatry. Available at: https://www.mcpap.com. Accessed September 8, 2019

254. Project Training and Education for the Advancement of Children's Health. Project TEACH (Training and Education for the Advancement of Children's Health). 2018. Available at: https://projectteachny.org/. Accessed September 8, 2019

255. Project Extension for Community Healthcare Outcomes. About ECHO. Available at: https://echo.unm.edu/about-echo/. Accessed September 8, 2019

256. Health Resources and Services Administration, Maternal and Child Health Bureau. Pediatric mental health care access program. Available at: https://mchb.hrsa.gov/training/projects.asp?program=34. Accessed July 2, 2019

257. National Network of Child Psychiatry Access Programs. Integrating mental and behavioral health care for every child. Available at: https://nncpap.org/. Accessed July 2, 2019

258. Horwitz SM, Storfer-Isser A, Kerker BD, et al. Barriers to the identification and management of psychosocial problems: changes from 2004 to 2013. *Acad Pediatr.* 2015;15(6):613–620

259. American Academy of Child and Adolescent Psychiatry Committee on Health Care Access and Economics Task Force on Mental Health. Improving mental health services in primary care: reducing administrative and financial barriers to access and collaboration [published correction appears in *Pediatrics. 2009;123(6):1611].* *Pediatrics.* 2009;123(4):1248–1251

260. Centers for Medicare and Medicaid Services. *Accountable Care Organizations (ACOs).* Baltimore, MD: Centers for Medicare and Medicaid Services; 2018. Available at: https://www.cms.gov/Medicare/Medicare-Fee-for-Service-Payment/ACO/. Accessed September 8, 2019

261. Fallu A, Dabouz F, Furtado M, Anand L, Katzman MA. A randomized, double-blind, cross-over, phase IV trial of oros-methylphenidate (CONCERTA(®)) and generic novo-methylphenidate ER-C (NOVO-generic). *Ther Adv Psychopharmacol.* 2016;6(4):237–251

262. Hagan JF, Shaw JS, Duncan PM, eds. *Bright Futures Guidelines for Health Supervision of Infants, Children, and Adolescents.* 4th ed. Elk Grove Village, IL: American Academy of Pediatrics; 2017

263. Foy JM, Kelleher KJ, Laraque D; American Academy of Pediatrics Task Force on Mental Health. Enhancing pediatric mental health care: strategies for preparing a primary care practice.*Pediatrics.* 2010;125(suppl 3): S87–S108

264. Allan C, Chacko A. Adverse events in behavioral parent training for children with ADHD: an under-appreciated phenomenon. *ADHD Rep.* 2018;26(1):4–9

265. US Department of Health and Human Services. Health information privacy. Available at: https://www.hhs.gov/hipaa/index.html. Accessed September 8, 2019

266. US Department of Education. *Family Educational Rights and Privacy Act (FERPA).* Washington, DC: Department of Education; 2018. Available at: https://www2.ed.gov/policy/gen/guid/fpco/ferpa/index.html. Accessed September 8, 2019

267. Epstein JN, Langberg JM, Lichtenstein PK, Kolb R, Altaye M, Simon JO. Use of an Internet portal to improve community-based pediatric ADHD care: a cluster randomized trial. *Pediatrics.* 2011;128(5). Available at: www.pediatrics.org/cgi/content/full/128/5/e1201

268. Centers for Medicare and Medicaid Services. *Electronic Health Records.* Baltimore, MD: Centers for Medicare and Medicaid Services; 2012. Available at: https://www.cms.gov/Medicare/E-Health/EHealthRecords/index.html. Accessed September 8, 2019

269. Ohno-Machado L. Electronic health record systems: risks and benefits. *J Am Med Inform Assoc.* 2014;21(e1):e1

270. Koppel R, Lehmann CU. Implications of an emerging EHR monoculture for hospitals and healthcare systems. *J Am Med Inform Assoc.* 2015;22(2):465–471

271. Babbott S, Manwell LB, Brown R, et al. Electronic medical records and physician stress in primary care: results from the MEMO Study. *J Am Med Inform Assoc.* 2014;21(e1):e100–e106

272. Burke BL Jr, Hall RW; Section on Telehealth Care. Telemedicine: pediatric applications. *Pediatrics.* 2015;136(1). Available at: www.pediatrics.org/cgi/content/full/136/1/e293

273. Marcin JP, Rimsza ME, Moskowitz WB; Committee on Pediatric Workforce. The use of telemedicine to address access and physician workforce shortages. *Pediatrics.* 2015;136(1): 202–209

274. Sibley MH, Comer JS, Gonzalez J. Delivering parent-teen therapy for ADHD through videoconferencing: a preliminary investigation. *J Psychopathol Behav Assess.* 2017; 39(3):467–485

275. Comer JS, Furr JM, Miguel EM, et al. Remotely delivering real-time parent training to the home: an initial randomized trial of Internet-delivered parent-child interaction therapy (I-PCIT). *J Consult Clin Psychol.* 2017;85(9): 909–917

276. American Academy of Child and Adolescent Psychiatry; American Academy of Pediatrics. HIPAA privacy rule and provider to provider communication. Available at: https://www.aap.org/en-us/advocacy-and-policy/aap-health-initiatives/Mental-Health/Pages/HIPAA-Privacy-Rule-and-Provider-to-Provider-Communication.aspx. Accessed September 8, 2019

277. Kolko DJ, Campo J, Kilbourne AM, Hart J, Sakolsky D, Wisniewski S. Collaborative care outcomes for

pediatric behavioral health problems: a cluster randomized trial. *Pediatrics*. 2014;133(4). Available at: www.pediatrics.org/cgi/content/full/133/4/e981

278. Pordes E, Gordon J, Sanders LM, Cohen E. Models of care delivery for children with medical complexity.

Pediatrics. 2018;141(suppl 3): S212–S223

279. Silverstein M, Hironaka LK, Walter HJ, et al. Collaborative care for children with ADHD symptoms: a randomized comparative effectiveness trial. *Pediatrics*. 2015;135(4). Available at:

www.pediatrics.org/cgi/content/full/135/4/e858

280. Liddle M, Birkett K, Bonjour A, Risma K. A collaborative approach to improving health care for children with developmental disabilities. *Pediatrics*. 2018;142(6):e20181136

SECTION 2
Adversity and Toxic Stress

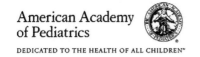

American Academy of Pediatrics
DEDICATED TO THE HEALTH OF ALL CHILDREN™

Organizational Principles to Guide and Define the Child
Health Care System and/or Improve the Health of all Children

POLICY STATEMENT

Early Childhood Adversity, Toxic Stress, and the Role of the Pediatrician: Translating Developmental Science Into Lifelong Health

abstract

Advances in a wide range of biological, behavioral, and social sciences are expanding our understanding of how early environmental influences (the ecology) and genetic predispositions (the biologic program) affect learning capacities, adaptive behaviors, lifelong physical and mental health, and adult productivity. A supporting technical report from the American Academy of Pediatrics (AAP) presents an integrated ecobiodevelopmental framework to assist in translating these dramatic advances in developmental science into improved health across the life span. Pediatricians are now armed with new information about the adverse effects of toxic stress on brain development, as well as a deeper understanding of the early life origins of many adult diseases. As trusted authorities in child health and development, pediatric providers must now complement the early identification of developmental concerns with a greater focus on those interventions and community investments that reduce external threats to healthy brain growth. To this end, AAP endorses a developing leadership role for the entire pediatric community—one that mobilizes the scientific expertise of both basic and clinical researchers, the family-centered care of the pediatric medical home, and the public influence of AAP and its state chapters—to catalyze fundamental change in early childhood policy and services. AAP is committed to leveraging science to inform the development of innovative strategies to reduce the precipitants of toxic stress in young children and to mitigate their negative effects on the course of development and health across the life span. *Pediatrics* 2012;129:e224–e231

INTRODUCTION

"It is easier to build strong children than to repair broken men."

Frederick Douglass (1817–1895)

From the time of its inception as a recognized specialty of medicine, the field of pediatrics has attached great significance to both the process of child development and the social/environmental context in which it unfolds. When the American Academy of Pediatrics (AAP) was founded in 1930, the acute health care needs of children were largely infectious in nature.[1] Over the ensuing 80 years, as increasingly effective vaccines, hygiene, and other public health initiatives produced dramatic gains, astute observers began to note that many noninfectious disease entities, such as developmental, behavioral, educational, and

COMMITTEE ON PSYCHOSOCIAL ASPECTS OF CHILD AND FAMILY HEALTH, COMMITTEE ON EARLY CHILDHOOD, ADOPTION, AND DEPENDENT CARE, AND SECTION ON DEVELOPMENTAL AND BEHAVIORAL PEDIATRICS

KEY WORDS
advocacy, brain development, ecobiodevelopmental framework, family pediatrics, health promotion, human capital investments, new morbidity, toxic stress, resilience

ABBREVIATIONS
AAP—American Academy of Pediatrics
EBD—ecobiodevelopmental

www.pediatrics.org/cgi/doi/10.1542/peds.2011-2662

doi:10.1542/peds.2011-2662

PEDIATRICS (ISSN Numbers: Print, 0031-4005; Online, 1098-4275).

family difficulties, were playing increasingly prominent roles in affecting child health and well-being.

In 1975, the term "new morbidity" was introduced to describe those non-infectious entities that appeared to be most prevalent.[2] This important conceptualization underscored a growing realization that significant societal changes (eg, increasing numbers of single parents and families with 2 working parents) were challenging pediatric health care providers to address complex concerns that were not strictly medical in nature. Although the impact of these "new" morbidities on pediatrics, public health, and society in general is no longer in question,[3–5] the professional training and practice of pediatricians continues to focus primarily on the acute medical needs of individual children. The pressing question now confronting contemporary pediatrics is how we can have a greater impact on improving the life prospects of children and families who face these increasingly complex and persistent threats to healthy development.

The need for creative, new strategies to confront these morbidities in a more effective way is essential to improve the physical and mental health of children, as well as the social and economic well-being of the nation.[6] Developmental, behavioral, educational, and family problems in childhood can have both lifelong and intergenerational effects.[7–18] Identifying and addressing these concerns early in life are essential for a healthier population and a more productive workforce.[5,6,19–21] Because the early roots or distal precipitants of problems in both learning and health typically lie beyond the walls of the medical office or hospital setting, the boundaries of pediatric concern must move beyond the acute medical care of children and expand into the larger ecology of the community, state, and society. Because this call for a broader, contextual approach to health is not new,[22] and the track record of matching rhetoric with effective action is limited, there is a compelling need for bold, new thinking to translate advances in developmental science into more effective interventions.

THE MERITS OF AN ECOBIODEVELOPMENTAL FRAMEWORK

The accompanying technical report[23] presents an ecobiodevelopmental (EBD) framework for understanding the promotion of health and prevention of disease across the life span that builds on advances in neuroscience, molecular biology, genomics, and the social sciences. Together, these diverse fields provide a remarkably convergent perspective on the inextricable interactions among the personal experiences (eg, family and social relationships), environmental influences (eg, exposures to toxic chemicals and inappropriate electronic media), and genetic predispositions that affect learning, behavior, and health across the life span. Applying this EBD framework to the challenges posed by significant childhood adversity reveals the powerful role that toxic stress can play in disrupting the architecture of the developing brain, thereby influencing behavioral, educational, economic, and health outcomes decades and generations later.[24] In contrast to positive or tolerable stress, toxic stress is defined as the excessive or prolonged activation of the physiologic stress response systems in the absence of the buffering protection afforded by stable, responsive relationships.[25] Within the ongoing interplay among assets for health and risks for illness, toxic stress early in life plays a critical role by disrupting brain circuitry and other important regulatory systems in ways that continue to influence physiology, behavior, and health decades later.[23] In short, an EBD approach to childhood adversity suggests that (1) early experiences with significant stress are critical, because they can undermine the development of those adaptive capacities and coping skills needed to deal with later challenges; (2) the roots of unhealthy lifestyles, maladaptive coping patterns, and fragmented social networks are often found in behavioral and physiologic responses to significant adversity that emerge in early childhood; and (3) the prevention of long-term, adverse consequences is best achieved by the buffering protection afforded by stable, responsive relationships that help children develop a sense of safety, thereby facilitating the restoration of their stress response systems to baseline.[25] An EBD approach recognizes that it is not adversity alone that predicts poor outcomes. It is the absence or insufficiency of protective relationships that reinforce healthy adaptations to stress, which, in the presence of significant adversity, leads to disruptive physiologic responses (ie, toxic stress) that produce "biological memories"[26] that increase the risk of health-threatening behaviors and frank disease later in life. The recent AAP technical report[23] summarizes the growing evidence base that links childhood toxic stress to the subsequent development of unhealthy lifestyles (eg, substance abuse, poor eating and exercise habits), persistent socioeconomic inequalities (eg, school failure and financial hardship), and poor health (eg, diabetes and cardiovascular disease). Given the extent to which costly health disparities in adults are rooted in these same unhealthy lifestyles and persistent inequalities,[5,9] the reduction of toxic stress in young children ought to be a high priority for medicine as a whole and for pediatrics in particular.

AN IMPORTANT ROLE FOR THE PEDIATRIC MEDICAL HOME

The effective reduction of toxic stress in young children could be advanced considerably by a broad-based, multisector commitment in which the profession of pediatrics plays an important role in designing, implementing, evaluating, refining, and advocating for a new generation of protective interventions. Pediatric providers are uniquely qualified and placed to assist in translating recent advances in developmental science into effective interventions for the home, the clinic, and the community. In addition to regular interactions with young children and an appreciation for the important role that families[27–29] and communities[30] play in determining child well-being, pediatricians bring several time-honored perspectives to this challenging task. These perspectives include a developmental approach to health, an understanding of the advantages of prevention over remediation, and an awareness of the critical importance of effective advocacy to promote changes in well-established systems that influence child health and development, even when those systems lie outside the traditional realm of pediatric practice.[31] In this context, it is essential that innovative and practical strategies continue to be developed that strengthen the capacity of the medical home to reduce sources of toxic stress and to mitigate their impact on the lives of young children. Rather than continuing the current trend of "doing more with less," as pediatricians take on a wide range of additional responsibilities, payment reforms should reflect the value of pediatricians' time and knowledge,

as well as the importance of a pediatrician-led medical home serving as a focal point for the reduction of toxic stress and for the support of child and family resiliency. This additional work and the reprioritization of efforts should reflect pediatricians' interest in preventive care that is more developmentally relevant,[32] parents' desire for a greater emphasis on their child's emerging skills and behavior,[33] the commitment to team-based services within the pediatric medical home,[28] and the growing evidence base that early developmental interventions can have significant effects on life-course trajectories.[34]

As the most logical candidate for a universal platform to promote healthy development and optimal life course trajectories, the pediatric medical home has become the focus of both increasing expectations and formidable challenges. High expectations are grounded in the public's deep respect for pediatricians as trusted guardians of child health. Compelling challenges include (1) the need for more extensive training for all health professionals on the adverse effects of excessive stress on the developing brain, as well as on the cardiovascular, immune, and metabolic regulatory systems (the technical report[23] is a start); (2) the significant constraints on existing, office-based approaches to fully address the new morbidities effectively; (3) the relatively limited availability of evidence-based strategies, within the medical home and across the full array of existing early childhood service systems, that have been shown to reduce sources of toxic stress in the lives of young children or mitigate their adverse consequences[35]; and (4) the financial difficulties associated with the incorporation of evidence-based developmental strategies into the pediatric medical home.

A Critical Assessment of Prevention at the Practice Level

From immunizations to seat belts to parenting education, the field of pediatrics has always embraced the centrality of prevention. That said, some degree of childhood adversity is inevitable, and dealing with manageable levels of stress is an important part of healthy development. Because the essence of toxic stress is the absence of buffers needed to return the physiologic stress response to baseline, the primary prevention of its adverse consequences includes those aspects of routine anticipatory guidance that strengthen a family's social supports, encourage a parent's adoption of positive parenting techniques, and facilitate a child's emerging social, emotional, and language skills. Examples include the promotion of the 7Cs of resilience (competence, confidence, connectedness, character, contribution, coping, and control),[36] optimism,[37] Reach Out and Read,[38–40] emotional coaching,[41–44] and numerous positive parenting programs (eg, Triple P,[45–47] Incredible Years,[48] Home visiting,[49,50] and Nurturing Parenting[51,52]). Although AAP resources, such as *Bright Futures*,[53] *Connected Kids*,[54] and the clinical report "The Pediatrician's Role in Child Maltreatment Prevention,"[55] already provide significant recommendations in this area, implementing a comprehensive, yet practical program of effective anticipatory guidance that nurtures the child's emerging social, emotional, and language skills and promotes positive parenting remains an ongoing challenge.

Beyond working to improve the impact of anticipatory guidance provided in the medical home, some motivated pediatric providers also advocate for a variety of community-based interventions that are implemented in homes,[56,57] preschools,[58] and schools,[59–61] as well as through an extended array of programs organized by faith-based organizations, social groups, and recreational centers. A more thorough description of the full range of practices designed to strengthen parenting skills and enhance child development can be found elsewhere.[35,62–64] Although most primary prevention programs have not been evaluated systematically, those that show promise should be assessed and, if found to be effective, replicated and taken to scale. As the number of evidence-based services increases, the pediatric community needs to continue to advocate for systemic changes in reimbursement strategies that incentivize collaboration among pediatric medical homes and the full range of effective community-based resources.[65]

Screening for Children and Families at Risk

Identifying children at high risk for toxic stress is the first step in providing targeted support for their parents and other caregivers. The challenges of developing secondary prevention strategies within the medical home begin with the implementation of practice-relevant screening and proceed through the complexities of diagnostic evaluations, sharing information, formulating joint action plans with parents, locating needed services beyond the medical home, arranging successful referrals, and conducting an ongoing monitoring and assessment of intervention impacts. That said, after several decades of prescriptive guidelines and outcome evaluations of a broad array of prevention strategies, the cumulative evidence of effectiveness is mixed. Some primary care practices have been successful in regularizing the identification and management of new morbidities within their daily routines.

Many continue to struggle with the basics of developmental screening, routine referral, and ongoing collaboration with community-based programs outside the medical system.[32] All confront the limited availability of accessible and affordable preventive supports for children and families experiencing significant adversity.

Within this highly variable and multidimensional context, the AAP and others have encouraged pediatric providers to develop a screening schedule that uses age-appropriate, standardized tools to identify risk factors that are highly prevalent or relevant to their particular practice setting.[29,66,67] In addition to the currently recommended screenings at 9, 18, and 24/36 months to assess children for developmental delays, pediatric practices have been asked to consider implementing standardized measures to identify other family- or community-level factors that put children at risk for toxic stress (eg, maternal depression, parental substance abuse, domestic or community violence, food scarcity, poor social connectedness). Pediatric providers have been encouraged to use *Current Procedural Terminology* code 99420 when they are assessing a child's risk and, if additional visits are needed to address any identified concerns, providers are encouraged to bill for that additional time by using codes 99401-4.[68] Continued advocacy at the national and state levels is needed, however, to ensure proper payment for the time needed for universal screening, problem identification, and ongoing assessments. More specific recommendations (regarding which screening tools should be used, when they should be administered, and how to secure reimbursement for their use) will be presented in a forthcoming AAP policy statement on social-emotional screening.

Collaborating With the Community

Routine screening for increased vulnerability is useful only if collaborative relationships exist with local services to address the identified concerns (as outlined in several previous reports[69–71]); moreover, it is also essential that those services demonstrate evidence of effectiveness. This is particularly important for the identification of young children experiencing toxic stress, given the limited proportion of community-based interventions for which significant, positive impacts have been documented in this domain, and the relatively modest magnitude of impact found for those that have been shown to be effective.

Rethinking Advocacy Beyond the Office Setting

Because so many of the origins and consequences of childhood toxic stress lie beyond the boundaries of the clinical setting, pediatric providers are often called on to work collaboratively with parents, social workers, teachers, coaches, civic leaders, policy makers, and other invested stakeholders to influence services that fall outside the traditional realm of clinical practice.[72] In many cases, these efforts extend even further afield, moving into the realm of ecologically based, public health initiatives that address the precipitants of toxic stress at the community, state, and national levels. Translating advances in developmental science into effective interventions and lifelong health will require a fundamental shift in the way the general public and policy makers view and invest in early childhood. Pediatric providers are integral to this effort, as they have a long history of advocating for systemic changes to advance child health and development.[31]

Examples of preventive interventions that could serve as targets for pediatrician-led advocacy campaigns include (1) education efforts focused on parents, foster parents, child care providers, and preschool teachers to increase awareness of the adverse consequences of toxic stress in early childhood for lifelong outcomes in learning, behavior, and health; (2) calls for investments in the development of creative, new strategies that can be incorporated into home-, school-, and center-based services to reduce sources of toxic stress and to strengthen the relationships that buffer children from the long-term consequences of significant adversity; (3) investments in community-based mentoring activities (eg, after-school programs, Big Brother/Big Sister, Little League, gymnastics, martial arts programs) that provide supportive relationships for vulnerable children that help them learn to cope with adversity in an adaptive manner; (4) investments in selected early-intervention programs, early-childhood mental health services, specialized family therapies, and medicolegal partnerships that have demonstrated evidence of positive impacts on vulnerable young children and families; (5) professional development programs that educate judges and other key participants in the juvenile court and foster care systems about the biology of adversity and its implications for case management, child custody, and foster care of children who have been abused or neglected; and (6) collaborative efforts with social workers, mental health providers, and other related professionals to address urgent needs as early as possible and to integrate effective services for the most vulnerable children and their families.

Treatment of Toxic Stress

Finally, the pediatric community must provide strong, proactive advocacy for more effective interventions for children with symptomatic evidence of toxic stress. These could include (1) the formation and/or continuous strengthening of local traumatic stress networks to treat children and families experiencing significant adversity; and (2) increasing the number of accessible, affordable, and culturally competent mental health professionals who are qualified to provide evidence-based treatments, such as trauma-based cognitive behavioral therapy and parent-child interaction therapy. In addition to the paucity of appropriately trained professionals in this area of significant unmet need, inadequate or inappropriate reimbursement mechanisms often block access to services for the most vulnerable young children. In such circumstances, pediatricians can be powerful advocates for expanded insurance coverage for childhood mental health services, even when they do not provide those services themselves.[73]

REAFFIRMING A COMMITMENT TO LEAD

This Policy Statement builds on numerous previous statements, including those regarding the new morbidities,[3] community pediatrics,[30] family-centered care,[27] home visitation,[49] and the prevention of child abuse.[55] The proposed EBD framework (1) incorporates growing evidence of the impact of toxic stress on the developing brain, (2) informs a deeper understanding of the early life origins of both educational failure and adult disease, and (3) underscores the need for collaborative efforts to prevent the long-term consequences of early adversity. The AAP is committed to leading an invigorated, science-based effort at transforming the way our society invests in the development of all children, particularly those who face significant adversity.[74]

RECOMMENDATIONS

1. All health care professionals should adopt the proposed EBD framework as a means of understanding the social, behavioral, and economic determinants of lifelong disparities in physical and mental health (see technical report[23]). Psychosocial problems and the new morbidities should no longer be viewed as categorically different from the causes and consequences of other biologically based health impairments.

2. The growing scientific knowledge base that links childhood toxic stress with disruptions of the developing nervous, cardiovascular, immune, and metabolic systems, and the evidence that these disruptions can lead to lifelong impairments in learning, behavior, and both physical and mental health, should be fully incorporated into the training of all current and future physicians (see technical report[23]).

3. Pediatricians should adopt a more proactive leadership role in educating parents, child care providers, teachers, policy makers, civic leaders, and the general public about the long-term consequences of toxic stress and the potential benefits of preventing or reducing sources of significant adversity in early childhood. Protecting young children from adversity is a promising, science-based strategy to address many of the most persistent and costly problems facing contemporary society, including limited educational achievement, diminished economic productivity, criminality, and disparities in health.

4. Pediatricians should be vocal advocates for the development and implementation of new, evidence-based interventions (regardless of the provider or venue) that reduce sources of toxic stress and/or

mitigate their adverse effects on young children, as they are likely to produce better outcomes and potentially be more cost-effective than trying to treat or remediate the numerous consequences of excessive childhood stress that reach far into adulthood. Such advocacy is particularly important when budget constraints force critical reassessments of public spending priorities.

5. Pediatric medical homes should (1) strengthen their provision of anticipatory guidance to support children's emerging social-emotional-linguistic skills and to encourage the adoption of positive parenting techniques; (2) actively screen for precipitants of toxic stress that are common in their particular practices; (3) develop, help secure funding, and participate in innovative service-delivery adaptations that expand the ability of the medical home to support children at risk; and (4) identify (or advocate for the development of) local resources that address those risks for toxic stress that are prevalent in their communities.

LEAD AUTHORS

Andrew S. Garner, MD, PhD
Jack P. Shonkoff, MD

COMMITTEE ON PSYCHOSOCIAL ASPECTS OF CHILD AND FAMILY HEALTH, 2010–2011

Benjamin S. Siegel, MD, Chairperson
Mary I. Dobbins, MD
Marian F. Earls, MD
Andrew S. Garner, MD, PhD
Laura McGuinn, MD
John Pascoe, MD, MPH
David L. Wood, MD

LIAISONS

Robert T. Brown, PhD
Society of Pediatric Psychology
Terry Carmichael, MSW
National Association of Social Workers
Mary Jo Kupst, PhD
Society of Pediatric Psychology
D. Richard Martini, MD
American Academy of Child and Adolescent Psychiatry
Mary Sheppard, MS, RN, PNP, BC
National Association of Pediatric Nurse Practitioners

CONSULTANT

George J. Cohen, MD

CONSULTANT AND CONTRIBUTING AUTHOR

Jack P. Shonkoff, MD

Center on the Developing Child at Harvard University

STAFF

Karen S. Smith

COMMITTEE ON EARLY CHILDHOOD, ADOPTION, AND DEPENDENT CARE, 2010–2011

Pamela C. High, MD, Chairperson
Elaine Donoghue, MD
Jill J. Fussell, MD
Mary Margaret Gleason, MD
Paula K. Jaudes, MD
Veronnie F. Jones, MD
David M. Rubin, MD
Elaine E. Schulte, MD, MPH

STAFF

Mary Crane, PhD, LSW

SECTION ON DEVELOPMENTAL AND BEHAVIORAL PEDIATRICS EXECUTIVE COMMITTEE, 2010–2011

Michelle M. Macias, MD, Chairperson
Carolyn Bridgemohan, MD
Jill Fussell, MD
Edward Goldson, MD
Laura J. McGuinn, MD
Carol Weitzman, MD
Lynn Mowbray Wegner, MD, Immediate Past Chairperson

STAFF

Linda B. Paul, MPH

REFERENCES

1. Baker JP, Pearson HA. *Dedicated to the Health of All Children.* Elk Grove Village, IL: The American Academy of Pediatrics; 2005

2. Haggerty RJ, Roghman RK, Pless IB. *Child Health and the Community.* New York, NY: John Wiley and Sons; 1975

3. Committee on Psychosocial Aspects of Child and Family Health. American Academy of Pediatrics. The new morbidity revisited: a renewed commitment to the psychosocial aspects of pediatric care. *Pediatrics.* 2001; 108(5):1227–1230

4. Dreyer BP. Mental health and child developmental problems: the "not-so-new morbidity". *Acad Pediatr.* 2009;9(4):206–208

5. Shonkoff JP, Boyce WT, McEwen BS. Neuroscience, molecular biology, and the childhood roots of health disparities: building a new framework for health promotion and

disease prevention. *JAMA.* 2009;301(21): 2252–2259

6. Knudsen EI, Heckman JJ, Cameron JL, Shonkoff JP. Economic, neurobiological, and behavioral perspectives on building America's future workforce. *Proc Natl Acad Sci U S A.* 2006;103(27):10155–10162

7. Anda RF, Dong M, Brown DW, et al. The relationship of adverse childhood experiences to a history of premature death of family members. *BMC Public Health.* 2009;9:106

8. Anda RF, Felitti VJ, Bremner JD, et al. The enduring effects of abuse and related adverse experiences in childhood. A convergence of evidence from neurobiology and epidemiology. *Eur Arch Psychiatry Clin Neurosci.* 2006;256(3):174–186

9. Braveman P, Barclay C. Health disparities beginning in childhood: a life-course

perspective. *Pediatrics.* 2009;124(Suppl 3): S163–S175

10. Chapman DP, Whitfield CL, Felitti VJ, Dube SR, Edwards VJ, Anda RF. Adverse childhood experiences and the risk of depressive disorders in adulthood. *J Affect Disord.* 2004;82 (2):217–225

11. Costello EJ, Compton SN, Keeler G, Angold A. Relationships between poverty and psychopathology: a natural experiment. *JAMA.* 2003;290(15):2023–2029

12. Danese A, Pariante CM, Caspi A, Taylor A, Poulton R. Childhood maltreatment predicts adult inflammation in a life-course study. *Proc Natl Acad Sci U S A.* 2007;104 (4):1319–1324

13. Dietz PM, Spitz AM, Anda RF, et al. Unintended pregnancy among adult women exposed to abuse or household dysfunction

during their childhood. *JAMA.* 1999;282(14): 1359–1364

14. Dong M, Giles WH, Felitti VJ, et al. Insights into causal pathways for ischemic heart disease: adverse childhood experiences study. *Circulation.* 2004;110(13):1761–1766

15. Dube SR, Anda RF, Felitti VJ, Chapman DP, Williamson DF, Giles WH. Childhood abuse, household dysfunction, and the risk of attempted suicide throughout the life span: findings from the Adverse Childhood Experiences Study. *JAMA.* 2001;286(24):3089–3096

16. Felitti VJ, Anda RF, Nordenberg D, et al. Relationship of childhood abuse and household dysfunction to many of the leading causes of death in adults. The Adverse Childhood Experiences (ACE) Study. *Am J Prev Med.* 1998;14(4):245–258

17. Kahn RS, Brandt D, Whitaker RC. Combined effect of mothers' and fathers' mental health symptoms on children's behavioral and emotional well-being. *Arch Pediatr Adolesc Med.* 2004;158(8):721–729

18. Wickrama KA, Conger RD, Lorenz FO, Jung T. Family antecedents and consequences of trajectories of depressive symptoms from adolescence to young adulthood: a life course investigation. *J Health Soc Behav.* 2008;49(4):468–483

19. Doyle O, Harmon CP, Heckman JJ, Tremblay RE. Investing in early human development: timing and economic efficiency. *Econ Hum Biol.* 2009;7(1):1–6

20. Heckman JJ. The economics, technology, and neuroscience of human capability formation. *Proc Natl Acad Sci U S A.* 2007;104 (33):13250–13255

21. Center on the Developing Child at Harvard University. *The Foundations of Lifelong Health are Built in Early Childhood.* Cambridge, MA: Center on the Developing Child at Harvard University; 2010. Available at www.developingchild.harvard.edu. Accessed March 8, 2011

22. Green M, Kessel SS. Diagnosing and treating health: bright futures. *Pediatrics.* 1993; 91(5):998–1000

23. Shonkoff JP, Garner AA and the American Academy of Pediatrics Committee on Psychosocial Aspects of Child and Family Health. Toxic stress, brain development, and the early childhood foundations of lifelong health. *Pediatrics.* 2011, In press

24. Shonkoff JP. Building a new biodevelopmental framework to guide the future of early childhood policy. *Child Dev.* 2010;81(1):357–367

25. National Scientific Council on the Developing Child. *Excessive Stress Disrupts the Architecture of the Developing Brain: Working Paper #3.* Cambridge, MA: National Scientific Council on the Developing Child, Center on the Developing Child at Harvard University; 2005. Available at www.developingchild.harvard.edu. Accessed March 8, 2011

26. National Scientific Council on the Developing Child. *Early experiences can alter gene expression and affect long-term development: Working Paper #10.* Cambridge, MA: National Scientific Council on the Developing Child, Center on the Developing Child at Harvard University; 2005. Available at www.developingchild.harvard.edu. Accessed March 8, 2011

27. Committee on Hospital Care. American Academy of Pediatrics. Family-centered care and the pediatrician's role. *Pediatrics.* 2003; 112(3 Pt 1):691–697

28. Rushton FE. *Family Support in Community Pediatrics: Confronting New Challenges.* Westport, CT: Praeger; 1998

29. Schor EL; American Academy of Pediatrics Task Force on the Family. Family pediatrics: report of the Task Force on the Family. *Pediatrics.* 2003;111(6 Pt 2):1541–1571

30. Rushton FE Jr; American Academy of Pediatrics Committee on Community Health Services. The pediatrician's role in community pediatrics. *Pediatrics.* 2005;115(4): 1092–1094

31. Palfrey J. *Child Health in America: Making a Difference Through Advocacy.* Baltimore, MD: Johns Hopkins University Press; 2006

32. Tanner JL, Stein MT, Olson LM, Frintner MP, Radecki L. Reflections on well-child care practice: a national study of pediatric clinicians. *Pediatrics.* 2009;124(3):849–857

33. Radecki L, Olson LM, Frintner MP, Tanner JL, Stein MT. What do families want from well-child care? Including parents in the rethinking discussion. *Pediatrics.* 2009;124 (3):858–865

34. Walker SP, Chang SM, Vera-Hernández M, Grantham-McGregor S. Early childhood stimulation benefits adult competence and reduces violent behavior. *Pediatrics.* 2011; 127(5):849–857

35. Regalado M, Halfon N. Primary care services promoting optimal child development from birth to age 3 years: review of the literature. *Arch Pediatr Adolesc Med.* 2001;155(12): 1311–1322

36. Ginsburg KR. *A Parent's Guide to Building Resilience in Children and Teens: Giving your child roots and wings.* Elk Grove Village, IL: The American Academy of Pediatrics; 2006

37. Seligman MEP, Reivich K, Jaycox L, Gillham J. *The Optimistic Child: A Proven Program To Safeguard Children Against Depression and Build Lifelong Resilience.* Boston, MA: Houghton Mifflin Co.; 2007

38. Berkule SB, Dreyer BP, Klass PE, Huberman HS, Yin HS, Mendelsohn AL. Mothers' expectations for shared reading after delivery: implications for reading activities at 6 months. *Ambul Pediatr.* 2008;8(3):169–174

39. Duursma E, Augustyn M, Zuckerman B. Reading aloud to children: the evidence. *Arch Dis Child.* 2008;93(7):554–557

40. Willis E, Kabler-Babbitt C, Zuckerman B. Early literacy interventions: reach out and read. *Pediatr Clin North Am.* 2007;54(3): 625–642, viii [viii.]

41. Gottman JM. *The Heart of Parenting: How to Raise an Emotionally Intelligent Child.* New York, NY: Simon and Schuster; 1997

42. Katz LF, Gottman JM. Buffering children from marital conflict and dissolution. *J Clin Child Psychol.* 1997;26(2):157–171

43. Katz LF, Hunter E, Klowden A. Intimate partner violence and children's reaction to peer provocation: the moderating role of emotion coaching. *J Fam Psychol.* 2008;22 (4):614–621

44. Katz LF, Windecker-Nelson B. Domestic violence, emotion coaching, and child adjustment. *J Fam Psychol.* 2006;20(1):56–67

45. de Graaf I, Speetjens P, Smit F, de Wolff M, Tavecchio L. Effectiveness of the Triple P Positive Parenting Program on behavioral problems in children: a meta-analysis. *Behav Modif.* 2008;32(5):714–735

46. Prinz RJ, Sanders MR, Shapiro CJ, Whitaker DJ, Lutzker JR. Population-based prevention of child maltreatment: the U.S. Triple p system population trial. *Prev Sci.* 2009;10 (1):1–12

47. Sanders MR, Markie-Dadds C, Tully LA, Bor W. The triple P-positive parenting program: a comparison of enhanced, standard, and self-directed behavioral family intervention for parents of children with early onset conduct problems. *J Consult Clin Psychol.* 2000;68(4):624–640

48. Webster-Stratton C, Mihalic SF. *The Incredible Years: Parent, Teacher and Child Training Series.* Boulder, CO: Center for the Study and Prevention of Violence, Institute of Behavioral Science, University of Colorado at Boulder; 2001

49. Council on Community Pediatrics. The role of preschool home-visiting programs in improving children's developmental and health outcomes. *Pediatrics.* 2009;123(2): 598–603

50. Kitzman HJ, Olds DL, Cole RE, et al. Enduring effects of prenatal and infancy home visiting by nurses on children: follow-up of a randomized trial among children at age

12 years. *Arch Pediatr Adolesc Med.* 2010; 164(5):412–418

51. Bavolek SJ. Nurturing Parenting Program. Asheville, NC and Park City, UT: Family Development Resources. Available at: www.nurturingparenting.com/npp/index.php. Accessed March8, 2011

52. Woods ER, Obeidallah-Davis D, Sherry MK, et al. The parenting project for teen mothers: the impact of a nurturing curriculum on adolescent parenting skills and life hassles. *Ambul Pediatr.* 2003;3(5):240–245

53. Hagan JF, Shaw JS, Duncan PM. *Bright Futures: Guidelines for Health Supervision of Infants, Children, and Adolescents.* 3rd ed. Elk Grove Village, IL: American Academy of Pediatrics; 2008

54. Committee on Injury, Violence, and Poison Prevention. Policy statement—Role of the pediatrician in youth violence prevention. *Pediatrics.* 2009;124(1):393–402

55. Flaherty EG, Stirling J Jr; American Academy of Pediatrics. Committee on Child Abuse and Neglect. Clinical report—the pediatrician's role in child maltreatment prevention. *Pediatrics.* 2010;126(4):833–841

56. Donelan-McCall N, Eckenrode J, Olds DL. Home visiting for the prevention of child maltreatment: lessons learned during the past 20 years. *Pediatr Clin North Am.* 2009; 56(2):389–403

57. Eckenrode J, Campa M, Luckey DW, et al. Long-term effects of prenatal and infancy nurse home visitation on the life course of youths: 19-year follow-up of a randomized trial. *Arch Pediatr Adolesc Med.* 2010;164 (1):9–15

58. Gordon M. Roots of empathy: responsive parenting, caring societies. *Keio J Med.* 2003;52(4):236–243

59. Illinois State Board of Education. Illinois Learning Standards: Social/Emotional Learning (SEL). Available at: www.isbe.state.il.us/ils/social_emotional/standards.htm. Accessed March 8, 2011

60. Payton J, Weissberg RP, Durlak JA, et al. *The Positive Impact of Social and Emotional Learning for Kindergarten to Eighth-Grade Students: Findings from Three Scientific Reviews.* Chicago, IL: Collaborative for Academic, Social and Emotional Learning; 2008. Available at: www.lpfch.org/sel/casel-fullreport.pdf. Accessed March 8, 2011

61. Durlak JA, Weissberg RP, Dymnicki AB, Taylor RD, Schellinger KB. The impact of enhancing students' social and emotional learning: a meta-analysis of school-based universal interventions. *Child Dev.* 2011;82(1):405–432

62. Isaacs J. *Impacts of Early Childhood Programs.* Washington, DC: First Focus and the Brookings Institution; 2008

63. Substance Abuse and Mental Health Services Administration. Promotion and Prevention in Mental Health; Strengthening Parenting and Enhancing Child Resilience. Rockville, MD: Department of Health and Human Services; 2007. DHHS Publication No. CMSH-SVP-0175

64. Center on the Developing Child at Harvard University. *A Science-based Framework for Early Childhood Policy: Using Evidence to Improve Outcomes in Learning, Behavior and Health for Vulnerable Children.* Cambridge, MA: Center on the Developing Child at Harvard University; 2007. Available at: www.developingchild.harvard.edu. Accessed March 8, 2011

65. American Academy of Pediatrics Council on Children with Disabilities. Care coordination in the medical home: integrating health and related systems of care for children with special health care needs. *Pediatrics.* 2005; 116(5):1238–1244

66. Council on Children With DisabilitiesSection on Developmental Behavioral Pediatrics-Bright Futures Steering CommitteeMedical Home Initiatives for Children With Special Needs Project Advisory Committee. Identifying infants and young children with developmental disorders in the medical home: an algorithm for developmental surveillance

and screening. *Pediatrics.* 2006;118(1):405–420

67. Garg A, Butz AM, Dworkin PH, Lewis RA, Thompson RE, Serwint JR. Improving the management of family psychosocial problems at low-income children's well-child care visits: the WE CARE Project. *Pediatrics.* 2007;120(3):547–558

68. Earls MF; Committee on Psychosocial Aspects of Child and Family Health American Academy of Pediatrics. Incorporating recognition and management of perinatal and postpartum depression into pediatric practice. *Pediatrics.* 2010;126(5):1032–1039

69. Committee on Psychosocial Aspects of Child and Family Health and Task Force on Mental Health. Policy statement—The future of pediatrics: mental health competencies for pediatric primary care. *Pediatrics.* 2009;124(1):410–421

70. Foy JM, Kelleher KJ, Laraque D; American Academy of Pediatrics Task Force on Mental Health. Enhancing pediatric mental health care: strategies for preparing a primary care practice. *Pediatrics.* 2010;125(Suppl 3): S87–S108

71. Foy JM, Perrin J; American Academy of Pediatrics Task Force on Mental Health. Enhancing pediatric mental health care: strategies for preparing a community. *Pediatrics.* 2010;125(Suppl 3):S75–S86

72. Ochoa ER, Jr, Nash C. Community engagement and its impact on child health disparities: building blocks, examples, and resources. *Pediatrics.* 2009;124(Suppl 3):S237–S245

73. American Academy of Child and Adolescent Psychiatry Committee on Health Care Access and Economics Task Force on Mental Health. Improving mental health services in primary care: reducing administrative and financial barriers to access and collaboration. *Pediatrics.* 2009;123(4):1248–1251

74. Shonkoff J. Protecting brains, not simply stimulating minds. *Science.* 2011;333(6045): 982–983

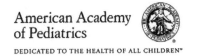

TECHNICAL REPORT

The Lifelong Effects of Early Childhood Adversity and Toxic Stress

abstract

Advances in fields of inquiry as diverse as neuroscience, molecular biology, genomics, developmental psychology, epidemiology, sociology, and economics are catalyzing an important paradigm shift in our understanding of health and disease across the lifespan. This converging, multidisciplinary science of human development has profound implications for our ability to enhance the life prospects of children and to strengthen the social and economic fabric of society. Drawing on these multiple streams of investigation, this report presents an ecobiodevelopmental framework that illustrates how early experiences and environmental influences can leave a lasting signature on the genetic predispositions that affect emerging brain architecture and long-term health. The report also examines extensive evidence of the disruptive impacts of toxic stress, offering intriguing insights into causal mechanisms that link early adversity to later impairments in learning, behavior, and both physical and mental well-being. The implications of this framework for the practice of medicine, in general, and pediatrics, specifically, are potentially transformational. They suggest that many adult diseases should be viewed as developmental disorders that begin early in life and that persistent health disparities associated with poverty, discrimination, or maltreatment could be reduced by the alleviation of toxic stress in childhood. An ecobiodevelopmental framework also underscores the need for new thinking about the focus and boundaries of pediatric practice. It calls for pediatricians to serve as both front-line guardians of healthy child development and strategically positioned, community leaders to inform new science-based strategies that build strong foundations for educational achievement, economic productivity, responsible citizenship, and lifelong health. *Pediatrics* 2012;129:e232–e246

INTRODUCTION

Of a good beginning cometh a good end.

John Heywood, *Proverbs* (1546)

The United States, like all nations of the world, is facing a number of social and economic challenges that must be met to secure a promising future. Central to this task is the need to produce a well-educated and healthy adult population that is sufficiently skilled to participate effectively in a global economy and to become responsible stakeholders in a productive society. As concerns continue to grow about the quality of public education and its capacity to prepare the nation's future workforce, increasing investments are being made in

Jack P. Shonkoff, MD, Andrew S. Garner, MD, PhD, and THE COMMITTEE ON PSYCHOSOCIAL ASPECTS OF CHILD AND FAMILY HEALTH, COMMITTEE ON EARLY CHILDHOOD, ADOPTION, AND DEPENDENT CARE, AND SECTION ON DEVELOPMENTAL AND BEHAVIORAL PEDIATRICS

KEY WORDS
ecobiodevelopmental framework, new morbidity, toxic stress, social inequalities, health disparities, health promotion, disease prevention, advocacy, brain development, human capital development, pediatric basic science

ABBREVIATIONS
ACE—adverse childhood experiences
CRH—corticotropin-releasing hormone
EBD—ecobiodevelopmental
PFC—prefrontal cortex

www.pediatrics.org/cgi/doi/10.1542/peds.2011-2663

doi:10.1542/peds.2011-2663

PEDIATRICS (ISSN Numbers: Print, 0031-4005; Online, 1098-4275).

the preschool years to promote the foundations of learning. Although debates about early childhood policy focus almost entirely on educational objectives, science indicates that sound investments in interventions that reduce adversity are also likely to strengthen the foundations of physical and mental health, which would generate even larger returns to all of society.[1,2] This growing scientific understanding about the common roots of health, learning, and behavior in the early years of life presents a potentially transformational opportunity for the future of pediatrics.

Identifying the origins of adult disease and addressing them early in life are critical steps toward changing our current health care system from a "sick-care" to a "well-care" model.[3–5] Although new discoveries in basic science, clinical subspecialties, and high-technology medical interventions continue to advance our capacity to treat patients who are ill, there is growing appreciation that a successful well-care system must expand its scope beyond the traditional realm of individualized, clinical practice to address the complex social, economic, cultural, environmental, and developmental influences that lead to population-based health disparities and unsustainable medical care expenditures.[2,6,7] The science of early childhood development has much to offer in the realization of this vision, and the well-being of young children and their families is emerging as a promising focus for creative investment.

The history of pediatrics conveys a rich narrative of empirical investigation and pragmatic problem solving. Its emergence as a specialized domain of clinical medicine in the late 19th century was dominated by concerns about nutrition, infectious disease, and premature death. In the middle of

the 20th century, as effective vaccines, antibiotics, hygiene, and other public health measures confronted the infectious etiologies of childhood illness, a variety of developmental, behavioral, and family difficulties became known as the "new morbidities."[8] By the end of the century, mood disorders, parental substance abuse, and exposure to violence, among other conditions, began to receive increasing attention in the pediatric clinical setting and became known as the "newer morbidities."[9] Most recently, increasingly complex mental health concerns; the adverse effects of television viewing; the influence of new technologies; epidemic increases in obesity; and persistent economic, racial, and ethnic disparities in health status have been called the "millennial morbidities."[10]

Advances in the biological, developmental, and social sciences now offer tools to write the next important chapter. The overlapping and synergistic characteristics of the most prevalent conditions and threats to child well-being—combined with the remarkable pace of new discoveries in developmental neuroscience, genomics, and the behavioral and social sciences—present an opportunity to confront a number of important questions with fresh information and a new perspective. What are the biological mechanisms that explain the well-documented association between childhood adversity and adult health impairment? As these causal mechanisms are better elucidated, what can the medical field, specifically, and society, more generally, do to reduce or mitigate the effects of disruptive early-life influences on the origins of lifelong disease? When is the optimal time for those interventions to be implemented?

This technical report addresses these important questions in 3 ways. First, it presents a scientifically grounded,

ecobiodevelopmental (EBD) framework to stimulate fresh thinking about the promotion of health and prevention of disease across the lifespan. Second, it applies this EBD framework to better understand the complex relationships among adverse childhood circumstances, toxic stress, brain architecture, and poor physical and mental health well into adulthood. Third, it proposes a new role for pediatricians to promote the development and implementation of science-based strategies to reduce toxic stress in early childhood as a means of preventing or reducing many of society's most complex and enduring problems, which are frequently associated with disparities in learning, behavior, and health. The magnitude of this latter challenge cannot be overstated. A recent technical report from the American Academy of Pediatrics reviewed 58 years of published studies and characterized racial and ethnic disparities in children's health to be extensive, pervasive, persistent, and, in some cases, worsening.[11] Moreover, the report found only 2 studies that evaluated interventions designed to reduce disparities in children's health status and health care that also compared the minority group to a white group, and none used a randomized controlled trial design.

The causal sequences of risk that contribute to demographic differences in educational achievement and physical well-being threaten our country's democratic ideals by undermining the national credo of equal opportunity. Unhealthy communities with too many fast food franchises and liquor stores, yet far too few fresh food outlets and opportunities for physical activity, contribute to an unhealthy population. Unemployment and forced mobility disrupt the social networks that stabilize communities and families and, thereby, lead to higher rates of violence and school dropout. The purpose of this technical report is to leverage new knowledge from the biological and social sciences to help achieve the positive life outcomes that could be accrued to all of society if more effective strategies were developed to reduce the exposure of young children to significant adversity.

A NEW FRAMEWORK FOR PROMOTING HEALTHY DEVELOPMENT

Advances in our understanding of the factors that either promote or undermine early human development have set the stage for a significant paradigm shift.[12] In simple terms, the process of development is now understood as a function of "nature dancing with nurture over time," in contrast to the longstanding but now outdated debate about the influence of "nature versus nurture."[13] That is to say, beginning prenatally, continuing through infancy, and extending into childhood and beyond, development is driven by an ongoing, inextricable interaction between biology (as defined by genetic predispositions) and ecology (as defined by the social and physical environment)[12,14,15] (see Fig 1).

Building on an ecological model that explains multiple levels of influence on psychological development,[16] and a recently proposed biodevelopmental framework that offers an integrated, science-based approach to coordinated, early childhood policy making and practice across sectors,[17] this technical report presents an EBD framework that draws on a recent report from the Center on the Developing Child at Harvard University to help physicians and policy makers think about how early childhood adversity can lead to lifelong impairments in learning, behavior, and both physical and mental health.[1,6]

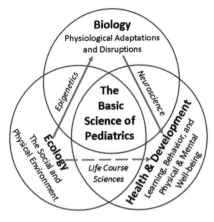

FIGURE 1

The basic science of pediatrics. An emerging, multidisciplinary science of development supports an EBD framework for understanding the evolution of human health and disease across the life span. In recent decades, epidemiology, developmental psychology, and longitudinal studies of early childhood interventions have demonstrated significant associations (hashed red arrow) between the ecology of childhood and a wide range of developmental outcomes and life course trajectories. Concurrently, advances in the biological sciences, particularly in developmental neuroscience and epigenetics, have made parallel progress in beginning to elucidate the biological mechanisms (solid arrows) underlying these important associations. The convergence of these diverse disciplines defines a promising new basic science of pediatrics.

Some of the most compelling new evidence for this proposed framework comes from the rapidly moving field of epigenetics, which investigates the molecular biological mechanisms (such as DNA methylation and histone acetylation) that affect gene expression without altering DNA sequence. For example, studies of maternal care in rats indicate that differences in the quality of nurturing affect neural function in pups and negatively affect cognition and the expression of psychopathology later in life. Moreover, rats whose mothers showed increased levels of licking and grooming during their first week of life also showed less exaggerated stress responses as adults compared with rats who were reared by mothers with a low level of licking and grooming, and the expression of mother-pup interactions in the pups

has been demonstrated to be passed on to the next generation.[18–22] This burgeoning area of research is challenging us to look beyond genetic predispositions to examine how environmental influences and early experiences affect when, how, and to what degree different genes are actually activated, thereby elucidating the mechanistic linkages through which gene-environment interaction can affect lifelong behavior, development, and health (see Fig 1).

Additional evidence for the proposed framework comes from insights accrued during the "Decade of the Brain" in the 1990s, when the National Institutes of Health invested significant resources into understanding both normal and pathologic neuronal development and function. Subsequent advances in developmental neuroscience have begun to describe further, in some cases at the molecular and cellular levels, how an integrated, functioning network with billions of neurons and trillions of connections is assembled. Because this network serves as the biological platform for a child's emerging social-emotional, linguistic, and cognitive skills, developmental neuroscience is also beginning to clarify the underlying causal mechanisms that explain the normative process of child development. In a parallel fashion, longitudinal studies that document the long-term consequences of childhood adversity indicate that alterations in a child's ecology can have measurable effects on his or her developmental trajectory, with lifelong consequences for educational achievement, economic productivity, health status, and longevity.[23–27]

The EBD framework described in this article presents a new way to think about the underlying biological mechanisms that explain this robust link between early life adversities (ie, the new morbidities of childhood) and important adult outcomes. The innovation of this approach lies in its mobilization of dramatic scientific advances in the service of rethinking basic notions of health promotion and disease prevention within a fully integrated, life span perspective from conception to old age.[6] In this context, significant stress in the lives of young children is viewed as a risk factor for the genesis of health-threatening behaviors as well as a catalyst for physiologic responses that can lay the groundwork for chronic, stress-related diseases later in life.

Understanding the Biology of Stress

Although genetic variability clearly plays a role in stress reactivity, early experiences and environmental influences can have considerable impact. Beginning as early as the prenatal period, both animal[28–30] and human[31,32] studies suggest that fetal exposure to maternal stress can influence later stress responsiveness. In animals, this effect has been demonstrated not only in the offspring of the studied pregnancy but also in subsequent generations. The precise biological mechanisms that explain these findings remain to be elucidated, but epigenetic modifications of DNA appear likely to play a role.[31,33,34] Early postnatal experiences with adversity are also thought to affect future reactivity to stress, perhaps by altering the developing neural circuits controlling these neuroendocrine responses.[34,35] Although much research remains to be performed in this area, there is a strong scientific consensus that the ecological context modulates the expression of one's genotype. It is as if experiences confer a "signature" on the genome to authorize certain characteristics and behaviors and to prohibit others. This concept

underscores the need for greater understanding of how stress "gets under the skin," as well as the importance of determining what external and internal factors can be mobilized to prevent that embedding process or protect against the consequences of its activation.

Physiologic responses to stress are well defined.[36–38] The most extensively studied involve activation of the hypothalamic-pituitary-adrenocortical axis and the sympathetic-adrenomedullary system, which results in increased levels of stress hormones, such as corticotropin-releasing hormone (CRH), cortisol, norepinephrine, and adrenaline. These changes co-occur with a network of other mediators that include elevated inflammatory cytokines and the response of the parasympathetic nervous system, which counterbalances both sympathetic activation and inflammatory responses. Whereas transient increases in these stress hormones are protective and even essential for survival, excessively high levels or prolonged exposures can be quite harmful or frankly toxic,[39–41] and the dysregulation of this network of physiologic mediators (eg, too much or too little cortisol; too much or too little inflammatory response) can lead to a chronic "wear and tear" effect on multiple organ systems, including the brain.[39–41] This cumulative, stress-induced burden on overall body functioning and the aggregated costs, both physiologic and psychological, required for coping and returning to homeostatic balance, have been referred to as "allostatic load."[38,42–44] The dynamics of these stress-mediating systems are such that their overactivation in the context of repeated or chronic adversity leads to alterations in their regulation.

The National Scientific Council on the Developing Child has proposed

a conceptual taxonomy comprising 3 distinct types of stress responses (in contrast to the actual stressors themselves) in young children—positive, tolerable, and toxic—on the basis of postulated differences in their potential to cause enduring physiologic disruptions as a result of the intensity and duration of the response.[17,45] A positive stress response refers to a physiologic state that is brief and mild to moderate in magnitude. Central to the notion of positive stress is the availability of a caring and responsive adult who helps the child cope with the stressor, thereby providing a protective effect that facilitates the return of the stress response systems back to baseline status. Examples of precipitants of a positive stress response in young children include dealing with frustration, getting an immunization, and the anxiety associated with the first day at a child care center. When buffered by an environment of stable and supportive relationships, positive stress responses are a growth-promoting element of normal development. As such, they provide important opportunities to observe, learn, and practice healthy, adaptive responses to adverse experiences.

A tolerable stress response, in contrast to positive stress, is associated with exposure to nonnormative experiences that present a greater magnitude of adversity or threat. Precipitants may include the death of a family member, a serious illness or injury, a contentious divorce, a natural disaster, or an act of terrorism. When experienced in the context of buffering protection provided by supportive adults, the risk that such circumstances will produce excessive activation of the stress response systems that leads to physiologic harm and long-term consequences for health and learning is greatly reduced. Thus, the essential characteristic that makes this form of stress response tolerable is the extent to which protective adult relationships facilitate the child's adaptive coping and a sense of control, thereby reducing the physiologic stress response and promoting a return to baseline status.

The third and most dangerous form of stress response, toxic stress, can result from strong, frequent, or prolonged activation of the body's stress response systems in the absence of the buffering protection of a supportive, adult relationship. The risk factors studied in the Adverse Childhood Experiences Study[23] include examples of multiple stressors (eg, child abuse or neglect, parental substance abuse, and maternal depression) that are capable of inducing a toxic stress response. The essential characteristic of this phenomenon is the postulated disruption of brain circuitry and other organ and metabolic systems during sensitive developmental periods. Such disruption may result in anatomic changes and/or physiologic dysregulations that are the precursors of later impairments in learning and behavior as well as the roots of chronic, stress-related physical and mental illness. The potential role of toxic stress and early life adversity in the pathogenesis of health disparities underscores the importance of effective surveillance for significant risk factors in the primary health care setting. More important, however, is the need for clinical pediatrics to move beyond the level of risk factor identification and to leverage advances in the biology of adversity to contribute to the critical task of developing, testing, and refining new and more effective strategies for reducing toxic stress and mitigating its effects as early as possible, before irrevocable damage is done. Stated simply, the next chapter of innovation in pediatrics remains to be written, but the outline and plot are clear.

Toxic Stress and the Developing Brain

In addition to short-term changes in observable behavior, toxic stress in young children can lead to less outwardly visible yet permanent changes in brain structure and function.[39,46] The plasticity of the fetal, infant, and early childhood brain makes it particularly sensitive to chemical influences, and there is growing evidence from both animal and human studies that persistently elevated levels of stress hormones can disrupt its developing architecture.[45] For example, abundant glucocorticoid receptors are found in the amygdala, hippocampus, and prefrontal cortex (PFC), and exposure to stressful experiences has been shown to alter the size and neuronal architecture of these areas as well as lead to functional differences in learning, memory, and aspects of executive functioning. More specifically, chronic stress is associated with hypertrophy and overactivity in the amygdala and orbitofrontal cortex, whereas comparable levels of adversity can lead to loss of neurons and neural connections in the hippocampus and medial PFC. The functional consequences of these structural changes include more anxiety related to both hyperactivation of the amygdala and less top-down control as a result of PFC atrophy as well as impaired memory and mood control as a consequence of hippocampal reduction.[47] Thus, the developing architecture of the brain can be impaired in numerous ways that create a weak foundation for later learning, behavior, and health.

Along with its role in mediating fear and anxiety, the amygdala is also an activator of the physiologic stress response. Its stimulation activates sympathetic activity and causes neurons in the hypothalamus to release CRH. CRH, in turn, signals the pituitary to release adrenocorticotropic hormone, which then stimulates the adrenal glands to increase serum cortisol concentrations. The amygdala contains large numbers of both CRH and glucocorticoid receptors, beginning early in life, which facilitate the establishment of a positive feedback loop. Significant stress in early childhood can trigger amygdala hypertrophy and result in a hyperresponsive or chronically activated physiologic stress response, along with increased potential for fear and anxiety.[48,49] It is in this way that a child's environment and early experiences get under the skin.

Although the hippocampus can turn off elevated cortisol, chronic stress diminishes its capacity to do so and can lead to impairments in memory and mood-related functions that are located in this brain region. Exposure to chronic stress and high levels of cortisol also inhibit neurogenesis in the hippocampus, which is believed to play an important role in the encoding of memory and other functions. Furthermore, toxic stress limits the ability of the hippocampus to promote contextual learning, making it more difficult to discriminate conditions for which there may be danger versus safety, as is common in posttraumatic stress disorder. Hence, altered brain architecture in response to toxic stress in early childhood could explain, at least in part, the strong association between early adverse experiences and subsequent problems in the development of linguistic, cognitive, and social-emotional skills, all of which are inextricably intertwined in the wiring of the developing brain.[45]

The PFC also participates in turning off the cortisol response and has an important role in the top-down regulation of autonomic balance (ie, sympathetic versus parasympathetic effects), as well as in the development of executive functions, such as decision-making, working memory, behavioral self-regulation, and mood and impulse control. The PFC is also known to suppress amygdala activity, allowing for more adaptive responses to potentially threatening or stressful experiences; however, exposure to stress and elevated cortisol results in dramatic changes in the connectivity within the PFC, which may limit its ability to inhibit amygdala activity and, thereby, impair adaptive responses to stress. Because the hippocampus and PFC both play a significant role in modulating the amygdala's initiation of the stress response, toxic stress–induced changes in architecture and connectivity within and between these important areas might account for the variability seen in stress-responsiveness.[50] This can then result in some children appearing to be both more reactive to even mildly adverse experiences and less capable of effectively coping with future stress.[36,37,45,51]

Toxic Stress and the Early Childhood Roots of Lifelong Impairments in Physical and Mental Health

As described in the previous section, stress-induced changes in the architecture of different regions of the developing brain (eg, amygdala, hippocampus, and PFC) can have potentially permanent effects on a range of important functions, such as regulating stress physiology, learning new skills, and developing the capacity to make healthy adaptations to future adversity.[52,53] As the scientific evidence for these associations has become better known and has been disseminated more widely, its implications for early childhood policy and programs have become increasingly

appreciated by decision makers across the political spectrum. Notwithstanding this growing awareness, however, discussions about early brain development in policy-making circles have focused almost entirely on issues concerned with school readiness as a prerequisite for later academic achievement and the development of a skilled adult workforce. Within this same context, the health dimension of early childhood policy has focused largely on the traditional components of primary pediatric care, such as immunizations, early identification of sensory impairments and developmental delays, and the prompt diagnosis and treatment of medical problems. That said, as advances in the biomedical sciences have generated growing evidence linking biological disruptions associated with adverse childhood experiences (ACE) to greater risk for a variety of chronic diseases well into the adult years, the need to reconceptualize the health dimension of early childhood policy has become increasingly clear.[1,6] Stated simply, the time has come to expand the public's understanding of brain development and shine a bright light on its relation to the early childhood roots of adult disease and to examine the compelling implications of this growing knowledge base for the future of pediatric practice.

The potential consequences of toxic stress in early childhood for the pathogenesis of adult disease are considerable. At the behavioral level, there is extensive evidence of a strong link between early adversity and a wide range of health-threatening behaviors. At the biological level, there is growing documentation of the extent to which both the cumulative burden of stress over time (eg, from chronic maltreatment) and the timing of specific environmental insults during

sensitive developmental periods (eg, from first trimester rubella or prenatal alcohol exposure) can create structural and functional disruptions that lead to a wide range of physical and mental illnesses later in adult life.[1,6] A selective overview of this extensive scientific literature is provided below.

The association between ACE and unhealthy adult lifestyles has been well documented. Adolescents with a history of multiple risk factors are more likely to initiate drinking alcohol at a younger age and are more likely to use alcohol as a means of coping with stress than for social reasons.[54] The adoption of unhealthy lifestyles as a coping mechanism might also explain why higher ACE exposures are associated with tobacco use, illicit drug abuse, obesity, and promiscuity,[55,56] as well as why the risk of pathologic gambling is increased in adults who were maltreated as children.[57] Adolescents and adults who manifest higher rates of risk-taking behaviors are also more likely to have trouble maintaining supportive social networks and are at higher risk of school failure, gang membership, unemployment, poverty, homelessness, violent crime, incarceration, and becoming single parents. Furthermore, adults in this high-risk group who become parents themselves are less likely to be able to provide the kind of stable and supportive relationships that are needed to protect their children from the damages of toxic stress. This intergenerational cycle of significant adversity, with its predictable repetition of limited educational achievement and poor health, is mediated, at least in part, by the social inequalities and disrupted social networks that contribute to fragile families and parenting difficulties.[7,58,59]

The adoption of unhealthy lifestyles and associated exacerbation of socioeconomic inequalities are potent risk factors for poor health. Up to 40% of early deaths have been estimated to be the result of behavioral or lifestyle patterns,[3] and 1 interpretation of the ACE study data is that toxic stress in childhood is associated with the adoption of unhealthy lifestyles as a coping mechanism.[60] An additional 25% to 30% of early deaths are thought to be attributable to either inadequacies in medical care[3] or socioeconomic circumstances, many of which are known to contribute to health care–related disparities.[61–67]

Beyond its strong association with later risk-taking and generally unhealthy lifestyles, it is critically important to underscore the extent to which toxic stress in early childhood has also been shown to cause physiologic disruptions that persist into adulthood and lead to frank disease, even in the absence of later health-threatening behaviors. For example, the biological manifestations of toxic stress can include alterations in immune function[68] and measurable increases in inflammatory markers,[69–72] which are known to be associated with poor health outcomes as diverse as cardiovascular disease,[69,70,73] viral hepatitis,[74] liver cancer,[75] asthma,[76] chronic obstructive pulmonary disease,[77] autoimmune diseases,[78] poor dental health,[72] and depression.[79–81] Thus, toxic stress in early childhood not only is a risk factor for later risky behavior but also can be a direct source of biological injury or disruption that may have lifelong consequences independent of whatever circumstances might follow later in life. In such cases, toxic stress can be viewed as the precipitant of a physiologic memory or biological signature that confers lifelong risk well beyond its time of origin.[38,42–44]

Over and above its toll on individuals, it is also important to address the enormous social and economic costs of toxic stress and its consequences for all of society. The multiple dimensions of these costs extend from differential levels of civic participation and their impacts on the quality of community life to the health and skills of the nation's workforce and its ability to participate successfully in a global economy. In the realm of learning and behavior, economists argue for early and sustained investments in early care and education programs, particularly for children whose parents have limited education and low income, on the basis of persuasive evidence from cost-benefit analyses that reveal the costs of incarceration and diminished economic productivity associated with educational failure.[82–86] In view of the relatively scarce attention to health outcomes in these long-term follow-up studies, the full return on investments that reduce toxic stress in early childhood is likely to be much higher. Health care expenditures that are paying for the consequences of unhealthy lifestyles (eg, obesity, tobacco, alcohol, and substance abuse) are enormous, and the costs of chronic diseases that may have their origins early in life include many conditions that consume a substantial percentage of current state and federal budgets. The potential savings in health care costs from even small, marginal reductions in the prevalence of cardiovascular disease, hypertension, diabetes, and depression are, therefore, likely to dwarf the considerable economic productivity and criminal justice benefits that have been well documented for effective early childhood interventions.

In summary, the EBD approach to childhood adversity discussed in this report has 2 compelling implications for a full, life span perspective on health promotion and disease prevention. First, it postulates that toxic stress in early childhood plays an important causal role in the intergenerational transmission of disparities in educational achievement and health outcomes. Second, it underscores the need for the entire medical community to focus more attention on the roots of adult diseases that originate during the prenatal and early childhood periods and to rethink the concept of preventive health care within a system that currently perpetuates a scientifically untenable wall between pediatrics and internal medicine.

THE NEED FOR A NEW PEDIATRIC PARADIGM TO PROMOTE HEALTH AND PREVENT DISEASE

In his 1966 Aldrich Award address, Dr Julius Richmond identified child development as the basic science of pediatrics.[87] It is now time to expand the boundaries of that science by incorporating more than 4 decades of transformational research in neuroscience, molecular biology, and genomics, along with parallel advances in the behavioral and social sciences (see Fig 1). This newly augmented, interdisciplinary, basic science of pediatrics offers a promising framework for a deeper understanding of the biology and ecology of the developmental process. More importantly, it presents a compelling opportunity to leverage these rapidly advancing frontiers of knowledge to formulate more effective strategies to enhance lifelong outcomes in learning, behavior, and health.

The time has come for a coordinated effort among basic scientists, pediatric subspecialists, and primary care clinicians to develop more effective strategies for addressing the origins of social class, racial, and ethnic disparities in health and development. To this end, a unified, science-based approach to early childhood policy and practice across multiple sectors (including primary health care, early care and education, and child welfare, among many others) could provide a compelling framework for a new era in community-based investment in which coordinated efforts are driven by a shared knowledge base rather than distracted by a diversity of traditions, approaches, and funding streams.

Recognizing both the critical value and clear limitations of what can be accomplished within the constraints of an office visit, 21st century pediatrics is well positioned to serve as the primary engine for a broader approach to health promotion and disease prevention that is guided by cutting-edge science and expanded in scope beyond individualized health care.[88,89] The pediatric medical home of the future could offer more than the early identification of concerns and timely referral to available programs, as enhanced collaboration between pediatricians and community-based agencies could be viewed as a vehicle for testing promising new intervention strategies rather than simply improving coordination among existing services. With this goal in mind, science tells us that interventions that strengthen the capacities of families and communities to protect young children from the disruptive effects of toxic stress are likely to promote healthier brain development and enhanced physical and mental well-being. The EBD approach proposed in this article is adapted from a science-based framework created by the Center on the Developing Child at Harvard University to advance early childhood policies and programs that support this vision (see Fig 2).[1] Its rationale, essential elements, and implications for pediatric practice are summarized below.

Broadening the Framework for Early Childhood Policy and Practice

Advances across the biological, behavioral, and social sciences support 2 clear and powerful messages for leaders who are searching for more effective ways to improve the health of the nation.[6] First, current health promotion and disease prevention policies focused largely on adults would be more effective if evidence-based investments were also made to strengthen the foundations of health in the prenatal and early childhood periods. Second, significant reductions in chronic disease could be achieved across the life course by decreasing the number and severity of adverse experiences that threaten the well-being of young children and by strengthening the protective relationships that help mitigate the harmful effects of toxic stress. The multiple domains that affect the biology of health and development—including the foundations of healthy development, caregiver and community capacities, and public and private sector policies and programs—provide a rich array of targeted opportunities for the introduction of innovative interventions, beginning in the earliest years of life.[1]

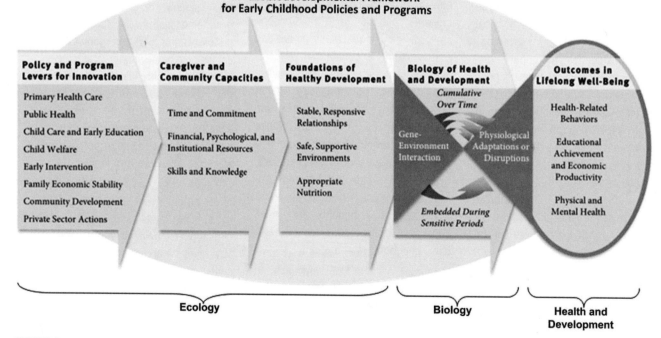

FIGURE 2
An ecobiodevelopmental framework for early childhood policies and programs. This was adapted from ref 1. See text for details.

The biology of health and development explains how experiences and environmental influences get under the skin and interact with genetic predispositions, which then result in various combinations of physiologic adaptation and disruption that affect lifelong outcomes in learning, behavior, and both physical and mental well-being. These findings call for us to augment adult-focused approaches to health promotion and disease prevention by addressing the early childhood origins of lifelong illness and disability.

The foundations of healthy development refers to 3 domains that establish a context within which the early roots of physical and mental well-being are nourished. These include (1) a stable and responsive environment of relationships, which provides young children with consistent, nurturing, and protective interactions with adults to enhance their learning and help them develop adaptive capacities that promote well-regulated stress-response systems; (2) safe and supportive physical, chemical, and built environments, which provide physical and emotional spaces that are free from toxins and fear, allow active exploration without significant risk of harm, and offer support for families raising young children; and (3) sound and appropriate nutrition, which includes health-promoting food intake and eating habits, beginning with the future mother's preconception nutritional status.

Caregiver and community capacities to promote health and prevent disease and disability refers to the ability of family members, early childhood program staff, and the social capital provided through neighborhoods, voluntary associations, and the parents' workplaces to play a major supportive role in strengthening the foundations of child health. These capacities can be grouped into 3 categories: (1) time

and commitment; (2) financial, psychological, social, and institutional resources; and (3) skills and knowledge.

Public and private sector policies and programs can strengthen the foundations of health through their ability to enhance the capacities of caregivers and communities in the multiple settings in which children grow up. Relevant policies include both legislative and administrative actions that affect systems responsible for primary health care, public health, child care and early education, child welfare, early intervention, family economic stability (including employment support for parents and cash assistance), community development (including zoning regulations that influence the availability of open spaces and sources of nutritious food), housing, and environmental protection, among others. It is also important to underscore the role that the private sector can play in strengthening the capacities of families to raise healthy and competent children, particularly through supportive workplace policies (such as paid parental leave, support for breastfeeding, and flexible work hours to attend school activities and medical visits).

Defining a Distinctive Niche for Pediatrics Among Multiple Early Childhood Disciplines and Services

Notwithstanding the important goal of ensuring a medical home for all children, extensive evidence on the social determinants of health indicates that the reduction of disparities in physical and mental well-being will depend on more than access to high-quality medical care alone. Moreover, as noted previously, experience tells us that continuing calls for enhanced coordination of effort across service systems are unlikely to be sufficient if the systems are guided by different

values and bodies of knowledge and the effects of their services are modest. With these caveats in mind, pediatricians are strategically situated to mobilize the science of early childhood development and its underlying neurobiology to stimulate fresh thinking about both the scope of primary health care and its relation to other programs serving young children and their families. Indeed, every system that touches the lives of children—as well as mothers before and during pregnancy—offers an opportunity to leverage this rapidly growing knowledge base to strengthen the foundations and capacities that make lifelong healthy development possible. Toward this end, explicit investments in the early reduction of significant adversity are particularly likely to generate positive returns.

The possibilities and limitations of well-child care within a multidimensional health system have been the focus of a spirited and enduring discussion within the pediatric community.[88,90,91] Over more than half a century, this dialogue has focused on the need for family-centered, community-based, culturally competent care for children with developmental disabilities, behavior problems, and chronic health impairments, as well as the need for a broader contextual approach to the challenges of providing more effective interventions for children living under conditions of poverty, with or without the additional complications of parental mental illness, substance abuse, and exposure to violence.[10] As the debate has continued, the gap between the call for comprehensive services and the realities of day-to-day practice has remained exceedingly difficult to reduce. Basic recommendations for routine developmental screening and referrals to appropriate community-based services have been particularly difficult to implement.[92] The obstacles to progress in this area have been formidable at both ends of the process—beginning with the logistical and financial challenges of conducting routine developmental screening in a busy office setting and extending to significant limitations in access to evidence-based services for children and families who are identified as having problems that require intervention.

Despite long-standing calls for an explicit, community-focused approach to primary care, a recent national study of pediatric practices identified persistent difficulties in achieving effective linkages with community-based resources as a major challenge.[92] A parallel survey of parents also noted the limited communication that exists between pediatric practices and community-based services, such as Supplemental Nutrition Program for Women, Infants, and Children; child care providers; and schools.[93] Perhaps most important, both groups agreed that pediatricians cannot be expected to meet all of a child's needs. This challenge is further complicated by the marked variability in quality among community-based services that are available—ranging from evidence-based interventions that clearly improve child outcomes to programs that appear to have only marginal effects or no measurable impacts. Thus, although chronic difficulty in securing access to indicated services is an important problem facing most practicing pediatricians, the limited evidence of effectiveness for many of the options that are available (particularly in rural areas and many states in which public investment in such services is more limited) presents a serious problem that must be acknowledged and afforded greater attention.

At this point in time, the design and successful implementation of more effective models of health promotion and disease prevention for children experiencing significant adversity will require more than advocacy for increased funding. It will require a deep investment in the development, testing, continuous improvement, and broad replication of innovative models of cross-disciplinary policy and programmatic interventions that are guided by scientific knowledge and led by practitioners in the medical, educational, and social services worlds who are truly ready to work together (and to train the next generation of practitioners) in new ways.[88,89] The sheer number and complexity of under-addressed threats to child health that are associated with toxic stress demands bold, creative leadership and the selection of strategic priorities for focused attention. To this end, science suggests that 2 areas are particularly ripe for fresh thinking: the child welfare system and the treatment of maternal depression.

For more than a century, child welfare services have focused on physical safety, reduction of repeated injury, and child custody. Within this context, the role of the pediatrician is focused largely on the identification of suspected maltreatment and the documentation and treatment of physical injuries. Advances in our understanding of the impact of toxic stress on lifelong health now underscore the need for a broader pediatric approach to meet the needs of children who have been abused or neglected. In some cases, this could be provided within a medical home by skilled clinicians with expertise in early childhood mental health. In reality, however, the magnitude of needs in this area generally exceeds the capacity of most primary care practice settings. A report from the Institute of Medicine and National Research Council[15] stated that these needs could be addressed through regularized referrals from the child welfare system to the early intervention system for children with developmental delays or disabilities; subsequent federal reauthorizations of the Keeping Children and Families Safe Act and the Individuals with Disabilities Education Act (Part C) both included requirements for establishing such linkages. The implementation of these federal requirements, however, has moved slowly.

The growing availability of evidence-based interventions that have been shown to improve outcomes for children in the child welfare system[94] underscores the compelling need to transform "child protection" from its traditional concern with physical safety and custody to a broader focus on the emotional, social, and cognitive costs of maltreatment. The Centers for Disease Control and Prevention has taken an important step forward by promoting the prevention of child maltreatment as a public health concern.[95,96] The pediatric community could play a powerful role in leading the call for implementation of the new requirement for linking child welfare to early intervention programs, as well as bringing a strong, science-based perspective to the collaborative development and implementation of more effective intervention models.

The widespread absence of attention to the mother-child relationship in the treatment of depression in women with young children is another striking example of the gap between science and practice that could be reduced by targeted pediatric advocacy.[97] Extensive research has demonstrated the extent to which maternal depression compromises the contingent reciprocity between a mother and her young child that is essential for healthy cognitive, linguistic, social, and emotional development.[98] Despite that well-documented observation, the treatment of depression in women with young children is typically viewed as an adult mental health service and rarely includes an explicit focus on the mother-child relationship. This serious omission illustrates a lack of understanding of the consequences for the developing brain of a young child when the required "serve and return" reciprocity of the mother-child relationship is disrupted or inconsistent. Consequently, and not surprisingly, abundant clinical research indicates that the successful treatment of a mother's depression does not generally translate into comparable recovery in her young child unless there is an explicit therapeutic focus on their dyadic relationship.[98] Pediatricians are the natural authorities to shed light on this current deficiency in mental health service delivery. Advocating for payment mechanisms that require (or provide incentives for) the coordination of child and parent medical services (eg, through automatic coverage for the parent-child dyad linked to reimbursement for the treatment of maternal depression) offers 1 promising strategy that American Academy of Pediatrics state chapters could pursue. As noted previously, although some medical homes may have the expertise to provide this kind of integrative treatment, most pediatricians rely on the availability of other professionals with specialized skills who are often difficult to find. Whether such services are provided within or connected to the medical home, it is clear that standard pediatric practice must move beyond screening for maternal depression and invest greater energy in securing the provision of appropriate and effective treatment that meets the needs of both mothers and their young children.

The targeted messages conveyed in these 2 examples are illustrative of the kinds of specific actions that offer promising new directions for the pediatric community beyond general calls for comprehensive, family-centered, community-based services. Although the practical constraints of office-based practice make it unlikely that many primary care clinicians will ever play a lead role in the treatment of children affected by maltreatment or maternal depression, pediatricians are still the best positioned among all the professionals who care for young children to provide the public voice and scientific leadership needed to catalyze the development and implementation of more effective strategies to reduce adversities that can lead to lifelong disparities in learning, behavior, and health.

A great deal has been said about how the universality of pediatric primary care makes it an ideal platform for coordinating the services needed by vulnerable, young children and their families. In this respect, the medical home is strategically positioned to play 2 important roles. The first is to ensure that needs are identified, state-of-the-art management is provided as indicated, and credible evaluation is conducted to assess the effects of the services that are being delivered. The second and, ultimately, more transformational role is to mobilize the entire pediatric community (including both clinical specialists and basic scientists) to drive the design and testing of much-needed, new, science-based interventions to reduce the sources and consequences of significant adversity in the lives of young children.[99] To this end, a powerful new role awaits a new breed of pediatricians who are prepared to build on the best of existing community-based services and to work closely with creative leaders from a range of disciplines and sectors to inform innovative approaches to health promotion and disease prevention that generate greater effects than existing efforts.

No other profession brings a comparable level of scientific expertise, professional stature, and public trust—and nothing short of transformational thinking beyond the hospital and office settings is likely to create the magnitude of breakthroughs in health promotion that are needed to match the dramatic advances that are currently emerging in the treatment of disease. This new direction must be part of the new frontier in pediatrics —a frontier that brings cutting-edge scientific thinking to the multidimensional world of early childhood policy and practice for children who face significant adversity. Moving that frontier forward will benefit considerably from pediatric leadership that provides an intellectual and operational bridge connecting the basic sciences of neurobiology, molecular genetics, and developmental psychology to the broad and diverse landscape of health, education, and human services.

SUMMARY

A vital and productive society with a prosperous and sustainable future is built on a foundation of healthy child development. Health in the earliest years—beginning with the future mother's well-being before she becomes pregnant—lays the groundwork for a lifetime of the physical and mental vitality that is necessary for a strong workforce and responsible participation in community life. When developing biological systems are strengthened by positive early experiences, children are more likely to thrive and grow up to be healthy, contributing adults. Sound health in early childhood provides a foundation for the construction of sturdy brain architecture and the achievement of a broad range of skills and learning capacities. Together these constitute the building blocks for a vital and sustainable society that invests in its human capital and values the lives of its children.

Advances in neuroscience, molecular biology, and genomics have converged on 3 compelling conclusions: (1) early experiences are built into our bodies; (2) significant adversity can produce physiologic disruptions or biological memories that undermine the development of the body's stress response systems and affect the developing brain, cardiovascular system, immune system, and metabolic regulatory controls; and (3) these physiologic disruptions can persist far into adulthood and lead to lifelong impairments in both physical and mental health. This technical report presents a framework for integrating recent advances in our understanding of human development with a rich and growing body of evidence regarding the disruptive effects of childhood adversity and toxic stress. The EBD framework that guides this report suggests that many adult diseases are, in fact, developmental disorders that begin early in life. This framework indicates that the future of pediatrics lies in its unique leadership position as a credible and respected voice on behalf of children, which provides a powerful platform for translating scientific advances into more effective strategies and creative interventions to reduce the early childhood adversities that lead to lifelong impairments in learning, behavior, and health.

CONCLUSIONS

1. Advances in a broad range of interdisciplinary fields, including developmental neuroscience, molecular biology, genomics, epigenetics, developmental psychology, epidemiology, and economics, are converging on an integrated, basic science of pediatrics (see Fig 1).

2. Rooted in a deepening understanding of how brain architecture is shaped by the interactive effects of both genetic predisposition and environmental influence, and how its developing circuitry affects a lifetime of learning, behavior, and health, advances in the biological sciences underscore the foundational importance of the early years and support an EBD framework for understanding the evolution of human health and disease across the life span.

3. The biology of early childhood adversity reveals the important role of toxic stress in disrupting developing brain architecture and adversely affecting the concurrent development of other organ systems and regulatory functions.

4. Toxic stress can lead to potentially permanent changes in learning (linguistic, cognitive, and social-emotional skills), behavior (adaptive versus maladaptive responses to future adversity), and physiology (a hyperresponsive or chronically activated stress response) and can cause physiologic disruptions that result in higher levels of stress-related chronic diseases and increase the prevalence of unhealthy lifestyles that lead to widening health disparities.

5. The lifelong costs of childhood toxic stress are enormous, as manifested in adverse impacts on learning, behavior, and health, and effective early childhood interventions provide critical opportunities to prevent these undesirable outcomes and generate large economic returns for all of society.

6. The consequences of significant adversity early in life prompt an urgent call for innovative strategies to reduce toxic stress within the context of a coordinated system of policies and services guided by an integrated science of early childhood and early brain development.

7. An EBD framework, grounded in an integrated basic science, provides a clear theory of change to help leaders in policy and practice craft new solutions to the challenges of societal disparities in health, learning, and behavior (see Fig 2).

8. Pediatrics provides a powerful yet underused platform for translating scientific advances into innovative early childhood policies, and practicing pediatricians are ideally positioned to participate "on the ground" in the design, testing, and refinement of new models of disease prevention, health promotion, and developmental enhancement beginning in the earliest years of life.

LEAD AUTHORS

Jack P. Shonkoff, MD
Andrew S. Garner, MD, PhD

COMMITTEE ON PSYCHOSOCIAL ASPECTS OF CHILD AND FAMILY HEALTH, 2010–2011

Benjamin S. Siegel, MD, Chairperson
Mary I. Dobbins, MD
Marian F. Earls, MD
Andrew S. Garner, MD, PhD
Laura McGuinn, MD
John Pascoe, MD, MPH
David L. Wood, MD

LIAISONS

Robert T. Brown, PhD — *Society of Pediatric Psychology*
Terry Carmichael, MSW — *National Association of Social Workers*
Mary Jo Kupst, PhD — *Society of Pediatric Psychology*
D. Richard Martini, MD — *American Academy of Child and Adolescent Psychiatry*
Mary Sheppard, MS, RN, PNP, BC — *National Association of Pediatric Nurse Practitioners*

CONSULTANT

George J. Cohen, MD

CONSULTANT AND LEAD AUTHOR

Jack P. Shonkoff, MD

STAFF

Karen S. Smith

REFERENCES

1. Center on the Developing Child at Harvard University. The foundations of lifelong health are built in early childhood. Available at: www.developingchild.harvard.edu. Accessed March 8, 2011

2. Knudsen EI, Heckman JJ, Cameron JL, Shonkoff JP. Economic, neurobiological, and behavioral perspectives on building America's future workforce. *Proc Natl Acad Sci U S A.* 2006;103(27):10155–10162

3. McGinnis JM, Williams-Russo P, Knickman JR. The case for more active policy attention to health promotion. *Health Aff (Millwood).* 2002;21(2):78–93

4. Schor EL, Abrams M, Shea K. Medicaid: health promotion and disease prevention for school readiness. *Health Aff (Millwood).* 2007;26(2):420–429

5. Wen CP, Tsai SP, Chung WS. A 10-year experience with universal health insurance in Taiwan: measuring changes in health and health disparity. *Ann Intern Med.* 2008;148(4):258–267

6. Shonkoff JP, Boyce WT, McEwen BS. Neuroscience, molecular biology, and the childhood roots of health disparities: building a new framework for health promotion and disease prevention. *JAMA.* 2009;301(21):2252–2259

7. Braveman P, Barclay C. Health disparities beginning in childhood: a life-course perspective. *Pediatrics.* 2009;124(suppl 3):S163–S175

8. Haggerty RJRK, Pless IB. *Child Health and the Community.* New York, NY: John Wiley and Sons; 1975

9. Committee on Psychosocial Aspects of Child and Family Health; American Academy of Pediatrics. The new morbidity revisited: a renewed commitment to the psychosocial aspects of pediatric care. *Pediatrics.* 2001;108(5):1227–1230

10. Palfrey JS, Tonniges TF, Green M, Richmond J. Introduction: addressing the millennial morbidity—the context of community pediatrics. *Pediatrics.* 2005;115(suppl 4):1121–1123

11. Flores G, ; Committee On Pediatric Research. Technical report—racial and ethnic disparities in the health and health care of children. *Pediatrics.* 2010;125(4). Available at: www.pediatrics.org/cgi/content/full/125/4/e979

12. Bronfenbrenner U. *The Ecology of Human Development: Experiments by Nature and Design.* Cambridge, MA: Harvard University Press; 1979

13. Sameroff A. A unified theory of development: a dialectic integration of nature and nurture. *Child Dev.* 2010;81(1):6–22

14. Sameroff AJ, Chandler MJ. Reproductive risk and the continuum of caretaking causality. In: Horowitz FD, Hetherington M, Scarr-Salapatek S, Siegel G, eds. *Review of Child Development Research.* Chicago, IL: University of Chicago; 1975:187–244

15. National Research Council, Institute of Medicine, Committee on Integrating the Science of Early Childhood Development; Shonkoff JP, Phillips D, eds. *From Neurons to Neighborhoods: The Science of Early Childhood Development.* Washington, DC: National Academies Press; 2000

16. Bronfenbrenner U. *Making Human Beings Human: Bioecological Perspectives on Human Development.* Thousand Oaks, CA: Sage Publications; 2005

17. Shonkoff JP. Building a new biodevelopmental framework to guide the future of early childhood policy. *Child Dev.* 2010;81(1):357–367

18. Bagot RC, Meaney MJ. Epigenetics and the biological basis of gene × environment interactions. *J Am Acad Child Adolesc Psychiatry.* 2010;49(8):752–771

19. National Scientific Council on the Developing Child. Early experiences can alter gene expression and affect long-term development: working paper #10. Available at: www.developingchild.net. Accessed March 8, 2011

20. Meaney MJ. Epigenetics and the biological definition of gene × environment interactions. *Child Dev.* 2010;81(1):41–79

21. Meaney MJ, Szyf M. Environmental programming of stress responses through DNA methylation: life at the interface between a dynamic environment and a fixed genome. *Dialogues Clin Neurosci.* 2005;7(2):103–123

22. Szyf M, McGowan P, Meaney MJ. The social environment and the epigenome. *Environ Mol Mutagen.* 2008;49(1):46–60

23. Felitti VJ, Anda RF, Nordenberg D, et al. Relationship of childhood abuse and household dysfunction to many of the leading causes of death in adults. The Adverse Childhood Experiences (ACE) Study. *Am J Prev Med.* 1998;14(4):245–258

24. Schweinhart LJ. *Lifetime Effects: The High/Scope Perry Preschool Study Through Age 40.* Ypsilanti, MI: High/Scope Press; 2005

25. Flaherty EG, Thompson R, Litrownik AJ, et al. Effect of early childhood adversity on child health. *Arch Pediatr Adolesc Med.* 2006;160(12):1232–1238

26. Koenen KC, Moffitt TE, Poulton R, Martin J, Caspi A. Early childhood factors associated with the development of post-traumatic stress disorder: results from a longitudinal birth cohort. *Psychol Med.* 2007;37(2):181–192

27. Flaherty EG, Thompson R, Litrownik AJ, et al. Adverse childhood exposures and reported child health at age 12. *Acad Pediatr.* 2009;9(3):150–156

28. Cottrell EC, Seckl JR. Prenatal stress, glucocorticoids and the programming of adult disease. *Front Behav Neurosci.* 2009;3:19

29. Darnaudéry M, Maccari S. Epigenetic programming of the stress response in male and female rats by prenatal restraint stress. *Brain Res Brain Res Rev.* 2008;57(2):571–585

30. Seckl JR, Meaney MJ. Glucocorticoid "programming" and PTSD risk. *Ann N Y Acad Sci.* 2006;1071:351–378

31. Oberlander TF, Weinberg J, Papsdorf M, Grunau R, Misri S, Devlin AM. Prenatal exposure to maternal depression, neonatal methylation of human glucocorticoid receptor gene (NR3C1) and infant cortisol

stress responses. *Epigenetics.* 2008;3(2): 97–106

32. Brand SR, Engel SM, Canfield RL, Yehuda R. The effect of maternal PTSD following in utero trauma exposure on behavior and temperament in the 9-month-old infant. *Ann N Y Acad Sci.* 2006;1071:454–458

33. Murgatroyd C, Patchev AV, Wu Y, et al. Dynamic DNA methylation programs persistent adverse effects of early-life stress. *Nat Neurosci.* 2009;12(12):1559–1566

34. Roth TL, Lubin FD, Funk AJ, Sweatt JD. Lasting epigenetic influence of early-life adversity on the BDNF gene. *Biol Psychiatry.* 2009;65(9):760–769

35. Szyf M. The early life environment and the epigenome. *Biochim Biophys Acta.* 2009; 1790(9):878–885

36. Compas BE. Psychobiological processes of stress and coping: implications for resilience in children and adolescents—comments on the papers of Romeo & McEwen and Fisher et al. *Ann N Y Acad Sci.* 2006; 1094:226–234

37. Gunnar M, Quevedo K. The neurobiology of stress and development. *Annu Rev Psychol.* 2007;58:145–173

38. McEwen BS. Physiology and neurobiology of stress and adaptation: central role of the brain. *Physiol Rev.* 2007;87(3):873–904

39. McEwen BS. Stressed or stressed out: what is the difference? *J Psychiatry Neurosci.* 2005;30(5):315–318

40. McEwen BS, Seeman T. Protective and damaging effects of mediators of stress. Elaborating and testing the concepts of allostasis and allostatic load. *Ann N Y Acad Sci.* 1999;896:30–47

41. McEwen BS. Protective and damaging effects of stress mediators. *N Engl J Med.* 1998;338(3):171–179

42. Korte SM, Koolhaas JM, Wingfield JC, McEwen BS. The Darwinian concept of stress: benefits of allostasis and costs of allostatic load and the trade-offs in health and disease. *Neurosci Biobehav Rev.* 2005;29 (1):3–38

43. McEwen BS. Mood disorders and allostatic load. *Biol Psychiatry.* 2003;54(3):200–207

44. McEwen BS. Stress, adaptation, and disease. Allostasis and allostatic load. *Ann N Y Acad Sci.* 1998;840:33–44

45. National Scientific Council on the Developing Child. *Excessive Stress Disrupts the Architecture of the Developing Brain: Working Paper #3.* Available at: developingchild.harvard.edu/resources/reports_and_working_papers/. Accessed March 8, 2011

46. McEwen BS. Protective and damaging effects of stress mediators: central role of

the brain. *Dialogues Clin Neurosci.* 2006;8 (4):367–381

47. McEwen BS, Gianaros PJ. Stress- and allostasis-induced brain plasticity. *Annu Rev Med.* 2011;62:431–445

48. National Scientific Council on the Developing Child. Persistent fear and anxiety can affect young children's learning and development: working paper #9. Available at: www.developingchild.net. Accessed March 8, 2011

49. Tottenham N, Hare TA, Quinn BT, et al. Prolonged institutional rearing is associated with atypically large amygdala volume and difficulties in emotion regulation. *Dev Sci.* 2010;13(1):46–61

50. Boyce WT, Ellis BJ. Biological sensitivity to context: I. An evolutionary-developmental theory of the origins and functions of stress reactivity. *Dev Psychopathol.* 2005;17 (2):271–301

51. Francis DD. Conceptualizing child health disparities: a role for developmental neurogenomics. *Pediatrics.* 2009;124(suppl 3): S196–S202

52. Juster RP, McEwen BS, Lupien SJ. Allostatic load biomarkers of chronic stress and impact on health and cognition. *Neurosci Biobehav Rev.* 2010;35(1):2–16

53. McEwen BS, Gianaros PJ. Central role of the brain in stress and adaptation: links to socioeconomic status, health, and disease. *Ann N Y Acad Sci.* 2010;1186:190–222

54. Rothman EF, Edwards EM, Heeren T, Hingson RW. Adverse childhood experiences predict earlier age of drinking onset: results from a representative US sample of current or former drinkers. *Pediatrics.* 2008;122(2). Available at: www.pediatrics.org/cgi/content/full/122/2/e298

55. Anda RF, Croft JB, Felitti VJ, et al. Adverse childhood experiences and smoking during adolescence and adulthood. *JAMA.* 1999;282 (17):1652–1658

56. Anda RF, Felitti VJ, Bremner JD, et al. The enduring effects of abuse and related adverse experiences in childhood. A convergence of evidence from neurobiology and epidemiology. *Eur Arch Psychiatry Clin Neurosci.* 2006;256(3):174–186

57. Scherrer JF, Xian H, Kapp JM, et al. Association between exposure to childhood and lifetime traumatic events and lifetime pathological gambling in a twin cohort. *J Nerv Ment Dis.* 2007;195(1):72–78

58. Wickrama KA, Conger RD, Lorenz FO, Jung T. Family antecedents and consequences of trajectories of depressive symptoms from adolescence to young adulthood: a life course investigation. *J Health Soc Behav.* 2008;49(4):468–483

59. Kahn RS, Brandt D, Whitaker RC. Combined effect of mothers' and fathers' mental health symptoms on children's behavioral and emotional well-being. *Arch Pediatr Adolesc Med.* 2004;158(8):721–729

60. Felitti VJ. Adverse childhood experiences and adult health. *Acad Pediatr.* 2009;9(3): 131–132

61. Althoff KN, Karpati A, Hero J, Matte TD. Secular changes in mortality disparities in New York City: a reexamination. *J Urban Health.* 2009;86(5):729–744

62. Cheng TL, Jenkins RR. Health disparities across the lifespan: where are the children? *JAMA.* 2009;301(23):2491–2492

63. DeVoe JE, Tillotson C, Wallace LS. Uninsured children and adolescents with insured parents. *JAMA.* 2008;300(16):1904–1913

64. Due P, Merlo J, Harel-Fisch Y, et al. Socioeconomic inequality in exposure to bullying during adolescence: a comparative, cross-sectional, multilevel study in 35 countries. *Am J Public Health.* 2009;99(5):907–914

65. Reid KW, Vittinghoff E, Kushel MB. Association between the level of housing instability, economic standing and health care access: a meta-regression. *J Health Care Poor Underserved.* 2008;19(4):1212–1228

66. Stevens GD, Pickering TA, Seid M, Tsai KY. Disparities in the national prevalence of a quality medical home for children with asthma. *Acad Pediatr.* 2009;9(4):234–241

67. Williams DR, Sternthal M, Wright RJ. Social determinants: taking the social context of asthma seriously. *Pediatrics.* 2009;123 (suppl 3):S174–S184

68. Bierhaus A, Wolf J, Andrassy M, et al. A mechanism converting psychosocial stress into mononuclear cell activation. *Proc Natl Acad Sci U S A.* 2003;100(4):1920–1925

69. Araújo JP, Lourenço P, Azevedo A, et al. Prognostic value of high-sensitivity C-reactive protein in heart failure: a systematic review. *J Card Fail.* 2009;15(3):256–266

70. Galkina E, Ley K. Immune and inflammatory mechanisms of atherosclerosis (*). *Annu Rev Immunol.* 2009;27:165–197

71. Miller GE, Chen E. Harsh family climate in early life presages the emergence of a proinflammatory phenotype in adolescence. *Psychol Sci.* 2010;21(6):848–856

72. Poulton R, Caspi A, Milne BJ, et al. Association between children's experience of socioeconomic disadvantage and adult health: a life-course study. *Lancet.* 2002;360 (9346):1640–1645

73. Ward JR, Wilson HL, Francis SE, Crossman DC, Sabroe I. Translational mini-review series on immunology of vascular disease: inflammation, infections and Toll-like

receptors in cardiovascular disease. *Clin Exp Immunol.* 2009;156(3):386–394

74. Heydtmann M, Adams DH. Chemokines in the immunopathogenesis of hepatitis C infection. *Hepatology.* 2009;49(2):676–688

75. Berasain C, Castillo J, Perugorria MJ, Latasa MU, Prieto J, Avila MA. Inflammation and liver cancer: new molecular links. *Ann N Y Acad Sci.* 2009;1155:206–221

76. Chen E, Miller GE. Stress and inflammation in exacerbations of asthma. *Brain Behav Immun.* 2007;21(8):993–999

77. Yao H, Rahman I. Current concepts on the role of inflammation in COPD and lung cancer. *Curr Opin Pharmacol.* 2009;9(4):375–383

78. Li M, Zhou Y, Feng G, Su SB. The critical role of Toll-like receptor signaling pathways in the induction and progression of autoimmune diseases. *Curr Mol Med.* 2009;9(3):365–374

79. Danese A, Moffitt TE, Pariante CM, Ambler A, Poulton R, Caspi A. Elevated inflammation levels in depressed adults with a history of childhood maltreatment. *Arch Gen Psychiatry.* 2008;65(4):409–415

80. Danese A, Pariante CM, Caspi A, Taylor A, Poulton R. Childhood maltreatment predicts adult inflammation in a life-course study. *Proc Natl Acad Sci U S A.* 2007;104(4):1319–1324

81. Howren MB, Lamkin DM, Suls J. Associations of depression with C-reactive protein, IL-1, and IL-6: a meta-analysis. *Psychosom Med.* 2009;71(2):171–186

82. Cuhna F, Heckman JJ, Lochner LJ, Masterov DV. Interpreting the evidence on life cycle skill formation. In: Hanushek EA, Welch F, eds. *Handbook of the Economics of Education.* Amsterdam, Netherlands: North-Holland; 2006: 697–812

83. Heckman JJ, Stixrud J, Urzua S. The effects of cognitive and non-cognitive abilities on labor market outcomes and social behavior. *J Labor Econ.* 2006;24:411–482

84. Heckman JJ. Role of income and family influence on child outcomes. Ann N Y Acad Sci. 2008;1136:307–323

85. Heckman JJ. The case for investing in disadvantaged young children. Available at: www.firstfocus.net/sites/default/files/r.2008-9.15.ff_.pdf. Accessed March 8, 2011

86. Heckman JJ, Masterov DV. The productivity argument for investing in young children. Available at: http://jenni.uchicago.edu/human-inequality/papers/Heckman_final_all_wp_2007-03-22c_jsb.pdf. Accessed March 8, 2011

87. Richmond JB. Child development: a basic science for pediatrics. *Pediatrics.* 1967;39(5):649–658

88. Leslie LK, Slaw KM, Edwards A, Starmer AJ, Duby JC, ; Members of Vision of Pediatrics 2020 Task Force. Peering into the future: pediatrics in a changing world. *Pediatrics.* 2010;126(5):982–988

89. Starmer AJ, Duby JC, Slaw KM, Edwards A, Leslie LK, ; Members of Vision of Pediatrics 2020 Task Force. Pediatrics in the year 2020 and beyond: preparing for plausible futures. *Pediatrics.* 2010;126(5):971–981

90. Halfon N, DuPlessis H, Inkelas M. Transforming the U.S. child health system. *Health Aff (Millwood).* 2007;26(2):315–330

91. Schor EL. The future pediatrician: promoting children's health and development. *J Pediatr.* 2007;151(suppl 5):S11–S16

92. Tanner JL, Stein MT, Olson LM, Frintner MP, Radecki L. Reflections on well-child care practice: a national study of pediatric clinicians. *Pediatrics.* 2009;124(3):849–857

93. Radecki L, Olson LM, Frintner MP, Tanner JL, Stein MT. What do families want from well-child care? Including parents in the rethinking discussion. *Pediatrics.* 2009;124(3):858–865

94. Fisher PA, Gunnar MR, Dozier M, Bruce J, Pears KC. Effects of therapeutic interventions for foster children on behavioral problems, caregiver attachment, and stress regulatory neural systems. *Ann N Y Acad Sci.* 2006;1094:215–225

95. Mercy JA, Saul J. Creating a healthier future through early interventions for children. *JAMA.* 2009;301(21):2262–2264

96. Middlebrooks JS, Audage NC. The effects of childhood stress on health across the lifespan. Available at: www.cdc.gov/ncipc/pub-res/pdf/Childhood_Stress.pdf. Accessed July 20, 2009

97. Earls MF, ; Committee on Psychosocial Aspects of Child and Family Health; American Academy of Pediatrics. Incorporating recognition and management of perinatal and postpartum depression into pediatric practice. *Pediatrics.* 2010;126(5):1032–1039

98. Center on the Developing Child at Harvard University. Maternal depression can undermine the development of young children: working paper #8. Available at: www.developingchild.harvard.edu. Accessed March 8, 2011

99. Shonkoff J. Protecting brains, not simply stimulating minds. *Science.* 2011;333(6045):982–983

SECTION 3
Depression and Bipolar Disorder

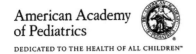

American Academy of Pediatrics
DEDICATED TO THE HEALTH OF ALL CHILDREN™

Guidance for the Clinician in
Rendering Pediatric Care

CLINICAL REPORT

Collaborative Role of the Pediatrician in the Diagnosis and Management of Bipolar Disorder in Adolescents

Benjamin N. Shain, MD, PhD and COMMITTEE ON ADOLESCENCE

KEY WORDS
adolescent bipolar disorder, interview guidelines, psychiatric diagnosis, psychotropic medication, collaboration

ABBREVIATIONS
ADHD—attention-deficit/hyperactivity disorder
DSM-IV-TR—*Diagnostic and Statistical Manual of Mental Disorders, Fourth Edition, Text Revision*
FDA—US Food and Drug Administration
OCD—obsessive-compulsive disorder
SMD—severe mood dysregulation

The guidance in this report does not indicate an exclusive course of treatment or serve as a standard of medical care. Variations, taking into account individual circumstances, may be appropriate.

www.pediatrics.org/cgi/doi/10.1542/peds.2012-2756

doi:10.1542/peds.2012-2756

All clinical reports from the American Academy of Pediatrics automatically expire 5 years after publication unless reaffirmed, revised, or retired at or before that time.

PEDIATRICS (ISSN Numbers: Print, 0031-4005; Online, 1098-4275).

abstract

Despite the complexity of diagnosis and management, pediatricians have an important collaborative role in referring and partnering in the management of adolescents with bipolar disorder. This report presents the classification of bipolar disorder as well as interviewing and diagnostic guidelines. Treatment options are described, particularly focusing on medication management and rationale for the common practice of multiple, simultaneous medications. Medication adverse effects may be problematic and better managed with collaboration between mental health professionals and pediatricians. Case examples illustrate a number of common diagnostic and management issues. *Pediatrics* 2012;130:e1725–e1742

Pediatricians are faced with increasing numbers of patients diagnosed with bipolar disorder and taking multiple psychotropic medications. In addition, pediatricians may be seeing these patients long before they are diagnosed and treated by a child and adolescent psychiatrist or other mental health professional. Pediatric bipolar disorder, once thought to be rare in adolescents and nearly nonexistent in younger children, has been diagnosed increasingly over the past decade.[1–3] In 2004, bipolar disorder accounted for 26% of primary discharge diagnoses among psychiatrically hospitalized adolescents in the United States.[3] Bipolar spectrum disorders,[4] encompassing the several types of bipolar disorder, have an estimated prevalence of 4% of children and adolescents in the general population.[5] The diagnosis remains controversial, and there has been a shift in how the diagnosis has been defined in youth.[1]

Associated impairments may include severe depression, high risk of suicide, psychosis, impulsive and dangerous behaviors, social and cognitive deficits, and frequent comorbidity with other psychiatric disorders, including substance use disorders, attention-deficit/hyperactivity disorder (ADHD), anxiety disorders, oppositional defiant disorder, and conduct disorder. Insight is frequently diminished, with youth vehemently blaming others for their difficulties and having little recognition of their own disruptive symptoms.[1] Management of these youth is additionally complicated by medication limitations, including troublesome adverse effects, lack of full response and the resultant common prescription of multiple medications, and incomplete prevention of relapse.[1] Not surprisingly, poor adherence to prescribed dosing is common.[6]

This report is not expected to give general pediatricians the tools necessary to diagnose and manage these complex cases independently. Some specific techniques are described with the intent of facilitating partnerships between pediatricians and child and adolescent psychiatrists and other mental health professionals. Additional goals include improved understanding of diagnosis and treatment; earlier referral of new, suspected cases, and patients with symptom relapse or worsening; and assistance in recognizing and managing medication adverse effects.

The focus of this report is diagnosis and management of adolescents with bipolar disorder. Children are mentioned as well when the subject matter applies to them.

CLASSIFICATION

The Diagnostic and Statistical Manual of Mental Disorders, Fourth Edition, Text Revision (DSM-IV-TR)[7] describes 4 types of bipolar disorders, all without age limitations: bipolar I disorder, bipolar II disorder, cyclothymic disorder, and bipolar disorder not otherwise specified. Manic symptoms are the key feature of these diagnoses; Tables 1, 2, and 3 provide criteria for mania, hypomania, and mixed episodes.[7] A key criterion is duration: the minimum duration for mania and mixed episodes is 7 days and for hypomania is 4 days.

Bipolar I Disorder

Bipolar I disorder is the "classic" form of the disorder and requires a current or past manic or mixed episode. At any given time, the patient may be in a manic, hypomanic, mixed, or major depressive episode or may have fully or partially recovered from the last mood episode. Notably, this is a historical diagnosis because the patient may be in any current mood state and

TABLE 1 Diagnostic Criteria for a Manic Episode

A. A distinct period of abnormally and persistently elevated, expansive, or irritable mood, lasting at least 1 wk (or for any duration if hospitalization is necessary)
B. During the period of mood disturbance, 3 (or more) of the following symptoms have persisted (4 if the mood is only irritable) and have been present to a significant degree
 1. Inflated self-esteem or grandiosity
 2. Decreased need for sleep (eg, feels rested after only 3 h)
 3. More talkative than usual or pressure to keep talking
 4. Flight of ideas or subjective experience that thoughts are racing
 5. Distractibility (ie, attention too easily drawn to unimportant or irrelevant external stimuli)
 6. Increase in goal-directed activity (either socially, at work or school, or sexually) or psychomotor agitation
 7. Excessive involvement in pleasurable activities that have a high potential for painful consequences (eg, engaging in unrestrained buying sprees, sexual indiscretions, or foolish business investments)
C. The symptoms do not meet criteria for a mixed episode
D. The mood disturbance is sufficiently severe to cause marked impairment in occupational functioning or in usual social activities or relationships with others or to necessitate hospitalization to prevent harm to self or others, or there are psychotic features
E. The symptoms are not due to the direct physiologic effects of a substance (eg, a drug of abuse, a medication, or other treatment) or a general medical condition (eg, hyperthyroidism)

Reprinted with permission from American Psychiatric Association. *Diagnostic and Statistical Manual of Mental Disorders, Fourth Edition, Text Revision (DSM-IV-TR).* Washington, DC: American Psychiatric Association; 2000.

still meet this criterion. History of a depressive episode is common but not required. Other criteria are that the mood symptoms cause significant distress or impaired functioning; are not better accounted for by schizoaffective disorder or superimposed on schizophrenia, schizophreniform disorder, delusional disorder, or psychotic disorder not otherwise specified; and are not the effect of a substance (including medications) or general medical condition.

TABLE 2 Diagnostic Criteria for a Hypomanic Episode

A. A distinct period of persistently elevated, expansive, or irritable mood, lasting throughout at least 4 d, that is clearly different from the usual nondepressed mood
B. Same as manic episode "B" (Table 1)
C. The episode is associated with an unequivocal change in functioning that is uncharacteristic of the person when not symptomatic
D. The disturbance in mood and the change in functioning are observable by others
E. The episode is not severe enough to cause marked impairment in social or occupational functioning or to necessitate hospitalization, and there are no psychotic features
F. Same as manic episode "E" (Table 1)

DSM-IV-TR asks for specification of certain patterns, including longitudinal course as with or without full interepisode recovery and/or rapid cycling. Rapid cycling is defined as more than 4 mood changes in a year. Researchers have defined patterns that commonly apply to pediatric bipolar disorder, including ultrarapid cycling, episodes lasting a few days to a few weeks, and ultradian cycling, variation occurring within a 24-hour period.[8,9]

Bipolar II Disorder

Depression typically is the major problem in bipolar II disorder. A current or at least 1 past major depressive episode is required, and the patient must have a current or past episode of hypomania with no manic or mixed episodes at any time. That is, currently or historically, a patient with bipolar I disorder has big "ups" (mania) and may or may not have "downs" (depression). A patient with bipolar II disorder has little "ups" (hypomania) plus big "downs" (major depression).

Cyclothymic Disorder

Cyclothymic disorder is characterized by relatively mild but chronic symptoms (hypomanic and depressive symptoms) that last at least 2 years (1 year with children and adolescents) before any full manic, mixed, or major depressive

TABLE 3 Diagnostic Criteria for a Mixed Episode

A. The criteria are met for both a manic episode and a major depressive episode (except for duration) nearly every day during at least a 1-wk period
B. Same as manic episode "D" (Table 1)
C. Same as manic episode "E" (Table 1)

episodes. These patients have little "ups" (hypomania) and little "downs" (dysthymia), but the disorder is chronic.

Bipolar Disorder Not Otherwise Specified

DSM-IV-TR describes the category of bipolar disorder not otherwise specified as including, "disorders with bipolar features that do not meet criteria for any specific bipolar disorder."[7] The American Academy of Child and Adolescent Psychiatry recommends using this diagnosis for youth with manic symptoms lasting hours to days or for those with chronic maniclike symptoms.[1] These youth may be significantly impaired and constitute the majority of those referred to mental health professionals.[10] Emerging evidence suggests that this disorder is on a continuum with bipolar I disorder,[11,12] and 45% of patients converted to bipolar I or bipolar II disorder at follow-up an average of 5 years later, particularly patients with a family history of bipolar disorder.[13]

Beyond DSM-IV-TR

Akiskal and Pinto described a bipolar spectrum in adults, ranging from bipolar I disorder to hyperthymic temperament.[4] The disorders and conditions on the spectrum share symptom characteristics that generally responded better to mood-stabilizing medication than to antidepressant medication.

Leibenluft et al suggested research diagnostic criteria for 3 clinical phenotypes of pediatric bipolar disorder: narrow, intermediate, and broad[14]

(Tables 4, 5, and 6). These criteria are included in this report to illustrate important features of diagnosis that are not present in DSM-IV-TR; they should not be construed as generally accepted by physicians or researchers. Narrow phenotype refers to a disorder in which, for at least 1 episode, full DSM-IV-TR criteria are met, including duration criteria, and elation and/or grandiosity also is present. Elation and grandiosity were argued by Geller et al[9] to be core bipolar features. Intermediate phenotype refers to patients with episodes that met full DSM-IV-TR criteria but lacked duration criteria (episodes too short) or had mania/hypomania that

TABLE 4 Research Criteria for the Narrow Phenotype of Juvenile Mania

A. Modification to the DSM-IV-TR criteria for manic episode
 a. The child must exhibit either elevated/expansive mood or grandiosity while also meeting the other DSM-IV-TR criteria for a (hypo)manic episode
B. Guidelines for applying the DSM-IV-TR criteria
 a. Episodes must meet the full duration criteria (ie, at least 7 d for mania and at least 4 d for hypomania) and be demarcated by switches from other mood states (depression, mixed state, euthymic).
 b. Episodes are characterized by a change from baseline in the patient's mood and, simultaneously, by the presence of the associated symptoms.
 c. Decreased need for sleep should be distinguished from insomnia.
 d. Poor judgment is not a diagnostic criterion unless it is in the context of "increased goal-directed activity" or "excessive involvement in pleasurable activities that have a high potential for painful consequences."

TABLE 5 Research Criteria for the Intermediate Phenotypes of Juvenile Mania

A. The child meets the criteria for the narrow phenotype except:
 a. (Hypo)manic episodes are 1 to 3 d in duration OR
 b. The (hypo)manic episodes include exclusively irritable, not elevated or expansive, mood, and DSM-IV-TR duration criteria are met

was irritable rather than euphoric. This phenotype still includes mood cycling as a required feature. Broad phenotype refers to a disorder characterized by chronic irritability and hyperarousal and does not include mood cycling. Compared with their peers, children and adolescents who have the broad phenotype show markedly increased reactivity to negative emotional stimuli. The broad phenotype has been referred to as severe mood dysregulation (SMD).

SMD among children 9 to 19 years of age has a lifetime prevalence of 3.3%, with most affected children having comorbid psychiatric disorders, most frequently disruptive behavior disorders (ADHD, conduct disorder, and oppositional defiant disorder).[15] Children with SMD were 7 times more likely to develop depression as young adults compared with those without SMD. Compared with children with narrow phenotype bipolar disorder, subjects with SMD had different psychopathological measures and were less likely to have parents with bipolar disorder,[16] suggesting that SMD is a disorder distinct from narrow phenotype bipolar disorder.

Mood diagnoses continue to evolve. The development web site for the forthcoming *Diagnostic and Statistical Manual of Mental Disorders, Fifth Edition,* lists an additional proposed mood diagnosis of "disruptive mood dysregulation disorder,"[17] characterized by severe recurrent temper outbursts in response to common stressors and similar to the broad phenotype. Characteristics for this diagnosis as well as others on the development Web site have been changing in response to public feedback. The *Diagnostic and Statistical Manual of Mental Disorders, Fifth Edition,* is expected to be published in May 2013. Because the final version may be fairly different, this report

TABLE 6 Research Criteria for Broad Phenotype of Juvenile Mania: Severe Mood and Behavioral Dysregulation

A. Inclusion criteria
  a. Age 7–17 y, with onset of symptoms before age 12
  b. Abnormal mood present at least half of the day most days and of sufficient severity to be noticeable by people in the child's environment
  c. Hyperarousal, as defined by at least 3 of the following symptoms: insomnia, agitation, distractibility, racing thoughts or flight of ideas, pressured speech, intrusiveness
  d. Compared with his/her peers, the child exhibits markedly increased reactivity to negative emotional stimuli that is manifest verbally or behaviorally
  e. The symptoms noted in the previous 3 items are currently present and have been present for at least 12 mo without any symptom-free periods exceeding 2 mo in duration
  f. The symptoms are severe in at least 1 setting and at least mild symptoms in a second setting
B. Exclusion criteria
  a. The individual exhibits any of the cardinal bipolar symptoms: elevated or expansive mood, grandiosity or inflated self-esteem, episodically decreased need for sleep
  b. The symptoms occur in distinct periods lasting more than 4 d
  c. The individual meets criteria for schizophrenia, schizoaffective illness, pervasive developmental disorder, or posttraumatic stress disorder
  d. The individual has met the criteria for substance abuse disorder in the past 3 mo
  e. IQ <80
  f. The symptoms are attributable to the direct physiologic effects of a drug of abuse or to a general medical or neurologic condition

does not include additional mention of diagnoses listed on the development web site.

The balance of this report refers to *DSM-IV-TR* as well as proposed research diagnoses. Pediatricians should be aware, however, of the changing classification of bipolar and related disorders.

INTERVIEWING FOR MANIA

The presence or history of mania of some sort is the determining factor for a diagnosis of bipolar disorder. Typi-cally, depressive symptoms are also present at some point in the illness and may be the major concern, but depression is not required to be present either currently or historically for a bipolar diagnosis. Depressed patients with bipolar disorder, par-ticularly those with the narrow or in-termediate phenotype, may require different medication from those with depression alone, so it is important for the pediatrician or mental health professional to attempt to make this differentiation before initiating phar-macotherapy.

Challenges in Diagnosing Mania

At a minimum, a full psychiatric evalu-ation should be performed to determine diagnosis.[1] A significant problem is that the diagnosis of mania typically is his-torical. Even with a patient who dem-onstrates manic symptoms during the interview, the interviewer still needs to determine that the symptoms represent a change, interfere with functioning, and are associated with less evident manic symptoms. Much more often, however, the patient presents as depressed or euthymic, leaving it for the interviewer to tease out groups of symptoms that occur together in episodes and are different from "normal adolescence." Adolescents and parents may tend to minimize these symptoms, wanting the trouble to be something less serious or, conversely, may tend to exaggerate, grasping at a bipolar diagnosis as a means of explaining a range of diffi-culties. Much of the public now has some education about bipolar disorder, often just enough to produce mis-conceptions about the diagnosis and associated symptoms, thus complicat-ing the job of the interviewer.

Simplifications

Without specific training in this area, the general pediatrician should not attempt initiation of treatment in newly diagnosed cases. The goal for the pediatrician in identification, there-fore, should be reasonable suspicion rather than diagnosis, followed by referral or seeking an appropriate mental health professional as partner. The balance of this section discusses several historical symptoms that may be considered red flags for the di-agnosis. The clear presence of any of these should be considered sufficient for reasonable suspicion.

Red Flag Symptoms

Rage Outbursts or Verbal or Physical Aggression

Rage is not a bipolar symptom per se but is common with adolescents ex-periencing episodic irritable mania or chronic severe mood dysregulation. In both cases, the adolescent is edgy and easily frustrated and provoked. Ques-tions the interviewer may ask include, "Do you lose your temper?" If so, the adolescent should be asked about frequency, duration, what happens, and what the triggers are (see Table 7 for a summary of examples of in-terview questions).

Episodes of Requiring Little Sleep

Requiring little sleep needs to be distinguished from going to bed late and getting up late and from receiving less sleep and consequently being tired the next day. Staying up late for 1 night during a sleepover or for a concert also does not count. Ado-lescents with this symptom have the experience of having high energy, receiving at least 2 hours less sleep per night, and remaining full of en-ergy often after several nights of this.[18] Questions include, "Do you ever have nights when you have lots of energy, do not need to sleep much, and do lots of things?" If so, "Are you tired the next day?"

TABLE 7 Examples of Interview Questions

Symptom	Question examples
Rage outbursts	"Do you lose your temper?" If so, ask about frequency, duration, what happens, what the triggers are.
Episodes of requiring little sleep	"Do you ever have nights when you have lots of energy, do not need to sleep much, and do lots of things?" If so, "Are you tired the next day?"
Spontaneous mood shifts	"Do you find yourself suddenly angry or extremely happy for no apparent reason?" If so, ask about frequency and duration of the moods.
Running away, sneaking out at night, spending money, hypersexuality	"Have you even run away or snuck out of the house at night?" "Do you have time when you spend a lot of money or when you feel that you cannot control your sexual urges?"
Grandiosity	"Do you have times when you feel that nothing can happen to you?" "Do you have times when you greatly overestimate your talents or abilities?"
Agitation or mania with antidepressant	"Have you ever taken medication for depression?" If so, "Did you have any side effects?" "Did you ever become very edgy or much more happy or angry than is typical for you?"

Spontaneous Mood Shifts

The adolescent experiences sudden mood shifts between euthymic, giddy, depressed, or angry, with no evident circumstantial trigger. The giddy, depressed, or angry mood state should significantly interfere with functioning, such as making concentration in school or appropriate behavior with friends much more difficult. A mood shift may happen multiple times per day. Questions include, "Do you find yourself suddenly angry or extremely happy for no apparent reason?" If so, ask about frequency and duration of the moods.

Running Away, Sneaking Out at Night, Spending Money, Hypersexuality

These activities may be categorized as "excessive involvement in pleasurable activities that have a high potential for painful consequences" (Table 1).[7] Running away also may be an example of an impulsive activity related to severe irritability. Questions include, "Have you ever run away or snuck out of the house at night?" "Do you have times when you spend a lot of money or when you feel that you cannot control your sexual urges?"

Grandiosity

Grandiosity is a grossly inflated belief in oneself having special talents or abilities, such as never being in danger regardless of the activity or being the best at a certain sport, or endless talk about a real talent. This must be a change from baseline and does not include a consistent picture of boastfulness or failure to appreciate consequences. Questions include, "Do you have times when you feel that nothing can happen to you?" "Do you have times when you greatly overestimate your talents or abilities?"

Agitation or Mania With Antidepressant

Adverse effects for a patient under the influence of antidepressant medication may be edginess, agitation, or less commonly, frank mania. By definition, a cluster of manic symptoms resulting from a medication or substance is not mania. It is, however, a risk factor for mania either continuing once the medication is withdrawn or mania at another time. Questions include, "Have you ever taken medication for depression?" If so, "Did you have any side effects?" "Did you ever become

very edgy or much more happy or angry than is typical for you?"

Any or all of these symptoms may be present currently, recently, or in the more distant past.

TREATMENT

Psychotherapy

Psychotherapeutic interventions are an important component of an overall treatment plan.[1] Interventions should be targeted to the following areas.

Psychoeducation

Information is provided to patient and family on the illness, treatment options, impact on functioning, and heritability. Relapse prevention typically is an important issue. Education is provided regarding importance of treatment adherence, avoidance of precipitating factors, and early recognition of symptoms. The illness may result in a dramatic tendency to blame others and minimize one's own symptoms and limitations, making engagement in the treatment plan difficult. For some individuals and families, education regarding relapse prevention is the key intervention.

Individual Psychotherapy

Cognitive-behavioral psychotherapy and interpersonal therapy support emotional and cognitive development, coping, and symptom monitoring.

Social and Family Functioning

Interventions aimed at communication and problem solving are needed to address disruptions in family and social relationships.

Academic and Occupational Functioning

Educational planning, specialized educational programs, and occupational training and support may be needed to address disruption of functioning in school or work from ongoing or intermittent symptoms.

Treatment of Comorbidities

Psychosocial interventions should be aimed at treatment of pre- or coexisting substance abuse disorders, behavioral disorders, anxiety disorders, learning problems, and confounding social issues.

Inpatient Psychiatric Hospitalization

Inpatient care typically is aimed at preventing imminent harm to self and others as well as allowing for treatment that could not be accomplished in a less restrictive setting.[19] A common reason for admission is suicidality, including suicidal ideation or a recent attempt. To be at high risk of suicide, the patient need not be thinking of suicide at the time of admission. Mood and behavior may have considerable day-to-day or even minute-to-minute variation; therefore, judgment as to safety should be based on recent thoughts, moods, and behaviors rather than just the current ones and on near-future projection on the basis of possible and sudden occurrence of common adolescent stressors. For example, in an adolescent with recent suicidal behavior and a history of grossly overreacting to negative circumstances, a romantic breakup could be lethal.

Other common reasons for psychiatric hospitalization for harm prevention are recent episodes of severe rage, agitation, or aggression attributable to mood symptoms or manic symptoms accompanied by severe impulsivity in areas that could inadvertently result in self-harm, such as running away or sexual activity with multiple partners. Patients with florid mania or acute psychosis typically require hospitalization even in the absence of overtly dangerous behaviors or ideation be-

cause of the high unpredictability of the behavior of afflicted individuals as well as difficulty with treatment adherence at a time when vigorous treatment is indicated.

Partial hospitalization[20] or hospital day treatment is used as a less restrictive, step-down treatment from inpatient care or as step-up treatment from mental health office services. Partial hospitalization does not afford the 24-hour monitoring and harm prevention provided with inpatient services but is less disruptive to the patient's life, less expensive, and gives the patient and family more responsibility for the patient's care while still providing intensive psychotherapeutic and medical management.

Residential treatment[21] is longer-term, 24-hour-a-day care in a less intensive, typically nonhospital setting, and may be a month to a year or more in duration. Residential care is designed for patients who cannot be safely managed otherwise despite adequate treatment or who have symptoms that require long-term behavioral intervention to effect improvement.

Psychopharmacology

Medication management is an important component of treatment of youth with bipolar disorder and is the primary treatment in cases of well-defined mania.[1,5] The primary medications used to treat patients with bipolar disorder are mood stabilizers, such as lithium; certain anticonvulsant medications, including divalproex, lamotrigine, carbamazepine, oxcarbazepine, gabapentin, and topiramate; and atypical antipsychotics, including aripiprazole, olanzapine, quetiapine, risperidone, ziprasidone, paliperidone, clozapine, asenapine, and iloperidone. Adjunctive medications include antidepressant medications and "typical" antipsychotics, as well as medications for ADHD, anxiety, and insomnia; more

information is available from the American Academy of Child and Adolescent practice parameters.[1,22–25]

The American Academy of Child and Adolescent Psychiatry[1] recommends basing the medication choice on the following: evidence of efficacy, phase of illness, type of presentation (eg, with psychotic symptoms), safety and adverse effect profile, history of medication response, and patient or family preference. Medication combinations are common, with some patients on 5 or more drugs. See Kowatch et al[5] for a suggested prescribing algorithm.

Efficacy Studies

Currently, lithium, aripiprazole, risperidone, olanzapine, and quetiapine are approved by the US Food and Drug Administration (FDA) for use in adolescents with bipolar disorder (Table 8).[26] In addition, divalproex, lamotrigine, carbamazepine, oxcarbazepine, gabapentin, and topiramate have nonmental health pediatric indications, and divalproex, lamotrigine, ziprasidone, and asenapine have indications for treatment of adults with bipolar disorder. Published studies have had mixed results (Tables 9, 10, and 11). Not all studies are available, because pharmaceutical companies are not required to publish their studies even when submitted to the FDA as part of an application for an indication. Lithium, aripiprazole, and olanzapine showed efficacy in published, double-blind, placebo-controlled studies, with open-label, chart review, and comparison studies giving support for use of divalproex, lamotrigine, clozapine, risperidone, quetiapine, and carbamazepine. Notably, divalproex and oxcarbazepine each failed to show efficacy in a double-blind, placebo-controlled study, but given the heterogeneity of this disorder, 1 negative study is not conclusive. Divalproex, lamotrigine, lithium, aripiprazole,

TABLE 8 FDA Indications for Oral Formulations of Mood Stabilizers and Atypical Antipsychotics

Medication	Bipolar disorder	Schizophrenia	Irritability associated with autism	Nonmental health	All adult mental health
Mood stabilizer					
Lithium (Eskalith)	Mania, ages 12–17				Mania
Divalproex (Depakote)				Seizures, ages 0–17	Mania
Lamotrigine (Lamictal)				Seizures, ages 2–17	Bipolar maintenance
Carbamazepine (Tegretol)				Seizures, ages 0–17; trigeminal neuralgia	
Oxcarbazepine (Trileptal)				Seizures, ages 2–17	
Gabapentin (Neurontin)				Seizures, ages 3–17	
Topiramate (Topamax)				Seizures, ages 2–17	
Atypical antipsychotics					
Aripiprazole (Abilify)	Manic and mixed episodes, ages 10–17	Ages 13–17	Ages 6–17		Bipolar mania, schizophrenia, adjunctive for major depression
Risperidone (Risperdal)	Manic and mixed episodes, ages 10–17	Ages 13–17	Ages 5–16		Schizophrenia, bipolar manic and mixed episodes
Olanzapine (Zyprexa)	Manic and mixed episodes, ages 13–17	Ages 13–17			Schizophrenia, bipolar manic and mixed episodes, bipolar and resistant depression (in combination with fluoxetine)
Quetiapine (Seroquel)	Manic episodes, ages 10–17	Ages 13–17			Schizophrenia, bipolar mania, bipolar depression
Ziprasidone (Geodon)					Schizophrenia, bipolar manic and mixed episodes, bipolar maintenance
Paliperidone (Invega)					Schizophrenia, schizoaffective disorder
Clozapine (Clozaril)					Schizophrenia, schizoaffective disorder
Asenapine (Saphris)					Schizophrenia, bipolar manic and mixed episodes
Iloperidone (Fanapt)					Schizophrenia
Lurasidone (Latuda)					Schizophrenia

quetiapine, risperidone, and topiramate have shown efficacy in medication combination studies. Kowatch et al[27] found a medication combination response rate of 80% among patients who did not respond to monotherapy with a mood stabilizer.

Adverse Effects

Mood stabilizer (Table 12)[5] and atypical antipsychotic (Table 13)[28,29] medications have a variety of adverse effects, interactions, and safety concerns. Pediatricians probably need to be most aware of weight gain and metabolic effects common with the atypical antipsychotics, although weight gain is also commonly associated with valproate and, to a lesser extent, lithium. Prescription of atypical antipsychotics in youth for bipolar disorder as well as for psychosis, disruptive behavior disorders, and other mood disorders has increased drastically in recent years.[30] Children and adolescents may be more vulnerable than adults to weight gain from these medications and, thus, likely to be at higher risk of glucose and lipid abnormalities.[31] Weight management potentially can be addressed with suggestions of diet and exercise as well as changing the dose and/or type of medication. Use of metformin may be of some help.[32,33] Stable patients should be seen by their pediatrician every 4 to 6 months, with more frequent visits when there are active adverse effects, interactions, or safety issues.

The American Diabetes Association[34] published a protocol for use in monitoring for weight gain and metabolic changes in adults treated with atypical antipsychotics, including obtaining personal and family history of related disorders, determining weight and height, determining waist circumference, taking blood pressure, and measuring fasting plasma glucose and fasting lipid profile. Weight should

TABLE 9 Published Studies of Efficacy of Mood Stabilizers With Pediatric Bipolar Disorder[a]

Medication	Study	Ages	Type	Results	Comments
Divalproex	Wagner et al (2002)[41]	7–19; n = 40	Open-label trial	Response rate 61% with manic symptoms	Manic, mixed, or hypomanic
Divalproex	Henry et al (2003)[42]	4–18; n = 15	Records review	Response rate 53% after 1 y	Divalproex alone and as add-on
Divalproex	Wagner et al (2009)[43]	10–17; n = 150	Double-blind	No significant difference from placebo	Manic or mixed
Lamotrigine	Chang et al (2006)[44]	12–17; n = 20	Open-label trial	Significant decreases in depression, mania, and aggression	Lamotrigine alone and in combination with other medication
Lamotrigine	Pavuluri et al (2009)[45]	8–18; n = 46	Open-label trial	Response rate 72% with manic symptoms and 82% with depressive symptoms	Monotherapy
Lithium	Strober et al (1990)[46]	13–17, n = 37	Naturalistic prospective follow-up	Relapse rate 3 times higher when lithium discontinued	Lithium alone and in combination with other medication
Lithium	Geller et al (1998)[47]	12–18; n = 25	Double-blind	Significant response rate difference, 46% versus 8% of placebo group	Bipolar disorder with secondary substance dependence
Lithium	Kafantaris et al (2003)[48]	12–18; n = 100	Open-label trial	Response rate 63% with manic symptoms	Acute mania
Lithium	Kafantaris, et al (2004)[49]	12–18; n = 40	Double-blind discontinuation	No significant difference from placebo	Mania with or without psychosis or aggression
Lithium	Patel et al (2006)[50]	12–18; n = 27	Open-label trial	Response rate 48% with depressive symptoms	Acute bipolar depression
Oxcarbazepine	Wagner et al (2006)[51]	7–18; n = 116	Double-blind	No significant difference from placebo	Manic or mixed
Topiramate	Del Bello et al (2002)[52]	5–20; n = 26	Chart review	Response rate 73% for mania and 62% for overall illness	Outpatient with acute manic, mixed, or depressive episode; adjunctive or monotherapy
Topiramate	Barzman et al (2005)[53]	7–20; n = 25	Chart review	Response rate 64%	Hospitalized with acute manic, mixed, or depressive episode; adjunctive or monotherapy
Topiramate	DelBello, et al (2005)[54]	6–17; n = 56	Double-blind	Mixed results	Inconclusive; study stopped early when early adult studies failed to show efficacy

[a] Includes only the most recent studies of divalproex and lithium.

TABLE 10 Published Studies of Efficacy of Atypical Antipsychotics for Pediatric Bipolar Disorder

Medication	Study	Ages	Type	Results	Comments
Aripiprazole	Barzman et al (2004)[55]	5–19; n = 30	Chart review	Response rate 67%	Bipolar or schizoaffective; adjunctive or monotherapy
Aripiprazole	Biederman et al (2005)[56]	4–17; n = 41	Records review	71% improvement of manic symptoms	Aripiprazole alone and as add-on
Aripiprazole	Biederman et al (2007)[57]	6–17; n = 19	Open-label trial	Significant improvement	Mania
Aripiprazole	Tramontina et al (2007)[58]	8–17; n = 10	Open-label trial	Significant improvement	Comorbid bipolar and ADHD; improved both mania and ADHD symptoms
Aripiprazole	Findling et al (2009)[59]	10–17; n = 296	Double-blind	Significant response rate difference, 44% (10 mg), 64% (30 mg), 26% (placebo)	Manic or mixed
Aripiprazole	Tramontina et al (2009)[60]	8–17; n = 43	Double-blind	Significant response rate difference, 89% vs 52% of placebo group	Manic or mixed comorbid with ADHD
Clozapine	Masi et al (2002)[61]	12–17; n = 10	Open-label trial	Significant improvement	Severe treatment-resistant manic or mixed
Olanzapine	Frazier et al (2001)[62]	5–14; n = 23	Open-label trial	Response rate 61%	Acute mania
Olanzapine	Tohen et al (2007)[63]	13–17; n = 161	Double-blind	Significant response rate difference, 45% vs 19% of placebo group	Acute manic or mixed
Olanzapine	Joshi et al (2010)[64]	4–17; n = 52	Open-label trial; secondary analysis of 2 trials	Significantly less antimanic response with comorbid OCD	Bipolar disorder
Quetiapine	Del Bello et al (2007)[65]	12–18; n = 20	Single-blind, open label	Response rate 87% with mood symptoms	Patients at high risk for bipolar I
Quetiapine	Del Bello et al (2009)[66]	12–18; n = 32	Double-blind	No significant difference from placebo	Bipolar depression
Quetiapine	Scheffer et al (2010)[67]	6–16; n = 75	Open-label trial	94% much improved at 8 wk; rapid loading tolerated well	Bipolar disorder
Risperidone	Frazier et al (1999)[68]	4–17; n = 28	Records review	Response rate 82% with manic and aggressive symptoms	Mixed or hypomanic
Risperidone	Biederman et al (2005)[69]	6–17; n = 30	Open-label trial	Response rate 70% with manic symptoms	Manic, mixed, or hypomanic
Risperidone	Haas et al (2009)[70]	10–17; n = 169	Double-blind	Significant response rate difference, 59% (0.5–2.5 mg), 63% (3–6 mg), 26% (placebo)	Acute manic or mixed
Risperidone	Carlson et al (2010)[71]	5–12; n = 151	Chart review	Reduced duration and rages	Hospitalized children with possible bipolar disorder
Risperidone	Krieger et al (2011)[72]	7–17; n = 21	Open-label trial	Significant reduction of irritability, depression, ADHD symptoms, and global functioning	Severe mood dysregulation
Ziprasidone	Biederman et al (2007)[73]	6–17; n = 21	Open-label trial	Response rate 71% with manic symptoms	Mania

be reassessed monthly for 3 months and then quarterly. Lipids and fasting plasma glucose may be measured after 3 months and then every 6 months. There is no a protocol currently for children and adolescents.[28]

When medications are prescribed by a physician other than the pediatrician, the decision of which physician monitors the patient's weight and metabolic consequences of the medication may be a matter of practicality. Certain measurements, such as vital signs, height, weight, and waist size, are easily and routinely obtained in a pediatrician's office but much more difficult to obtain in a psychiatrist's office, because it typically is not set up with the proper equipment and usually does not have a nurse on staff. In addition, at times, the patients may perceive these measurements to be physically intrusive when obtained by the psychiatrist. The pediatrician should collaborate with the prescribing physician in monitoring for and managing these medication adverse effects.

Other Medication Caution

A number of medications should be used with care because they may increase mood cycling (Table 14).[18] In particular, antidepressant medications are commonly prescribed, because bipolar disorder usually includes depression, and depression is the most common reason for the initial referral for treatment. Antidepressant induction of mania may be less frequent than once thought,[35] but common practice is to start with a mood stabilizer or atypical antipsychotic (or combination) and add an antidepressant to the mix only if there is insufficient response.

Few studies have addressed the use of mood stabilizers and atypical antipsychotics with pediatric bipolar depression. Lithium and lamotrigine

TABLE 11 Published Comparison Studies of Efficacy of Mood Stabilizers and Atypical Antipsychotics With Pediatric Bipolar Disorder

Medication	Study	Ages	Type	Results	Comments
Lithium, Divalproex, Carbamazepine	Kowatch et al (2000)[74]	6–18; n = 42	Open-label trial	Large effect size for all 3 medications; response rate with manic symptoms of divalproex 53%, lithium 38%, and carbamazepine 38%	Manic or mixed
Quetiapine, Divalproex	Del Bello et al (2002)[75]	12–18; n = 30	Double-blind	Significant response rate difference, 87% vs 53% of placebo group	Manic or mixed; divalproex plus quetiapine versus divalproex plus placebo
Risperidone, Lithium, Divalproex	Pavuluri et al (2004)[76]	5–18; n = 37	Open-label trial	Response rate 80% for risperidone plus divalproex and 82% for risperidone plus lithium	Manic or mixed
Lithium, Divalproex	Findling et al (2005)[77]	5–17; n = 60	Double-blind; no placebo group	No significant difference between the groups	Stabilized on lithium plus divalproex and then compared maintenance monotherapy with one or the other
Quetiapine, Divalproex	Del Bello et al (2006)[78]	12–18; n = 50	Double-blind, no placebo group	Significant improvement in both groups; no significant difference in amount of improvement but significantly faster improvement in quetiapine group	Manic or mixed; compared quetiapine and divalproex
Risperidone, Divalproex	MacMillan et al (2008)[79]	5–14; n = 28	Records review	Risperidone group showed significantly faster decrease of symptoms than divalproex group	More wt gain with risperidone
Risperidone, Divalproex	Pavuluri et al (2010)[80]	8–18; n = 66	Double-blind, no placebo group	More rapid improvement in risperidone group but no difference in final scores	No significant wt gain in either group; better retention of subjects in risperidone group

have shown efficacy in open-label trials (Table 9) and quetiapine was not significantly better than placebo (Table 10).

Medication Combinations

Adolescents with bipolar disorder may have a range of symptoms within the disorder, including symptoms of mania or hypomania, depression, and psychosis, and commonly have comorbidities with a variety of other psychiatric disorders, including ADHD, generalized anxiety disorder, obsessive-compulsive disorder (OCD), posttraumatic stress disorder, and others.[5] These comorbidities can lead to a complexity of symptoms and often difficult choices for medication management. As a result, use of multiple medications is common in treating adolescents with bipolar disorder, who often are prescribed 2 to 5, or more, simultaneous medications. Even in a research setting using algorithms designed to limit the number of medications, only 28% of patients were able to remain on monotherapy for >6 months.[36]

Reasons for combining medications include the following:

- Partial response. A group of symptoms, such as expansive mood, grandiosity, and pleasure-seeking behaviors, may have improved with a particular medication (with adequate dose and time), but symptoms continue sufficiently to cause distress and/or impairment of functioning. A second (or sometimes third) medication is then added as an "augmentation agent" to improve response. Another type of partial response is when some symptoms improve and others do not (eg, symptoms of mania improve but the patient still suffers from intermittent or persistent depression).

- Target specific symptom. There may be a particular troublesome and/or easily treated symptom, such as

TABLE 12 Adverse Effects and Possible Monitoring of Mood Stabilizers

Medication	Summary of adverse effects	Suggested monitoring
Lithium	Reduced renal function, hypothyroidism, nausea, diarrhea, abdominal distress, sedation, tremor, polyuria, wt gain, acne, cardiac conduction problems, hypoparathyroidism	Baseline: serum electrolytes, creatinine, BUN, calcium, CBC count, TFTs, EKG, pregnancy test (sexually active female patients)
	Wt gain may be additive when combined with an atypical antipsychotic[28]	Ongoing: lithium level, renal function, thyroid function, calcium
	Toxic levels may produce confusion, ataxia, dysarthria, seizures, coma, death	
Divalproex	Polycystic ovaries, nausea, increased appetite, wt gain, sedation, thrombocytopenia, hair loss, tremor, vomiting, rare pancreatitis or liver failure	Baseline: height and wt, pregnancy test (sexually active female patients), liver function tests, CBC
	Wt gain may be additive when combined with an atypical antipsychotic[28]	Every 6 mo: divalproex level, liver function tests, CBC
Carbamazepine	Multiple medication interactions (decrease or increase the other medication levels including oral contraceptive failure), sedation, ataxia, dizziness, blurred vision, nausea, vomiting, aplastic anemia, hyponatremia, Stevens-Johnson	Baseline: CBC Every 6 mo: carbamazepine level, CBC
Lamotrigine	Severe cutaneous reactions (risk 3 times greater <16), dizziness, tremor, sedation, asthenia, headache, interactions with oral contraceptives; case reports of leucopenia, agranulocytosis, hepatic failure, multiorgan failure	Baseline: CBC and liver function tests
Oxcarbazepine	Hyponatremia, oral contraceptive failure, cutaneous reactions, cognitive symptoms, sedation, coordination difficulties, nausea, vomiting, asthenia, headache, dizziness[26]	Baseline and periodic: serum sodium
Gabapentin	Mostly benign; most common are sedation, dizziness, tremor, headache, ataxia, fatigue, wt gain	None
Topiramate	Oral contraceptive failure, sedation, fatigue, impaired concentration, psychomotor slowing, word-finding difficulties, nephrolithiasis	Baseline and periodic: serum bicarbonate

BUN, blood urea nitrogen; CBC, complete blood cell (count); EKG, electrocardiogram; TFT, thyroid function test.

insomnia, that is treated with a medication just for that symptom.

- Cross-taper. When a medication is thought to be working poorly or not at all, a decision may be to replace it with another medication. The cleanest way to do so is to taper down the dose of the first medication, wait for a period of time for medication "wash out," and then start the second medication at a low dose with subsequent appropriate increases. This approach may be problematic at times if, in retrospect, the first medication is discovered to have been more effective than previously thought, but regardless, the patient goes longer without an effective medication. The likelihood of a relapse is higher, and depending on the patient's history, relapse may be debilitating or life-threatening or may interfere with a planned transition, such as starting school or leaving the hospital. The way to decrease the likelihood of relapse and treat current symptoms more quickly is to "cross-taper," for example, starting the second medication with the full dose of the first medication, and then, if the second medication is tolerated and appears to be adding incremental benefit, the second medication gradually is increased while the first medication is decreased.

- Treat comorbid disorders. Additional medications may be used to treat symptoms of comorbid disorders, such as inattentiveness with ADHD or worrying with an anxiety disorder.

PRESCRIBING GUIDELINES

The process of medicating is stepwise, with few patients having a full, lasting response to all symptoms with the first dose of the first medication. Each step is the opportunity for the physician to make a change (add or stop a medication or change a dose) or continue the current regimen as is (eg, the patient is stable or improving or needs a longer amount of time for a medication to work or for an adverse effect to resolve). Each patient becomes an individual study, with the result sometimes being good efficacy with odd-appearing or counterintuitive medication combinations. A number of issues may guide the decision at each step:

- **One Change at a Time.** With multiple medications, knowing which medication is causing positive effects or adverse effects may be difficult. Making 1 change at a time and then observing the effect can help deal with this problem, although this guideline may be discontinued at times for the sake of urgency or when there is little expected overlap in effects and

TABLE 13 Adverse Effects and Possible Monitoring of Atypical Antipsychotics

Adverse effect	Time course	Suggested monitoring	Medications most likely to cause
Anticholinergic	Early		Clozapine, olanzapine
Acute parkinsonism	Early	During titration, at 3 mo and annually	Paliperidone, risperidone
Akathisia	Early/intermediate	During titration, at 3 mo and annually	Aripiprazole
Cardiovascular events	Not known	EKG at baseline if taking ziprasidone or clozapine and during titration if taking ziprasidone	
Diabetes	Late	Fasting blood glucose at 3 mo and then every 6 mo	Clozapine, olanzapine (but problem for all)
Increased lipids	Early?	Lipids at 3 mo and then every 6 mo	Clozapine, olanzapine (but problem for all)
Neutropenia	Most likely within first 6 mo	Clozapine registry recommended CBC monitoring	Clozapine
Orthostasis	Early	Orthostatic blood pressure and pulse if symptomatic; blood pressure and pulse at 3 mo and annually	Clozapine, olanzapine, quetiapine
Increased prolactin and sexual dysfunction	Early	Sexual history during titration and then every 3 mo; prolactin level only if symptomatic	Paliperidone, risperidone, olanzapine
Decreased prolactin	Early	Prolactin level only if symptomatic	Aripiprazole
Increased QTc interval	Not known	EKG at baseline if taking ziprasidone or clozapine and during titration if taking ziprasidone	Ziprasidone
Sedation	Early	Each visit	Clozapine, olanzapine, quetiapine (but problem for all)
Seizures	During titration		Clozapine
Tardive dyskinesia	Late	At 3 mo and annually (abnormal involuntary movement scale)	Lower risk compared with first generation antipsychotics
Withdrawal dyskinesia	Early during fast switch	During titration	Aripiprazole, paliperidone
Wt gain	First 3–6 mo	Height, wt, BMI percentile, BMI z score each visit	All, but clozapine and olanzapine highest and aripiprazole and ziprasidone least
Other laboratories		Electrolytes, CBC, renal function test annually, and liver function tests at 3 mo and annually	

TABLE 14 Medications That May Increase Mood Cycling in Children and Adolescents

Antidepressants
   Tricyclic antidepressants
   Selective serotonin reuptake inhibitors
   Serotonin-norepinephrine reuptake inhibitors
Aminophylline
Oral or intravenous corticosteroids
Sympathomimetic amines (eg, pseudoephedrine)
Antibiotics (eg, clarithromycin, erythromycin, and
   amoxicillin)

adverse effects of medications in a particular combination. .

- **Important Cluster of Symptoms.** When a group of symptoms is causing severe impairment and distress, such as full-fledged ma-

nia or acute psychosis, it must be addressed first.

- **Treat the Most Troublesome Symptoms First.** A more common situation is that there is no group of symptoms that is overwhelming. In that case, first treat the group of symptoms that is causing the most distress or impairment. For example, moderate depression is treated before mild to moderate inattentiveness.

- **Opportunity to Reduce the Number of Medications That Eventually Will Be Needed.** A medication may be used that may not be the

best for any particular group of symptoms but has the potential to treat ≥2 groups of symptoms.

- **Manage an Adverse Effect.** Depending on the urgency of the need for clinical effect and the troublesomeness of the adverse effect, an adverse effect may temporarily halt the search for an effective regimen until it can be resolved or reduced to an acceptable level.

- **Treat a "Lynchpin" Symptom.** At times, a symptom seems to be the basis for other symptoms, for example, an anxious and inattentive adolescent who goes into a rage attempting to complete homework. As an alternative to using a medication that works to reduce rage, using a medication to reduce anxiety or to increase attentiveness may be at least as effective (of course, the prescriber may choose to do both to potentially increase the effect).

- **Preference for a Medication That Works Quickly.** At times, a medication is chosen over another one for a particular effect because it works quickly. The thinking is that if it then does not work, less time is lost in pursuing the other medication, thus increasing the chance of finding an effective medication in a given period of time.

An example that illustrates the use of several of these guidelines is a patient with insomnia in the context of depression. Choices for the first medication(s) include (1) a mood agent to treat the depression (the more impairing symptom) while waiting for the insomnia to resolve as the depression improves, (2) a hypnotic to treat the insomnia because the response is likely to be quick and the patient's mood may improve once he or she no longer is sleep deprived, (3) combination of a hypnotic with an optimal mood agent for this patient, or (4) a sedating mood agent that may treat both the depression and the insomnia. For a particular patient, these may all be reasonable options, or there may be other factors, such as treatment history, that favor one option over others.

CONCURRENT MEDICAL CONDITIONS

Scheffer and Linden[37] divided medical conditions concurrent with pediatric bipolar disorder into 4 types: (1) conditions related to bipolar disorder

or its treatment, (2) conditions that mimic mania, (3) conditions that occur more commonly in patients with bipolar disorder that appear unrelated to its treatment, and (4) conditions related to risk behaviors associated with bipolar disorder. The authors noted that little has been published specifically with regard to pediatric bipolar disorder and concurrent medical conditions, but a number of reports that focused on adults included pediatric subjects.

Tables 12 and 13 summarize medical adverse effects from medications commonly used to treat bipolar disorder. Pediatricians should familiarize themselves with these and monitor for them. Lithium treatment can result in hypothyroidism and, regardless of the cause, hypothyroidism can make bipolar disorder more difficult to treat.[37] Elevated prolactin levels, typically from certain atypical antipsychotics, are associated with low bone mass for chronologic age, sexual dysfunction, menstrual irregularities, gynecomastia, galactorrhea, and retrograde ejaculation. Cardiovascular disease[38] and type 2 diabetes mellitus[39] may be associated with the illness itself. Conditions that may mimic mania are listed in Table 15.[5,37] Unrelated conditions more common in patients with bipolar disorder[37] include migraine headaches, epilepsy, and at least in 1 large family, autosomal dominant medullary cystic kidney disease. Conditions associated with bipolar risk behaviors[37] include complications of substance use and abuse, sexually transmitted diseases, and traumatic brain injury.

CASE VIGNETTES

The following fictitious cases are conglomerates based on the authors' clinical experience and are designed to illustrate common diagnostic and treatment issues.

Case 1

Mary is a 16-year-old girl who presents for admission to psychiatry inpatient after sudden onset 1 week previously of euphoric and giddy mood, talking rapidly and jumping from topic to topic, and little sleep with almost none over the past 3 days. She has spent most of her time since then at her health club trying to "pick up" male patrons, a behavior very out of character for her. Before age 14, she was high achieving and well adjusted, earning mostly A's in school, socially active, and described by her parents as a "model daughter." At age 14, she broke up with a boyfriend and became severely depressed, responding after 2 months to a combination of sertraline and psychotherapy. She discontinued both treatments 4 months later because she had been doing well. She continued to do well until 1 year ago, when she developed an episode similar to the current one, but her behavior was controlled, and she was managed outside the hospital, responding after 2 weeks to a combination of lithium and psychotherapy. She had difficulty with moodiness and functioning in school for the next 6 months and again stopped the treatments. She then continued about the same until this current episode.

Mary is diagnosed with bipolar I disorder, current episode manic, severe, and without psychotic features. She has the narrow phenotype. She is restarted on lithium and also is started on quetiapine for sleeping, calming, and additional mood stabilization. Lithium is chosen because of her past response to this medication. Her psychiatrist decides to combine this with quetiapine immediately, despite treatment algorithms suggesting starting with monotherapy,[5,18] for 2 reasons: (1) previous treatment with lithium yielded a good acute response but only a partial response long-term, even before she stopped the medication and (2)

TABLE 15 Medical Conditions That May Mimic Mania

Hyperthyroidism
Closed or open head injury
Temporal lobe epilepsy
Multiple sclerosis
Systemic lupus erythematosus
Fetal alcohol spectrum disorder/alcohol-related neurodevelopmental disorder
Wilson disease
HIV
Lyme disease
Dementia
Fibromyalgia
Niemann-Pick disease
Familial leukoencephalopathy

lithium can easily take 1 week or more to be effective, and Mary needs something with more immediate effect for calming and sleeping.

Mary is in a relatively consistent (abnormal) mood state. The primary treatment goals are, therefore, to help her out of this state, return her to a euthymic mood, and prevent the next mood episode. If her current mood state were depression instead of mania, mood-stabilizing medication would still be the first choice, but often, antidepressant medication is cautiously added should the depression prove resistant to the mood stabilizing medication alone. The caution is related to the possibility that the antidepressant could make it easier for her to go into a manic episode, even when combined with the mood-stabilizing medication. In addition, during the time she is in a manic state, an antidepressant is generally not recommended.

Case 2

Charles is a 15-year-old boy who presents to the psychiatrist's office for his first mental health visit with the complaint of increasing, severe depression over the past month. He feels that the depression started 3 years ago when his parents divorced and he moved with his mother and siblings to a new city and new school.

Additional questions reveal that depression probably existed on and off for quite some time before the divorce. Furthermore, the depression is not continuous. Even over the past week, he reports having 1 or 2 days at a time of feeling great and "energized," spending most of the night playing an online game with little fatigue the next day, talking more, having racing thoughts, and having a more difficult time focusing on school work. He has other times, up to 2 days at a time, of being easily angered, punching a wall at times, ruminating about slights from peers and parents, and generally feeling "edgy."

Charles is diagnosed with bipolar disorder not otherwise specified and the intermediate phenotype. He does not meet duration criteria for mania (7 days) or hypomania (4 days). Key features are the spontaneous and frequent changes of mood symptoms, unrelated or only very loosely related to environmental circumstances, and the lack of distinct, continuous manic or hypomanic states for even 4 days.

Medication management for Charles is similar to that for Mary in case 1; the primary initial objective is mood stabilization with ≥1 mood stabilizers and/or atypical antipsychotics. A difference is that Charles's mood symptoms are not stable. He only has to wait a few days or less to switch to a different group of symptoms. Despite depression being the primary concern, antidepressants may make his condition worse by increasing the frequency or intensity of mood changes or undermining the effects of the mood-stabilizing medication. Even for treating the depression symptoms, the preference is typically to find more effective mood stabilizing medication rather than add an antidepressant. Exceptions are common, however, with the treatment of bipolar illness.

Cases 1 and 2 illustrate the findings of a recent study showing that in 90% of

cases the first mood episode in pediatric bipolar disorder is depression.[40]

Case 3

Dan is a 17-year-old boy who presents for psychiatric inpatient admission after damaging his father's car with a crow bar and threatening to kill his parents and then himself after parents took away his cell phone. The patient reports having had difficulty with temper outbursts for years. This is the worst such episode, but the patient commonly yells or leaves the house when upset and tends to overreact to his parents' attempts to set limits. Both patient and parents report that he does "fine" most of the time and just overreacts to frustration. He was diagnosed with ADHD in the third grade and has been on and off treatment for that (currently off). He has had mild to moderate depression at times but not recently. On interview, the patient reports that the incident with the car was "not a big deal" and says that he currently feels "fine," although he appears quite edgy and becomes frustrated with the interviewer for "asking too many questions."

The patient is diagnosed with mood disorder not otherwise specified and meets criteria for bipolar spectrum broad phenotype or severe mood dysregulation. He shows no evidence for mood cycling, except for the history of depression, but his mood changes quickly with minor provocation, and he is highly sensitive to frustrating circumstances.

Common practice is to treat the rage symptoms and edginess with mood stabilizers and/or atypical antipsychotics. Treatment of rage and edginess in this population has been poorly studied, but risperidone and aripiprazole are approved by the FDA for the treatment of irritability associated with autism (Table 8). With some patients, these symptoms may respond to ≥1 medications for depression, anxiety, or ADHD.

Case 4

Claire is a 13-year-old girl who presents to the psychiatrist's office because of daily episodes of rage, which have been present for years but increasing over the past year. She has the rage only at home and does well academically and socially. She denies any history of significant depression, although she does report a strong tendency to worry and has had this for most of her life. With further questioning, she reports multiple different ritualistic behaviors, such as needing to touch the doorframe in a certain way before going through it and needing to do household tasks in groups of 3. She becomes enraged when parents inadvertently interfere with her ability to complete a behavior.

Claire is diagnosed with OCD as well as generalized anxiety disorder. She does not have a mood disorder despite the rage outbursts. The rage would probably diminish with a mood stabilizer or atypical antipsychotic, but a better treatment is medication and psychotherapy for OCD and anxiety.

Case 5

George is a 14-year-old boy who presents to the pediatrician having recently moved from another state. According to his mother, he has been doing fairly well for the past 6 months and has been diagnosed with bipolar disorder and ADHD. He is currently taking lithium, methylphenidate, quetiapine, aripiprazole, sertraline, and clonazepam. He last saw his previous psychiatrist 2 months ago, and the mother requests a refill for his medications, because he does not have a psychiatrist currently. George's mother said that he has been in general good health but gained 40 pounds over the past year. George's mother attributes this to the medication. In addition to her routine for a new

patient visit, the pediatrician does the following:

- Asks more questions to confirm clinical stability, such as potential adverse effects of the medications and clinical course, including depression, suicidality, and behavioral problems.

- Asks about medication dosing adherence.

- Contacts the previous psychiatrist to confirm medications and doses, obtain history, and obtain the psychiatrist's opinion on recent stability.

- Orders laboratory studies, including lithium concentration 12 hours after last dose, electrolytes, thyroid studies, calcium, lipids, and glucose (a fasting glucose may be ordered later if the random one is abnormal).

- Performs physical examination, including vital signs, height, and weight, and calculates BMI percentile.

- Refers George to a local child and adolescent psychiatrist for ongoing mental health care and arranges to partner with the out-of-state psychiatrist for care in the meantime.

- Renews the current medications unless there is a compelling reason otherwise. Given 6 months of stability, a slow medication taper may be safe, but this should be conducted under psychiatric supervision. Not renewing the medications is dangerous, because it may precipitate a major relapse as well as withdrawal symptoms.

- Refers George to a dietitian, recommends an exercise program, and plans to work with the psychiatrist on adjusting medications to reduce weight.

If it were determined that George may not be stable in some respect, resources include phone consultations with the out-of-state psychiatrist (and the out-of-

state therapist, if there was one), urgent referral to a local child and adolescent psychiatrist, urgent referral to a local psychologist or other therapist for psychotherapy, and evaluation at a local hospital emergency department.

SUMMARY

Pediatricians have a collaborative role in diagnosis and management of adolescents with bipolar disorder, a common and often debilitating illness. Interviewing for current or past mania or hypomania, the defining feature of bipolar disorder, may be challenging but may be simplified by asking about red flag symptoms that, when present in the history, signal reasonable suspicion of bipolar disorder. In suspected or previously diagnosed cases of bipolar disorder, patients with current or recent symptoms or impairments should be referred for treatment. Pediatricians can actively monitor for and manage medication adverse effects, particularly weight gain, hyperlipidemia, and diabetes mellitus.

ADVICE FOR PEDIATRICIANS

1. Have some familiarity with diagnostic criteria and different types of bipolar disorder.

2. Maintain communication with child and adolescent psychiatrists and other mental health professionals.

3. Maintain familiarity with adverse effects and suggested monitoring protocols for mood-stabilizing and atypical antipsychotic medications.

4. Assist in monitoring for and managing medication adverse effects, particularly weight gain, hyperlipidemia, and diabetes mellitus.

5. Carefully and thoroughly document all recommendations, including referrals, medications prescribed, and instructions for observing and reporting adverse reactions.

LEAD AUTHOR

Benjamin Shain, MD, PhD

COMMITTEE ON ADOLESCENCE, 2011–2012

Paula K. Braverman, MD, Chairperson
William P. Adelman, MD
Cora C. Breuner, MD, MPH
David A. Levine, MD

Arik V. Marcell, MD
Pamela J. Murray, MD, MPH
Rebecca F. O'Brien, MD

LIAISONS

Loretta E. Gavin, PhD, MPH — *Centers for Disease Control and Prevention*
Rachel J. Miller, MD — *American College of Obstetricians and Gynecologists*

Hatim A. Omar, MD — *AAP Section on Adolescent Health*
Jorge L. Pinzon, MD — *Canadian Pediatric Society*
Benjamin Shain, MD, PhD — *American Academy of Child and Adolescent Psychiatry*

STAFF

Karen Smith
Mark Del Monte, JD

REFERENCES

1. American Academy of Child and Adolescent Psychiatry. Practice parameters for the assessment and treatment of children and adolescents with bipolar disorder. *J Am Acad Child Adolesc Psychiatry.* 2007;46(1):107–122

2. Carlson GA. Early onset bipolar disorder: clinical and research considerations. *J Clin Child Adolesc Psychol.* 2005;34(2):333–343

3. Blader JC, Carlson GA. Increased rates of bipolar disorder diagnoses among U.S. child, adolescent, and adult inpatients, 1996-2004. *Biol Psychiatry.* 2007;62(2):107–114

4. Akiskal HS, Pinto O. The evolving bipolar spectrum. Prototypes I, II, III, and IV. *Psychiatr Clin North Am.* 1999;22(3):517–534, vii

5. Kowatch RA, Fristad MA, Findling RL, eds. *Clinical Manual for Management of Bipolar Disorder in Children and Adolescents.* Washington, DC: American Psychiatric Publishing Inc; 2009

6. Drotar D, Greenley RN, Demeter CA, et al. Adherence to pharmacological treatment for juvenile bipolar disorder. *J Am Acad Child Adolesc Psychiatry.* 2007;46(7):831–839

7. American Psychiatric Association. *Diagnostic and Statistical Manual of Mental Disorders, Fourth Edition, Text Revision (DSM-IV-TR).* Washington, DC: American Psychiatric Association; 2000

8. Kramlinger KG, Post RM. Ultra-rapid and ultradian cycling in bipolar affective illness. *Br J Psychiatry.* 1996;168(3):314–323

9. Geller B, Williams M, Zimerman B, Frazier J, Beringer L, Warner KL. Prepubertal and early adolescent bipolarity differentiate from ADHD by manic symptoms, grandiose delusions, ultra-rapid or ultradian cycling. *J Affect Disord.* 1998;51(2):81–91

10. Pavuluri MN, Birmaher B, Naylor MW. Pediatric bipolar disorder: a review of the past 10 years. *J Am Acad Child Adolesc Psychiatry.* 2005;44(9):846–871

11. Axelson D, Birmaher B, Strober M, et al. Phenomenology of children and adolescents with bipolar spectrum disorders. *Arch Gen Psychiatry.* 2006;63(10):1139–1148

12. Birmaher B, Axelson D, Strober M, et al. Clinical course of children and adolescents with bipolar spectrum disorders. *Arch Gen Psychiatry.* 2006;63(2):175–183

13. Axelson DA, Birmaher B, Strober MA, et al. Course of subthreshold bipolar disorder in youth: diagnostic progression from bipolar disorder not otherwise specified. *J Am Acad Child Adolesc Psychiatry.* 2011;50(10):1001.e3–1016.e3

14. Leibenluft E, Charney DS, Towbin KE, Bhangoo RK, Pine DS. Defining clinical phenotypes of juvenile mania. *Am J Psychiatry.* 2003;160(3):430–437

15. Brotman MA, Schmajuk M, Rich BA, et al. Prevalence, clinical correlates, and longitudinal course of severe mood dysregulation in children. *Biol Psychiatry.* 2006;60(9):991–997

16. Brotman MA, Kassem L, Reising MM, et al. Parental diagnoses in youth with narrow phenotype bipolar disorder or severe mood dysregulation. *Am J Psychiatry.* 2007;164(8):1238–1241

17. American Psychiatric Association. D 00 disruptive mood dysregulation disorder. DSM-5 Development. Available at: www.dsm5.org/ProposedRevision/Pages/proposedrevision.aspx?rid=397#. Accessed February 14, 2012

18. Kowatch RA, Fristad M, Birmaher B, Wagner KD, Findling RL, Hellander M; Child Psychiatric Workgroup on Bipolar Disorder. Treatment guidelines for children and adolescents with bipolar disorder. *J Am Acad Child Adolesc Psychiatry.* 2005;44(3):213–235

19. Sederer LI, Summergrad P. Criteria for hospital admission. *Hosp Community Psychiatry.* 1993;44(2):116–118

20. Kiser LJ, Heston JD, Millsap PA, Pruitt DB. Treatment protocols in child and adolescent day treatment. *Hosp Community Psychiatry.* 1991;42(6):597–600

21. Teich JL, Ireys HT. A national survey of state licensing, regulating, and monitoring of residential facilities for children with mental illness. *Psychiatr Serv.* 2007;58(7):991–998

22. Connolly SD, Bernstein GA; Work Group on Quality Issues. Practice parameter for the assessment and treatment of children and adolescents with anxiety disorders. *J Am Acad Child Adolesc Psychiatry.* 2007;46(2):267–283

23. Birmaher B, Brent D, Bernet W, et al; AACAP Work Group on Quality Issues. Practice parameter for the assessment and treatment of children and adolescents with depressive disorders. *J Am Acad Child Adolesc Psychiatry.* 2007;46(11):1503–1526

24. Pliszka S; AACAP Work Group on Quality Issues. Practice parameter for the assessment and treatment of children and adolescents with attention-deficit/hyperactivity disorder. *J Am Acad Child Adolesc Psychiatry.* 2007;46(7):894–921

25. American Academy of Child and Adolescent Psychiatry. Practice parameter on the use of psychotropic medication in children and adolescents. *J Am Acad Child Adolesc Psychiatry.* 2009;48(9):961–973

26. US Food and Drug Administration. Drugs@FDA [database]. Available at: www.accessdata.fda.gov/scripts/cder/drugsatfda/index.cfm. Accessed February 14, 2012

27. Kowatch RA, Sethuraman G, Hume JH, Kromelis M, Weinberg WA. Combination pharmacotherapy in children and adolescents with bipolar disorder. *Biol Psychiatry.* 2003;53(11):978–984

28. Correll CU. Weight gain and metabolic effects of mood stabilizers and antipsychotics in pediatric bipolar disorder: a systematic review and pooled analysis of short-term trials. *J Am Acad Child Adolesc Psychiatry.* 2007;46(6):687–700

29. Correll CU. Antipsychotic use in children and adolescents: minimizing adverse

effects to maximize outcomes. *J Am Acad Child Adolesc Psychiatry.* 2008;47(1):9–20

30. Olfson M, Blanco C, Liu L, Moreno C, Laje G. National trends in the outpatient treatment of children and adolescents with antipsychotic drugs. *Arch Gen Psychiatry.* 2006;63(6):679–685

31. Patel NC, Hariparsad M, Matias-Akthar M, et al. Body mass indexes and lipid profiles in hospitalized children and adolescents exposed to atypical antipsychotics. *J Child Adolesc Psychopharmacol.* 2007;17(3):303–311

32. Klein DJ, Cottingham EM, Sorter M, Barton BA, Morrison JA. A randomized, double-blind, placebo-controlled trial of metformin treatment of weight gain associated with initiation of atypical antipsychotic therapy in children and adolescents. *Am J Psychiatry.* 2006;163(12):2072–2079

33. Shin L, Bregman H, Breeze JL, Noyes N, Frazier JA. Metformin for weight control in pediatric patients on atypical antipsychotic medication. *J Child Adolesc Psychopharmacol.* 2009;19(3):275–279

34. American Diabetes Association; American Psychiatric Association; American Association of Clinical Endocrinologists; North American Association for the Study of Obesity. Consensus development conference on antipsychotic drugs and obesity and diabetes. *J Clin Psychiatry.* 2004;65(2):267–272

35. Goldberg JF. Antidepressants in bipolar disorder: 7 myths and realities. *Curr Psychiatry.* 2010;9(5):41–48

36. Pavuluri MN, Henry DB, Devineni B, Carbray JA, Naylor MW, Janicak PG. A pharmacotherapy algorithm for stabilization and maintenance of pediatric bipolar disorder. *J Am Acad Child Adolesc Psychiatry.* 2004;43(7):859–867

37. Scheffer RE, Linden S. Concurrent medical conditions with pediatric bipolar disorder. *Curr Opin Psychiatry.* 2007;20(4):398–401

38. Weeke A. Juel Knud, Vaerth M. Cardiovascular death and manic-depressive psychosis. *J Affect Disord.* 1987;13(3):287–292

39. Taylor V, MacQueen G. Associations between bipolar disorder and metabolic syndrome: A review. *J Clin Psychiatry.* 2006;67(7):1034–1041

40. Duffy A, Alda M, Hajek T, Grof P. Early course of bipolar disorder in high-risk offspring: prospective study. *Br J Psychiatry.* 2009;195(5):457–458

41. Wagner KD, Weller EB, Carlson GA, et al. An open-label trial of divalproex in children and adolescents with bipolar disorder. *J Am Acad Child Adolesc Psychiatry.* 2002;41(10):1224–1230

42. Henry CA, Zamvil LS, Lam C, Rosenquist KJ, Ghaemi SN. Long-term outcome with divalproex in children and adolescents with bipolar disorder. *J Child Adolesc Psychopharmacol.* 2003;13(4):523–529

43. Wagner KD, Redden L, Kowatch RA, et al. A double-blind, randomized, placebo-controlled trial of divalproex extended-release in the treatment of bipolar disorder in children and adolescents. *J Am Acad Child Adolesc Psychiatry.* 2009;48(5):519–532

44. Chang K, Saxena K, Howe M. An open-label study of lamotrigine adjunct or monotherapy for the treatment of adolescents with bipolar depression. *J Am Acad Child Adolesc Psychiatry.* 2006;45(3):298–304

45. Pavuluri MN, Henry DB, Moss M, Mohammed T, Carbray JA, Sweeney JA. Effectiveness of lamotrigine in maintaining symptom control in pediatric bipolar disorder. *J Child Adolesc Psychopharmacol.* 2009;19(1):75–82

46. Strober M, Morrell W, Lampert C, Burroughs J. Relapse following discontinuation of lithium maintenance therapy in adolescents with bipolar I illness: a naturalistic study. *Am J Psychiatry.* 1990;147(4):457–461

47. Geller B, Cooper TB, Sun K, et al. Double-blind and placebo-controlled study of lithium for adolescent bipolar disorders with secondary substance dependency. *J Am Acad Child Adolesc Psychiatry.* 1998;37(2):171–178

48. Kafantaris V, Coletti DJ, Dicker R, Padula G, Kane JM. Lithium treatment of acute mania in adolescents: a large open trial. *J Am Acad Child Adolesc Psychiatry.* 2003;42(9):1038–1045

49. Kafantaris V, Coletti DJ, Dicker R, Padula G, Pleak RR, Alvir JM. Lithium treatment of acute mania in adolescents: a placebo-controlled discontinuation study. *J Am Acad Child Adolesc Psychiatry.* 2004;43(8):984–993

50. Patel NC, DelBello MP, Bryan HS, et al. Open-label lithium for the treatment of adolescents with bipolar depression. *J Am Acad Child Adolesc Psychiatry.* 2006;45(3):289–297

51. Wagner KD, Kowatch RA, Emslie GJ, et al. A double-blind, randomized, placebo-controlled trial of oxcarbazepine in the treatment of bipolar disorder in children and adolescents. *Am J Psychiatry.* 2006;163(7):1179–1186

52. DelBello MP, Kowatch RA, Warner J, et al. Adjunctive topiramate treatment for pediatric bipolar disorder: a retrospective chart review. *J Child Adolesc Psychopharmacol.* 2002;12(4):323–330

53. Barzman DH, DelBello MP, Kowatch RA, et al. Adjunctive topiramate in hospitalized children and adolescents with bipolar disorders. *J Child Adolesc Psychopharmacol.* 2005;15(6):931–937

54. Delbello MP, Findling RL, Kushner S, et al. A pilot controlled trial of topiramate for mania in children and adolescents with bipolar disorder. *J Am Acad Child Adolesc Psychiatry.* 2005;44(6):539–547

55. Barzman DH, DelBello MP, Kowatch RA, et al. The effectiveness and tolerability of aripiprazole for pediatric bipolar disorders: a retrospective chart review. *J Child Adolesc Psychopharmacol.* 2004;14(4):593–600

56. Biederman J, McDonnell MA, Wozniak J, et al. Aripiprazole in the treatment of pediatric bipolar disorder: a systematic chart review. *CNS Spectr.* 2005;10(2):141–148

57. Biederman J, Mick E, Spencer T, et al. An open-label trial of aripiprazole monotherapy in children and adolescents with bipolar disorder. *CNS Spectr.* 2007;12(9):683–689

58. Tramontina S, Zeni CP, Pheula GF, de Souza CK, Rohde LA. Aripiprazole in juvenile bipolar disorder comorbid with attention-deficit/hyperactivity disorder: an open clinical trial. *CNS Spectr.* 2007;12(10):758–762

59. Findling RL, Nyilas M, Forbes RA, et al. Acute treatment of pediatric bipolar I disorder, manic or mixed episode, with aripiprazole: a randomized, double-blind, placebo-controlled study. *J Clin Psychiatry.* 2009;70(10):1441–1451

60. Tramontina S, Zeni CP, Ketzer CR, Pheula GF, Narvaez J, Rohde LA. Aripiprazole in children and adolescents with bipolar disorder comorbid with attention-deficit/hyperactivity disorder: a pilot randomized clinical trial. *J Clin Psychiatry.* 2009;70(5):756–764

61. Masi G, Mucci M, Millepiedi S. Clozapine in adolescent inpatients with acute mania. *J Child Adolesc Psychopharmacol.* 2002;12(2):93–99

62. Frazier JA, Biederman J, Tohen M, et al. A prospective open-label treatment trial of olanzapine monotherapy in children and adolescents with bipolar disorder. *J Child Adolesc Psychopharmacol.* 2001;11(3):239–250

63. Tohen M, Kryzhanovskaya L, Carlson G, et al. Olanzapine versus placebo in the treatment of adolescents with bipolar mania. *Am J Psychiatry.* 2007;164(10):1547–1556

64. Joshi G, Mick E, Wozniak J, et al. Impact of obsessive-compulsive disorder on the antimanic response to olanzapine therapy in youth with bipolar disorder. *Bipolar Disord.* 2010;12(2):196–204

65. DelBello MP, Adler CM, Whitsel RM, Stanford KE, Strakowski SM. A 12-week single-blind trial of quetiapine for the treatment of mood symptoms in adolescents at high risk for developing bipolar I disorder. *J Clin Psychiatry.* 2007;68(5):789–795

66. DelBello MP, Chang K, Welge JA, et al. A double-blind, placebo-controlled pilot study of quetiapine for depressed adolescents with bipolar disorder. *Bipolar Disord.* 2009; 11(5):483–493

67. Scheffer RE, Tripathi A, Kirkpatrick FG, Schultz T. Rapid quetiapine loading in youths with bipolar disorder. *J Child Adolesc Psychopharmacol.* 2010;20(5):441–445

68. Frazier JA, Meyer MC, Biederman J, et al. Risperidone treatment for juvenile bipolar disorder: a retrospective chart review. *J Am Acad Child Adolesc Psychiatry.* 1999;38 (8):960–965

69. Biederman J, Mick E, Wozniak J, Aleardi M, Spencer T, Faraone SV. An open-label trial of risperidone in children and adolescents with bipolar disorder. *J Child Adolesc Psychopharmacol.* 2005;15(2):311–317

70. Haas M, Delbello MP, Pandina G, et al. Risperidone for the treatment of acute mania in children and adolescents with bipolar disorder: a randomized, double-blind, placebo-controlled study. *Bipolar Disord.* 2009;11(7):687–700

71. Carlson GA, Potegal M, Margulies D, Basile J, Gutkovich Z. Liquid risperidone in the treatment of rages in psychiatrically hospitalized children with possible bipolar disorder. *Bipolar Disord.* 2010;12(2):205–212

72. Krieger FV, Pheula GF, Coelho R, et al. An open-label trial of risperidone in children and adolescents with severe mood dysregulation. *J Child Adolesc Psychopharmacol.* 2011;21(3):237–243

73. Biederman J, Mick E, Spencer T, Dougherty M, Aleardi M, Wozniak J. A prospective open-label treatment trial of ziprasidone monotherapy in children and adolescents with bipolar disorder. *Bipolar Disord.* 2007; 9(8):888–894

74. Kowatch RA, Suppes T, Carmody TJ, et al. Effect size of lithium, divalproex sodium, and carbamazepine in children and adolescents with bipolar disorder. *J Am Acad Child Adolesc Psychiatry.* 2000;39(6):713–720

75. Delbello MP, Schwiers ML, Rosenberg HL, Strakowski SM. A double-blind, randomized, placebo-controlled study of quetiapine as adjunctive treatment for adolescent mania. *J Am Acad Child Adolesc Psychiatry.* 2002; 41(10):1216–1223

76. Pavuluri MN, Henry DB, Carbray JA, Sampson G, Naylor MW, Janicak PG. Open-label prospective trial of risperidone in combination with lithium or divalproex sodium in pediatric mania. *J Affect Disord.* 2004;82(suppl 1): S103–S111

77. Findling RL, McNamara NK, Youngstrom EA, et al. Double-blind 18-month trial of lithium versus divalproex maintenance treatment in pediatric bipolar disorder. *J Am Acad Child Adolesc Psychiatry.* 2005;44(5):409–417

78. DelBello MP, Kowatch RA, Adler CM, et al. A double-blind randomized pilot study comparing quetiapine and divalproex for adolescent mania. *J Am Acad Child Adolesc Psychiatry.* 2006;45(3):305–313

79. MacMillan CM, Withney JE, Korndörfer SR, Tilley CA, Mrakotsky C, Gonzalez-Heydrich JM. Comparative clinical responses to risperidone and divalproex in patients with pediatric bipolar disorder. *J Psychiatr Pract.* 2008;14(3):160–169

80. Pavuluri MN, Henry DB, Findling RL, et al. Double-blind randomized trial of risperidone versus divalproex in pediatric bipolar disorder. *Bipolar Disord.* 2010;12(6): 593–605

STATEMENT OF ENDORSEMENT

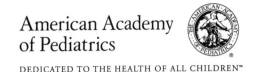

American Academy
of Pediatrics

DEDICATED TO THE HEALTH OF ALL CHILDREN™

Guidelines for Adolescent Depression in Primary Care (GLAD-PC): Part I. Practice Preparation, Identification, Assessment, and Initial Management

Rachel A. Zuckerbrot, MD,[a] Amy Cheung, MD,[b] Peter S. Jensen, MD,[c] Ruth E.K. Stein, MD,[d] Danielle Laraque, MD,[e] GLAD-PC STEERING GROUP

OBJECTIVES: To update clinical practice guidelines to assist primary care (PC) clinicians in the management of adolescent depression. This part of the updated guidelines is used to address practice preparation, identification, assessment, and initial management of adolescent depression in PC settings.

METHODS: By using a combination of evidence- and consensus-based methodologies, guidelines were developed by an expert steering committee in 2 phases as informed by (1) current scientific evidence (published and unpublished) and (2) draft revision and iteration among the steering committee, which included experts, clinicians, and youth and families with lived experience.

RESULTS: Guidelines were updated for youth aged 10 to 21 years and correspond to initial phases of adolescent depression management in PC, including the identification of at-risk youth, assessment and diagnosis, and initial management. The strength of each recommendation and its evidence base are summarized. The practice preparation, identification, assessment, and initial management section of the guidelines include recommendations for (1) the preparation of the PC practice for improved care of adolescents with depression; (2) annual universal screening of youth 12 and over at health maintenance visits; (3) the identification of depression in youth who are at high risk; (4) systematic assessment procedures by using reliable depression scales, patient and caregiver interviews, and *Diagnostic and Statistical Manual of Mental Disorders, Fifth Edition* criteria; (5) patient and family psychoeducation; (6) the establishment of relevant links in the community; and (7) the establishment of a safety plan.

CONCLUSIONS: This part of the guidelines is intended to assist PC clinicians in the identification and initial management of adolescents with depression in an era of great clinical need and shortage of mental health specialists, but they cannot replace clinical judgment; these guidelines are not meant to be the sole source of guidance for depression management in adolescents. Additional research that addresses the identification and initial management of youth with depression in PC is needed, including empirical testing of these guidelines.

abstract

[a]Division of Child and Adolescent Psychiatry, Department of Psychiatry, Columbia University Medical Center, and New York State Psychiatric Institute, New York, New York; [b]University of Toronto, Toronto, Canada; [c]University of Arkansas for Medical Science, Little Rock, Arkansas; [d]Albert Einstein College of Medicine, Bronx, New York, New York; and [e]State University of New York Upstate Medical University, Syracuse, New York

This document is copyrighted and is property of the American Academy of Pediatrics and its Board of Directors. All authors have filed conflict of interest statements with the American Academy of Pediatrics. Any conflicts have been resolved through a process approved by the Board of Directors. The American Academy of Pediatrics has neither solicited nor accepted any commercial involvement in the development of the content of this publication.

The guidance in this publication does not indicate an exclusive course of treatment or serve as a standard of medical care. Variations, taking into account individual circumstances, may be appropriate.

All statements of endorsement from the American Academy of Pediatrics automatically expire 5 years after publication unless reaffirmed, revised, or retired at or before that time.

DOI: https://doi.org/10.1542/peds.2017-4081

Address correspondence to Rachel A. Zuckerbrot, MD. E-mail: rachel.zuckerbrot@nyspi.columbia.edu

PEDIATRICS (ISSN Numbers: Print, 0031-4005; Online, 1098-4275).

Copyright © 2018 by the American Academy of Pediatrics

To cite: Zuckerbrot RA, Cheung A, Jensen PS, et al. Guidelines for Adolescent Depression in Primary Care (GLAD-PC): Part I. Practice Preparation, Identification, Assessment, and Initial Management. *Pediatrics.* 2018;141(3):e20174081

BACKGROUND

Major depression in adolescents is recognized as a serious psychiatric illness with extensive acute and chronic morbidity and mortality.[1–4] Research shows that only 50% of adolescents with depression are diagnosed before reaching adulthood.[5] In primary care (PC), as many as 2 in 3 youth with depression are not identified by their PC clinicians and fail to receive any kind of care.[6,7] Even when diagnosed by PC providers, only half of these patients are treated appropriately.[5] Furthermore, rates of completion of specialty mental health referral for youth with a recognized emotional disorder from general medical settings are low.[8]

In view of the shortage of mental health clinicians, the barriers to children's access to mental health professionals, the well-documented need for PC clinicians to learn how to manage this condition, the increasing evidence base that is available to guide clinical practice, the increased selective serotonin reuptake inhibitor–prescribing rates in pediatric PC,[9,10] and new evidence that a multifaceted approach with mental health consultation may improve the management of depression in PC settings,[8,10–16] guidance for the identification and management of depression in adolescents in PC were urgently needed. To address this gap as well as to meet the needs of PC clinicians and families who are on the front lines with few mental health resources available, in 2007, the Center for the Advancement of Children's Mental Health at Columbia University and the Sunnybrook Health Sciences Center at the University of Toronto joined forces with the New York Forum for Child Health, the New York District II Chapter 3 of the American Academy of Pediatrics (AAP),

and the Resource for Advancing Children's Health (REACH) Institute along with leading experts across the United States and Canada to address the need for a synthesis of knowledge in this area. The result of this initiative was the development of the Guidelines for Adolescent Depression in Primary Care (GLAD-PC). These guidelines are based on available research and the consensus of experts in depression and PC. The two companion articles[17,18] constituted the first-ever evidence- and expert consensus–derived guidelines to guide PC clinicians' management of adolescent depression. The guidelines were also accompanied by a tool kit (available at no cost for download at http://www.gladpc.org).

In this article, we present the updated recommendations on the identification, assessment, and initial management of depression in PC settings and new recommendations on practice preparations (not previously in the GLAD-PC). In the accompanying report, we present the results of the reviews and recommendations on treatment (psychotherapy, psychopharmacology, and pediatric counseling) and ongoing management.

Major depressive disorder (MDD) is a specific diagnosis described in the *Diagnostic and Statistical Manual of Mental Disorders, Fifth Edition* (DSM-5)[19] characterized by discrete episodes of at least 2 weeks' duration (although episodes can last considerably longer) and involving changes in affect, cognition and neurovegetative functions, and interepisode remissions. Other types of depression exist, such as persistent depressive disorder and premenstrual dysphoric disorder. It is important to note that depressive disorders have been separated from bipolar and related disorders in

the DSM-5. Although the evidence for the psychopharmacology recommendations in the accompanying article focuses exclusively on MDD, the recommendations around identification, assessment, and initial management can be applied to other forms of depression as well.

Our guidelines also distinguish between mild, moderate, and severe forms of MDD. The DSM-5 depression criteria include 9 specific symptoms that have been shown to cluster together, run in families, and have a genetic basis,[20–24] and a large body of evidence accumulated over time now supports the internal consistency of depressive symptoms and the validity of the major depression construct.[20] According to the DSM-5, the severity of depressive disorders can be based on symptom count, intensity of symptoms, and/or level of impairment. This commonly used method to define depression severity has been used in large population-based studies[25] and may be particularly relevant in PC settings, in which less severe clinical presentations of depression may be more common. Thus, mild depression may be characterized on the basis of lower scores on standardized depression scales with a shorter duration of symptoms or meeting minimal criteria for depression. Following the DSM-5, mild depression might be defined as 5 to 6 symptoms that are mild in severity. Furthermore, the patient might experience only mild impairment in functioning.

In contrast, depression might be deemed severe when a patient experiences all of the depressive symptoms listed in the DSM-5. Depression might also be considered severe if the patient experiences severe impairment in functioning. Moderate depression falls between these 2 categories.

In general, however, even if not all 9 DSM-5–defined symptoms of depression are present, for the purposes of these guidelines, an adolescent with at least 5 criteria of MDD should be considered in the severe category if he or she presents with a specific suicide plan, clear intent, or recent attempt; psychotic symptoms; family history of first-degree relatives with bipolar disorder; or severe impairment in functioning (such as being unable to leave home).

These guidelines were developed for PC clinicians who are in a position to identify and assist youth with depression in their practice settings. Although the age range of 10 to 21 years may encompass preteenagers, adolescents, and young adults in specific instances, this age range was chosen to include those who might be considered developmentally adolescent. Research that supports adult depression guidelines includes adults 18 years and older. Much of the adolescent depression research focuses on children 18 years and younger. However, because adolescent medicine clinicians and school health clinicians often see patients until they are 21 years old, we have included the older adolescents. Furthermore, a PC clinician faced with an adolescent between the ages of 18 and 21 years can choose to use either adult or adolescent depression guidelines on the basis of the developmental status of the adolescent and his or her own comfort and familiarity with each set of guidelines.

METHODS

The original GLAD-PC recommendations were developed on the basis of a synthesis of expert consensus– and evidence-based research review methodologies, as described in Zuckerbrot et al.[17] The 5-step process included conducting focus groups with PC clinicians, patients, and their families, a systematic literature review, a survey of depression experts to address questions that were not answered in the empirical literature,[26] an expert consensus workshop, and an iterative guideline drafting process with opportunity for input from all workshop attendees.

For the research update of the GLAD-PC, systematic literature reviews were conducted in the same 5 key areas of adolescent depression management in PC settings as the original guidelines: identification and assessment, initial management, safety planning, treatment, and ongoing management of youth depression. Consistent with the original review, the updated searches were conducted by using relevant databases (eg, Medline and PsycInfo), and all primary studies published since the original GLAD-PC reviews in 2005 and 2006 were examined. All update procedures were conducted with the input and guidance of the steering group, which is composed of clinical and research experts, organizational liaisons, and youth and families with lived experience. As in the original review, recommendations were graded on the basis of the University of Oxford's Centre for Evidence-Based Medicine grade of evidence (1–5) system, with 1 to 5 corresponding to the strongest to the weakest evidence respectively (see http://www.cebm.net/wp-content/uploads/2014/06/CEBM-Levels-of-Evidence-2.1.pdf). They were also rated on the basis of the strength of expert consensus among the steering group members that the recommended practice is appropriate. Recommendations with strong (>70%) or very strong (>90%) agreement are given here.

In addition, a new review on the topic of practice preparation was conducted given the emerging evidence for this area since the development of the original GLAD-PC guidelines. Electronic searches of relevant databases were conducted for English-language studies in which researchers examined practice preparation for treating youth depression in PC that were published between 1946 and September 2016. Search terms were grouped by categories and included the following: "child* or adolesc* or youth or teen* or juvenile" and "primary care or pediatr* or family prac* or general prac*" and "depress* or dysth* or mood or bipolar" and "collaborative care or integrat* health or medical-behavioral health care or behavioral health or medical home or shared care or facilita* or practice prepar*". Reference lists for relevant articles were also examined for additional studies that were not identified through search engines. A total of 135 abstracts were carefully examined. Studies that were conducted outside of PC facilities or that used solely adult populations were screened out, leaving a total of 8 relevant articles. A full report of all the literature reviews is available on request.

RESULTS

Literature Reviews

Practice Preparation

Once PC practices have buy-in from administrative and clinical staff to improve depression care for youth, 2 important steps are necessary. First, before practices embark on screening for or identifying youth who are at risk for depression, training in such issues as appropriate screening tools, assessment and diagnostic methods, safety planning, and so on is important. Second, it is necessary to have access to community resources, such as mental health specialists (mental health specialists can include child and adolescent psychiatrists, psychiatric nurse practitioners, and therapists), not just as a potential referral resource but also for as-needed consultation for case patients that the PC clinicians choose to manage. We review the available evidence pertaining to these 2 areas (provider training and specialty consultation) below.

Effective Training Methods

PC practices vary widely in their capacity to implement full-scale collaborative or integrative behavioral health programs to address psychological difficulties in youth. At minimum, providing PC providers with guidance, education, and training in key topic areas such as identification, evaluation of suicide risk, and initial management of adolescent depression can be a feasible and cost-efficient means of improving care delivery when comprehensive organizational restructuring efforts are out of reach. However, simply providing PC providers with relevant information is not enough because passive education strategies are usually inadequate for producing lasting change in provider behavior.[27]

Researchers in large-scale review studies suggest that the adoption of practice guidelines improves when training and implementation strategies are tailored to the PC practice (eg, training that is developed by primary mental health care specialists, such as the training provided by the REACH Institute [http://www.thereachinstitute.org/] and Child and Adolescent Psychology for Primary Care [http://www.cappcny.org/])[28] and/or use comprehensive training methods, such as varying information

delivery methods and skill-building exercises, such as role-playing.[27] Evidence regarding which specific theory-driven training strategies are most effective at eliciting behavior change with PC providers, particularly related to mental health, is sparse, but 1 promising framework leverages principles from the theories of reasoned action and planned behavior to inform training methodology (see Perkins et al[29] for explanation and review). This approach posits 3 primary determinants of PC behavior change: attitudes toward the practice innovation, the strength of intention to adopt the new practice(s), and sense of self-efficacy in one's ability to continue the new behavior. Although no randomized trials in which researchers use this or other systematic frameworks for PC provider–training methodologies were identified, researchers in preliminary studies offer support for training approaches that incorporate basic science–guided behavior change theory and methods. There is increasing evidence that quality-improvement strategies and techniques can change PC practitioner behavior both in mental health and in other arenas.[30,31] The REACH Institute (which is committed to renewing and improving techniques for professionals and parents to treat children with behavioral and emotional needs) has developed and widely implemented a 3-day intensive training on evidence-based pediatric mental health assessment, diagnosis, and treatment practices (including for youth depression) that is guided by basic science behavior change principles, demonstrating long-term practice changes (eg, increased use of symptom scales) as well as favorable PC provider attitudes toward, intentions to follow, and self-efficacy to adhere to the clinical guidelines up to 1 year

later.[32] In another study of the same training approach, participating PC providers showed higher levels of self-efficacy in diagnosing and managing youth depression and related disorders than those who received only more traditional continuing education programs (eg, lectures).[33]

An unrelated study demonstrated that provider attitudes toward youth mental health in PC impacts rates of identification. PC providers who viewed psychosocial treatment as burdensome were less likely to identify youth mental health problems.[34] A subsequent follow-up to the study revealed that providing PC staff with communication training enhanced their self-efficacy and willingness to discuss depression symptoms with patients and staff, and this was associated with long-term changes in practice behaviors, such as providing an agenda during the PC visit, querying for additional mental health concerns, and making encouraging statements to patients and families when symptoms are disclosed.[35] The small amount of available literature offers support for hands-on, interactive, and basic science theory–driven training strategies for PC clinicians, but more research is needed before a consensus can be reached on how best to optimize training and educational strategies for PC providers.

Access to Specialty Consultation

In addition to obtaining relevant training, PC providers will benefit from having access to ongoing consultation with mental health specialists.[36,37] Consultation after training allows learning to be tailored to the PC provider's actual practice[38] and can increase provider comfort with diagnosing and treating mental health issues.[33,39] More than 25 states have established programs to promote collaboration between PC providers and child psychiatrists by providing PC providers with education, rapid access to consultation, and referral options. Among the first psychiatric consultation programs was Targeted Child Psychiatry Services (TCPS) in the state of Massachusetts,[40,41] which offered regional providers access to real-time telephone consultation with a child psychiatrist and the option to refer a child to the psychiatry practice for a mental health evaluation, short-term psychosocial therapy, and/or pharmacotherapy. Program use data revealed that TCPS consultation support alone was sufficient to retain and treat in PC 43% of youth who potentially would have been referred to specialty services.[40] TCPS was subsequently expanded statewide and became known as the Massachusetts Child Psychiatry Access Project.[14] Similar programs in other states offer free training, telephone consultation, and referral advice to PC providers.[14,42,43] Participating PC providers consistently report being highly satisfied with the consultation they receive[14,42,43] and increasingly comfortable with treating mental health problems within the PC setting after consultation.[14,42,43] Additionally, consultation programs may improve access to mental health care not only by increasing its availability within PC but also by decreasing potentially unnecessary referrals to specialty care, which in turn makes specialty providers more available to treat complex or severe patients.[41,44]

Identification and Assessment

In 2009, after the publication of the GLAD-PC, the United States Preventive Services Task Force (USPSTF) endorsed universal adolescent depression screening in teenagers ages 12 to 18 years.[45] This recommendation was based on evidence that there are validated depression screening tools that work in an adolescent PC population and the evidence that there are treatments that work for the identified population.[45,46] On the basis of our review to date, no researchers in a randomized control trial (RCT) have compared functional or depressive outcomes in a cohort of adolescents who were screened in PC by the PC providers themselves versus a cohort of adolescents who were not screened. This lack of evidence, which is also mentioned in the Canadian review of the literature in 2005,[47] the 2009 Williams et al[46] review performed for the USPSTF, the updated 2016 Forman-Hoffman et al[48] review for the USPSTF, and a 2013 systematic literature review published in *Pediatrics*,[49] becomes less relevant as more evidence accumulates regarding the specific steps in the process, such as the validity of PC screening, the feasibility of PC screening, the feasibility of implementing treatment in those who are identified as having depression, and the efficacy of treatment of those who received evidence-based treatments in PC. In our updated review in this area, we found 8 new articles that provide some psychometric data regarding the use of depression screens in the pediatric PC population (Supplemental Table 1) and 38 other articles that touch on screening issues that range from whether screening is taking place and whether screening impacts follow-up procedures or treatment to the specifics of screening, such as the use of mobile devices or gated procedures (Supplemental Table 2). Supplemental Tables 1 and 2 present the new evidence as well as the limitations for existing screening tools and protocols. Please see our original 2007 guidelines for the past review of screening tools and protocols.

During the original GLAD-PC development process, secondary to the paucity of data on the validity of screening tools in the adolescent PC population, the original GLAD-PC guideline was used to review instruments that are used in community and psychiatric populations as well.[17] Given that those screens are still in use and that their psychometric data still apply, in this current review, we focus only on new screening data in PC. Eight of the articles present psychometric data, such as sensitivity, specificity, positive predictive value (PPV), negative predictive value (NPV), or area under the curve (Supplemental Table 1). Most relevant were the 2 publications by Richardson et al[56,57] in which they validated the Patient Health Questionnaire-2 (PHQ-2) and the Patient Health Questionnaire-9 (PHQ-9) in a PC sample against a gold standard diagnostic interview (the Diagnostic Interview Schedule for Children-IV [DISC-IV]). The PHQ-9, with a cut-point of 11, had a sensitivity and specificity of 89.5% and 77.5%, respectively, to DISC-IV MDD with a PPV of 15.2% and NPV of 99.4%. A PHQ-2 cut score of 3 had a sensitivity and specificity of 73.7% and 75.2%, respectively, to DISC-IV MDD.

Researchers have looked at brief depression-specific screening questions that stand alone (eg, the PHQ-2),[51,57,65,75,79,82,85] longer depression-specific scales that stand alone (eg, the PHQ-9, the Mood and Feelings Questionnaire, the Columbia Depression Scale, and the PHQ-9: Modified for Teens),[58,62,63,66,67,70,74,78,80–82,86–88] brief depression screening questions that are part of a larger psychosocial tool (eg, the Guidelines for Adolescent Preventive Services [GAPS] questionnaire and the Pediatric Symptom Checklist [PSC]),[53,54,64,68,69] and brief screening questions or longer depression-specific scales that are combined with other screens for either other psychiatric disorders (eg, Screen for Child Anxiety Related Disorders-5) and/ or screens for other high-risk behaviors (eg, substance use and sexual activity) to make a more multidimensional tool or packet in 1 (eg, the behavioral health screen [BHS]).[50,52,55,59–61,76,77,83,84,89] Not all of the screens in these studies have specific psychometric validation data (eg, 2 depression questions on the GAPS). Clinicians may also consider the use of tools that can be used to screen for depression and other risk behaviors or more disorders. Although no researchers have compared the functional or depressive outcomes of a cohort of adolescents who were initially screened only for depression with a cohort of adolescents who were initially screened for an array of high-risk behaviors and emotional issues, some hint at the possibility that too much information may overwhelm the clinician and result in positive depression screening questions being overlooked in the morass of issues needing to be addressed.[52,53,59–61,64,76,80,82–84,89] Therefore, clinicians should base the selection of a depression-specific tool versus a more general tool on their own expertise and clinical supports in their practices. For example, a solo practitioner starting to address depression care in his or her practice may choose to start with screening for depression alone before moving to more general screening for riskier behaviors or disorders.

There is limited evidence to evaluate whether one can use a general parent questionnaire as a gated entry for adolescent self-report depression screening. Researchers in 1 study of general mental health screening used the parent- or youth-completed Pediatric Symptom Checklist-35 alone to screen for internalizing disorders, but this provides no

psychometric data,[69] whereas others used the Parent Pediatric Symptom Checklist-17 (PSC-17) along with other, more depression-specific child and parent scales.[54,56,57,82] One of these studies reveals adequate psychometric data for the parent PSC-17 internalizing subscale as compared with the Kiddie Schedule for Affective Disorders and Schizophrenia (K-SADS) MDD module, performing as well as the Children's Depression Inventory but only with children aged 8 to 15 years.[54] Richardson et al[56,57,82] suggest some correlation with adolescent depression self-report tools, with the adolescent scores that are higher on the PHQ-9 or PHQ-2 being associated with higher mean on the parent PSC-17 internalizing subscale, with a correlation of 0.21 ($P = .02$). However, the data presented do reveal that some teenagers who scored above the cutoffs on the self-reports would have parents who score below the cutoff of 5 on the internalizing subscale of the PSC-17. The authors do not present the data regarding how many teenagers would be missed by using the internalizing subscale as a gate and whether those teenagers met DISC-IV MDD criteria. Lastly, researchers in 1 study looked at the correlation of the PSC-17 internalizing subscale between the parent- and youth-completed PSC-17 but only among subjects whose parents were already positive.[53] The data revealed low agreement, with a κ of 0.15 (95% confidence interval of 0.00–0.30). However, those adolescents who did match with their parents were of higher severity than those parents who were positive but did not match with their negative-scoring teenagers. In addition, the parent PSC-17 in general has usually been studied with the younger adolescent cohort and not the older adolescent cohort. Once again, there is no RCT in

which researchers compare the outcomes of a cohort of adolescents who were universally screened with an adolescent depression self-report versus a cohort that was only screened with self-reports after a positive parent PSC result. All of these data reveal that there is limited evidence in the older teenage cohort about using parent reports alone, that parent information may be helpful if used in conjunction with child reports when a clinician is available to resolve discrepant data, and that if used alone, parent reports may only account for the adolescents with the most severe conditions, but those data are unclear.

Researchers have also looked at paper screens, Internet-based screens, and electronic screens that are accessed through a mobile or personal digital assistant device. Although there appears to be no evidence of researchers comparing such screening methods to each other, all methods seem to be equally successful (in that adolescents rarely refuse screening) and equally problematic (obstacles to universal screening exist with every method). See Supplemental Tables 1 and 2 for more specific information.

Some researchers report adaptive (brief initial questions and, if gated questions have positive results, then automated additional questions)[61] as well as algorithmic screening, in which a positive PHQ-2 result or the equivalent triggers a person to then administer a PHQ-9 or the equivalent.[65,75,79,85] Although evidence for this type of gated screening is limited, researchers in 1 study compared the psychometric data of the PHQ-2 versus the PHQ-9 in the same population.[57]

One limitation of brief depression screening may be the loss of the suicide questions if one focuses only on brief questions on the basis of criterion A for MDD. The validation study of the PHQ-2 found that 19% of teenagers who did endorse suicidality did not screen positive on the PHQ-2, suggesting that in a real-world setting, they would have been missed.[57] Several studies in which researchers used brief or long depression-specific screenings that did not include a suicide question did add a suicide question for this reason.[60,70,83,84,89] In this review, we did not review the suicide screening in pediatric PC literature but are aware of the USPSTF decision not to endorse suicide screening secondary to its conclusion for the lack of evidence for PC intervention for suicidal adolescents.[90] However, we do note which depression screening studies also looked for suicide as well as the rates of suicidality that were found (Supplemental Tables 1 and 2).

One other area that was examined in the review is the definition of depression when screening for depression. The definition of depression affects the psychometric properties and evidence for the use of a screen given that trying to find only MDD versus trying to find any depressive symptoms requires different specificities and sensitivities, and using the same screens for both purposes would result in choosing different cutoffs. Again, whereas the USPSTF comments on screening for MDD, the screening literature seems to be more unfocused. Richardson et al[79] used a score of 2 as the initial gate and a score of 10 on the PHQ-9 as a positive score for entry into the next step. Forty percent of the sample did not meet the criteria for MDD but were deemed to be impaired enough with depressive symptoms to enter the study. When Lewandowski et al[74] studied the large-scale use of the PHQ-9 modified in the

health maintenance organization (HMO), they looked at whether any depressive disorder was identified, even adjustment disorder, rather than just MDD. The Youth Partners in Care (YPIC) intervention[11,58] also included teenagers without MDD who had clinically significant and current depressive symptoms. Van Voorhees et al,[91] in a series of small studies and now in a large RCT, have been purposely screening to account for depressive symptoms and depressive disorders other than MDD because the Competent Adulthood Transition with Cognitive-behavioral, Humanistic and Interpersonal Training (CATCH-IT) prevention model was developed for teenagers with depressive symptoms and disorders other than MDD.[65] Thus, the evidence for choosing instruments and cutoff scores may depend on what depression end point a PC provider is pursuing and what intervention the clinician wishes to put in place.

Although the USPSTF clearly endorsed screening at age 12 years, the literature in which researchers look at depression screening includes studies that have starting ages ranging from age 8 to 14 years and later ages ranging from 15 to 24 years. Most of the younger-age studies include depression as part of a broader psychosocial screening effort, with the researchers looking specifically at depression screening that focuses on some of the older age ranges (Supplemental Tables 1 and 2). With that said, there is no evidence to compare outcomes in a cohort of adolescents who were screened at age 11 years versus age 12 years versus age 13 years.

The last guideline review included the YPIC study, which did reveal that an identification program in PC, when combined with high-quality depression treatment,

actually yields better outcomes than treatment-as-usual conditions (when no high-quality depression treatment is available).[11] Two follow-up publications from the same intervention[58,87] are included in this review and once again show that identified youth who receive evidence-based treatment do have better outcomes. More recently, Richardson and colleagues, in their collaborative care for adolescent depression RCT, compared controls who screened positive and whose positive results were given to both parents and PC clinicians with subjects who were screened and placed in a collaborative care intervention.[79] Those in the collaborative care intervention had a greater chance of response and remission at 12 months and a greater likelihood of receiving evidence-based treatments. The researchers only tracked outcomes in those who were screened; although it is possible that those who were screened did better than those adolescents with depression who were not screened, the study does reveal that screening alone is not likely to improve outcomes by much given how much better those in the group that had screening combined with an intervention in place did and how much more likely they were to receive care than those who were only screened.

Although much of the literature on identification crosses both the area of screening and assessment in that the PC provider can use the screening tool to aid in the assessment, we found some studies that focused less on the screening tools and more on the assessment of depression in pediatric PC. These studies included those in which researchers used standardized patients to help with depression and suicide assessment as well as a protocol to teach PC clinicians how to do a therapeutic interview during the assessment process.[62,63,71–73]

In summary, no perfect depression screening and/or assessment tool exists, and no perfect screening algorithm or systematic protocol exists, but a number of adolescent depression assessment instruments do possess adequate psychometric properties to recommend their use in depression detection and assessment, and there is a limited amount of evidence to support some differing methods of implementation (Supplemental Table 3). Thus, it is reasonable to expect that depression detection in PC can be improved by the use of adolescent self-report checklists with or without parent self-reports. Reliance on adolescent self-report depression checklists alone will lead to substantial numbers of false-positive and false-negative cases. Screening and detection are only the first step to making a diagnosis. Instead, optimal diagnostic procedures should combine the use of depression-specific screening tools as diagnostic aids, buttressed by follow-up clinical interviews in which one obtains information from other informants (eg, parents) as legally permissible and uses either other tools or interviews to assess for other psychiatric diagnoses as well, reconciling discrepant information to arrive at an accurate diagnosis and impairment assessment before treatment. Although screening parents may not be required, gathering information from third-party collaterals to make a diagnosis is important. Teenagers should be encouraged to allow their parents to access their information, and the importance of including parents in the diagnostic discussion should be emphasized. For more information about rating scales and cutoff scores, please refer to the GLAD-PC tool kit.

Initial Management of Adolescent Depression

On behalf of the initial GLAD-PC team, Stein et al[92] reviewed the literature on psychosocial interventions for anticipatory guidance. No RCTs or evidence-based reviews were found. Citing earlier literature reviews in the area of injury prevention[93] and anticipatory guidance,[94] Stein et al[92] found some limited evidence that anticipatory guidance strategies, such as education and counseling, in the PC setting can be effective.

Another area reviewed by Stein et al[92] involved psychosocial interventions for improved adherence. In an evidence review on asthma adherence, Lemanek et al[95] suggested that some educational and behavioral strategies are probably efficacious in creating change. In addition, a study in which researchers used cognitive behavioral strategies revealed that diabetic adherence can also be improved.[95]

For this update, our team searched the Cochrane Database of Systematic Reviews for all types of interventions that were implemented in the adherence arena. These reviews[96–98] revealed that only complex, multifaceted approaches that include convenient care, patient education, reminders, reinforcement, counseling, and additional supervision by a member of the care team were effective in improving adherence in different chronic medical conditions, including asthma, hypertension, diabetes, and adult depression. In the pediatric literature, research regarding adherence commonly involved interventions that targeted both patients and their families.[99] Several key components have been identified that may improve compliance and/or adherence, including patient self-management and/or monitoring, patient and/or family education and/or support, and the setting and supervision of management goals.[100,101] The identification and periodic review of short- and long-term goals provides an individualized plan that both the provider and the patient and family can follow over time.[100,101] Specifically in the area of youth depression, however, current research evidence reveals that only more complex interventions are likely to have the greatest impact on both adherence and treatment outcomes. This kind of coordinated care, which is often described as collaborative care or integrated behavioral health, is discussed further in the accompanying report on depression treatment and ongoing management.[102]

Safety Planning

Safety planning with adolescent patients who have depression and are suicidal or potentially suicidal usually consists of instructing the family to remove lethal means, instructing the family to monitor for risk factors for suicide (including sexual orientation and intellectual disability), engaging the potentially suicidal adolescent in treatment, providing adolescents with mutually agreeable and available emergency contacts, and establishing clear follow-up. In our updated review of the literature, we found no trials in which researchers have studied the impact of or how to conduct any of these aspects of safety planning with adolescents with depression. Once again, no studies were found in which researchers examined the benefits or risks of a safety contract. Researchers in several articles reviewed what little literature is available regarding the use of suicide safety contracts, and all concluded that these should not be used in clinical practice because there is no empirical evidence that they actually prevent suicide.[103–107] Multiple authors also asserted that contracts have numerous flaws, which could actually be harmful to the clinician-patient alliance. Some alternatives to a contract have been proposed (for example, the commitment to treatment statement discussed by Rudd et al[107]), but none have been tested in a clinical trial. Some studies have suggested that limiting access to firearms or other lethal means can decrease suicide by those methods, but the evidence is still unclear as to whether, on a broader population level, restricting access to certain lethal methods results in an overall decrease of suicide rates.[108–116] In addition, Brent et al[117] found that the families of adolescents with depression are frequently noncompliant with recommendations to remove firearms from the house. Yet, a small prospective follow-up of patients who were seen in an emergency department (ED) for mental health concerns found that the majority of their families removed or secured lethal means (firearms, alcohol, prescription medications, and over the counter medications) after injury-prevention education in the ED.[117] Some limited evidence suggests that quick and consistent follow-up and/or treatment with a team approach will be most helpful in increasing compliance and engagement among patients who are suicidal.[118–120]

GUIDELINES

The strength of the evidence on which each recommendation is based has been rated 1 (strongest) through 5 (weakest) according to the Centre for Evidence-Based Medicine levels of evidence and paired with the strength of the recommendation (strong or very strong).

Practice Preparation

Recommendation 1:*PC clinicians are encouraged to seek training in depression assessment, identification, diagnosis, and treatment if they are not previously trained (grade of evidence: 5; strength of recommendation: very strong).*

Consistent with the original GLAD-PC guidelines, PC clinicians who manage adolescent depression are advised to pursue additional education in identification, assessment, diagnosis, treatment and follow-up, consent and confidentiality, safety risk assessment and management, liability, and billing practices. Appropriate training on the assessment, diagnosis, and treatment of adolescent depression enhances PC providers' attitudes and self-efficacy to treat youth depression within their practices, thereby making it more likely that psychological disorders will be identified in the patient population.[34] The REACH Institute and Child and Adolescent Psychology for Primary Care are examples of organizations that provide training opportunities to PC clinicians. In addition to high-quality content, studies of PC provider training reveal that effective information delivery methods are important to the successful uptake of new practice behaviors. Such training methods include a succinct presentation of high-priority information, interactive content delivery methods, hands-on learning activities (eg, role-plays), and cultivating peer leaders to champion new practices. Additionally, access to ongoing consultation after training allows learning to be tailored to the PC provider's actual practice[38] and can increase comfort with diagnosing and treating mental health issues.[33,39] Clinicians also need to practice self-care by using supports for themselves as they take on more responsibilities of caring for youth with depression because engaging with this population can prove to be emotionally challenging.

Recommendation 2: *PC clinicians should establish relevant referral and collaborations with mental health resources in the community, which may include patients and families who have dealt with adolescent depression and are willing to serve as a resource for other affected adolescents and their family members. Consultations should be pursued whenever*

available in initial cases until the PC clinician acquires confidence and skills and when challenging cases arise. In addition, whenever available, these resources may also include state-wide or regional child and adolescent psychiatry consultation programs (grade of evidence: 5; strength of recommendation: very strong).

The lack of linkages among relevant services within a system of care is a large gap in the management of chronic disorders in young people.[121] Furthermore, family-based interventions have been shown to help youth with mental illness.[122] Therefore, establishing mental health referral and collaboration resources in the local community for adolescents with depression and their families is essential to ensuring timely and effective access to needed services.[11,123] Such linkages may include mental health sites to which patients can be referred for specialty care services, such as comprehensive evaluations, psychosocial treatment, pharmacotherapy, and crises intervention services (in the event of suicidality). In highly underserved areas, these linkages may also include paraprofessionals who are tasked with providing the bulk of supportive counseling services to local residents. To reduce barriers to care, PC providers may arrange to have standing agreements with these practices regarding referral, the exchange of clinical information, points of contact, and so on. Schools play a critical role, especially if therapeutic support is available. Clinicians should connect to any available resources in the school system. PC providers should also work with the patient and/or family to establish an individual education plan to provide supports for the teenager in the school setting. Other linkages may include online or in-person support groups, advocacy groups (eg, the American

Foundation for Suicide Prevention), and family partner organizations (ie, patients and/or caregivers who have experience dealing with adolescent depression and serve as a resource for affected adolescents and families whenever these services are available).

To provide support to PC providers, >25 states have established programs to promote collaboration between PC providers and child psychiatrists by providing PC providers with education, rapid access to consultation, and referral options. PC sites may wish to search registries such as the National Network of Child Psychiatry Access Programs (www.nncpap.org) to identify any regional or state-wide programs that are available in their areas.

Identification and Surveillance

Recommendation 1: Adolescent patients ages 12 years and older should be screened annually for depression (MDD or depressive disorders) with a formal self-report screening tool either on paper or electronically (universal screening) (grade of evidence: 2; strength of recommendation: very strong).

Given the high prevalence of adolescent depression (lifetime prevalence is estimated to be ~ 20% by age 20 years), the evidence that adolescent depression can be persistent, the fact that adolescence is a time of significant brain maturation, and longitudinal studies that reveal that adolescents with depression have significant problems as adults, it is important to try to identify and treat adolescents with depression early in the course of the disorder. Although most PC clinicians believe it is their responsibility to identify depression in their adolescent patients, evidence suggests that only a fraction of these youth are identified when presenting in PC settings even after the USPSTF mandate on screening.[45] Extant

evidence does suggest that screening with a systematic tool will identify more adolescents with depressive disorders than not screening at all. Providers should choose a tool with at least minimal validation data. Given that more evidence is needed to guide the choice of a depression screening tool, at this point, providers should choose a depression-only tool or a combined tool, a short tool as a gate or a longer initial tool, and an adaptive screening or a paper screen on the basis of what they believe will work better for their practices, patients, and health organizations. Furthermore, the current literature does reveal that screening and scoring before the provider is in the room with the patient can be most helpful to the workflow. Although both the USPSTF and the AAP support the universal use of an adolescent self-report screen, using a parent-completed PSC as an initial gate may be acceptable given the limited evidence. However, 1 limitation to gated depression screening, using either a short self-report or a longer parent psychosocial report as the initial gate, is the loss of the suicide questions that are part of longer adolescent self-reports. Given the high rate of suicidal ideation and attempts among adolescents and the fact that not all adolescents who are suicidal will have MDD, it seems likely that screening for suicidality may be helpful as well, so providers should consider including suicide questions. Choosing a cutoff score for the selected tool will need to depend on the practice's expected prevalence rates as well as the practice's available and accepted pathways for intervention. Although there is no evidence to suggest how often a teenager should be screened, screening once per year seems reasonable until more evidence is amassed, whether this takes place at health maintenance visits or at the next available sick visit. Finally, this recommendation

should not discourage PC providers who regularly speak with their teenagers about their moods from continuing to do so and should not dissuade clinicians from learning how to better identify teens with depression through interview, but we merely endorse universal adolescent depression self-report instruments as an initial screening tool.

Recommendation 2: Patients with depression risk factors (eg, a history of previous depressive episodes, a family history, other psychiatric disorders, substance use, trauma, psychosocial adversity, frequent somatic complaints, previous high-scoring screens without a depression diagnosis, etc) should be identified (grade of evidence: 2; strength of recommendation: very strong) and systematically monitored over time for the development of a depressive disorder by using a formal depression instrument or tool (targeted screening) (grade of evidence: 2; strength of recommendation: very strong).

As part of overall health care, PC clinicians should routinely monitor the psychosocial functioning of all youth because problems in psychosocial functioning may be an early indication of a variety of problems, including depression. Risk factors that clinicians may use to identify those who are at high risk for depression include a previous history or family history of (1) depression, (2) bipolar disorder, (3) suicide-related behaviors, (4) substance use, and (5) other psychiatric illness; (6) significant psychosocial stressors, such as family crises, physical and sexual abuse, neglect, and other trauma history; (7) frequent somatic complaints; as well as (8) foster care and adoption.[124–126] Research evidence shows that patients who present with such risk factors are likely to experience future depressive episodes.[22,127–133] There are recent data as well that reveal that those who score high on depression screening instruments, even when they are not initially diagnosed with depression, may be at risk for a depression diagnosis within 6 months.[66] Although these at-risk teenagers may be screened annually as part of the practice's universal depression screening, they may also require a more frequent, systematic, targeted screening during other health care visits (ie, well-child visits and urgent care visits). Following the chronic care model, teens with depression, past depression, frequent somatization, or other risk factors may need to be included in a registry and managed more closely over time.

Assessment and/or Diagnosis

Recommendation 1: PC clinicians should evaluate for depression in those who screen positive on the formal screening tool (whether it is used as part of universal or targeted screening), in those who present with any emotional problem as the chief complaint, and in those in whom depression is highly suspected despite a negative screen result. Clinicians should assess for depressive symptoms on the basis of the diagnostic criteria established in theDSM-5 or the International Classification of Diseases, 10th Revision(grade of evidence: 3; strength of recommendation: very strong) and should use standardized depression tools to aid in the assessment (if they are not already used as part of the screening process) (grade of evidence: 1; strength of recommendation: very strong).

Scoring high on a screening tool alone does not make for a diagnosis of MDD, especially given that in a low-risk PC population, the PPV of a positive screen result may be low. However, as discussed earlier, a positive screen result can also indicate a different depressive disorder or subthreshold depression. On the other hand, in youth who are suspected of having depression on the basis of other initiating triggers, such as risk factors, somatic complaints, or other emotional chief complaints, assessing for depression (regardless of whether there is a positive screen result) may be in order. PC clinicians should probe for the presence of any of several depressive disorders, including MDD, persistent depressive disorder (dysthymia), and other specified or unspecified depressive disorders by using systematic, rigorous assessment methods. Although standardized instruments should be used to help with diagnosis, they should not replace direct interview by a clinician.[134–136] Because adolescents with depression may not be able to clearly identify depressed mood as their presenting complaint, providers need to be aware of common presenting symptoms that may signal MDD. These may include irritability, fatigue, insomnia or sleeping more, weight loss or weight gain, decline in academic functioning, family conflict, and other symptoms of depressive disorders.[137]

Recommendation 2: Assessment for depression should include direct interviews with the patients and families and/or caregivers (grade of evidence: 2; strength of recommendation: very strong) and should include the assessment of functional impairment in different domains (grade of evidence: 1; strength of recommendation: very strong) and other existing psychiatric conditions (grade of evidence: 1; strength of recommendation: very strong). Clinicians should remember to interview an adolescent alone.

Evidence of the core symptoms of depression and functional impairment should be obtained from the youth as well as from families and/or caregivers separately.[138–140] The involvement of the family is critical in all phases of management and should be included in the assessment for depressive disorders. If family involvement is determined to be detrimental, then involving another responsible adult would be appropriate. Family relationships may also affect the presentation of depression in adolescents. However, despite the importance of family involvement and the imperative to try to include family, adolescents value their sense of privacy, confidentiality, and individuality. It is important to remember that adolescents should be interviewed alone about their depressive symptoms, suicidality, and psychosocial risk factors and circumstances. The cultural backgrounds of the patients and their families should also be considered during the assessments because they can impact the presentation of core symptoms.[141] Collateral information from other sources (eg, teachers) may also be obtained to aid in the assessment. Given the high rates of comorbidities, clinicians should assess for the existence of comorbid conditions that may affect the diagnosis and treatment of the depressive disorder.[2,22,142,143] These comorbidities may include 1 or more of the following conditions: substance use, anxiety disorder, attention-deficit/hyperactivity disorder, bipolar disorder, physical abuse, and trauma. Instruments that assess for a range of common comorbid mental health conditions should be considered as well during this assessment phase if they were not used in the initial screening protocol. Clinicians should also assess for impairment in key areas of functioning, including school, home, and peer settings.[144] Subjective distress should be evaluated as well. Regardless of the diagnostic impression or any further treatment plans, a safety assessment, including for suicidality, should be completed by the clinician (see recommendation 3 in Initial Management of Depression).

Initial Management of Depression

Recommendation 1: Clinicians should educate and counsel families and patients about depression and options for the management of the disorder (grade of evidence: 5; strength of recommendation: very strong). Clinicians should also discuss the limits of confidentiality with the adolescent and family (grade of evidence: 5; strength of recommendation: very strong).

Management should be based on a plan that is developed with the understanding that depression is often a recurring condition. As seen in studies of depression interventions, families and patients need to be educated about the causes and symptoms of depression, impairments associated with it, and the expected outcomes of treatment.[145–148] Information should be provided at a developmentally appropriate level and in a way that the patient and family can understand the nature of the condition and the management plan. Communication that is developmentally appropriate should facilitate the ability of parents and patients to work with the clinicians to develop an effective and achievable treatment plan. To establish a strong therapeutic alliance, the clinicians should also take into account cultural factors that may affect the diagnosis and management of this disorder.[141] Clinicians should also be aware of the negative reactions of family members to a possible diagnosis of depression in a teen (ie, sadness, anger, and denial). Sample materials are available in the GLAD-PC and include resources for patients and parents. Because the symptoms of depression can also affect many areas of an adolescent's life, other

ongoing partnerships may need to be established with personnel in schools and other settings (eg, extracurricular activities). Confidentiality should also be discussed with the adolescent and his or her family. Adolescents and families should be aware of the limits of confidentiality, including the need to involve parents or legal authorities when the risk of harm to the adolescent or others may be imminent. Clinicians should be aware of state laws regarding confidentiality (for additional information, see www.advocatesforyouth.org).

Recommendation 2: After appropriate training, PC clinicians should develop a treatment plan with patients and families (grade of evidence: 5; strength of recommendation: very strong) and set specific treatment goals in key areas of functioning, including home, peer, and school settings (grade of evidence: 5; strength of recommendation: very strong).

From studies of chronic disorders in youth, it is suggested that better adherence to treatment is associated with the identification and tracking of specific treatment goals and outcomes. Written action plans in asthma management have some evidence for improved outcomes.[149] Similarly, studies of adolescents with depression reveal greater adherence and outcomes when they were assessed to be ready for change and received their treatment of choice.[11,86] If a patient presents with moderate-to-severe depression or has persistent depressive symptoms, treatment goals and outcomes should be identified and agreed on via close collaboration with the patient and family at the time of treatment initiation. Treatment goals may include the establishment of a regular exercise routine, adequate nutrition, and regular meetings to resolve issues at home. In the adult depression literature, monitoring appears to be most effective when it

is implemented through designated case managers who monitor patients' clinical status and treatment plan adherence.[12] The benefits of such programs may be enhanced through the use of electronic medical records (EMRs) and the development of patient registries. Technologies such as apps are being used more commonly in clinical practice, and there is emerging evidence for their effectiveness.[150]

Recommendation 3: All management should include the establishment of a safety plan, which includes restricting lethal means, engaging a concerned third party, and developing an emergency communication mechanism should the patient deteriorate, become actively suicidal or dangerous to others, or experience an acute crisis associated with psychosocial stressors, especially during the period of initial treatment, when safety concerns are the highest (grade of evidence: 3; strength of recommendation: very strong). The establishment and development of a safety plan within the home environment is another important management step.

Suicidality, including ideation, behaviors, and attempts, is common among adolescents with depression. In studies of completed suicide, more than 50% of the victims had a diagnosis of depression.[151] Therefore, clinicians who manage this disorder should develop an emergency communication mechanism for handling increased suicidality or acute crises. After assessing a patient for suicidality, the clinician should obtain information from a third party, assess that adequate adult supervision and support are available, have an adult agree to help remove lethal means (eg, medications and firearms) from the premises, warn the patient of the disinhibiting effects of drugs and alcohol, put contingency planning

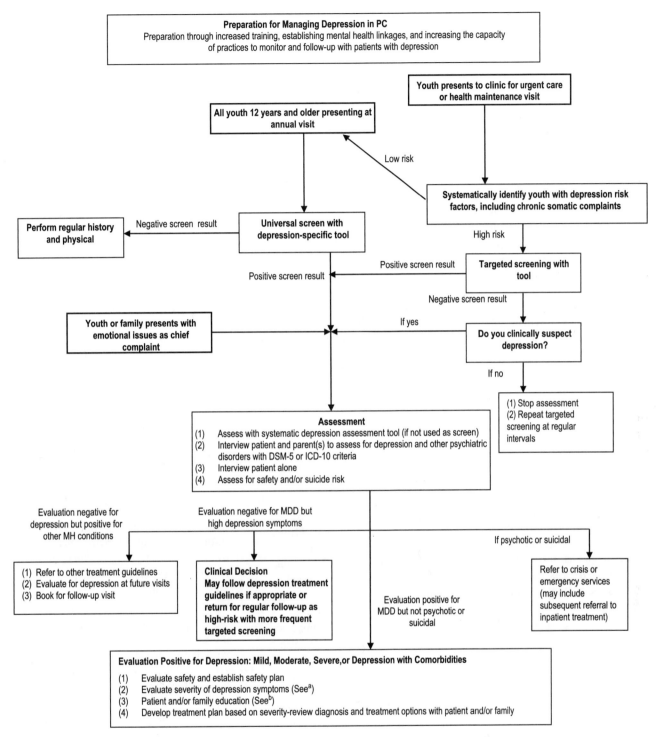

FIGURE 1

Clinical assessment flowchart. ICD-10, *International Classification of Diseases, 10th Revision*; MH, mental health. [a] See part I of the guidelines for definitions of mild, moderate, and severe depression. Please consult the tool kit for methods that are available to aid clinicians in distinguishing among mild, moderate, and severe depression. [b] Psychoeducation, supportive counseling, facilitation of parental and patient self-management, referring for peer support, and regular monitoring of depressive symptoms and suicidality.

in place, and establish follow-up within a reasonable period of time.[109,120,152,153] This plan should be developed with adolescents (and with their families and/or caregivers if possible) and should include a list of persons and/or services for the adolescent to contact in case of acute crisis or increased suicidality. The establishment of this plan is especially important during the period of diagnosis and initial treatment, when safety concerns are the highest. It is critical for PC clinicians to make linkages with their closest crisis support and hospital services so that they are supported in crisis situations when caring for youth with depression. Clinicians may also work with schools to develop an emergency plan for all students who may experience acute suicidal crises. This global approach may prevent, in some instances, having to label a specific child as suicidal when providers are merely trying to ensure that safety measures are in place in case the child decompensates. Components of a safety plan may also include a list of persons who are aware of the adolescents' issues and will be able to assist if contacted during an acute crisis (Fig 1).

DISCUSSION

Although not definitive and subject to modification on the basis of the ongoing accumulation of additional evidence, this part of the updated guidelines is intended to help address the lack of recommendations regarding practice preparation, screening, diagnosis, and initial management of depression in adolescents aged 10 to 21 years in PC settings in the United States and Canada. As such, these guidelines are intended to assist PC clinicians in family medicine, pediatrics, nursing, and internal medicine, who may be the first (and sometimes only) clinicians to identify, manage, and possibly treat adolescent depression. These guidelines may also be helpful to allied health professionals who care for adolescents.

Although not all the steps involved in identifying, diagnosing, and initially managing the care for adolescent depression in PC have been (or even can be) subject to rigorous RCTs, there is sound reason

to believe that existing tools and management protocols for adolescent depression can be applied in the PC setting. Although more research is needed, we suggest that these components of the identification and initial management of adolescent depression in PC can be done. The recommendations were developed and updated on the basis of areas that had at least strong agreement among experts.

Should These Guidelines Be Universally Deployed?

One might question whether PC clinicians should identify and diagnose the problem of adolescent depression if the lack of psychiatric services prevents them from referring these youth.[154] This caution notwithstanding, the increasingly prevailing recommendation is that at a minimum, PC clinicians should be provided the necessary guidance to support the initial management of adolescent depression.[155,156] Nonetheless, because practitioners and their clinical practice settings vary widely in their degree of readiness in identifying and managing adolescent depression, it is likely that a good deal of time and flexibility will be required before these guidelines are adopted systematically or as a universal requirement. It is conceivable that integrated health care systems with EMRs, tracking systems, and access to specialty mental health backup and consultation will be most ready and able to fully implement the guidelines. The second part of the guidelines, the companion article, addresses the treatment of depression. Practices that do identify adolescent depression and have nowhere to refer patients to may benefit from the guidance offered in the next set of recommendations.

Preparatory Steps

Because the management of adolescent depression may constitute a new or major challenge for some

PC practices, a number of important considerations should be kept in mind when preparing to implement the guidelines given the findings from studies in the adult literature; input from our focus groups of clinicians, families, and patients; and the experience of members of the GLAD-PC Steering Committee. Specifically, PC clinicians who manage adolescent depression should pursue the following: (1) additional training regarding issues such as advances in screening, diagnosis, treatment, follow-up, liability, consent, confidentiality, and billing; (2) practice and systems changes, such as office staff training and buy-in, EMRs, and automated tracking systems, whenever available; and (3) establishing linkages with mental health services.

Linkages with community mental health resources are necessary to both meet the learning needs of the PC clinicians and to facilitate consultation for and/or referral of difficult cases. Practice and systems changes are useful in increasing clinicians' capacity to facilitate monitoring and follow-up of patients with depression. For example, staff training may help prioritize calls from adolescent patients who may not state the nature of their call. Specific tools and/or templates have been developed that offer examples of how to efficiently identify, monitor, track, and refer teenagers with depression. These materials are available in the GLAD-PC tool kit. The tool kit addresses how each of the recommendations might be accomplished without each practice necessarily having to "reinvent the wheel."

CONCLUSIONS

Review of the evidence suggests that PC clinicians who have appropriate training and are attempting to deliver comprehensive health care should be able to identify and initiate the management of adolescent depression. This will likely require real changes in existing systems of care. As health care models such as the medical home indicate, comprehensive health care should include assessment and coordination of care for both physical and behavioral health issues. This first part of the guidelines for adolescent depression in PC may enable providers to pull together the current best evidence and deliver the best available, high-quality care even in instances when they are not in a position to treat such youth. Mounting evidence suggests that pediatric providers can and should identify and coordinate depression care in their adolescent populations.

APPENDIX: PART I TOOLKIT ITEMS

- Screening/assessment instruments (i.e., Columbia Depression Scale)

- Information sheet on the developmental considerations in the diagnosis of depression

- Assessment Algorithm/Flow Sheet (Fig 1)

- Fact sheet/family education materials

- Educational materials on suicide prevention/safety planning

LEAD AUTHORS

Rachel A. Zuckerbrot, MD
Amy Cheung, MD
Peter S. Jensen, MD
Ruth E.K. Stein, MD
Danielle Laraque, MD

GLAD-PC PROJECT TEAM

Peter S. Jensen, MD – Project Director, *University of Arkansas for Medical Science*
Amy Cheung, MD – Project Coordinator, *University of Toronto* and *Columbia University*
Rachel Zuckerbrot, MD – Project Coordinator, *Columbia University Medical Center* and *New York State Psychiatric Institute*

Anthony Levitt, MD – Project Consultant, *University of Toronto*

STEERING COMMITTEE MEMBERS

GLAD-PC Youth and Family Advisory Team
Joan Asarnow, PhD – *David Geffen School of Medicine, University of California, Los Angeles*
Boris Birmaher, MD – *Western Psychiatric Institute and Clinic, University of Pittsburgh*
John Campo, MD – *Ohio State University*
Greg Clarke, PhD – *Center for Health Research, Kaiser Permanente*
M. Lynn Crismon, PharmD – *The University of Texas at Austin*
Graham Emslie, MD – *University of Texas Southwestern Medical Center and Children's Health System Texas*
Miriam Kaufman, MD – *Hospital for Sick Children, University of Toronto*
Kelly J. Kelleher, MD – *Ohio State University*
Stanley Kutcher, MD – *Dalhousie Medical School*
Danielle Laraque, MD – *State University of New York Upstate Medical University*
Michael Malus, MD – *Department of Family Medicine, McGill University*
Diane Sacks, MD – *Canadian Paediatric Society*
Ruth E. K. Stein, MD – *Albert Einstein College of Medicine and Children's Hospital at Montefiore*
Barry Sarvet, MD – *Baystate Health, Massachusetts*
Bruce Waslick, MD – *Baystate Health Systems, Massachusetts, and University of Massachusetts Medical School*
Benedetto Vitiello, MD – *University of Turin and NIMH (former)*

ORGANIZATIONAL LIAISONS

Nerissa Bauer, MD – *AAP*
Diane Sacks, MD – *Canadian Paediatric Society*
Barry Sarvet, MD – *American Academy of Child and Adolescent Psychiatry*
Mary Kay Nixon, MD – *Canadian Academy of Child and Adolescent Psychiatry*
Robert Hilt, MD – *American Psychiatric Association*
Darcy Gruttadaro (former) – *National Alliance on Mental Illness*
Teri Brister – *National Alliance on Mental Illness*

ACKNOWLEDGMENTS

The authors wish to acknowledge research support from Justin Chee, Lindsay Williams, Robyn Tse, Isabella Churchill, Farid Azadian, Geneva Mason, Jonathan West, Sara Ho and Michael West. We are most grateful to the advice and guidance of Dr. Jeff Bridge, Dr. Purti Papneja, Dr. Elena Mann, Dr. Rachel Lynch, Dr. Marc Lashley, and Dr. Diane Bloomfield.

ABBREVIATIONS

AAP: American Academy of Pediatrics
BHS: Behavioral Health Screen
CATCH-IT: Competent Adulthood Transition with Cognitive-behavioral, Humanistic and Interpersonal Training
DISC-IV: Diagnostic Interview Schedule for Children-IV
DSM-5: *Diagnostic and Statistical Manual of Mental Disorders, Fifth Edition*
ED: emergency department
EMR: electronic medical record
GAPS: Guidelines for Adolescent Preventive Services
GLAD-PC: Guidelines for Adolescent Depression in Primary Care
HMO: health maintenance organization
K-SADS: Kiddie Schedule for Affective Disorders and Schizophrenia
MDD: major depressive disorder
NPV: negative predictive value
PC: primary care
PHQ-2: Patient Health Questionnaire-2
PHQ-9: Patient Health Questionnaire-9
PPV: positive predictive value
PSC: Pediatric Symptom Checklist
PSC-17: Pediatric Symptom Checklist-17
RCT: randomized controlled trial
REACH: Resource for Advancing Children's Health
TCPS: Targeted Child Psychiatry Services
USPSTF: United States Preventive Services Task Force
YPIC: Youth Partners in Care

FINANCIAL DISCLOSURE: In the past 2 years, Dr Jensen has received royalties from several publishing companies: Random House, Oxford University Press, and APPI Inc. He also is a part owner of a consulting company, CATCH Services LLC. He is the chief executive officer and president of a nonprofit organization, the Resource for Advancing Children's Health Institute, but receives no compensation; the other authors have indicated they have no financial relationships relevant to this article to disclose.

FUNDING: We thank the following organizations for their financial support of the Guidelines for Adolescent Depression in Primary Care project: the Resource for Advancing Children's Health Institute and the Bell Canada Chair in Adolescent Mood and Anxiety Disorders.

POTENTIAL CONFLICT OF INTEREST: Dr Zuckerbrot works for CAP PC, child and adolescent psychiatry for primary care, now a regional provider for Project TEACH in New York State. Dr Zuckerbrot is also on the steering committee as well as faculty for the REACH Institute. Both of these institutions are described in this publication. Drs Cheung and Zuckerbrot receive book royalties from Research Civic Institute.

COMPANION PAPER: A companion to this article can be found online at www.pediatrics.org/cgi/doi/10.1542/peds.2017-4082.

REFERENCES

1. Fleming JE, Offord DR, Boyle MH. Prevalence of childhood and adolescent depression in the community. Ontario Child Health Study. *Br J Psychiatry.* 1989;155(5):647–654

2. Birmaher B, Brent D, et al. Practice parameters for the assessment and treatment of children and adolescents with depressive disorders. AACAP. *J Am Acad Child Adolesc Psychiatry.* 1998;37(suppl 10):63S–83S

3. Copeland WE, Angold A, Shanahan L, Costello EJ. Longitudinal patterns of anxiety from childhood to adulthood: the Great Smoky Mountains Study. *J Am Acad Child Adolesc Psychiatry.* 2014;53(1):21–33

4. Mandoki MW, Tapia MR, Tapia MA, Sumner GS, Parker JL. Venlafaxine in the treatment of children and adolescents with major depression. *Psychopharmacol Bull.* 1997;33(1):149–154

5. Kessler RC, Avenevoli S, Ries Merikangas K. Mood disorders in children and adolescents: an epidemiologic perspective. *Biol Psychiatry.* 2001;49(12):1002–1014

6. Burns BJ, Costello EJ, Angold A, et al. Children's mental health service use across service sectors. *Health Aff (Millwood).* 1995;14(3):147–159

7. Leaf PJ, Alegria M, Cohen P, et al. Mental health service use in the community and schools: results from the four-community MECA Study. Methods for the Epidemiology of Child and Adolescent Mental Disorders Study. *J Am Acad Child Adolesc Psychiatry.* 1996;35(7):889–897

8. Martini R, Hilt R, Marx L, et al. *Best Principles for Integration of Child Psychiatry Into the Pediatric Health Home.* Washington, DC: American Academy for Child and Adolescent Psychiatry; 2012

9. Rushton JL, Clark SJ, Freed GL. Pediatrician and family physician prescription of selective serotonin reuptake inhibitors. *Pediatrics.* 2000;105(6). Available at: www.pediatrics.org/cgi/content/full/105/6/e82

10. Zito JM, Safer DJ, DosReis S, et al. Rising prevalence of antidepressants among US youths. *Pediatrics.* 2002;109(5):721–727

11. Asarnow JR, Jaycox LH, Duan N, et al. Effectiveness of a quality improvement intervention for adolescent depression in primary care clinics: a randomized controlled trial. *JAMA.* 2005;293(3):311–319

12. Gilbody S, Whitty P, Grimshaw J, Thomas R. Educational and organizational interventions to improve the management of depression in primary care: a systematic review. *JAMA.* 2003;289(23):3145–3151

13. Scott J, Thorne A, Horn P. Quality improvement report: effect of a multifaceted approach to detecting and managing depression in primary care. *BMJ.* 2002;325(7370):951–954

14. Sarvet B, Gold J, Bostic JQ, et al. Improving access to mental health care for children: the Massachusetts Child Psychiatry Access Project. *Pediatrics.* 2010;126(6):1191–1200

15. Kolko DJ, Campo J, Kilbourne AM, Hart J, Sakolsky D, Wisniewski S. Collaborative care outcomes for pediatric behavioral health problems: a cluster randomized trial. *Pediatrics.* 2014;133(4). Available at: www.pediatrics.org/cgi/content/full/133/4/e981

16. Kolko DJ, Perrin E. The integration of behavioral health interventions in children's health care: services, science, and suggestions. *J Clin Child Adolesc Psychol.* 2014;43(2):216–228

17. Zuckerbrot RA, Cheung AH, Jensen PS, Stein RE, Laraque D; GLAD-PC Steering Group. Guidelines for Adolescent Depression in Primary Care (GLAD-PC): I. Identification, assessment, and initial management. *Pediatrics.* 2007;120(5). Available at: www.pediatrics.org/cgi/content/full/120/5/e1299

18. Cheung AH, Zuckerbrot RA, Jensen PS, Ghalib K, Laraque D, Stein REK; GLAD-PC Steering Group. Guidelines for Adolescent Depression in Primary Care (GLAD-PC): II. Treatment and ongoing management [published correction appears in *Pediatrics.* 2008;121(1):227]. *Pediatrics.* 2007;120(5). Available at: www.pediatrics.org/cgi/content/full/120/5/e1313

19. American Psychiatric Association. *Diagnostic and Statistical Manual of Mental Disorders (DSM-5).* 5th ed. Washington, DC: American Psychiatric Association; 2013

20. Robins E, Guze SB. Establishment of diagnostic validity in psychiatric illness: its application to schizophrenia. *Am J Psychiatry.* 1970;126(7):983–987

21. Feighner JP, Robins E, Guze SB, Woodruff RA Jr, Winokur G, Munoz R. Diagnostic criteria for use in psychiatric research. *Arch Gen Psychiatry.* 1972;26(1):57–63

22. Lewinsohn PM, Essau CA. Depression in adolescents. In: Gotlib IH, Hammen CL, eds. *Handbook of Depression*. New York, NY: Guilford Press; 2002:541–559

23. Costello EJ, Mustillo S, Erkanli A, Keeler G, Angold A. Prevalence and development of psychiatric disorders in childhood and adolescence. *Arch Gen Psychiatry*. 2003;60(8):837–844

24. Keller MB, Klein DN, Hirschfeld RM, et al. Results of the DSM-IV mood disorders field trial. *Am J Psychiatry*. 1995;152(6):843–849

25. Cuijpers P, de Graaf R, van Dorsselaer S. Minor depression: risk profiles, functional disability, health care use and risk of developing major depression. *J Affect Disord*. 2004;79(1–3):71–79

26. Cheung AH, Zuckerbrot RA, Jensen PS, Stein REK, Laraque D; GLAD-PC Steering Committee. Expert survey for the management of adolescent depression in primary care. *Pediatrics*. 2008;121(1). Available at: www.pediatrics.org/cgi/content/full/121/1/e101

27. Oxman AD, Thomson MA, Davis DA, Haynes RB. No magic bullets: a systematic review of 102 trials of interventions to improve professional practice. *CMAJ*. 1995;153(10):1423–1431

28. Baskerville NB, Liddy C, Hogg W. Systematic review and meta-analysis of practice facilitation within primary care settings. *Ann Fam Med*. 2012;10(1):63–74

29. Perkins MB, Jensen PS, Jaccard J, et al. Applying theory-driven approaches to understanding and modifying clinicians' behavior: what do we know? *Psychiatr Serv*. 2007;58(3):342–348

30. Rinke ML, Driscoll A, Mikat-Stevens N, et al. A quality improvement collaborative to improve pediatric primary care genetic services. *Pediatrics*. 2016;137(2):e20143874

31. Chauhan BF, Jeyaraman MM, Mann AS, et al. Behavior change interventions and policies influencing primary healthcare professionals' practice-an overview of reviews [published correction appears in *Implement Sci*. 2017;12(1):38]. *Implement Sci*. 2017;12(1):3

32. Humble C, Domino M, Jensen P, et al. Changes in perceptions of guideline-level care for ADHD in North Carolina. In: *American Public Health Association Annual Meeting*; October 27–31, 2012; San Francisco, CA

33. Hargrave TM, Fremont W, Cogswell A, et al. Helping primary care clinicians give mental health care: what works? In: *Annual Meeting of the American Academy of Child and Adolescent Psychiatry*; October 20–25, 2014; San Antonio, TX

34. Brown JD, Riley AW, Wissow LS. Identification of youth psychosocial problems during pediatric primary care visits. *Adm Policy Ment Health*. 2007;34(3):269–281

35. Brown JD, Wissow LS, Cook BL, Longway S, Caffery E, Pefaure C. Mental health communications skills training for medical assistants in pediatric primary care. *J Behav Health Serv Res*. 2013;40(1):20–35

36. Craven MA, Bland R. Better practices in collaborative mental health care: an analysis of the evidence base. *Can J Psychiatry*. 2006;51(6, suppl 1):7S–72S

37. Gillies D, Buykx P, Parker AG, Hetrick SE. Consultation liaison in primary care for people with mental disorders. *Cochrane Database Syst Rev*. 2015;(9):CD007193

38. Powell BJ, McMillen JC, Proctor EK, et al. A compilation of strategies for implementing clinical innovations in health and mental health. *Med Care Res Rev*. 2012;69(2):123–157

39. Kaye D, Fornari V, Scharf M, et al. Learn then apply: increased impact of formal education with consultation support on PCP knowledge, skills, and confidence in child mental health care. *J Am Acad Child Adolesc Psychiatry*. 2016;55(10):S210–S211

40. Connor DF, McLaughlin TJ, Jeffers-Terry M, et al. Targeted child psychiatric services: a new model of pediatric primary clinician–child psychiatry collaborative care. *Clin Pediatr (Phila)*. 2006;45(5):423–434

41. Aupont O, Doerfler L, Connor DF, Stille C, Tisminetzky M, McLaughlin TJ. A collaborative care model to improve access to pediatric mental health services. *Adm Policy Ment Health*. 2013;40(4):264–273

42. Gadomski AM, Wissow LS, Palinkas L, Hoagwood KE, Daly JM, Kaye DL. Encouraging and sustaining integration of child mental health into primary care: interviews with primary care providers participating in Project TEACH (CAPES and CAP PC) in NY. *Gen Hosp Psychiatry*. 2014;36(6):555–562

43. Hilt RJ, Romaire MA, McDonell MG, et al. The Partnership Access Line: evaluating a child psychiatry consult program in Washington state. *JAMA Pediatr*. 2013;167(2):162–168

44. Ivbijaro GO, Enum Y, Khan AA, Lam SS, Gabzdyl A. Collaborative care: models for treatment of patients with complex medical-psychiatric conditions. *Curr Psychiatry Rep*. 2014;16(11):506

45. US Preventive Services Task Force. Screening and treatment for major depressive disorder in children and adolescents: US Preventive Services Task Force recommendation statement. *Pediatrics*. 2009;123(4):1223–1228

46. Williams SB, O'Connor EA, Eder M, Whitlock EP. Screening for child and adolescent depression in primary care settings: a systematic evidence review for the US Preventive Services Task Force. *Pediatrics*. 2009;123(4). Available at: www.pediatrics.org/cgi/content/full/123/4/e716

47. MacMillan HL, Patterson CJ, Wathen CN, et al; Canadian Task Force on Preventive Health Care. Screening for depression in primary care: recommendation statement from the Canadian Task Force on Preventive Health Care. *CMAJ*. 2005;172(1):33–35

48. Forman-Hoffman V, McClure E, McKeeman J, et al. Screening for major depressive disorder in children and adolescents: a systematic review for the U.S. Preventive Services Task Force. *Ann Intern Med*. 2016;164(5):342–349

49. Lewandowski RE, Acri MC, Hoagwood KE, et al. Evidence for the management of adolescent depression. *Pediatrics*. 2013;132(4). Available at: www.pediatrics.org/cgi/content/full/132/4/e996

50. Bevans KB, Diamond G, Levy S. Screening for adolescents'

internalizing symptoms in primary care: item response theory analysis of the behavior health screen depression, anxiety, and suicidal risk scales. *J Dev Behav Pediatr.* 2012;33(4):283–290

51. Borner I, Braunstein JW, St Victor R, Pollack J. Evaluation of a 2-question screening tool for detecting depression in adolescents in primary care. *Clin Pediatr (Phila).* 2010;49(10):947–953

52. Diamond G, Levy S, Bevans KB, et al. Development, validation, and utility of Internet-based, behavioral health screen for adolescents. *Pediatrics.* 2010;126(1). Available at: www.pediatrics.org/cgi/content/full/126/1/e163

53. Duke N, Ireland M, Borowsky IW. Identifying psychosocial problems among youth: factors associated with youth agreement on a positive parent-completed PSC-17. *Child Care Health Dev.* 2005;31(5):563–573

54. Gardner W, Lucas A, Kolko DJ, Campo JV. Comparison of the PSC-17 and alternative mental health screens in an at-risk primary care sample. *J Am Acad Child Adolesc Psychiatry.* 2007;46(5):611–618

55. Katon W, Russo J, Richardson L, McCauley E, Lozano P. Anxiety and depression screening for youth in a primary care population. *Ambul Pediatr.* 2008;8(3):182–188

56. Richardson LP, McCauley E, Grossman DC, et al. Evaluation of the Patient Health Questionnaire-9 Item for detecting major depression among adolescents. *Pediatrics.* 2010;126(6):1117–1123

57. Richardson LP, Rockhill C, Russo JE, et al. Evaluation of the PHQ-2 as a brief screen for detecting major depression among adolescents. *Pediatrics.* 2010;125(5). Available at: www.pediatrics.org/cgi/content/full/125/5/e1097

58. Asarnow JR, Jaycox LH, Tang L, et al. Long-term benefits of short-term quality improvement interventions for depressed youths in primary care. *Am J Psychiatry.* 2009;166(9):1002–1010

59. Bakken S, Jia H, Chen ES, et al. The effect of a mobile health decision support system on diagnosis and management of obesity, tobacco use, and depression in adults and children. *J Nurse Pract.* 2014;10(10):774–780

60. Chisolm DJ, Klima J, Gardner W, Kelleher KJ. Adolescent behavioral risk screening and use of health services. *Adm Policy Ment Health.* 2009;36(6):374–380

61. Dumont IP, Olson AL. Primary care, depression, and anxiety: exploring somatic and emotional predictors of mental health status in adolescents. *J Am Board Fam Med.* 2012;25(3):291–299

62. Fallucco EM, Seago RD, Cuffe SP, Kraemer DF, Wysocki T. Primary care provider training in screening, assessment, and treatment of adolescent depression. *Acad Pediatr.* 2015;15(3):326–332

63. Fallucco EM, Conlon MK, Gale G, Constantino JN, Glowinski AL. Use of a standardized patient paradigm to enhance proficiency in risk assessment for adolescent depression and suicide. *J Adolesc Health.* 2012;51(1):66–72

64. Gadomski AM, Scribani MB, Krupa N, Jenkins PL. Do the Guidelines for Adolescent Preventive Services (GAPS) facilitate mental health diagnosis? *J Prim Care Community Health.* 2014;5(2):85–89

65. Gladstone TG, Marko-Holguin M, Rothberg P, et al. An internet-based adolescent depression preventive intervention: study protocol for a randomized control trial. *Trials.* 2015;16:203

66. Gledhill J, Garralda ME. Sub-syndromal depression in adolescents attending primary care: frequency, clinical features and 6 months' outcome. *Soc Psychiatry Psychiatr Epidemiol.* 2013;48(5):735–744

67. Gledhill J, Garralda ME. The short-term outcome of depressive disorder in adolescents attending primary care: a cohort study. *Soc Psychiatry Psychiatr Epidemiol.* 2011;46(10):993–1002

68. Grasso DJ, Connor DF, Scranton V, Macary S, Honigfeld L. Implementation of a computerized algorithmic support tool for identifying depression and anxiety at the pediatric well-child visit. *Clin Pediatr (Phila).* 2015;54(8):796–799

69. Hacker K, Arsenault L, Franco I, et al. Referral and follow-up after mental health screening in commercially insured adolescents. *J Adolesc Health.* 2014;55(1):17–23

70. John R, Buschman P, Chaszar M, Honig J, Mendonca E, Bakken S. Development and evaluation of a PDA-based decision support system for pediatric depression screening. *Stud Health Technol Inform.* 2007;129(pt 2):1382–1386

71. Kramer T, Iliffe S, Bye A, Miller L, Gledhill J, Garralda ME; TIDY Study Team. Testing the feasibility of therapeutic identification of depression in young people in British general practice. *J Adolesc Health.* 2013;52(5):539–545

72. Kramer T, Iliffe S, Gledhill J, Garralda ME. Recognising and responding to adolescent depression in general practice: developing and implementing the Therapeutic Identification of Depression in Young people (TIDY) programme. *Clin Child Psychol Psychiatry.* 2012;17(4):482–494

73. Iliffe S, Gallant C, Kramer T, et al. Therapeutic identification of depression in young people: lessons from the introduction of a new technique in general practice. *Br J Gen Pract.* 2012;62(596):e174–e182

74. Lewandowski RE, O'Connor B, Bertagnolli A, et al. Screening for and diagnosis of depression among adolescents in a large health maintenance organization. *Psychiatr Serv.* 2016;67(6):636–641

75. Libby JM, Stuart-Shor E, Patankar A. The implementation of a clinical toolkit and adolescent depression screening program in primary care. *Clin Pediatr (Phila).* 2014;53(14):1336–1344

76. Olson AL, Gaffney CA, Hedberg VA, Gladstone GR. Use of inexpensive technology to enhance adolescent health screening and counseling. *Arch Pediatr Adolesc Med.* 2009;163(2):172–177

77. Ozer EM, Zahnd EG, Adams SH, et al. Are adolescents being screened for emotional distress in primary care? *J Adolesc Health.* 2009;44(6):520–527

78. Rausch J, Hametz P, Zuckerbrot R, Rausch W, Soren K. Screening

for depression in urban Latino adolescents. *Clin Pediatr (Phila)*. 2012;51(10):964–971

79. Richardson LP, Ludman E, McCauley E, et al. Collaborative care for adolescents with depression in primary care: a randomized clinical trial. *JAMA*. 2014;312(8):809–816

80. Richardson LP, Russo JE, Lozano P, McCauley E, Katon W. Factors associated with detection and receipt of treatment for youth with depression and anxiety disorders. *Acad Pediatr*. 2010;10(1):36–40

81. Richardson L, McCauley E, Katon W. Collaborative care for adolescent depression: a pilot study. *Gen Hosp Psychiatry*. 2009;31(1):36–45

82. Rockhill CM, Katon W, Richards J, et al. What clinical differences distinguish depressed teens with and without comorbid externalizing problems? *Gen Hosp Psychiatry*. 2013;35(4):444–447

83. Stevens J, Klima J, Chisolm D, Kelleher KJ. A trial of telephone services to increase adolescent utilization of health care for psychosocial problems. *J Adolesc Health*. 2009;45(6):564–570

84. Stevens J, Kelleher KJ, Gardner W, et al. Trial of computerized screening for adolescent behavioral concerns. *Pediatrics*. 2008;121(6):1099–1105

85. Sudhanthar S, Thakur K, Sigal Y, Turner J. Improving validated depression screen among adolescent population in primary care practice using electronic health records (EHR). *BMJ Qual Improv Rep*. 2015;4(1):u209517.w3913

86. Tanielian T, Jaycox LH, Paddock SM, Chandra A, Meredith LS, Burnam MA. Improving treatment seeking among adolescents with depression: understanding readiness for treatment. *J Adolesc Health*. 2009;45(5):490–498

87. Wells KB, Tang L, Carlson GA, Asarnow JR. Treatment of youth depression in primary care under usual practice conditions: observational findings from Youth Partners in Care. *J Child Adolesc Psychopharmacol*. 2012;22(1):80–90

88. Zuckerbrot RA, Maxon L, Pagar D, Davies M, Fisher PW, Shaffer D. Adolescent depression screening in primary care: feasibility

and acceptability. *Pediatrics*. 2007;119(1):101–108

89. Gardner W, Klima J, Chisolm D, et al. Screening, triage, and referral of patients who report suicidal thought during a primary care visit. *Pediatrics*. 2010;125(5):945–952

90. LeFevre ML; US Preventive Services Task Force. Screening for suicide risk in adolescents, adults, and older adults in primary care: U.S. Preventive Services Task Force recommendation statement. *Ann Intern Med*. 2014;160(10):719–726

91. Van Voorhees BW, Vanderplough-Booth K, Fogel J, et al. Integrative Internet-based depression prevention for adolescents: a randomized clinical trial in primary care for vulnerability and protective factors. *J Can Acad Child Adolesc Psychiatry*. 2008;17(4):184–196

92. Stein RE, Zitner LE, Jensen PS. Interventions for adolescent depression in primary care. *Pediatrics*. 2006;118(2):669–682

93. Bass JL, Christoffel KK, Widome M, et al. Childhood injury prevention counseling in primary care settings: a critical review of the literature. *Pediatrics*. 1993;92(4):544–550

94. Nelson CS, Wissow LS, Cheng TL. Effectiveness of anticipatory guidance: recent developments. *Curr Opin Pediatr*. 2003;15(6):630–635

95. Lemanek KL, Kamps J, Chung NB. Empirically supported treatments in pediatric psychology: regimen adherence. *J Pediatr Psychol*. 2001;26(5):253–275

96. Haynes RB, McDonald H, Garg AX, Montague P. Interventions for helping patients to follow prescriptions for medications. *Cochrane Database Syst Rev*. 2002;(2):CD000011

97. Haynes RB, Yao X, Degani A, Kripalani S, Garg A, McDonald HP. Interventions to enhance medication adherence. *Cochrane Database Syst Rev*. 2005;(4):CD000011

98. Roter DL, Hall JA, Merisca R, Nordstrom B, Cretin D, Svarstad B. Effectiveness of interventions to improve patient compliance: a meta-analysis. *Med Care*. 1998;36(8):1138–1161

99. Blum RW. Compliance in the adolescent with chronic illness. *Semin Adolesc Med*. 1987;3(2):157–162

100. La Greca AM. It's "all in the family": responsibility for diabetes care. *J Pediatr Endocrinol Metab*. 1998;11(suppl 2):379–385

101. La Greca AM, Bearman KJ. Commentary: if "an apple a day keeps the doctor away," why is adherence so darn hard? *J Pediatr Psychol*. 2001;26(5):279–282

102. Cooley WC. Redefining primary pediatric care for children with special health care needs: the primary care medical home. *Curr Opin Pediatr*. 2004;16(6):689–692

103. Edwards SJ, Sachmann MD. No-suicide contracts, no-suicide agreements, and no-suicide assurances: a study of their nature, utilization, perceived effectiveness, and potential to cause harm. *Crisis*. 2010;31(6):290–302

104. Garvey KA, Penn JV, Campbell AL, Esposito-Smythers C, Spirito A. Contracting for safety with patients: clinical practice and forensic implications. *J Am Acad Psychiatry Law*. 2009;37(3):363–370

105. McMyler C, Pryjmachuk S. Do 'no-suicide' contracts work? *J Psychiatr Ment Health Nurs*. 2008;15(6):512–522

106. Lewis LM. No-harm contracts: a review of what we know. *Suicide Life Threat Behav*. 2007;37(1):50–57

107. Rudd MD, Mandrusiak M, Joiner TE Jr. The case against no-suicide contracts: the commitment to treatment statement as a practice alternative. *J Clin Psychol*. 2006;62(2):243–251

108. Brent DA, Perper JA, Allman CJ, Moritz GM, Wartella ME, Zelenak JP. The presence and accessibility of firearms in the homes of adolescent suicides. A case-control study. *JAMA*. 1991;266(21):2989–2995

109. Brent DA, Perper JA, Moritz G, Baugher M, Schweers J, Roth C. Firearms and adolescent suicide. A community case-control study. *Am J Dis Child*. 1993;147(10):1066–1071

110. Shah S, Hoffman RE, Wake L, Marine WM. Adolescent suicide and household access to firearms in Colorado: results

of a case-control study. *J Adolesc Health.* 2000;26(3):157–163

111. Hawton K, Townsend E, Deeks J, et al. Effects of legislation restricting pack sizes of paracetamol and salicylate on self poisoning in the United Kingdom: before and after study. *BMJ.* 2001;322(7296):1203–1207

112. Sinyor M, Levitt AJ. Effect of a barrier at Bloor Street Viaduct on suicide rates in Toronto: natural experiment. *BMJ.* 2010;341:c2884

113. Sinyor M, Howlett A, Cheung AH, Schaffer A. Substances used in completed suicide by overdose in Toronto: an observational study of coroner's data. *Can J Psychiatry.* 2012;57(3):184–191

114. Sinyor M, Schaffer A, Redelmeier DA, et al. Did the suicide barrier work after all? Revisiting the Bloor Viaduct natural experiment and its impact on suicide rates in Toronto. *BMJ Open.* 2017;7(5):e015299

115. Hawton K, Bergen H, Simkin S, et al. Effect of withdrawal of co-proxamol on prescribing and deaths from drug poisoning in England and Wales: time series analysis. *BMJ.* 2009;338:b2270

116. Hawton K, Bergen H, Simkin S, et al. Long term effect of reduced pack sizes of paracetamol on poisoning deaths and liver transplant activity in England and Wales: interrupted time series analyses. *BMJ.* 2013;346:f403

117. Brent DA, Baugher M, Birmaher B, Kolko DJ, Bridge J. Compliance with recommendations to remove firearms in families participating in a clinical trial for adolescent depression. *J Am Acad Child Adolesc Psychiatry.* 2000;39(10):1220–1226

118. Brent DA. Assessment and treatment of the youthful suicidal patient. *Ann N Y Acad Sci.* 2001;932:106–128; discussion 128–131

119. Stewart SE, Manion IG, Davidson S. Emergency management of the adolescent suicide attempter: a review of the literature. *J Adolesc Health.* 2002;30(5):312–325

120. Asarnow JR, Berk M, Hughes JL, Anderson NL. The SAFETY Program: a treatment-development trial of a cognitive-behavioral family treatment for adolescent suicide attempters. *J Clin Child Adolesc Psychol.* 2015;44(1):194–203

121. Stroul B, Friedman RM. *A System of Care for Children and Youth With Severe Emotional Disturbances.* Washington, DC: CASSP Technical Assistance Center, Center for Child Health and Mental Health Policy, Georgetown University Child Development Center; 1994

122. Hoagwood KE. Family-based services in children's mental health: a research review and synthesis. *J Child Psychol Psychiatry.* 2005;46(7):690–713

123. Heflinger CA, Sonnichsen SE, Brannan AM. Parent satisfaction with children's mental health services in a children's mental health managed care demonstration. *J Ment Health Adm.* 1996;23(1):69–79

124. Slap G, Goodman E, Huang B. Adoption as a risk factor for attempted suicide during adolescence. *Pediatrics.* 2001;108(2). Available at: www.pediatrics. org/cgi/content/full/108/2/e30

125. Bruskas D. Children in foster care: a vulnerable population at risk. *J Child Adolesc Psychiatr Nurs.* 2008;21(2):70–77

126. Lehmann SH, Havik OE, Havik T, Heiervang ER. Mental disorders in foster children: a study of prevalence, comorbidity and risk factors. *Child Adolesc Psychiatry Ment Health.* 2013;7(1):39

127. Fergusson DM, Horwood LJ, Lynskey MT. Maternal depressive symptoms and depressive symptoms in adolescents. *J Child Psychol Psychiatry.* 1995;36(7):1161–1178

128. Fergusson DM, Horwood LJ, Lynskey MT. Childhood sexual abuse and psychiatric disorder in young adulthood: II. Psychiatric outcomes of childhood sexual abuse. *J Am Acad Child Adolesc Psychiatry.* 1996;35(10):1365–1374

129. Fergusson DM, Woodward LJ, Horwood LJ. Risk factors and life processes associated with the onset of suicidal behaviour during adolescence and early adulthood. *Psychol Med.* 2000;30(1):23–39

130. Goodwin RD, Fergusson DM, Horwood LJ. Early anxious/withdrawn behaviours predict later internalising disorders. *J Child Psychol Psychiatry.* 2004;45(4):874–883

131. Weissman MM, Wickramaratne P, Nomura Y, et al. Families at high and low risk for depression: a 3-generation study. *Arch Gen Psychiatry.* 2005;62(1):29–36

132. Weissman MM, Wickramaratne P, Nomura Y, Warner V, Pilowsky D, Verdeli H. Offspring of depressed parents: 20 years later. *Am J Psychiatry.* 2006;163(6):1001–1008

133. Nomura Y, Wickramaratne PJ, Warner V, Mufson L, Weissman MM. Family discord, parental depression, and psychopathology in offspring: ten-year follow-up. *J Am Acad Child Adolesc Psychiatry.* 2002;41(4):402–409

134. Piacentini J, Shaffer D, Fisher P, Schwab-Stone M, Davies M, Gioia P. The diagnostic interview schedule for children-revised version (DISC-R): III. Concurrent criterion validity. *J Am Acad Child Adolesc Psychiatry.* 1993;32(3):658–665

135. Cox A, Hopkinson K, Rutter M. Psychiatric interviewing techniques II. Naturalistic study: eliciting factual information. *Br J Psychiatry.* 1981;138:283–291

136. Cox A, Rutter M, Holbrook D. Psychiatric interviewing techniques V. Experimental study: eliciting factual information. *Br J Psychiatry.* 1981;139:29–37

137. Ryan ND, Puig-Antich J, Ambrosini P, et al. The clinical picture of major depression in children and adolescents. *Arch Gen Psychiatry.* 1987;44(10):854–861

138. Costello EJ, Angold A, Burns BJ, et al. The Great Smoky Mountains Study of youth. Goals, design, methods, and the prevalence of DSM-III-R disorders. *Arch Gen Psychiatry.* 1996;53(12):1129–1136

139. Schwab-Stone ME, Shaffer D, Dulcan MK, et al. Criterion validity of the NIMH diagnostic interview schedule for children version 2.3 (DISC-2.3). *J Am Acad Child Adolesc Psychiatry.* 1996;35(7):878–888

140. Jensen PS, Rubio-Stipec M, Canino G, et al. Parent and child contributions

to diagnosis of mental disorder: are both informants always necessary? *J Am Acad Child Adolesc Psychiatry*. 1999;38(12):1569–1579

141. Manson S, Shore J, Bloom J. The depressive experience in American Indian communities: a challenge for psychiatric theory and diagnosis. In: Kleinman A, Good B, eds. *Culture and Depression*. Berkeley, CA: University of California Press; 1985:331–368

142. Treatment for Adolescents With Depression Study Team. The treatment for adolescents with depression study (TADS): demographic and clinical characteristics. *J Am Acad Child Adolesc Psychiatry*. 2005;44(1):28–40

143. Kovacs M, Obrosky DS, Sherrill J. Developmental changes in the phenomenology of depression in girls compared to boys from childhood onward. *J Affect Disord*. 2003;74(1):33–48

144. Curry J, Rohde P, Simons A, et al; TADS Team. Predictors and moderators of acute outcome in the Treatment for Adolescents with Depression Study (TADS). *J Am Acad Child Adolesc Psychiatry*. 2006;45(12):1427–1439

145. Brooks SJ, Kutcher S. Diagnosis and measurement of adolescent depression: a review of commonly utilized instruments. *J Child Adolesc Psychopharmacol*. 2001;11(4):341–376

146. Emslie GJ, Findling RL, Yeung PP, Kunz NR, Li Y. Venlafaxine ER for the treatment of pediatric subjects with depression: results of two placebo-controlled trials. *J Am Acad Child Adolesc Psychiatry*. 2007;46(4):479–488

147. Clarke GN, Rohde P, Lewinsohn PM, Hops H, Seeley JR. Cognitive-behavioral treatment of adolescent depression: efficacy of acute group treatment and booster sessions. *J Am Acad Child Adolesc Psychiatry*. 1999;38(3):272–279

148. Mufson L, Dorta KP, Wickramaratne P, Nomura Y, Olfson M, Weissman MM. A randomized effectiveness trial of interpersonal psychotherapy for depressed adolescents. *Arch Gen Psychiatry*. 2004;61(6):577–584

149. Bhogal S, Zemek R, Ducharme FM. Written action plans for asthma in children. *Cochrane Database Syst Rev*. 2006;(3):CD005306

150. Boydell KM, Hodgins M, Pignatiello A, Teshima J, Edwards H, Willis D. Using technology to deliver mental health services to children and youth: a scoping review. *J Can Acad Child Adolesc Psychiatry*. 2014;23(2):87–99

151. Shaffer D, Fisher P, Dulcan MK, et al. The NIMH diagnostic interview schedule for children version 2.3 (DISC-2.3): description, acceptability, prevalence rates, and performance in the MECA study. Methods for the Epidemiology of Child and Adolescent mental disorders study. *J Am Acad Child Adolesc Psychiatry*. 1996;35(7):865–877

152. American Academy of Child and Adolescent Psychiatry. Summary of the practice parameters for the assessment and treatment of children and adolescents with suicidal behavior. *J Am Acad Child Adolesc Psychiatry*. 2001;40(4):495–499

153. Berk MS, Asarnow JR. Assessment of suicidal youth in the emergency department. *Suicide Life Threat Behav*. 2015;45(3):345–359

154. Asarnow JR, Jaycox LH, Anderson M. Depression among youth in primary care models for delivering mental health services. *Child Adolesc Psychiatr Clin N Am*. 2002;11(3):477–497, viii

155. Olin SC, Hoagwood K. The surgeon general's national action agenda on children's mental health. *Curr Psychiatry Rep*. 2002;4(2):101–107

156. Coyle JT, Pine DS, Charney DS, et al; Depression and Bipolar Support Alliance Consensus Development Panel. Depression and bipolar support alliance consensus statement on the unmet needs in diagnosis and treatment of mood disorders in children and adolescents. *J Am Acad Child Adolesc Psychiatry*. 2003;42(12):1494–1503

STATEMENT OF ENDORSEMENT

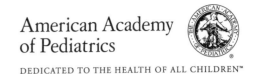

American Academy
of Pediatrics

DEDICATED TO THE HEALTH OF ALL CHILDREN™

Guidelines for Adolescent Depression in Primary Care (GLAD-PC): Part II. Treatment and Ongoing Management

Amy H. Cheung, MD,[a] Rachel A. Zuckerbrot, MD,[b] Peter S. Jensen, MD,[c] Danielle Laraque, MD,[d] Ruth E.K. Stein, MD,[e] GLAD-PC STEERING GROUP

OBJECTIVES: To update clinical practice guidelines to assist primary care (PC) in the screening and assessment of depression. In this second part of the updated guidelines, we address treatment and ongoing management of adolescent depression in the PC setting.

METHODS: By using a combination of evidence- and consensus-based methodologies, the guidelines were updated in 2 phases as informed by (1) current scientific evidence (published and unpublished) and (2) revision and iteration among the steering committee, including youth and families with lived experience.

RESULTS: These updated guidelines are targeted for youth aged 10 to 21 years and offer recommendations for the management of adolescent depression in PC, including (1) active monitoring of mildly depressed youth, (2) treatment with evidence-based medication and psychotherapeutic approaches in cases of moderate and/or severe depression, (3) close monitoring of side effects, (4) consultation and comanagement of care with mental health specialists, (5) ongoing tracking of outcomes, and (6) specific steps to be taken in instances of partial or no improvement after an initial treatment has begun. The strength of each recommendation and the grade of its evidence base are summarized.

CONCLUSIONS: The Guidelines for Adolescent Depression in Primary Care cannot replace clinical judgment, and they should not be the sole source of guidance for adolescent depression management. Nonetheless, the guidelines may assist PC clinicians in the management of depressed adolescents in an era of great clinical need and a shortage of mental health specialists. Additional research concerning the management of depressed youth in PC is needed, including the usability, feasibility, and sustainability of guidelines, and determination of the extent to which the guidelines actually improve outcomes of depressed youth.

abstract

[a]University of Toronto, Toronto, Ontario, Canada; [b]Division of Child and Adolescent Psychiatry, Department of Psychiatry, Columbia University Medical Center and New York State Psychiatric Institute, New York, New York; [c]University of Arkansas for Medical Sciences, Little Rock, Arkansas; [d]State University of New York Upstate Medical University, Syracuse, New York; and [e]Albert Einstein College of Medicine, Bronx, New York

This document is copyrighted and is property of the American Academy of Pediatrics and its Board of Directors. All authors have filed conflict of interest statements with the American Academy of Pediatrics. Any conflicts have been resolved through a process approved by the Board of Directors. The American Academy of Pediatrics has neither solicited nor accepted any commercial involvement in the development of the content of this publication.

The guidance in this document does not indicate an exclusive course of treatment or serve as a standard of medical care. Variations, taking into account individual circumstances, may be appropriate.

All statements of endorsement from the American Academy of Pediatrics automatically expire 5 years after publication unless reaffirmed, revised, or retired at or before that time.

DOI: https://doi.org/10.1542/peds.2017-4082

Address correspondence to Amy H. Cheung, MD. E-mail: amy.cheung@sunnybrook.ca

PEDIATRICS (ISSN Numbers: Print, 0031-4005; Online, 1098-4275).

FINANCIAL DISCLOSURE: In the past 2 years, Dr Jensen has received royalties from the following publishing companies: Random House, Oxford, and APPI, Inc. He also is a part owner of a consulting company,

To cite: Cheung AH, Zuckerbrot RA, Jensen PS, et al. Guidelines for Adolescent Depression in Primary Care (GLAD-PC): Part II. Treatment and Ongoing Management. *Pediatrics.* 2018;141(3):e20174082

BACKGROUND

Studies have revealed that up to 9% of teenagers meet criteria for depression at any one time, with as many as 1 in 5 teenagers having a history of depression at some point during adolescence.[1–7] In primary care (PC) settings, point prevalence rates are likely higher, with rates up to 28%.[8–12] Taken together, in epidemiologic and PC-specific studies it is suggested that despite relatively high rates, major depressive disorder (MDD) in youth is underidentified and undertreated in PC settings.[13,14]

Because adolescents face barriers to receive specialty mental health services, only a small percentage of depressed adolescents are treated by mental health professionals.[15] As a result, PC settings have become the de facto mental health clinics for this population, although most PC clinicians feel inadequately trained, supported, or reimbursed for the management of depression.[14–21] Although MDD management guidelines have been developed for specialty care settings (eg, the American Academy of Child and Adolescent Psychiatry[22]) or related problems such as suicidal ideation or attempts,[23] it is clear that significant practice and clinician differences exist between the primary and specialty care settings that do not allow a simple transfer of guidelines from one setting to another.

Recognizing this gap in clinical guidance for PC providers, in 2007, a group of researchers and clinical experts from the United States and Canada established Guidelines for Adolescent Depression in Primary Care (GLAD-PC), a North American collaborative, to develop guidelines for the management of adolescent depression in the PC setting. The development process of GLAD-PC is described in detail in Part I of the original GLAD-PC articles.[24,25] In this article, we describe the updated recommendations regarding treatment, ongoing management, and

follow-up, along with the supporting empirical evidence for these recommendations. In our companion article, we provide a detailed description of the update process as well as the corresponding updated recommendations for GLAD-PC regarding practice preparation, depression identification, assessment, and diagnosis, and initial management before formal treatment.

METHODS

A full description of the methodology used for the update of GLAD-PC is included in our companion article. In brief, the expert collaborative used a mix of qualitative (expert consensus) and quantitative (literature reviews) methods to inform the update of GLAD-PC. In view of space limitations, only the methods and results of the updated literature reviews regarding available evidence for treatment and ongoing management are presented in this article.

The following 3 literature reviews were conducted for the updated GLAD-PC recommendations: (1) nonspecific psychosocial interventions in pediatric PC, including studies pertaining to integrated behavioral health and collaborative care models; (2) antidepressant treatment; and (3) psychotherapy interventions.

For the first review, we searched the literature (PubMed, PsycInfo, and the Cochrane Database) for articles published from 2005 to the present in which researchers examined evidence for psychosocial interventions delivered in the PC setting to update the previous review conducted by Stein et al.[26] The "related articles" function was used to search for articles similar to Asarnow et al[14] and Richardson et al.[27] In addition, reference lists of all relevant articles were also examined for other relevant studies.

In the second updated review, we examined the efficacy and safety of antidepressant medications in the pediatric population (under the age of 18 years). This review was used to update the findings from the US Food and Drug Administration (FDA) safety report[28] and the previously published GLAD-PC review on antidepressants in youth depression.[29] Studies in which researchers examined the management of depression with the use of antidepressants as both monotherapy and combination therapy were included.

In the third review, we searched the literature for depression trials in which researchers examined the efficacy of psychotherapy for the management of depression in children and adolescents. The search included all forms of psychotherapy, including both individual and group-based therapies. We not only identified both individual studies but also high-quality systematic reviews, given the extensive empirical literature in this area. In both the second and third reviews, the literature searches were conducted by using Medline and PsycInfo to find studies published between 2005 to the present. To ensure additional articles were not missed, reference lists of included articles were hand-searched for other relevant studies. A full description of the 3 reviews is available on request.

RESULTS

Organizational Adoption of Integrative Care

Within the past decade, there has been a shift in medicine and in mental health away from the "traditional" model of autonomous individual providers and toward delivering empirically supported interventions in a team-based manner. This followed a growing recognition that complex chronic conditions, such as depression, are more successfully managed with proactive, multidisciplinary patient-centered care teams. Ongoing changes in the health care landscape helped to solidify support for this revolution. Systems are enacting top-down changes designed to make the entire delivery system (organizations, clinics, and providers) more effective, efficient, safe, and satisfying to both patients and providers.

Proposed integrated care models include "chronic care management," "integrated behavioral health care," "collaborative care," and "medical home." Here, the term "integrative care" will be used to collectively refer to models such as these. These complex care models share multiple features, such as an emphasis on systematically identifying and tracking target populations, multidisciplinary patient care, structured protocols for symptom management, regular follow-ups, decreasing fragmentation across the care team, and enhancing the patient's ability to self-manage their condition.[30] The following list represents many of the components described in 1 or more of these health care models:

1. a treatment team that includes the patient, the family, and access to mental health expertise;

2. education (including decision tools) for PC providers, patients, and family;

3. tools and/or procedures to systematically identify, assess, and diagnose patients who are at risk or are currently experiencing depressive symptoms;

4. a care plan for target patients (which may involve the family when possible and includes resources at other agencies or in the community);

5. improved communication and coordination of care across providers and/or between patient, family, and provider;

6. case management and/or patient and family support;

7. routine tracking of patient progress, with appropriate follow-up action as needed;

8. routine evaluation of staff performance metrics to inform ongoing quality improvement efforts; and

9. increased patient and family motivation and capacity to self-manage symptoms, including education, feedback, etc.

A variety of integrative care models have been proposed or discussed in the literature,[31,32] but few studies have actually been conducted to examine whether they ultimately improve care for children and adolescents with mental health disorders, broadly speaking, or depression, specifically. In the present review, only 3 randomized clinical trials were identified. In the first, Asarnow et al[14] found that adolescents treated for depression at PC clinics engaging in a quality improvement initiative received higher rates of mental health care and psychosocial therapy, endorsed fewer depressive symptoms, reported a greater quality of life, and expressed greater satisfaction with their care than comparison adolescents in a usual care condition. In a second study, researchers examined the additive benefits of providing brief (4-session) cognitive behavioral therapy (CBT) for depression in conjunction with antidepressant medication compared with medication alone in a collaborative care practice with embedded care managers and found a weak but positive benefit for adjunctive CBT.[33] Finally, Richardson et al[27] randomly assigned adolescents to either an integrative care condition, in which patients chose from a treatment menu of antidepressant medication alone, brief CBT alone, or a combination of the 2, versus usual care. Results

revealed that integrative care was associated with significant decreases in depression scores and improved response and remission rates at 12 months compared with treatment as usual.[27] The results of a cost-effectiveness analysis of this trial revealed that the integrative care condition was more effective at reducing depression symptoms for adolescents, resulting in incremental cost savings given the quality of life years gained from improved functioning.[34]

Although research studies offer support for the impact of integrative or collaborative health care delivery models as a whole,[35] multiple changes to the practice setting are being evaluated simultaneously. The components of integrative health care models have largely been identified through practice-based research[36] or "best ideas" about how to solve identified problems, without a clear theoretical or empirical basis for these components individually or in combination. Thus, it is unknown what "active ingredients" account for the greatest proportion of variance in patient improvement because no dismantling studies have been conducted in which the relative impact of the individual components was examined. Given that integrated health care approaches are resource-intensive to implement and maintain, it may not be feasible for many PC practices to fully adopt such a model. Some states and communities have attempted to implement "wraparound services" under the "systems of care model"; however, unfortunately, these services are usually restricted to severely impaired children with chronic mental health problems. Nonetheless, such services are available if PC providers are interested.[37,38] Unfortunately, there is relatively little information to help guide prioritization and decision-making for PC clinics that wish to improve patient care within the constraints of highly limited human and/or financial resources.

Antidepressant Treatment

The updated treatment review for antidepressant safety and efficacy included randomized controlled trials (RCTs) of antidepressants in youth with depression. In this GLAD-PC review, we identified 27 peer-reviewed articles in this area, including trials with fluoxetine, sertraline, citalopram, paroxetine, duloxetine, and venlafaxine. In addition, in several studies, the switch from a selective serotonin reuptake inhibitor (SSRI) to venlafaxine, a serotonin norepinephrine reuptake inhibitor, was explored.[39–41] Older antidepressants (ie, monoamine oxidase inhibitors, tricyclic antidepressants) were not included in our updated review because of several reasons. First, the 2004 FDA review that was used for the development of the guidelines only involved newer classes of antidepressants. Second, older antidepressants are not used because of the lack of efficacy demonstrated in clinical trials data for other classes of older antidepressants.[42]

Overall, both individual clinical trial evidence and evidence from systematic reviews still support the use of antidepressants in adolescents with MDD. Bridge et al[43] conducted a meta-analysis of the clinical trials data and calculated the numbers needed to treat and numbers needed to harm. They concluded that 6 times more teenagers would benefit from treatment with antidepressants than would be harmed.[43] In reviewing the individual studies, the percentage of subjects who responded to antidepressants ranged from 47% to 69% and from 33% to 57% for those on placebo (see Table 1). The majority of these studies revealed a significant difference between those on medication versus those on placebo. Similarly, on the basis of the

TABLE 1 Response Rates in RCTs of Antidepressants Based on Clinical Global Impression

Medication	Drug, %	Placebo, %	P
Fluoxetine[45,a]	56	33	.02
Fluoxetine[46]	52	37	.03
Fluoxetine[47]	61	35	.001
Paroxetine[48,b]	66	48	.02
Paroxetine[49]	69	57	NS
Paroxetine[49]	65	46	.005
Citalopram[50]	47	45	NS
Citalopram[51]	51	53	NS
Sertraline[52]	63	53	.05
Escitalopram[53]	63	52	.14
Escitalopram[54]	64	53	.03

NS, not significant.
[a] Fluoxetine alone compared with placebo.
[b] Paroxetine compared with placebo.

updated review, fluoxetine still has the most evidence to support its use in the adolescent population.[44]

The largest study, the Treatment of Adolescent Depression Study, involved subjects who were randomly assigned to receive placebo, CBT alone, fluoxetine alone, or a combination treatment of CBT with fluoxetine.[45] Subjects assigned to receive combination treatment or fluoxetine alone showed significantly greater improvement in their depressive symptoms compared with those on placebo or those treated with CBT alone (also see subsection "CBT"). There is also a more rapid initial response when medication is initiated first or in combination with therapy.[55] The superiority of combination therapy is also demonstrated in adolescents with anxiety.[56,57] However, a few trials have revealed little extra benefit to combination therapy, but these findings might be confounded by the control therapy intervention (ie, routine specialist care).[58–60]

Combination therapy has also been evaluated in adolescents with treatment-resistant depression. In the Treatment of SSRI-resistant Depression in Adolescents study, researchers examined treatment options for adolescents aged 12 to 18 whose depression had not improved after 1 adequate trial of an SSRI.[39–41,49,61–63] Subjects were randomly assigned to 4 possible

interventions: (1) switch to a different SSRI (citalopram, fluoxetine, paroxetine), (2) switch to a second SSRI in combination with CBT, (3) switch to venlafaxine, or (4) switch to venlafaxine in combination with CBT. Patients who received CBT and changed their medication to a second SSRI or venlafaxine had a higher response rate (54.8%; 95% confidence interval [CI]: 47%–62%) than changing the medication alone (40.5%; 95% CI: 33%–48%; $P = .009$). Additionally, there was no difference in response rate between venlafaxine and a second SSRI (48.2%; 95% CI: 41%–56%; and 47%; 95% CI: 40%–55%; $P = .83$) as well as no significant differences among Children's Depression Rating Scale–Revised improvements between treatment options.

Finally, with available evidence from RCTs, it is suggested that adverse effects do emerge in depressed youth who are treated with antidepressants.[45] Adverse effects (ie, nausea, headaches, behavioral activation, etc) were found to occur in most adolescents treated with antidepressants, with duloxetine, venlafaxine, and paroxetine as the most intolerable.[45] Therefore, routine monitoring of the development of adverse events is critical for depressed youth treated with antidepressants.

The most significant adverse effect of antidepressants is the emergence of new onset or worsening suicidality, which was demonstrated in the FDA review in 2004.[29] The estimated risk of suicidality is 4% in those on medication versus 2% in those on placebo. However, further analyses of clinical trials data revealed that there is overall improvement in suicidality in subjects treated with antidepressants, with only a few subjects reporting worsening or new onset suicidality.[49] In the FDA review, it was also suggested that paroxetine and venlafaxine have a significantly higher risk for suicidality compared with other serotonergic antidepressants.

The doubling of risk of suicidality was also confirmed in population level studies.[63] However, studies have also revealed that almost all adolescents who die by suicide do not test positive for antidepressants in postmortem toxicology tests despite being prescribed these drugs.[64] Furthermore, Olfson et al[65] found an inverse relationship between rates of SSRI prescriptions and rates of suicide in adolescent populations.

Psychotherapy

In the third review conducted, we examined the efficacy of psychotherapy, such as CBT, interpersonal psychotherapy for adolescents (IPT-A), as well as nonspecific interventions such as counseling and support. Through our search, we were able to identify both individual studies as well as several high-quality meta-analyses and/or reviews that were recently conducted to examine the efficacy of psychotherapy in adolescent depression.

CBT

Numerous meta-analyses and reviews have been conducted on CBT in the treatment of adolescent depression and showed improved outcomes for subjects treated with CBT.[66–68] There are also several ongoing studies in which researchers

are evaluating CBT in youth up to age 21.[69]

The effectiveness of CBT for adolescents with moderate to moderately severe depression was also evaluated in Treatment of Adolescent Depression Study, in which researchers randomly assigned 439 12- to 17-year-olds who were depressed to treatment with CBT, fluoxetine, CBT plus fluoxetine, or placebo.[45,70] According to Clinical Global Impressions severity scores, the posttreatment response rate to 15 sessions of CBT over 12 weeks (43.2%; 95% CI: 34%–52%) was not significantly different ($P = .40$) from placebo (34.8%; 95% CI: 26%–44%). The authors attributed this relatively low response rate, in part, to the fact that the study population suffered from more severe and chronic depression than participants in previous studies and to a high rate of psychiatric comorbidity in their study participants. Along with the fairly robust placebo-response rate, it is also possible that the nonspecific therapeutic aspects of the medication management could have successfully competed with the specific effects of the CBT intervention. As a consequence, one cannot and should not conclude that CBT is ineffective.

In another study with adolescents with depression, Fleming et al[71] evaluated the effectiveness of a computerized cognitive behavioral therapy (CCBT) intervention called SPARX in treating adolescents aged 13 to 16 years excluded from mainstream education ($n = 20$). After randomly assigning them to CCBT or the waitlist control, it was found that there were significantly greater reductions in Children's Depression Rating Scale and Reynolds Adolescent Depression Scale scores from baseline to week 5 for the intervention group compared with those who waited. In addition, the SPARX group was significantly more likely to be in remission or have a significant reduction in symptoms.

In several other studies, researchers have evaluated CCBT interventions and have also found similar results, with 1 study conducted in the PC setting.[72,73]

IPT-A

In terms of IPT-A, only a handful of studies have been conducted. First, Tang et al[74] randomly assigned 347 adolescents who were depressed to receive IPT-A in schools or treatment as usual. IPT-A was found to have significantly higher effects on reducing severity of depression, suicidal ideation, and hopelessness compared with treatment as usual. In Gunlicks-Stoessel et al's[75] study, 63 adolescents who were depressed were randomly assigned to IPT-A or treatment as usual. Adolescents who were depressed who reported higher baseline levels of interpersonal difficulties showed a greater and more rapid reduction in depressive symptoms if treated with IPT-A compared with treatment as usual. In the most recent study,[76] 57 adolescents with depressive symptoms were randomly assigned to receive either 8 weeks of interpersonal therapy–adolescent skills training or supportive school counseling. Adolescents who were treated with interpersonal therapy–adolescent skills training showed significantly greater rates of change compared with adolescents who received school counseling on the Center for Epidemiologic Studies Depression Scale ($t[215] = -2.56$, $P = .01$), Children's Depression Rating Scale-Revised ($t[169] = -3.09$, $P < .01$), and the Children's Global Assessment Scale ($t[168] = 3.24$, $P < .01$).

GUIDELINES

Each of the recommendations below was graded on the basis of the level of supporting research evidence from the literature and the extent to which experts agreed that it is highly appropriate in PC. The level of supporting evidence for each recommendation is based on the Oxford Centre for Evidence-Based Medicine grades of evidence[1-5] system, with 1 to 5 corresponding to strongest to weakest evidence (see http://www.cebm.net/wp-content/uploads/2014/06/CEBM-Levels-of-Evidence-2.1.pdf/).

Recommendation strength based on expert consensus was rated in 4 categories: very strong (>90% agreement), strong (>70% agreement), fair (>50% agreement), and weak (<50% agreement). The recommendations in the guidelines were developed only in areas of management that had at least a "strong agreement" among experts (see Fig 1 for the treatment algorithm).

Treatment

Recommendation 1: PC clinicians should work with administration to organize their clinical settings to reflect best practices in integrated and/or collaborative care models (eg, facilitating contact with psychiatrists, case managers, embedded therapists). (grade of evidence: 4; strength of recommendation: very strong).

There is a growing recognition that complex chronic conditions, such as depression, are most successfully managed with proactive, multidisciplinary, patient-centered care teams.[77,78] Proposed integrated care models include chronic care management, integrated behavioral health care, collaborative care, and medical home. These complex care models have been shown to be more effective in improving outcomes and share multiple features, such as an emphasis on systematically identifying and tracking target populations, decreasing fragmentation across the care team, and enhancing the patient's ability to self-manage their condition.

Recommendation 2: After initial diagnosis, in cases of mild depression, clinicians should consider a period of active support and monitoring before starting evidence-based treatment (grade of evidence: 3; strength of recommendation: very strong).

After a preliminary diagnostic assessment, in cases of mild depression, clinicians should consider a period of active support and monitoring before recommending treatment (from 6 to 8 weeks of weekly or biweekly visits for active monitoring). Evidence from RCTs with antidepressants and CBT show that a sizable percentage of patients respond to nondirective supportive therapy and regular symptom monitoring.[42,43,45,48,50,70,79] However, if symptoms persist, treatment with antidepressants or psychotherapy should be offered, whether provided by PC or mental health. Active support and monitoring is also essential in cases in which depressed patients and/or their families and/or caregivers refuse other treatments. Active support and counseling for adolescents by pediatric PC clinicians have been evaluated for several different disorders, including substance abuse and sleep disorders.[22]

Furthermore, expert opinion based on extensive clinical experience and qualitative research with families, patients, and clinicians indicates that these strategies are a crucial component of management by PC clinicians. For further guidance on how to provide active support, please refer to the GLAD-PC toolkit (http://www.gladpc.org).

For moderate or severe cases, the clinician should recommend treatment; crisis intervention; patient and family support services, such as in-home or skill-building services (as indicated); and mental health consultation immediately, without a period of active monitoring.

Recommendation 3: If a PC clinician identifies an adolescent with moderate or severe depression or complicating factors and/or conditions such as coexisting substance abuse or psychosis, consultation with a mental health specialist should be considered (grade of evidence: 5; strength of recommendation: strong). Appropriate roles and responsibilities for ongoing comanagement by the PC clinician and mental health clinician(s) should be communicated and agreed on (grade of evidence: 5; strength of recommendation: strong). The patient and family should be active team members and approve the roles of the PC and mental health clinicians (grade of evidence: 5; strength of recommendation: strong).

In adolescents with severe depression or comorbidities, such as substance abuse, clinicians should consider consultation with mental health professionals and refer to such professionals when deemed necessary. In cases of moderate depression with or without comorbid anxiety, clinicians should consider consultation by mental health and/or treatment in the PC setting. Although the access barriers to mental health services need to be addressed by policy makers to make mental health consultations more feasible, available, and affordable in underserved areas, clinical judgment should prevail in the meantime; thus, the need for consultation should be based on the clinician's judgment. PC providers should also take into consideration the treatment preferences of patients and/or families, the severity and urgency of the case presentation, and the PC provider's level of training and experience.

Active support and treatment should also be started in cases in which there is a lengthy waiting list for mental health services. Once a

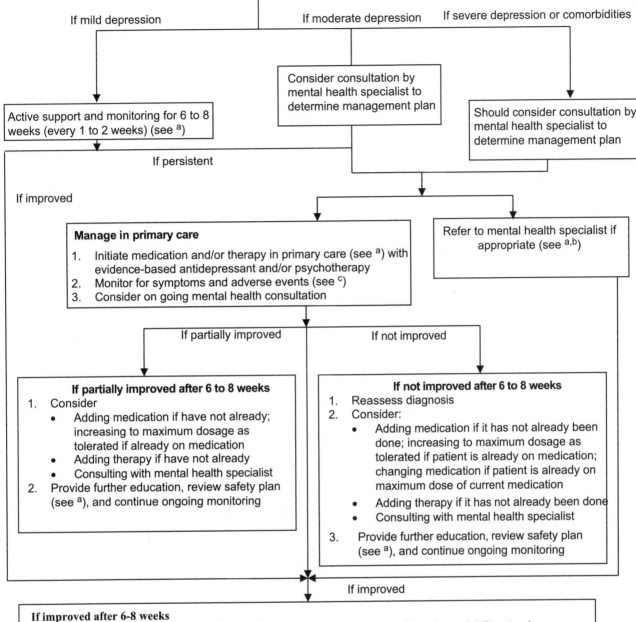

FIGURE 1

Clinical management flowchart. [a]Psychoeducation, supportive counseling, facilitate parental and patient self-management, refer for peer support, and regular monitoring of depressive symptoms and suicidality. [b]Negotiate roles and/or responsibilities between PC and mental health and designate case coordination responsibilities. Continue to monitor in PC after referral and maintain contact with mental health. [c]Clinicians should monitor for changes in symptoms and emergence of adverse events, such as increased suicidal ideation, agitation, or induction of mania. For monitoring guidelines, please refer to the guidelines and/or toolkit. AACAP, American Academy of Child and Adolescent Psychiatry.

referral is made, comanagement of treatment should take place with the PC clinician remaining involved in follow-up. In particular, roles and responsibilities should be agreed on between the PC clinician and mental health clinician(s), including the designation of case coordination responsibilities.[48,50,77,78,80,81] It is critical for PC clinicians to make linkages with their closest crisis support and hospital services so that they are supported in crisis situations when caring for depressed youth.

Recommendation 4: PC clinicians should recommend scientifically tested and proven treatments (ie, psychotherapies, such as CBT or IPT-A, and/or antidepressant treatment, such as SSRIs) whenever possible and appropriate to achieve the goals of the treatment plan[82] (grade of evidence: 1; strength of recommendation: very strong).

After providing education and support to the patient and family, the range of effective treatment options, including medications, psychotherapies, and family support should be considered. The patient and family should be assisted to arrive at a treatment plan that is both acceptable and implementable, taking into account their preferences and the availability of treatment services. The treatment plan should be customized according to the severity of disease, risk of suicide, and the existence of comorbid conditions. The GLAD-PC toolkit (www.gladpc. org) provides more detailed guidance around the factors that may influence treatment choices (ie, a patient with psychomotor retardation may not be able to actively engage in psychotherapy). A "common factors" approach is focused on evidence-based practices, which are common across therapies. Common factors include better communication skills, to be supportive, to take advantage of therapeutic alliance, and to engage in shared decision-making.[83] Common sense approaches such as the prescription of physical exercise, sleep hygiene, and adequate nutrition should also be used in the management of these patients.

As an aside, the majority of CBT and IPT-A studies in which researchers included patients with MDD also included patients with depression not otherwise specified, subthreshold depressive symptoms, or dysthymic disorder. In contrast, medication RCTs for depression in adolescents

TABLE 2 Components of CBT and IPT-A

Therapy	Key Components
CBT	Thoughts influence behaviors and feelings and vice versa. Treatment targets patient's thoughts and behaviors to improve his or her mood. Essential elements of CBT include increasing pleasurable activities (behavioral activation), reducing negative thoughts (cognitive restructuring), and improving assertiveness and problem-solving skills to reduce feelings of hopelessness. CBT for adolescents may include sessions with parents and/or caregivers to review progress and to increase compliance with CBT-related tasks.
IPT-A	Interpersonal problems may cause or exacerbate depression, and that depression, in turn, may exacerbate interpersonal problems. Treatment targets patient's interpersonal problems to improve both interpersonal functioning and his or her mood. Essential elements of interpersonal therapy include identifying an interpersonal problem area, improving interpersonal problem-solving skills, and modifying communication patterns. Parents and/or caregivers are involved in sessions during specific phases of the therapy.

generally only included subjects with MDD. Thus, although the general treatment of depression is addressed in these guidelines, medication-specific guidelines apply only to fully expressed MDD.

Psychotherapies

Both CBT and IPT-A have been adapted to address depression in adolescents and have been shown to be effective in treating adolescents with MDD in tertiary care as well as community settings.[57,84] CBT has been used in the PC setting with preliminary positive results.[33,35] Also suggested in emerging evidence is the superior efficacy of combination therapy (medication and CBT) versus CBT alone.[43] For a brief description of the 2 therapies, see Table 2.

Antidepressant Treatment

Previous research has shown that up to 25% of pediatric PC clinicians and 42% of family physicians in the United States had recently prescribed SSRIs for more than 1 adolescent under the age of 18.[15] When indicated by clinical presentation (ie, clear diagnosis of MDD with no comorbid conditions) and patient and/or family preference, an SSRI should be used. The selection of the specific SSRI should be based on the optimum combination of safety and efficacy data. Deliberate self-harm and/or suicide risk is more likely to occur if the SSRI is started at higher doses

(rather than normal starting doses).[85] The patient and family should be informed about the possible adverse effects (clinicians may use checklist), including possible switch to mania or the development of behavioral activation or suicide-related events. Once the antidepressant is started, and if tolerated, the clinician should support an adequate trial up to the maximum dose and duration.

In Table 3, recommended antidepressants and dosages for use in adolescents with depression are listed. These recommendations are based on the updated literature review and reviewed by the GLAD-PC Steering Committee. Generally, the effective dosages for antidepressants in adolescents are lower than would be found in adult guidelines. Note that only fluoxetine has been approved by the FDA for use in children and adolescents with depression, and only escitalopram has been approved for use in adolescents aged 12 years and older. Clinicians should know the potential drug interactions with SSRIs. Further information on the use of antidepressants is described in the GLAD-PC toolkit (www.gladpc.org). In addition, all SSRIs should be slowly tapered when discontinued because of risk of withdrawal effects. Details regarding the initial selection of a specific SSRI and possible reasons for initial drug choice can be found in the GLAD-PC toolkit.

TABLE 3 SSRI Titration Schedule

Medication	Starting Dose (qd/od), mg	Increments, mg	Effective Dose, mg	Maximum Dosage, mg	Contraindicated
Citalopram	10	10	20	60	MAOIs
Fluoxetine	10	10–20	20	60	MAOIs
Fluvoxamine	50	50	150	300	MAOIs
Paroxetine[a]	10	10	20	60	MAOIs
Sertraline	25	12.5–25	50	200	MAOIs
Escitalopram	10	5	10	20	MAOIs

MAOI, monoamine oxidase inhibitor; qd/od, every day once daily.

[a] Not recommended to be started in PC.

Contact (either in person or by telephone with either the clinician or member of the clinical staff) should take place after the initiation of treatment to review the patient's and family's understanding of and adherence to the treatment plan. Issues such as the current status of the patient and the patient and/or family's access to educational materials regarding depression should be discussed during follow-up conversations. For relevant educational resources for patients and/or families, please refer to the GLAD-PC toolkit (www.gladpc.org).

Recommendation 5: PC clinicians should monitor for the emergence of adverse events during antidepressant treatment (SSRIs) (grade of evidence: 3; strength of recommendation: very strong).[82]

Re-analysis of safety data from clinical trials of antidepressants led to a black-box warning from the FDA regarding the use of these medications in children and adolescents in 2004 and a recommendation for close monitoring. The exact wording of the FDA recommendation is:

All pediatric patients being treated with antidepressants for any indication should be observed closely for clinical worsening, suicidality, and unusual changes in behavior, especially during the initial few months of a course of drug therapy, or at times of dose changes, either increases or decreases.

It should be noted, however, that there is no empirical evidence to support the requirement of face-to-face meetings per se. In fact, evidence from large population-based surveys reveals high reliability of telephone interviews with adolescent subjects for the diagnosis of depression.[86,87] Although obtaining a diagnosis is not the same as the elicitation of adverse events while in treatment, with this evidence, it is suggested that telephone contact may be just as effective in monitoring for adverse events. More importantly, a regular and frequent monitoring schedule should be developed, taking care to obtain input from the adolescents and families to ensure compliance with the monitoring strategy.[88,89] This may include monitoring of depressive symptoms, risky behaviors, and also functioning in the school setting, especially if an individualized education program is in place. Working closely with the family will ensure appropriate monitoring and help-seeking by caregivers.

Ongoing Management

The strength of evidence on which each recommendation is based has been rated 1 (strongest) through 5 (weakest), according to the Oxford Centre for Evidence-Based Medicine levels of evidence, and paired with the strength of recommendation (Very strong [>90% agreement]), Strong [>70% agreement], Fair [>50% agreement], Weak [<50% agreement]).

Recommendation 1: Systematic and regular tracking of goals and outcomes from treatment should be performed, including assessment of depressive symptoms and *functioning in several key domains. These include home, school, and peer settings (grade of evidence: 4; strength of recommendation: very strong).*

Goals should include both improvement in functioning and resolution of depressive symptoms. Tracking of goals and outcomes from treatment should include function in several important domains (ie, home, school, peers). Evidence from large RCTs reveals that depressive symptoms and functional impairments may not improve at the same rate with treatment.[28,70] Therefore, symptoms and functioning should be tracked regularly during the course of treatment with information gathered from both the patients and their families when possible.

According to expert consensus, it is ideal that patients are assessed in person within 1 week of the initiation of treatment. At every assessment, clinicians should inquire about each of the following: (1) ongoing depressive symptoms, (2) risk of suicide, (3) possible adverse effects from treatment (including the use of specific adverse-effect scales), (4) adherence to treatment, and (5) new or ongoing environmental stressors. In several studies, researchers have examined medication maintenance after response.[90–93] Emslie et al[93] randomly assigned pediatric patients who had responded to fluoxetine by 19 weeks to placebo or to medication continuation for an additional 32 weeks. Of the 20 subjects randomly assigned to the 32-week medication relapse-prevention arm, 10 were exposed to fluoxetine for 51 weeks. Significantly fewer relapses occurred in the group randomly assigned to medication maintenance, which suggests that longer medication continuation periods, possibly 1 year, may be necessary for relapse prevention. In addition, Emslie et al[93] found the greatest risk of relapse to be in the first 8 to 12 weeks after discontinuing medication, which suggests that after stopping an antidepressant, close follow-up should be encouraged for at least 2 to 3 months. Other studies have revealed similar benefits of prolonged treatment after acute response.[90–93]

With the limited evidence in children and adolescents and the emerging evidence in the adult literature in which it is suggested that antidepressant medication should be continued for 1 year after remission, both GLAD-PC and the American Academy of Child and Adolescent Psychiatry concluded that medication be maintained for 6 to 12 months after the full resolution of depressive symptoms.[22,90–93]

However, regardless of the length of treatment, all patients should be monitored on a monthly basis for 6 to 12 months after the full resolution of symptoms.[22,93,94] If the depressive episode is a recurrence, clinicians are encouraged to monitor patients for up to 2 years given the high rates of recurrence as demonstrated in the adult literature in which maintenance treatment in those with recurrent depression continues for up to 2 years after the full resolution of symptoms. Clinicians should obtain consultation from mental health professionals if a teenager develops psychosis, suicidal or homicidal ideation, and new or worsening of comorbid conditions.

Recommendation 2: Diagnosis and initial treatment should be reassessed if no improvement is noted after 6 to 8 weeks of treatment (grade of evidence: 4; strength of recommendation: very strong). Mental health consultation should be considered (grade of evidence: 4; strength of recommendation: very strong).

If improvement is not seen within 6 to 8 weeks of treatment, mental health consultation should be considered. Evidence of improvement may include reduction in the number of depressive symptoms, improved functioning in social or school settings, or improvement spontaneously reported by the adolescent and/or parent or caregiver. The clinician should also reassess the initial diagnosis, choice and adequacy of initial treatment, adherence to treatment plan, presence of comorbid conditions (eg, substance abuse) or bipolar symptoms that may influence treatment effectiveness, and new external stressors. If a patient has no response to a maximum therapeutic dose of an antidepressant medication, the clinician should consider changing the medication. Alternatively, if the patient has failed to improve on antidepressant medication or therapy alone, the addition of or switch to the other modality should be considered.

Recommendation 3: For patients achieving only partial improvement after PC diagnostic and therapeutic approaches have been exhausted (including exploration of poor adherence, comorbid disorders, and ongoing conflicts or abuse), a mental health consultation should be considered (grade of evidence: 4; strength of recommendation: very strong).

If a patient only partially improves with treatment, mental health consultation should be considered. The clinician should also review the diagnosis and explore possible causes of partial response, such as poor adherence to treatment, comorbid disorders, or ongoing conflicts and/or abuse. These causes may need to be managed first before changes to the treatment plan are made.

If a patient has been treated with a SSRI (maximum tolerated dosage) and has shown only partial improvement, the addition of an evidence-based psychotherapy should be considered, if not previously initiated. Other considerations may include the addition of another medication, an increase of the dosage above FDA-approved ranges, or a switch to another medication as suggested in the Treatment of SSRI-resistant Depression in Adolescents study,[39] preferably done in consultation with a mental health professional. Likewise, if a patient's condition fails to improve after a trial of either CBT or IPT-A and has not yet begun medication, the clinician should consider a trial of SSRI antidepressant treatment. Strong consideration should also be given to a referral to mental health services.

Recommendation 4: PC clinicians should actively support depressed adolescents referred to mental health services to ensure adequate management (grade of evidence: 5; strength of recommendation: very strong). PC clinicians may also consider sharing care with mental health agencies and/ or professionals where possible (grade of evidence: 1; strength of recommendation: very strong). Appropriate roles and responsibilities regarding the provision and comanagement of care should be communicated and agreed on by the PC clinician and the mental health clinician(s) (grade of evidence: 4; strength of recommendation: very strong).

PC clinicians should continue follow-up with adolescents with depression who have been referred to mental health services for assessment and/or management.[95] Where possible, PC clinicians may consider sharing management of depressed adolescents with mental health agencies and/or professionals. There is emerging evidence from the literature about the greater effectiveness of "shared-care" models for the management of depression in the PC setting.[27,31,95–97] There is also increasing evidence to support that quality improvement strategies and techniques can change PC practitioner behavior both in mental health and in other arenas.[98, 99]

DISCUSSION

The recommendations regarding treatment and ongoing management highlight the need for PC providers to become familiar with the use of empirically tested treatments for adolescent depression, including both antidepressants and psychotherapy. In particular, antidepressant treatments can be useful in certain clinical situations in the PC setting. In many of these clinical scenarios, PC providers should schedule systematic and routine follow-up, including mental health support when appropriate. The need for systematic follow-up, whether by PC provider or by mental health provider, is especially important in light of the FDA black-box warnings regarding the emergence of adverse events with antidepressant treatment.

Psychotherapy is also recommended as first-line treatment of adolescents who are depressed in the PC setting. Although the provision of psychotherapy may be less feasible and practical within the constraints (ie, time, availability of trained staff) of PC settings, there is some evidence to support that quality improvement projects involving psychotherapy can improve the care of adolescents who are depressed.[35]

GLAD-PC was developed and now updated on the basis of the needs of PC clinicians who are faced with the challenge of caring for depressed adolescents as well as many barriers, including the shortage of mental health resources in most community settings. Although it is clear that more evidence and research in this area are needed, these updated guidelines represent a necessary step toward improving the care of depressed adolescents in the PC setting. Similar guidelines have also been produced for other health care contexts, such as in the United

Kingdom (https://www.nice.org.uk/guidance/cg28). The updated GLAD-PC guidelines and the toolkit (www.gladpc.org) reflect the coming together of available evidence and the consensus of experts representing a broad spectrum of specialties and advocacy organizations within the North American health care context. However, no improvements in care will be achieved if changes do not occur in the health care systems that would allow for increased training in mental health for PC clinicians and in collaborative models for both primary and specialty care clinicians. Therefore, it is critical that training programs for PC providers increase their focus on mental health issues and that trainees in both PC and specialty care areas be helped to hone their skills in working in collaborative care models[89] (see http://www.aap.org/en-us/advocacy-and-policy/aap-health-initiatives/Mental-Health/Pages/implementing_mental_health_priorities_in_practice.aspx). For providers who are currently practicing, continuing education should strengthen skills in collaborative work, and specifically, for PC providers, increase skills and knowledge in the management of depression.

LIMITATIONS

Although the guidelines covered a range of issues regarding the management of adolescent depression in the PC setting, there were other controversial areas that were not addressed in these recommendations. These included such issues as the use of augmenting agents and treatment of subthreshold symptoms. New emerging evidence may impact on the inclusion of such areas in future iterations of the guidelines and the toolkit (available for download at www.gladpc.org). Many of these recommendations are made in the face of an absence

of evidence or at lower levels of evidence.

FUTURE DIRECTIONS

Ample evidence exists to support the notion that guidelines alone are insufficient in closing the gaps between recommended versus actual practices.[100,101] Thus, it will be necessary to identify effective methods for disseminating information and provide assistance to PC clinicians in changing practice. Researchers should build on this work by piloting and evaluating methods, tools, and strategies to facilitate the adoption of these guidelines for the management of adolescent depression in PC settings. Researchers should also explore optimal methods for helping clinicians and their clinical settings address the range of obstacles that may interfere with the adoption of necessary practices to yield sustainable management of adolescent depression in PC settings.

Many jurisdictions have recognized the need to increase collaborative care to address the care of adolescents with mental illness. In Canada and the United States, models of care involving mental health and PC are being implemented (National Network of Child Psychiatry Access Programs: www.nncpap.org; Massachusetts Child Psychiatry Access Program: https://www.mcpap.com/; Partnership Access Line; Training and Education for the Advancement of Children's Health).[102–106] However, the empirical support for these models is modest internationally; therefore, additional research is urgently needed.

ACKNOWLEDGEMENTS

The authors wish to acknowledge research support from Justin Chee, Lindsay Williams, Robyn Tse, Isabella Churchill, Farid Azadian, Geneva

Mason, Jonathan West, Sara Ho and Michael West. We are most grateful to the advice and guidance of Dr Joan Asarnow, Dr Jeff Bridge, Dr Purti Papneja, Dr Elena Mann, Dr Rachel Lynch, Dr Marc Lashley, Dr Diane Bloomfield, and Dr Cori Green.

LEAD AUTHORS

Amy Cheung, MD
Rachel A. Zuckerbrot, MD
Peter S. Jensen, MD
Danielle Laraque, MD
Ruth E.K. Stein, MD

GLAD-PC PROJECT TEAM

Peter S. Jensen, MD, Project Director – *University of Arkansas for Medical Science*
Amy Cheung, MD, Project Coordinator – *University of Toronto and Columbia University*
Rachel Zuckerbrot, MD, Project Coordinator – *Columbia University*
Anthony Levitt, MD, Project Consultant – *University of Toronto*

STEERING COMMITTEE MEMBERS

GLAD-PC Youth and Family Advisory Team
Joan Asarnow, PhD – *David Geffen School of Medicine, University of California Los Angeles*
Boris Birmaher, MD – *Western Psychiatric Institute and Clinic, University of Pittsburgh*

John Campo, MD – *Ohio State University*
Greg Clarke, PhD – *Center for Health Research, Kaiser Permanente*
M. Lynn Crimson, Pharm.D – *The University of Texas at Austin*
Graham Emslie, MD – *University of Texas Southwestern Medical Center and Children's Health System Texas*
Miriam Kaufman, MD – *Hospital for Sick Children, University of Toronto*
Kelly J. Kelleher, MD – *Ohio State University*
Stanley Kutcher, MD – *Dalhousie Medical School*
Danielle Laraque, MD – *State University of New York Upstate Medical University*
Michael Malus, MD – *Department of Family Medicine, McGill University*
Diane Sacks, MD – *Canadian Pediatric Society*
Ruth E.K. Stein, MD – *Albert Einstein College of Medicine and Children's Hospital at Montefiore*
Barry Sarvet, MD – *Baystate Health Systems, MA*
Bruce Waslick, MD – *Baystate Health Systems, MA and University of Massachusetts Medical School*
Benedetto Vitiello, MD – *University of Turin and NIHM (former)*

ORGANIZATIONAL LIAISONS

Nerissa Bauer, MD – *American Academy of Pediatrics*
Diane Sacks, MD – *Canadian Pediatric Society*
Barry Sarvet, MD – *American Academy of Child and Adolescent Psychiatry*

Mary Kay Nixon, MD – *Canadian Academy of Child Psychiatry*
Robert Hilt, MD – *American Psychiatric Association*
Darcy Gruttadaro – *National Alliance on Mental Illness*
Teri Brister – *National Alliance on Mental Illness*

ABBREVIATIONS

CBT: cognitive behavioral therapy
CCBT: computerized cognitive behavioral therapy
CI: confidence interval
FDA: Food and Drug Administration
GLAD-PC: Guidelines for Adolescent Depression in Primary Care
IPT-A: interpersonal psychotherapy for adolescents
MDD: major depressive disorder
PC: primary care
RCT: randomized controlled trial
SSRI: selective serotonin reuptake inhibitor

CATCH Services, LLC. He is the chief executive officer and president of a nonprofit organization, the REACH Institute, but receives no compensation; the other authors have indicated they have no financial relationships relevant to this article to disclose.

FUNDING: We thank the following organizations for financial support of the GLAD-PC project: REACH Institute, and Bell Canada.

POTENTIAL CONFLICT OF INTEREST: In the past 2 years, Dr Jensen has received royalties from several publishing companies: Random House, Oxford University Press, and APPI Inc. He also is part owner of a consulting company, CATCH Services LLC. He is the chief executive officer and president of a nonprofit organization, the Resource for Advancing Children's Health Institute, but receives no compensation. Dr Zuckerbrot works for CAP PC, child and adolescent psychiatry for primary care, now a regional provider for Project TEACH in New York State. Dr Zuckerbrot is also on the steering committee as well as faculty for the REACH Institute. Both of these institutions are described in this publication. Drs Cheung and Zuckerbrot receive book royalties from Research Civic Institute.

COMPANION PAPER: A companion to this article can be found online at www.pediatrics.org/cgi/doi/10.1542/peds.2017-4081.

REFERENCES

1. Costello EJ, He JP, Sampson NA, Kessler RC, Merikangas KR. Services for adolescents with psychiatric disorders: 12-month data from the National Comorbidity Survey-Adolescent. *Psychiatr Serv.* 2014;65(3):359–366

2. Merikangas KR, He JP, Burstein M, et al. Lifetime prevalence of mental disorders in US adolescents: results from the National Comorbidity Survey Replication–Adolescent Supplement (NCS-A). *J Am Acad Child Adolesc Psychiatry.* 2010;49(10):980–989

3. Fleming JE, Offord DR, Boyle MH. Prevalence of childhood and adolescent depression in the community. Ontario Child Health Study. *Br J Psychiatry.* 1989;155:647–654

4. Shaffer D, Gould MS, Fisher P, et al. Psychiatric diagnosis in child and adolescent suicide. *Arch Gen Psychiatry.* 1996;53(4):339–348

5. Garrison CZ, Addy CL, Jackson KL, McKeown RE, Waller JL. Major depressive disorder and dysthymia in young adolescents. *Am J Epidemiol.* 1992;135(7):792–802

6. Lewinsohn PM, Hops H, Roberts RE, Seeley JR, Andrews JA. Adolescent psychopathology: I. Prevalence and incidence of depression and other DSM-III-R disorders in high school students [published correction appears in *J Abnorm Psychol.* 1993;102(4):517]. *J Abnorm Psychol.* 1993;102(1):133–144

7. Whitaker A, Johnson J, Shaffer D, et al. Uncommon troubles in young people: prevalence estimates of selected

psychiatric disorders in a nonreferred adolescent population. *Arch Gen Psychiatry.* 1990;47(5):487–496

8. Johnson JG, Harris ES, Spitzer RL, Williams JB. The patient health questionnaire for adolescents: validation of an instrument for the assessment of mental disorders among adolescent primary care patients. *J Adolesc Health.* 2002;30(3):196–204

9. Bartlett JA, Schleifer SJ, Johnson RL, Keller SE. Depression in inner city adolescents attending an adolescent medicine clinic. *J Adolesc Health.* 1991;12(4):316–318

10. Schubiner H, Robin A. Screening adolescents for depression and parent-teenager conflict in an ambulatory medical setting: a preliminary investigation. *Pediatrics.* 1990;85(5):813–818

11. Winter LB, Steer RA, Jones-Hicks L, Beck AT. Screening for major depression disorders in adolescent medical outpatients with the Beck Depression Inventory for Primary Care. *J Adolesc Health.* 1999;24(6):389–394

12. Rifkin A, Wortman R, Reardon G, Siris SG. Psychotropic medication in adolescents: a review. *J Clin Psychiatry.* 1986;47(8):400–408

13. Kessler RC, Avenevoli S, Ries Merikangas K. Mood disorders in children and adolescents: an epidemiologic perspective. *Biol Psychiatry.* 2001;49(12):1002–1014

14. Asarnow JR, Jaycox LH, Duan N, et al. Effectiveness of a quality improvement intervention for adolescent depression in primary care clinics: a randomized controlled trial. *JAMA.* 2005;293(3):311–319

15. Rushton J, Bruckman D, Kelleher K. Primary care referral of children with psychosocial problems. *Arch Pediatr Adolesc Med.* 2002;156(6):592–598

16. Rushton JL, Clark SJ, Freed GL. Pediatrician and family physician prescription of selective serotonin reuptake inhibitors. *Pediatrics.* 2000;105(6). Available at: www.pediatrics.org/cgi/content/full/105/6/e82

17. Zito JM, Safer DJ, DosReis S, et al. Rising prevalence of antidepressants among US youths. *Pediatrics.* 2002;109(5):721–727

18. Costello EJ, Edelbrock C, Costello AJ, Dulcan MK, Burns BJ, Brent D. Psychopathology in pediatric primary care: the new hidden morbidity. *Pediatrics.* 1988;82(3, pt 2):415–424

19. Briggs-Gowan MJ, Horwitz SM, Schwab-Stone ME, Leventhal JM, Leaf PJ. Mental health in pediatric settings: distribution of disorders and factors related to service use. *J Am Acad Child Adolesc Psychiatry.* 2000;39(7):841–849

20. Jensen PS. Closing the evidence-based treatment gap for children's mental health services: what we know vs. what we do. *Rep Emotional Behav Disord Youth.* 2002;2(2):43-47

21. Olin SC, Hoagwood K. The surgeon general's national action agenda on children's mental health. *Curr Psychiatry Rep.* 2002;4(2):101–107

22. Birmaher B, Brent D, Bernet W, et al; AACAP Work Group on Quality Issues. Practice parameter for the assessment and treatment of children and adolescents with depressive disorders. *J Am Acad Child Adolesc Psychiatry.* 2007;46(11):1503–1526

23. Shain BN; American Academy of Pediatrics Committee on Adolescence. Suicide and suicide attempts in adolescents. *Pediatrics.* 2007;120(3):669–676

24. Zuckerbrot RA, Cheung AH, Jensen PS, Stein RE, Laraque D; GLAD-PC Steering Group. Guidelines for Adolescent Depression in Primary Care (GLAD-PC): I. Identification, assessment, and initial management. *Pediatrics.* 2007;120(5). Available at: www.pediatrics.org/cgi/content/full/120/5/e1299

25. Cheung AH, Zuckerbrot RA, Jensen PS, Ghalib K, Laraque D, Stein RE; GLAD-PC Steering Group. Guidelines for Adolescent Depression in Primary Care (GLAD-PC): II. Treatment and ongoing management [published correction appears in *Pediatrics.* 2008;121(1):227]. *Pediatrics.* 2007;120(5). Available at: www.pediatrics.org/cgi/content/full/120/5/e1313

26. Stein REK, Zitner LE, Jensen PS. Interventions for adolescent depression in primary care. *Pediatrics.* 2006;118(2):669–682

27. Richardson LP, Ludman E, McCauley E, et al. Collaborative care for adolescents with depression in primary care: a randomized clinical trial. *JAMA.* 2014;312(8):809–816

28. Cheung AH, Emslie GJ, Mayes TL. Review of the efficacy and safety of antidepressants in youth depression. *J Child Psychol Psychiatry.* 2005;46(7):735–754

29. Hammad TA, Laughren T, Racoosin J. Suicidality in pediatric patients treated with antidepressant drugs. *Arch Gen Psychiatry.* 2006;63(3):332–339

30. Coventry PA, Hudson JL, Kontopantelis E, et al. Characteristics of effective collaborative care for treatment of depression: a systematic review and meta-regression of 74 randomised controlled trials. *PLoS One.* 2014;9(9):e108114

31. Kolko DJ, Campo J, Kilbourne AM, Hart J, Sakolsky D, Wisniewski S. Collaborative care outcomes for pediatric behavioral health problems: a cluster randomized trial. *Pediatrics.* 2014;133(4). Available at: www.pediatrics.org/cgi/content/full/133/4/e981

32. Lewandowski RE, Acri MC, Hoagwood KE, et al. Evidence for the management of adolescent depression. *Pediatrics.* 2013;132(4). Available at: www.pediatrics.org/cgi/content/full/132/4/e996

33. Clarke G, Debar L, Lynch F, et al. A randomized effectiveness trial of brief cognitive-behavioral therapy for depressed adolescents receiving antidepressant medication. *J Am Acad Child Adolesc Psychiatry.* 2005;44(9):888–898

34. Wright DR, Haaland WL, Ludman E, McCauley E, Lindenbaum J, Richardson LP. The costs and cost-effectiveness of collaborative care for adolescents with depression in primary care settings: a randomized clinical trial. *JAMA Pediatr.* 2016;170(11):1048–1054

35. Asarnow JR, Rozenman M, Wiblin J, Zeltzer L. Integrated medical-behavioral care compared with usual primary care for child and adolescent behavioral health: a meta-analysis. *JAMA Pediatr.* 2015;169(10):929–937

36. Ladden MD, Bodenheimer T, Fishman NW, et al. The emerging primary care

workforce: preliminary observations from the primary care team: learning from effective ambulatory practices project. *Acad Med.* 2013;88(12):1830–1834

37. Goldman SK. The conceptual framework for wraparound. In: Burns BJ, Goldman SK, eds. *Promising Practices in Wraparound for Children With Severe Emotional Disorders and Their Families. Systems of Care: Promising Practices in Children's Mental Health.* 1998 series.Vol 4. Washington, DC: Center for Effective Collaboration and Practice; 1999:27–34

38. Winters NC, Metz WP. The wraparound approach in systems of care. *Psychiatr Clin North Am.* 2009;32(1):135–151

39. Brent D, Emslie G, Clarke G, et al. Switching to another SSRI or to venlafaxine with or without cognitive behavioral therapy for adolescents with SSRI-resistant depression: the TORDIA randomized controlled trial. *JAMA.* 2008;299(8):901–913

40. Brent DA, Emslie GJ, Clarke GN, et al. Predictors of spontaneous and systematically assessed suicidal adverse events in the treatment of SSRI-resistant depression in adolescents (TORDIA) study. *Am J Psychiatry.* 2009;166(4):418–426

41. Shamseddeen W, Clarke G, Wagner KD, et al. Treatment-resistant depressed youth show a higher response rate if treatment ends during summer school break. *J Am Acad Child Adolesc Psychiatry.* 2011;50(11):1140–1148

42. Mandoki MW, Tapia MR, Tapia MA, Sumner GS, Parker JL. Venlafaxine in the treatment of children and adolescents with major depression. *Psychopharmacol Bull.* 1997;33(1):149–154

43. Bridge JA, Salary CB, Birmaher B, Asare AG, Brent DA. The risks and benefits of antidepressant treatment for youth depression. *Ann Med.* 2005;37(6):404–412

44. Cipriani A, Zhou X, Del Giovane C, et al. Comparative efficacy and tolerability of antidepressants for major depressive disorder in children and adolescents: a network meta-analysis. *Lancet.* 2016;388(10047):881–890

45. March J, Silva S, Petrycki S, et al; Treatment for Adolescents With Depression Study (TADS) Team. Fluoxetine, cognitive-behavioral therapy, and their combination for adolescents with depression: Treatment for Adolescents with Depression Study (TADS) randomized controlled trial. *JAMA.* 2004;292(7):807–820

46. Emslie GJ, Rush AJ, Weinberg WA, et al. A double-blind, randomized, placebo-controlled trial of fluoxetine in children and adolescents with depression. *Arch Gen Psychiatry.* 1997;54(11):1031–1037

47. Emslie GJ, Heiligenstein JH, Wagner KD, et al. Fluoxetine for acute treatment of depression in children and adolescents: a placebo-controlled, randomized clinical trial. *J Am Acad Child Adolesc Psychiatry.* 2002;41(10):1205–1215

48. Keller MB, Ryan ND, Strober M, et al. Efficacy of paroxetine in the treatment of adolescent major depression: a randomized, controlled trial. *J Am Acad Child Adolesc Psychiatry.* 2001;40(7):762–772

49. Emslie G, Kratochvil C, Vitiello B, et al; Columbia Suicidality Classification Group; TADS Team. Treatment for Adolescents with Depression Study (TADS): safety results. *J Am Acad Child Adolesc Psychiatry.* 2006;45(12):1440–1455

50. Wagner KD, Robb AS, Findling RL, Jin J, Gutierrez MM, Heydorn WE. A randomized, placebo-controlled trial of citalopram for the treatment of major depression in children and adolescents. *Am J Psychiatry.* 2004;161(6):1079–1083

51. von Knorring AL, Olsson GI, Thomsen PH, Lemming OM, Hultén A. A randomized, double-blind, placebo-controlled study of citalopram in adolescents with major depressive disorder. *J Clin Psychopharmacol.* 2006;26(3):311–315

52. Wagner KD, Ambrosini P, Rynn M, et al Sertraline Pediatric Depression Study Group. Efficacy of sertraline in the treatment of children and adolescents with major depressive disorder: two randomized controlled trials. *JAMA.* 2003;290(8):1033–1041

53. Wagner KD, Jonas J, Findling RL, Ventura D, Saikali K. A double-blind, randomized, placebo-controlled trial of escitalopram in the treatment of pediatric depression. *J Am Acad Child Adolesc Psychiatry.* 2006;45(3):280–288

54. Emslie GJ, Ventura D, Korotzer A, Tourkodimitris S. Escitalopram in the treatment of adolescent depression: a randomized placebo-controlled multisite trial. *J Am Acad Child Adolesc Psychiatry.* 2009;48(7):721–729

55. March JS, Silva S, Petrycki S, et al. The Treatment for Adolescents with Depression Study (TADS): long-term effectiveness and safety outcomes. *Arch Gen Psychiatry.* 2007;64(10):1132–1143

56. Ginsburg GS, Kendall PC, Sakolsky D, et al. Remission after acute treatment in children and adolescents with anxiety disorders: findings from the CAMS. *J Consult Clin Psychol.* 2011;79(6):806–813

57. Walkup JT, Albano AM, Piacentini J, et al. Cognitive behavioral therapy, sertraline, or a combination in childhood anxiety. *N Engl J Med.* 2008;359(26):2753–2766

58. Wilkinson P, Dubicka B, Kelvin R, Roberts C, Goodyer I. Treated depression in adolescents: predictors of outcome at 28 weeks. *Br J Psychiatry.* 2009;194(4):334–341

59. Goodyer I, Dubicka B, Wilkinson P, et al. Selective serotonin reuptake inhibitors (SSRIs) and routine specialist care with and without cognitive behaviour therapy in adolescents with major depression: randomised controlled trial. *BMJ.* 2007;335(7611):142

60. Cox GR, Callahan P, Churchill R, et al. Psychological therapies versus antidepressant medication, alone and in combination for depression in children and adolescents. *Cochrane Database Syst Rev.* 2014;30(11):CD008324

61. Asarnow JR, Porta G, Spirito A, et al. Suicide attempts and nonsuicidal self-injury in the treatment of resistant depression in adolescents: findings from the TORDIA study. *J Am Acad Child Adolesc Psychiatry.* 2011;50(8):772–781

62. Asarnow JR, Emslie G, Clarke G, et al. Treatment of selective serotonin

reuptake inhibitor-resistant depression in adolescents: predictors and moderators of treatment response. *J Am Acad Child Adolesc Psychiatry.* 2009;48(3):330–339

63. Barbui C, Esposito E, Cipriani A. Selective serotonin reuptake inhibitors and risk of suicide: a systematic review of observational studies. *CMAJ.* 2009;180(3):291–297

64. Leon AC, Marzuk PM, Tardiff K, Bucciarelli A, Markham Piper T, Galea S. Antidepressants and youth suicide in New York City, 1999-2002. *J Am Acad Child Adolesc Psychiatry.* 2006;45(9):1054–1058

65. Olfson M, Shaffer D, Marcus SC, Greenberg T. Relationship between antidepressant medication treatment and suicide in adolescents. *Arch Gen Psychiatry.* 2003;60(10):978–982

66. Reinecke MA, Ryan NE, DuBois DL. Cognitive-behavioral therapy of depression and depressive symptoms during adolescence: a review and meta-analysis. *J Am Acad Child Adolesc Psychiatry.* 1998;37(1):26–34

67. Harrington R, Campbell F, Shoebridge P, Whittaker J. Meta-analysis of CBT for depression in adolescents. *J Am Acad Child Adolesc Psychiatry.* 1998;37(10):1005–1007

68. Compton SN, March JS, Brent D, Albano AM V, Weersing R, Curry J. Cognitive-behavioral psychotherapy for anxiety and depressive disorders in children and adolescents: an evidence-based medicine review. *J Am Acad Child Adolesc Psychiatry.* 2004;43(8):930–959

69. Stikkelbroek Y, Bodden DH, Deković M, van Baar AL. Effectiveness and cost effectiveness of cognitive behavioral therapy (CBT) in clinically depressed adolescents: individual CBT versus treatment as usual (TAU). *BMC Psychiatry.* 2013;13:314

70. March J, Silva S, Curry J, et al; Treatment for Adolescents With Depression Study (TADS) Team. The Treatment for Adolescents with Depression Study (TADS): outcomes over 1 year of naturalistic follow-up. *Am J Psychiatry.* 2009;166(10):1141–1149

71. Fleming T, Dixon R, Frampton C, Merry S. A pragmatic randomized controlled trial of computerized CBT (SPARX) for symptoms of depression among adolescents excluded from mainstream education. *Behav Cogn Psychother.* 2012;40(5):529–541

72. Van Voorhees BW, Fogel J, Reinecke MA, et al. Randomized clinical trial of an Internet-based depression prevention program for adolescents (Project CATCH-IT) in primary care: 12-week outcomes. *J Dev Behav Pediatr.* 2009;30(1):23–37

73. Stice E, Rohde P, Seeley JR, Gau JM. Brief cognitive-behavioral depression prevention program for high-risk adolescents outperforms two alternative interventions: a randomized efficacy trial. *J Consult Clin Psychol.* 2008;76(4):595–606

74. Tang TC, Jou SH, Ko CH, Huang SY, Yen CF. Randomized study of school-based intensive interpersonal psychotherapy for depressed adolescents with suicidal risk and parasuicide behaviors. *Psychiatry Clin Neurosci.* 2009;63(4):463–470

75. Gunlicks-Stoessel M, Mufson L, Jekal A, Turner JB. The impact of perceived interpersonal functioning on treatment for adolescent depression: IPT-A versus treatment as usual in school-based health clinics. *J Consult Clin Psychol.* 2010;78(2):260–267

76. Young JF, Mufson L, Gallop R. Preventing depression: a randomized trial of interpersonal psychotherapy-adolescent skills training. *Depress Anxiety.* 2010;27(5):426–433

77. Wells KB, Sherbourne C, Schoenbaum M, et al. Impact of disseminating quality improvement programs for depression in managed primary care: a randomized controlled trial [published correction appears in *JAMA.* 2000;283(24):3204]. *JAMA.* 2000;283(2):212–220

78. Katon W, Von Korff M, Lin E, et al. Stepped collaborative care for primary care patients with persistent symptoms of depression: a randomized trial. *Arch Gen Psychiatry.* 1999;56(12):1109–1115

79. Tavernier LA. The fifteen minute hour: applied psychotherapy for the primary care physician, 2nd ed. *Prim Care Companion J Clin Psychiatry.* 1999;1(6):194–195

80. Lang AJ, Norman GJ, Casmar PV. A randomized trial of a brief mental health intervention for primary care patients. *J Consult Clin Psychol.* 2006;74(6):1173–1179

81. Unützer J, Katon W, Callahan CM, et al; IMPACT Investigators; Improving Mood-Promoting Access to Collaborative Treatment. Collaborative care management of late-life depression in the primary care setting: a randomized controlled trial. *JAMA.* 2002;288(22):2836–2845

82. Riddle MA. *Pediatric Psychopharmacology for Primary Care.* Elk Grove Village, IL: AAP Publishing; 2016

83. Wissow L, Anthony B, Brown J, et al. A common factors approach to improving the mental health capacity of pediatric primary care. *Adm Policy Ment Health.* 2008;35(4):305–318

84. Mufson L, Weissman MM, Moreau D, Garfinkel R. Efficacy of interpersonal psychotherapy for depressed adolescents. *Arch Gen Psychiatry.* 1999;56(6):573–579

85. Miller M, Swanson SA, Azrael D, Pate V, Stürmer T. Antidepressant dose, age, and the risk of deliberate self-harm. *JAMA Intern Med.* 2014;174(6):899–909

86. Rohde P, Lewinsohn PM, Seeley JR. Comparability of telephone and face-to-face interviews in assessing axis I and II disorders. *Am J Psychiatry.* 1997;154(11):1593–1598

87. Simon GE, Revicki D, VonKorff M. Telephone assessment of depression severity. *J Psychiatr Res.* 1993;27(3):247–252

88. Greenhill LL, Vitiello B, Riddle MA, et al. Review of safety assessment methods used in pediatric psychopharmacology. *J Am Acad Child Adolesc Psychiatry.* 2003;42(6):627–633

89. Greenhill LL, Vitiello B, Fisher P, et al. Comparison of increasingly detailed elicitation methods for the assessment of adverse events in pediatric psychopharmacology. *J Am Acad Child Adolesc Psychiatry.* 2004;43(12):1488–1496

90. Cheung A, Mayes T, Levitt A, et al. Anxiety as a predictor of treatment outcome in children and adolescents with depression. *J Child Adolesc Psychopharmacol.* 2010;20(3):211–216

91. Cheung A, Levitt A, Cheng M, et al. A pilot study of citalopram treatment in preventing relapse of depressive episode after acute treatment. *J Can Acad Child Adolesc Psychiatry.* 2016;25(1):11–16

92. Kennard BD, Emslie GJ, Mayes TL, et al. Sequential treatment with fluoxetine and relapse–prevention CBT to improve outcomes in pediatric depression. *Am J Psychiatry.* 2014;171(10):1083–1090

93. Emslie GJ, Heiligenstein JH, Hoog SL, et al. Fluoxetine treatment for prevention of relapse of depression in children and adolescents: a double-blind, placebo-controlled study. *J Am Acad Child Adolesc Psychiatry.* 2004;43(11):1397–1405

94. Cheung A, Kusumakar V, Kutcher S, et al. Maintenance study for adolescent depression. *J Child Adolesc Psychopharmacol.* 2008;18(4):389–394

95. Raney LE. Integrating primary care and behavioral health: the role of the psychiatrist in the collaborative care model. *Am J Psychiatry.* 2015;172(8):721–728

96. Sarvet B, Gold J, Bostic JQ, et al. Improving access to mental health care for children: the Massachusetts Child Psychiatry Access Project. *Pediatrics.* 2010;126(6):1191–1200

97. Kolko DJ, Perrin E. The integration of behavioral health interventions in children's health care: services, science, and suggestions. *J Clin Child Adolesc Psychol.* 2014;43(2):216–228

98. Chauhan BF, Jeyaraman MM, Mann AS, et al. Behavior change interventions and policies influencing primary healthcare professionals' practice-an overview of reviews [published correction appears in *Implement Sci.* 2017;12(1):38]. *Implement Sci.* 2017;12(1):3

99. Rinke ML, Singh H, Ruberman S, et al. Primary care pediatricians' interest in diagnostic error reduction. *Diagnosis (Berl).* 2016;3(2):65–69

100. Davis DA, Taylor-Vaisey A. Translating guidelines into practice. A systematic review of theoretic concepts, practical experience and research evidence in the adoption of clinical practice guidelines. *CMAJ.* 1997;157(4):408–416

101. Oxman AD, Thomson MA, Davis DA, Haynes RB. No magic bullets: a systematic review of 102 trials of interventions to improve professional practice. *CMAJ.* 1995;153(10):1423–1431

102. Connor DF, McLaughlin TJ, Jeffers-Terry M, et al. Targeted child psychiatric services: a new model of pediatric primary clinician–child psychiatry collaborative care. *Clin Pediatr (Phila).* 2006;45(5):423–434

103. Aupont O, Doerfler L, Connor DF, Stille C, Tisminetzky M, McLaughlin TJ. A collaborative care model to improve access to pediatric mental health services. *Adm Policy Ment Health.* 2013;40(4):264–273

104. Kerker BD, Chor KH, Hoagwood KE, et al. Detection and treatment of mental health issues by pediatric PCPs in New York State: an evaluation of Project TEACH. *Psychiatr Serv.* 2015;66(4):430–433

105. Gadomski AM, Wissow LS, Palinkas L, Hoagwood KE, Daly JM, Kaye DL. Encouraging and sustaining integration of child mental health into primary care: interviews with primary care providers participating in Project TEACH (CAPES and CAP PC) in NY. *Gen Hosp Psychiatry.* 2014;36(6):555–562

106. Hilt RJ, Romaire MA, McDonell MG, et al. The partnership access line: evaluating a child psychiatry consult program in Washington State. *JAMA Pediatr.* 2013;167(2):162–168

POLICY STATEMENT Organizational Principles to Guide and Define the Child Health Care System and/or Improve the Health of all Children

American Academy of Pediatrics

DEDICATED TO THE HEALTH OF ALL CHILDREN™

Incorporating Recognition and Management of Perinatal Depression Into Pediatric Practice

Marian F. Earls, MD, MTS, FAAP,[a,b] Michael W. Yogman, MD, FAAP,[c] Gerri Mattson, MD, MSPH, FAAP,[d,e] Jason Rafferty, MD, MPH, EdM, FAAP,[f,g,h] COMMITTEE ON PSYCHOSOCIAL ASPECTS OF CHILD AND FAMILY HEALTH

abstract

Perinatal depression (PND) is the most common obstetric complication in the United States. Even when screening results are positive, mothers often do not receive further evaluation, and even when PND is diagnosed, mothers do not receive evidence-based treatments. Studies reveal that postpartum depression (PPD), a subset of PND, leads to increased costs of medical care, inappropriate medical treatment of the infant, discontinuation of breastfeeding, family dysfunction, and an increased risk of abuse and neglect. PPD, specifically, adversely affects this critical early period of infant brain development. PND is an example of an adverse childhood experience that has potential long-term adverse health complications for the mother, her partner, the infant, and the mother-infant dyad. However, PND can be treated effectively, and the stress on the infant can be buffered. Pediatric medical homes should coordinate care more effectively with prenatal providers for women with prenatally diagnosed maternal depression; establish a system to implement PPD screening at the 1-, 2-, 4-, and 6-month well-child visits; use community resources for the treatment and referral of the mother with depression; and provide support for the maternal-child (dyad) relationship, including breastfeeding support. State chapters of the American Academy of Pediatrics, working with state departments of public health, public and private payers, and maternal and child health programs, should advocate for payment and for increased training for PND screening and treatment. American Academy of Pediatrics recommends advocacy for workforce development for mental health professionals who care for young children and mother-infant dyads, and for promotion of evidence-based interventions focused on healthy attachment and parent-child relationships.

[a]Community Care of North Carolina, Raleigh, North Carolina; [b]Department of Pediatrics at the School of Medicine, University of North Carolina, Chapel Hill, North Carolina; [c]Department of Pediatrics, Harvard Medical School, Boston, Massachusetts; [d]Department of Maternal and Child Health at the Gillings School of Global Public Health, Chapel Hill, North Carolina; [e]Wake County Health and Human Services, Raleigh, North Carolina; [f]Department of Pediatrics, Thundermist Health Centers, Woonsocket, Rhode Island; [g]Department of Child Psychiatry, Emma Pendleton Bradley Hospital, East Providence, Rhode Island; and [h]Department of Psychiatry and Human Behavior, Warren Alpert Medical School of Brown University, Providence, Rhode Island

Drs Earls, Yogman, Mattson, and Rafferty conceptualized the statement, drafted the initial manuscript, reviewed and revised the manuscript, approved the final manuscript as submitted, and agree to be accountable for all aspects of the work.

Policy statements from the American Academy of Pediatrics benefit from expertise and resources of liaisons and internal (AAP) and external reviewers. However, policy statements from the American Academy of Pediatrics may not reflect the views of the liaisons or the organizations or government agencies that they represent.

The guidance in this statement does not indicate an exclusive course of treatment or serve as a standard of medical care. Variations, taking into account individual circumstances, may be appropriate.

To cite: Earls MF, Yogman MW, Mattson G, et al; AAP Committee on Psychosocial Aspects of Child and Family Health. Incorporating Recognition and Management of Perinatal Depression Into Pediatric Practice. *Pediatrics.* 2019;143(1):e20183259

BACKGROUND INFORMATION

A 2010 clinical report from the American Academy of Pediatrics (AAP) described the rationale and need for screening for postpartum depression (PPD) in pediatric primary care.[1] Although primary care clinicians (PCCs) have improved the rates of integrating screening in practice since then, according to the 2013 periodic survey of AAP members, less than half of pediatricians screened mothers for depression. The expanding understanding of the effects of adverse childhood experiences, the recognition of screening as an evidence-based recommendation by the US Preventive Services Task Force (USPSTF),[2,3] and the statement of the Centers for Medicare and Medicaid Services (CMS)[4,5] for support of the coverage of PPD screening under Early and Periodic Screening, Diagnostic and Treatment services have emphasized that it is time to close the gap in rates of screening.

Maternal depression affects the whole family.[6] This policy statement focuses specifically on the effects of maternal depression on the young infant and the role of the pediatric PCC (physician, nurse practitioner, or physician assistant) in identifying PPD and referring the mother-infant dyad for treatment. Perinatal depression (PND) is a major or minor depressive disorder, with an episode occurring during pregnancy or within the first year after the birth of a child. A family history of depression, substance use, marital discord, family violence, isolation, poverty, difficult infant temperament, young maternal age, chronic illness, and a personal history of depression increase the risk of PND.[7] In addition, the risk is also higher with multiple births, preterm birth, and congenital or acquired physical or neurodevelopmental deficits in the infant. Stressful transitions, such as returning to work, may also be a risk factor. Minority, immigrant, and refugee populations are especially at risk because they face the added stress of adjusting to and learning to function in a new environment without as much local family support and with added financial concerns or cultural barriers (language or not asking for help because of cultural norms or lack of awareness of resources).[8,9]

Pediatric PCCs are in a good position to recognize the signs of PPD because they are in frequent contact with parents of infants. PND peaks in women 18 to 44 years of age. In general, as many as 12% of all women who are pregnant or in the postpartum period experience depression in a given year, and 11% to 18% of women report postpartum depressive symptoms. The prevalence in women with low income is estimated to be double at 25%. Moreover, adolescent mothers with low income report depressive symptoms at a rate of 40% to 60%.[1] Minor depression peaks at 2 to 3 months postpartum, and the peak for major depression is at 6 weeks postpartum. There is another peak for depression at 6 months postpartum. Depression in a parent is known to have a profound effect on infants and other children in the family. A growing understanding of early brain development reveals the ecobiodevelopmental factors that determine lifelong physical and mental health. In fact, according to a study by the Centers for Disease Control and Prevention, PPD is 1 of the most common adverse childhood experiences that are associated with the costliest adverse adult health outcomes.[10]

Studies have documented that maternal health care costs associated with PPD are 90% higher than those for comparison groups of women who are postpartum and do not have PPD; the difference is attributable to increased use of mental health services and emergency department visits by both mothers and children. Overall, costs to employers for US workers with PPD, including worker absence and lost productivity, are $44 billion per year and $12.4 billion in health care costs.[11,12]

PPD has a spectrum ranging from milder symptoms of "postpartum blues" to PPD and postpartum psychosis (PPP). It is estimated that 50% to 80% of all mothers experience postpartum blues after childbirth. These symptoms are transient (beginning a few days after childbirth and lasting up to 2 weeks), but they do not impair function. Symptoms include crying, depressed mood, irritability, anxiety, and confusion.

PPD meets the criteria of the *Diagnostic and Statistical Manual of Mental Disorders, Fifth Edition* as a major depressive disorder. Anxiety is a common component of PPD.[13] If a woman experiences PPD, she is likely to experience it with subsequent pregnancies. However, PPD can also affect mothers with subsequent pregnancies even without a previous history with earlier births.

PPP is a relatively rare event. Only 1 to 2 per 1000 women experience PPP after childbirth. Occurring in the first 4 weeks after childbirth, impairment is serious and may include paranoia, mood shifts, hallucinations and/or delusions, and suicidal and/or homicidal thoughts. PPP requires immediate medical attention.

Fathers also suffer from PPD, with a prevalence rate that varies from 2% to as high as 25%, with an increase to 50% when the mother experiences PPD.[14–19] Although the rate of paternal depression is higher when the mother has PPD (which compounds the effect on children), a father who is not depressed is 1 protective factor for children of mothers with depression. Fathers are less likely to seek help. They are more likely to present with symptoms of substance use, domestic violence, and undermining breastfeeding instead of sadness.[20]

IMPACT ON THE INFANT, DYAD, AND FAMILY

Research on early brain development, toxic stress, epigenetics, and adverse childhood experiences has revealed the physiologic effect of the infant's environment on health, development, and learning in the short- and long-term.[21] An infant in the environment of significant maternal depression is at risk for toxic stress and its consequences. Toxic stress is an unhealthy prolonged activation of the stress response unbuffered by a caregiver. Physiologic responses to stress in the infant's environment affect the infant's social-emotional development. The infant, therefore, is at risk for impaired social interaction and delays in language, cognitive, and social-emotional development.

Sequelae of untreated maternal PPD include failure to implement the injury-prevention components from anticipatory guidance (eg, car safety seats and electrical plug covers),[22] failure to implement preventive health practices for the child (eg, Back to Sleep campaign),[22–25] and difficulty managing chronic health conditions (such as asthma or disabilities) in the young child.[23,26] Families with a parent who is depressed (ie, any parental depression) overuse health care and emergency facilities, often presenting with somatic complaints.[26]

Untreated PPD can lead to impaired parent-child interaction, discontinuation of breastfeeding, child abuse and neglect, and family dysfunction.[27] In extreme situations, it can result in suicide or infanticide. With PPD, there is potential immediate impairment of parenting. PPD can:

- hinder bonding, reciprocal interaction, and healthy attachment;

- distort perception of the infant's behavior;

- cause the mother to be less sensitive and attuned, indifferent, or more controlling; and

- impair the mother's attention to, and judgment for, health and safety.

Because maternal depression compromises bonding, the mother-child relationship may create an environment in which the infant withdraws from daily activities and may avoid interaction. In this situation, the infant is at risk for failure to thrive and attachment disorders of infancy (reactive attachment disorder or other trauma, stress and deprivation disorder, or relationship-specific disorder of infancy and early childhood, as defined in the *Diagnostic Classification of Mental Health and Developmental Disorders of Infancy and Early Childhood*).[28]

Early response to PPD is urgent. If the mother continues to experience depression and there is no intervention for the mother-infant relationship, the child's developmental issues are likely to persist and be less responsive to intervention over time. Long-term effects extend to preschoolers and older children. Maternal depression in infancy also is predictive of cortisol levels in preschoolers, and these changes in levels are linked with anxiety, social wariness, and withdrawal.[29–32] As they age, children of mothers who are untreated for PPD often have poor self-control, poor peer relationships, school problems, and aggression. These children may need special education services, can experience grade retention, and may exit school

early.[33] Attachment disorders, behavior problems, and depression and other mood disorders can occur into childhood and adolescence.[34]

THE ROLE OF THE MEDICAL HOME

PCCs caring for infants have crucial opportunities to promote healthy social-emotional development, to prevent (beginning at prenatal visits) and/or ameliorate the effects of toxic stress,[35] and to provide routine screening for PPD in early infancy. Pediatric PCCs also have the opportunity to perform depression screening in pregnant mothers at sibling visits. Pediatric medical homes can establish a system to implement screening and to identify and use community resources for the further assessment and treatment of the mother with depression as well as for the support of the mother-child dyad. Identification and coordinating access to treatment of PPD are evidence-based examples of the successful buffering of toxic stress or an adverse childhood experience by pediatricians. Despite previous recommendations, less than half of pediatricians screened mothers for maternal depression in the 2013 periodic survey of AAP members, and it is now time to close the gap.[36,37]

There is much support for primary care incorporating these approaches. The AAP policy statement "The Future of Pediatrics: Mental Health Competencies for Pediatric Primary Care" recognizes the unique advantage the PCC has for surveillance, screening, and working with families to improve mental health outcomes.[38] The AAP Task Force on Mental Health promotes the use of a common-factors approach to engage families and build an alliance for addressing mental health issues. *Bright Futures: Guidelines for Health Supervision of Infants, Children, and Adolescents, fourth Edition*[39] places particular emphasis on engaging families in identifying parental strengths and discussing social determinants of health. Screening for PPD in the medical home is consistent with this 2-generation emphasis.

IMPLEMENTATION

The infant and the mother-infant dyad relationship are the primary concerns of the pediatric PCC. Treatment, when focused solely on the adult, is often less effective than treatment that is focused on the mother-infant dyad. Apart from the adolescent mother who is a patient of the pediatric practice, the mother is generally not the pediatric PCC's patient, but concern extends to the mother herself as well as to her partner. Using a validated tool to screen for depression is 1 of the ways PCCs engage families about psychosocial risks. PCCs (often using a formal surveillance tool or standardized questions) also ask about homelessness, food insecurity, domestic violence, tobacco use, substance use, guns in the home, etc, so they can link the family with community resources, if needed, to reduce the risk for the child. The pediatric PCC also manages the child closely to monitor the possible effects of these risk factors. Referral and follow-up for the infant and mother-infant dyad are the major areas of focus for the pediatric PCC, but knowledge of community resources to which to refer the parent, including knowing how to access community mental health crisis services, is essential to implementing an office process for screening. Implementation often requires a quality improvement approach to office process.

Concerns may be raised regarding liability for the pediatric PCC because the mother is not the patient of that visit. Screening for PPD is performed for the benefit of the infant because the well-being of the infant is inextricably linked to the mother-infant dyad. The pediatric PCC's focus is the dyad, and the PCC is facilitating referral for the mother, not providing treatment.

Surveillance and Screening

Over the course of routine well-child care, the pediatric PCC and the family are developing a longitudinal relationship. A crucial part of this relationship is eliciting parent, family, and child strengths and risks. Psychosocial screening and surveillance for risk and protective factors is an integral part of routine care. Pediatric PCCs need to be aware of and promote protective factors, such as parental knowledge and skills about child development and caregiving, good parental or caregiver physical and mental health, positive father or partner involvement, strong emotional bonding or attachment between infant or child and parent or caregiver, and social supports (ie, friends, neighbors, relatives, faith-based groups, and other agencies). According to resilience theory, an individual's resilience is determined by balancing risk and protective factors in the face of adversity.[40] Promotion of family protective factors promotes resiliency. For example, a father who is not depressed is one protective factor for infants of mothers with depression.

The prenatal visit to the pediatric office is an excellent opportunity for the pediatric PCC and expectant parent(s) to discuss strengths and stressors during pregnancy, including depression.[35] The pediatric PCC may be able to provide anticipatory guidance and to initiate supportive strategies for the mother for the benefit of the infant, even before the infant's birth. Obstetricians and other obstetric providers who identify depression during pregnancy can be especially encouraged to refer prospective parents to pediatricians prenatally so that postpartum management of PND is coordinated. Communication between the obstetrician and pediatric PCC is desirable for this reason. The American College of Obstetricians and Gynecologists specifically recommends this collaboration between obstetricians and their pediatric colleagues.[41] In turn, pediatric PCCs would encourage communication on behalf of the infant.

On the basis of knowledge regarding peak occurrence times for PPD, routine screening in which a validated screening tool is used should occur at well-infant visits at 1, 2, 4, and 6 months. Repeated screening at these visits allows for a mother who may not be comfortable disclosing initially to do so at a later visit, and it maximizes the opportunity to engage a dyad that may miss 1 or more of the recommended well-infant visits. Components of documentation in the infant's chart include the type of screening tool used, results, discussion with the mother or parents (whether positive or negative), and a follow-up and referral plan if indicated. There is no reason to open a chart on the mother because she is not receiving treatment. Although not the focus of this statement, it should also be noted that there are recommendations that PPD screening should be performed for the parents of infants who are hospitalized and the parents of infants up to 1 year of age seen in the emergency department.[42,43]

Pediatricians should be encouraged to consider screening the partner as well at the 6-month visit with the Edinburgh Postpartum Depression Scale (EPDS), either in person if the partner is present or by having the partner fill out the screen at home and mail it back. If the partner is male, this process is more feasible if the pediatrician has identified referral resources when he screens positive for depression.

Screening tools for PPD include the EPDS (note that the EPDS is now included within the Survey of Well-being of Young Children [SWYC]) or the Patient Health Questionnaire. The EPDS is completed by the mother, and a score of 10 or greater indicates possible depression. The EPDS also contains 2 questions regarding anxiety. Screening for PPD by using the EPDS has now been validated for men as well as women.[20]

It should be noted that screening is not diagnostic. A positive screen result indicates a risk that depression is present, and the purpose of referral is to clarify the diagnosis and offer the indicated treatment.

As with other screening implementations, it is essential for the practice to understand and prepare for referral and linkages with appropriate resources for children and/or families who are identified as at risk.

Follow-up, Referral, Treatment

When screening reveals a concern, next steps include communication and demystification, support, identification of community and family resources, and referrals as indicated.

Immediate action is necessary if question 10 on the EPDS is positive (indicating possible suicidality), if question 9 on the Patient Health Questionnaire 9 is positive (indicating possible suicidality), if the mother expresses concern about her or her infant's safety, or if the PCC suspects that the mother is suicidal, homicidal, severely depressed, manic, or psychotic. As with any mental health crisis in which suicidality is a concern, referral to emergency mental health services (most communities have mental health crisis teams or services) is needed, and the mother should only leave

with her support person or under the care of community resources, such as mental health crisis services or emergency medical services.

When a depression screen result is positive, management will vary according to the degree of concern and need. Because the mother is not the patient of the pediatrician, a detailed discussion of treatment of the mother is outside the scope of this article, but a Cochrane review of a few studies of mothers with PPD revealed that there is no difference between the effectiveness of antidepressants and psychological and/or psychosocial treatments.[44] At the very least, management will require support and demystification. Management of PPD includes:

- demystification (reducing guilt and shame by emphasizing how common these feelings are);
- support resources (family and community); and
- referrals for the mother (to a mental health professional or the mother's PCC or obstetrician), for the mother-infant dyad, for the child (for targeted promotion of social-emotional development and early intervention [EI]), and for the mother who is breastfeeding (for lactation support from an experienced provider).

Regardless of the referral arrangement, a key component is a follow-up with the mother to be certain that she is receiving treatment and that depressive symptoms are decreased. Such follow-up could be conducted by a designated referral person on the practice staff.

Demystification removes the mystery about maternal depression, acknowledging that PPD happens to many women, that the mother is not at fault or a "bad" mother, that depression is treatable, and that the PCC is a resource. A brief intervention at the visit would involve:

- promoting the strength of the mother-infant relationship;
- encouraging the mother and reassuring her regarding any concerns about breastfeeding;
- encouraging understanding and responding to the infant's cues;
- encouraging reading and talking to the infant;
- encouraging routines for predictability and security, sleep, diet, exercise, and stress relief;
- promoting realistic expectations and prioritizing important things; and
- encouraging social connections.

To follow-up on the impact on the infant and dyad, use of a screening tool for infant social-emotional development is appropriate. One such tool, the Baby Pediatric Symptom Checklist, is brief and in the public domain as part of the SWYC. It screens for irritability, inflexibility, and difficulty with routines. The Ages & Stages Questionnaires: Social-Emotional, Second Edition is another infant social-emotional screening tool (not in the public domain). It is completed by the parent, has a single cutoff score, and screens affect, self-regulation, adaptive functioning, autonomy, compliance, and communication.[45–47]

If there are concerns about attachment and bonding, the dyad needs referral to a mental health professional with expertise in the treatment of young children. Evidence-based interventions for the dyad (child's age 0–5 years) include child-parent psychotherapy, Circle of Security (www.circleofsecurityinternational.com), and Attachment and Biobehavioral Catch-up.[46,47] These interventions are used to address the dyadic relationship in high-risk families and are often used in situations of abuse and neglect or interpersonal violence, and with Circle of Security, in the setting of PND. A key component of follow-up is comanagement (and standardized communication) with the mental health professional serving the dyad.

If the practice has an integrated mental health professional, such as a licensed clinical social worker or counselor, that team member can provide immediate triage for a positive screen, administer secondary screens, offer support and follow-up, facilitate referrals, and coordinate follow-up with the PCC.

Referral to EI services for children from birth to 3 years of age through Part C of the Individuals with Disabilities Education Act is also important to address the dyad relationship.[48–50] EI in the home can provide modeling for interaction and play to prevent toxic stress and promote healthy development. However, in many states, it is difficult to access EI services because of eligibility processes. This difficulty is attributable in part to funding limitations, leading to more restrictive eligibility, but the crucial issue is that the domain of social-emotional development may not be included in eligibility criteria. Given the inextricable connection of social-emotional development to cognitive and language development, such eligibility policies can be detrimental to children and families.

Community resources include Early Head Start, Healthy Start, home visiting programs, and other community organizations. Other community resources for the family include public health nurses, lactation specialists, parent educators, parent support groups, parent-child groups, and postpartum support groups.

Coding and Billing

The AAP, along with the USPSTF[2,3] and the CMS,[4,5] recognizes that PPD screens are a measure of risk in the infant's environment, and therefore, billing is appropriate at the infant's visit, with the infant as the patient. *Current Procedural Terminology* code 96161 (effective as of January 2017)

allows reporting of the administration of a caregiver-focused health risk assessment (eg, parent depression screen) for the benefit of the patient. However, because billing codes may vary by payer and by state, PCCs are advised to consult AAP state chapter pediatric councils and payers for updated coding guidance. When a screen result is positive, the PCC should be familiar with coding on the basis of counseling time and complexity when indicated.

CONCLUSIONS

The 2010 AAP clinical report[1] acknowledged that PPD leads to adverse effects on infant brain development, family dysfunction, cessation of breastfeeding, inappropriate medical treatment of the infant, and increased costs of medical care. Since that time, PCCs in several states have successfully implemented screening and have built referral relationships for evidence-based interventions, for community resources for the treatment and referral of the mother with depression, and for resources to support the mother-child (dyad) relationship.

National recognition of toxic stress, adverse childhood experiences, and the importance of trauma-informed care has led to recommendations for recognition and intervention from professional and policy organizations, including the USPSTF and CMS as well as the AAP. Recognizing and building resilience against toxic stress, education, and advocacy has been a focus of the national advocacy campaign of the AAP Section on Pediatric Trainees (https://www.aap.org/en-us/advocacy-and-policy/aap-health-initiatives/resilience/Pages/default.aspx).[51]

The pediatric PCC has a unique opportunity to identify PPD and help prevent untoward developmental and mental health outcomes for the infant and family. Screening has proven

successful in several initiatives and locations and can be implemented in office workflow by PCCs caring for infants and their families. Intervention and referral are optimized by collaborative relationships with community resources and/or by collocated and/or integrated mental health in primary care.

RECOMMENDATIONS

Routine screening for PPD should be integrated into well-child visits at 1, 2, 4, and 6 months of age. This screening schedule is recommended in *Bright Futures: Guidelines for Health Supervision of Infants, Children, and Adolescents, Fourth Edition*.[39] PPD screening has also been recognized as evidence based according to the USPSTF (Grade B recommendation; see accompanying technical report[52]). Training and continuing medical education programs should be available for all pediatric providers on the subject of PPD screening and referral.[4]

OPPORTUNITIES FOR ADVOCACY

1. AAP chapters, other stakeholders, and state public health agencies and officials can increase awareness of the need for PND screening as outlined in the obstetric and pediatric periodicity of care schedules. Advocacy should be conducted with commercial payers to ensure payment for PND screening and related services.

2. In keeping with current CMS recommendations, state Medicaid programs may pay for PPD screening under Early and Periodic Screening, Diagnostic and Treatment using a validated screening instrument, such as the EPDS, Patient Health Questionnaire, or the SWYC.

3. The AAP can collaborate with the American College of

Obstetricians and Gynecologists to encourage prenatal referral of all mothers to the PCC of the infant so that care is coordinated and integrated for families at a high risk for PPD.[53]

4. Screening of mothers for PPD by pediatricians at least once during the first 6 months after birth should be part of quality metrics used for payment.

5. Establishment of consultation and referral resources to improve access to treatment of mothers identified with PPD should be advocated.

6. Workforce development should be promoted for mental health providers who care for young children and the parent-infant dyad.

7. Evidence-based interventions focused on healthy attachment and parent-child relationships should be promoted.

8. Federal funding should be advocated for states to establish, improve, or maintain programs for screening, assessment, and treatment services for women who are pregnant or who have given birth within the preceding 12 months, as required under the 21st Century Cures Act of 2016 (Public Law 114–255).

9. Inclusion of social-emotional development as a domain for eligibility in Part C programs should be supported.

10. Creation of postpartum support networks in local communities should be encouraged by partnering with local businesses and nonprofits.

11. Media campaigns and messaging to counteract stigma associated with PND should be encouraged.

LEAD AUTHORS

Marian Earls, MD, FAAP
Michael Yogman, MD, FAAP
Gerri Mattson, MD, MSPH, FAAP
Jason Rafferty, MD, MPH, EdM

COMMITTEE ON PSYCHOSOCIAL ASPECTS OF CHILD AND FAMILY HEALTH, 2016–2017

Michael Yogman, MD, FAAP Chairperson
Rebecca Baum, MD, FAAP
Thresia Gambon, MD, FAAP
Arthur Lavin, MD, FAAP
Gerri Mattson, MD, MSPH, FAAP
Jason Rafferty, MD, MPH, EdM
Lawrence Wissow, MD, MPH, FAAP

LIAISONS

Sharon Berry, PhD – *Society of Pediatric Psychology*
Terry Carmichael, MSW – *National Association of Social Workers*
Edward R. Christopherson, PhD, FAAP (hon) – *Society of Pediatric Psychology*
Norah Johnson, PhD, RN, CPNP-PC – *National Association of Pediatric Nurse Practitioners*
L. Read Sulik, MD, FAAP – *American Academy of Child and Adolescent Psychiatry*

STAFF

Stephanie Domain, MS

ABBREVIATIONS

AAP:	American Academy of Pediatrics
CMS:	Centers for Medicare and Medicaid Services
EI:	early intervention
EPDS:	Edinburgh Postpartum Depression Scale
PCC:	primary care clinician
PND:	perinatal depression
PPD:	postpartum depression
PPP:	postpartum psychosis
SWYC:	Survey of Well-being of Young Children
USPSTF:	US Preventive Services Task Force

All policy statements from the American Academy of Pediatrics automatically expire 5 years after publication unless reaffirmed, revised, or retired at or before that time.

DOI: https://doi.org/10.1542/peds.2018-3259

Address Correspondence to Marian Earls, MD, MTS, FAAP. Email: mearls@communitycarenc.org

PEDIATRICS (ISSN Numbers: Print, 0031-4005; Online, 1098-4275).

FINANCIAL DISCLOSURE: The authors have indicated they have no financial relationships relevant to this article to disclose.

FUNDING: No external funding.

POTENTIAL CONFLICT OF INTEREST: The authors have indicated they have no potential conflicts of interest to disclose.

REFERENCES

1. Earls MF; Committee on Psychosocial Aspects of Child and Family Health; American Academy of Pediatrics. Incorporating recognition and management of perinatal and postpartum depression into pediatric practice. *Pediatrics.* 2010;126(5):1032–1039

2. US Preventive Services Task Force. Final recommendation statement. Depression in adults: screening. 2016. Available at: https://www.uspreventiveservicestaskforce.org/Page/Document/RecommendationStatementFinal/depression-in-adults-screening1. Accessed February 2, 2018

3. Siu AL, Bibbins-Domingo K, Grossman DC, et al; US Preventive Services Task Force (USPSTF). Screening for depression in adults: US Preventive Services Task Force recommendation statement. *JAMA.* 2016;315(4):380–387

4. Centers for Medicare and Medicaid Services. CMCS Informational Bulletin,

May 11, 2016. Maternal depression screening and treatment: a critical role for Medicaid in the care of mothers and children. Available at: https://www.medicaid.gov/federal-policy-guidance/downloads/cib051116.pdf. Accessed July 22, 2018

5. Olin SS, McCord M, Stein REK, et al. Beyond Screening: A Stepped Care Pathway for Managing Postpartum Depression in Pediatric Settings. *J Womens Health (Larchmt)*. 2017;26(9):966–975

6. Isaacs M. *Community Care Networks for Depression in Low-Income Communities and Communities of Color: A Review of the Literature*. Washington, DC: Howard University School of Social Work and National Alliance of Multiethnic Behavioral Health Associations; 2004

7. Kahn RS, Wise PH, Wilson K. Maternal smoking, drinking and depression: a generational link between socioeconomic status and child behavior problems [abstract]. *Pediatr Res*. 2002;51(pt 2):191A

8. Doe S, LoBue S, Hamaoui A, Rezai S, Henderson CE, Mercado R. Prevalence and predictors of positive screening for postpartum depression in minority parturients in the South Bronx. *Arch Womens Ment Health*. 2017;20(2):291–295

9. Cebollos M, Wallace G, Goodwin G. Postpartum depression among African-American and Latina mothers living in small cities, towns, and rural communities. *J Racial Ethn Health Disparities*. 2017;4(5):916–927

10. Felitti VJ, Anda RF, Nordenberg D, et al. Relationship of childhood abuse and household dysfunction to many of the leading causes of death in adults. The Adverse Childhood Experiences (ACE) study. *Am J Prev Med*. 1998;14(4):245–258

11. Witters D, Liu D, Agrawal S. Depression costs U.S. workplaces $23 billion in absenteeism. 2013. Available at: http://news.gallup.com/poll/163619/depression-costs-workplaces-billion-absenteeism.aspx. Accessed February 2, 2018

12. Dagher RK, McGovern PM, Dowd BE, Gjerdingen DK. Postpartum depression and health services expenditures among employed women. *J Occup Environ Med*. 2012;54(2):210–215

13. Ross LE, McLean LM. Anxiety disorders during pregnancy and the postpartum period: a systematic review. *J Clin Psychiatry*. 2006;67(8):1285–1298

14. Davis RN, Davis MM, Freed GL, Clark SJ. Fathers' depression related to positive and negative parenting behaviors with 1-year-old children. *Pediatrics*. 2011;127(4):612–618

15. Chang JJ, Halpern CT, Kaufman JS. Maternal depressive symptoms, father's involvement, and the trajectories of child problem behaviors in a US national sample. *Arch Pediatr Adolesc Med*. 2007;161(7):697–703

16. Goodman JH. Paternal postpartum depression, its relationship to maternal postpartum depression, and implications for family health. *J Adv Nurs*. 2004;45(1):26–35

17. Edmondson OJ, Psychogiou L, Vlachos H, Netsi E, Ramchandani PG. Depression in fathers in the postnatal period: assessment of the Edinburgh Postnatal Depression Scale as a screening measure. *J Affect Disord*. 2010;125(1–3):365–368

18. Ramchandani PG, Psychogiou L, Vlachos H, et al. Paternal depression: an examination of its links with father, child and family functioning in the postnatal period. *Depress Anxiety*. 2011;28(6):471–477

19. Paulson JF, Bazemore SD. Prenatal and postpartum depression in fathers and its association with maternal depression: a meta-analysis. *JAMA*. 2010;303(19):1961–1969

20. Rochlen AB. Men in (and out of) therapy: central concepts, emerging directions, and remaining challenges. *J Clin Psychol*. 2005;61(6):627–631

21. Garner AS, Shonkoff JP; Committee on Psychosocial Aspects of Child and Family Health; Committee on Early Childhood, Adoption, and Dependent Care; Section on Developmental and Behavioral Pediatrics. Early childhood adversity, toxic stress, and the role of the pediatrician: translating developmental science into lifelong health. *Pediatrics*. 2012;129(1). Available at: www.pediatrics.org/cgi/content/full/129/1/e224

22. McLennan JD, Kotelchuck M. Parental prevention practices for young children in the context of maternal depression. *Pediatrics*. 2000;105(5):1090–1095

23. Chung EK, McCollum KF, Elo IT, Lee HJ, Culhane JF. Maternal depressive symptoms and infant health practices among low-income women. *Pediatrics*. 2004;113(6). Available at: www.pediatrics.org/cgi/content/full/113/6/e523

24. Kavanaugh M, Halterman JS, Montes G, Epstein M, Hightower AD, Weitzman M. Maternal depressive symptoms are adversely associated with prevention practices and parenting behaviors for preschool children. *Ambul Pediatr*. 2006;6(1):32–37

25. Paulson JF, Dauber S, Leiferman JA. Individual and combined effects of postpartum depression in mothers and fathers on parenting behavior. *Pediatrics*. 2006;118(2):659–668

26. Sills MR, Shetterly S, Xu S, Magid D, Kempe A. Association between parental depression and children's health care use. *Pediatrics*. 2007;119(4). Available at: www.pediatrics.org/cgi/content/full/119/4/e829

27. Ip S, Chung M, Raman G, et al. *Breastfeeding and Maternal and Infant Health Outcomes in Developed Countries*. Rockville, MD: Agency for Health Research and Quality; 2007:130–131

28. Zero to Three. *DC:0-5: Diagnostic Classification of Mental Health and Developmental Disorders of Infancy and Early Childhood*. Washington, DC: Zero to Three; 2016

29. Beardslee WR, Versage EM, Gladstone TR. Children of affectively ill parents: a review of the past 10 years. *J Am Acad Child Adolesc Psychiatry*. 1998;37(11):1134–1141

30. Smider NA, Essex MJ, Kalin NH, et al. Salivary cortisol as a predictor of socioemotional adjustment during kindergarten: a prospective study. *Child Dev*. 2002;73(1):75–92

31. Essex MJ, Klein MH, Cho E, Kalin NH. Maternal stress beginning in infancy may sensitize children to later stress exposure: effects on cortisol and behavior. *Biol Psychiatry*. 2002;52(8):776–784

32. Essex MJ, Klein MH, Miech R, Smider NA. Timing of initial exposure to maternal major depression and children's mental health symptoms in kindergarten. *Br J Psychiatry.* 2001;179:151–156

33. Lahti M, Savolainen K, Tuovinen S, et al. Maternal depressive symptoms during and after pregnancy and psychiatric problems in children. *J Am Acad Child Adolesc Psychiatry.* 2017;56(1):30–39. e7

34. Netsi E, Pearson RM, Murray L, Cooper P, Craske MG, Stein A. Association of persistent and severe postnatal depression with child outcomes. *JAMA Psychiatry.* 2018;75(3):247–253

35. Yogman M, Lavin A, Cohen G; Committee on Psychosocial Aspects of Child and Family Health. The prenatal visit. *Pediatrics.* 2018;142(1):e20181218

36. Kerker BD, Storfer-Isser A, Stein RE, et al. Identifying maternal depression in pediatric primary care: changes over a decade. *J Dev Behav Pediatr.* 2016;37(2):113–120

37. Yogman MW. Postpartum depression screening by pediatricians: time to close the gap. *J Dev Behav Pediatr.* 2016;37(2):157

38. Committee on Psychosocial Aspects of Child and Family Health; Task Force on Mental Health. Policy statement–the future of pediatrics: mental health competencies for pediatric primary care. *Pediatrics.* 2009;124(1):410–421

39. Hagan J, Shaw JS, Duncan PM, eds. *Bright Futures: Guidelines for Health Supervision of Infants, Children, and Adolescents.* 4th ed. Elk Grove Village, IL: American Academy of Pediatrics; 2017

40. Luthar SS, Cicchetti D, Becker B. The construct of resilience: a critical evaluation and guidelines for future work. *Child Dev.* 2000;71(3):543–562

41. Committee on Obstetric Practice. The American College of Obstetricians and Gynecologists Committee opinion no. 630. Screening for perinatal depression. *Obstet Gynecol.* 2015;125(5):1268–1271

42. Trost MJ, Molas-Torreblanca K, Man C, Casillas E, Sapir H, Schrager SM. Screening for maternal postpartum depression during infant hospitalizations. *J Hosp Med.* 2016;11(12):840–846

43. Emerson BL, Bradley ER, Riera A, Mayes L, Bechtel K. Postpartum depression screening in the pediatric emergency department. *Pediatr Emerg Care.* 2014;30(11):788–792

44. Molyneaux E, Howard LM, McGeown HR, Karia AM, Trevillion K. Antidepressant treatment for postnatal depression. *Cochrane Database Syst Rev.* 2014;(9):CD002018

45. Weitzman C, Wegner L; Section on Developmental and Behavioral Pediatrics; Committee on Psychosocial Aspects of Child and Family Health; Council on Early Childhood; Society for Developmental and Behavioral Pediatrics; American Academy of Pediatrics. Promoting optimal development: screening for behavioral and emotional problems [published correction appears in *Pediatrics.* 2015;135(5):946]. *Pediatrics.* 2015;135(2):384–395

46. Gleason MM, Goldson E, Yogman MW; Council on Early Childhood; Committee on Psychosocial Aspects of Child and Family Health; Section on Developmental and Behavioral Pediatrics. Addressing early childhood emotional and behavioral problems. *Pediatrics.* 2016;138(6):e20163025

47. Council on Early Childhood; Committee on Psychosocial Aspects of Child and Family Health; Section on Developmental and Behavioral Pediatrics. Addressing early childhood emotional and behavioral problems. *Pediatrics.* 2016;138(6):e20163023

48. Pilowsky DJ, Wickramaratne P, Talati A, et al. Children of depressed mothers 1 year after the initiation of maternal treatment: findings from the STAR*D-Child Study. *Am J Psychiatry.* 2008;165(9):1136–1147

49. Foster CE, Webster MC, Weissman MM, et al. Remission of maternal depression: relations to family functioning and youth internalizing and externalizing symptoms. *J Clin Child Adolesc Psychol.* 2008;37(4):714–724

50. Cicchetti D, Rogosch FA, Toth SL. The efficacy of toddler-parent psychotherapy for fostering cognitive development in offspring of depressed mothers. *J Abnorm Child Psychol.* 2000;28(2):135–148

51. American Academy of Pediatrics. Resilience project. Available at: https://www.aap.org/en-us/advocacy-and-policy/aap-health-initiatives/resilience/Pages/default.aspx. Accessed July 22, 2018

52. Rafferty J, Mattson G, Earls M, Yogman M; Committee on Psychosocial Aspects of Child and Family Health. Incorporating recognition and management of perinatal depression into pediatric practice. *Pediatrics.* 2018;143(1):e20183260

53. American College of Obstetricians and Gynecologists' Committee on Obstetric Practice; Association of Women's Health, Obstetric and Neonatal Nurses. Committee opinion no. 666: optimizing postpartum care. *Obstet Gynecol.* 2016;127(6):e187–e192

TECHNICAL REPORT

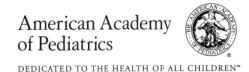

American Academy
of Pediatrics

DEDICATED TO THE HEALTH OF ALL CHILDREN™

Incorporating Recognition and Management of Perinatal Depression Into Pediatric Practice

Jason Rafferty, MD, MPH, EdM, FAAP,[a,b,c] Gerri Mattson, MD, MSPH, FAAP,[d,e] Marian F. Earls, MD, MTS, FAAP,[f,g] Michael W. Yogman, MD, FAAP,[h] COMMITTEE ON PSYCHOSOCIAL ASPECTS OF CHILD AND FAMILY HEALTH

abstract

Perinatal depression is the most common obstetric complication in the United States, with prevalence rates of 15% to 20% among new mothers. Untreated, it can adversely affect the well-being of children and families throught increasing the risk for costly complications during birth and lead to deterioration of core supports, including partner relationships and social networks. Perinatal depression contributes to long-lasting, and even permanent, consequences for the physical and mental health of parents and children, including poor family functioning, increased risk of child abuse and neglect, delayed infant development, perinatal obstetric complications, challenges with breastfeeding, and costly increases in health care use. Perinatal depression can interfere with early parent-infant interaction and attachment, leading to potentially long-term disturbances in the child's physical, emotional, cognitive, and social development. Fortunately, perinatal depression is identifiable and treatable. The US Preventive Services Task Force, Centers for Medicare and Medicaid Services, and many professional organizations recommend routine universal screening for perinatal depression in women to facilitate early evidence-based treatment and referrals, if necessary. Despite significant gains in screening rates from 2004 to 2013, a minority of pediatricians routinely screen for postpartum depression, and many mothers are still not identified or treated. Pediatric primary care clinicians, with a core mission of promoting child and family health, are in an ideal position to implement routine postpartum depression screens at several well-child visits throughout infancy and to provide mental health support through referrals and/or the interdisciplinary services of a pediatric patient-centered medical home model.

[a]Department of Pediatrics, Thundermist Health Centers, Providence, Rhode Island; [b]Department of Child Psychiatry, Emma Pendeltom Bradley Hospital, East Providence, Rhode Island; [c]Department of Psychiatry and Human Behavior, Warren Alpert Medical School of Brown University, Providence, Rhode Island; [d]Wake County Health and Human Services, Raleigh, North Carolina; [e]Department of Maternal and Child Health, Gillings School of Global Public Health, and [f]Department of Pediatrics, School of Medicine, University of North Carolina, Chapel Hill, North Carolina; [g]Community Care of North Carolina, Raleigh, North Carolina; and [h]Department of Pediatrics, Harvard Medical School, Boston, Massachusetts

Drs Rafferty, Mattson, Earls, and Yogman conceptualized the statement and drafted, reviewed, and revised the initial manuscript; and all authors approved the final manuscript as submitted and agree to be accountable for all aspects of the work.

Technical reports from the American Academy of Pediatrics benefit from expertise and resources of liaisons and internal (AAP) and external reviewers. However, technical reports from the American Academy of Pediatrics may not reflect the views of the liaisons or the organizations or government agencies that they represent.

The guidance in this report does not indicate an exclusive course of treatment or serve as a standard of medical care. Variations, taking into account individual circumstances, may be appropriate.

To cite: Rafferty J, Mattson G, Earls MF, et al. Incorporating Recognition and Management of Perinatal Depression Into Pediatric Practice. *Pediatrics.* 2019;143(1):e20183260

BACKGROUND

Depression is experienced by women most often during their childbearing years.[1] Over the last several decades, research has revealed that untreated maternal depression during pregnancy or the first year after childbirth can have significant adverse effects on the well-being of women, infants, and their families. Maternal depression experienced around the time of childbirth can increase the risk for costly complications during birth and can contribute to long-lasting and even permanent effects on the child's development.[2] Only in the last decade has universal screening for maternal depressive symptoms during the perinatal period been recommended by professional health care associations, including the American College of Obstetricians and Gynecologists (ACOG),[3] American Academy of Family Physicians (AAFP),[4] and American Academy of Pediatrics (AAP).[1] However, screening remains far from universal. In 1 study, nearly 6 out of 10 women screening positive on the Edinburgh Postnatal Depression Scale (EPDS) had not spoken to a health care professional about their symptoms or concerns.[5] It is estimated that 50% of women who are depressed during and after pregnancy have their depression go undiagnosed and untreated, which makes it the most underdiagnosed and undertreated obstetric complication.[6] However, most mothers (80%) report being comfortable with the idea of being screened for depression.[7] Among pediatricians, 90% in 1 study reported assuming responsibility for identifying maternal depression, but most (71%) rarely or never assessed for it, and almost all (93%) reported having never or rarely provided mental health referrals.[8] From 2004 to 2013, screening rates by pediatricians for maternal depression increased from 13% to only 44% in periodic surveys by a number of organizations, including the AAP.[9] Inadequate perinatal depression screening rates and limited access to evidence-based treatment are attributable to the stigma associated with mental health, patient apprehension about openly admitting to emotional struggles, limits in provider education and skill sets, and systemic limitations around delivery of and payment for screening.[7,10,11]

There has been increased attention given to perinatal depression, including the release of the US Surgeon General's Report on Mental Health in 2000 in which postpartum depression and psychosis was mentioned,[12] the 2000 report of the US Surgeon General's Conference on Children's Mental Health,[13] and a recent review article in the *New England Journal of Medicine*.[14] Congress designated increased funding to address screening and treatment of perinatal depression through the Health Resources and Services Administration's Maternal and Child Health Bureau in 2004.[2] In 2018, Congress designated $5 million for programs used to address maternal perinatal depression in the 2018 Omnibus Funding Bill (public law 114–255). This funding will be used to support state grants primarily aimed at establishing, improving, and maintaining programs to train professionals to screen and treat for maternal perinatal depression.

The most recent update of the AAP's *Bright Futures: Guidelines for Health Supervision of Infants, Children, and Adolescents, Fourth Edition* includes a recommendation for pediatric providers to screen for postpartum depression at 4 well-child visits in the first 6 months of life and refer to appropriate evaluation and treatment services for the mother and infant when indicated.[15] In 2009, the AAP released a policy statement, "The Future of Pediatrics: Mental Health Competencies for Pediatric Primary Care," emphasizing the unique role pediatric providers have in screening for mental health concerns in children and families, including parental depressive symptoms, and working with families to improve mental health outcomes.[16] The National Academy of Sciences published its report on parental depression in 2009, emphasizing the role of the AAP Medical Home Initiative in reducing perinatal depression occurrence.[17,18] It was followed by a clinical report from the AAP that was focused on recognition and management of perinatal and postpartum depression in 2010[1] and the US Healthy People 2020 objectives to reduce the proportion of mothers experiencing perinatal depression (maternal, infant, and child health objective 34) and to improve overall maternal and child perinatal health.[19] It is within this context that the National Institute for Health Care Management released a report concluding:

The consequences of allowing maternal depression to go underdiagnosed and untreated are detrimental to the health of all mothers and their children. Knowing a woman's risk of developing depression peaks during her childbearing years, it is vital for all health care providers to recognize the symptoms of depression and understand the risk factors associated with maternal depression to identify and treat depression as soon as possible.[2]

In 2016, the US Preventive Services Task Force (USPSTF) reviewed available research and asserted that direct and indirect evidence shows a "moderate net benefit" to screening for perinatal depression because it contributes to a significant reduction in overall prevalence of depression and associated morbidities.[20,21] In addition, in 2016, the Centers for Medicare and Medicaid Services (CMS) sent a directive to all state Medicaid directors clarifying that maternal postpartum depression screening can be billed under well-infant visits as a "screening of the caregiver."[22] Both the USPSTF and CMS encourage universal maternal postpartum depression screening by pediatric providers, with appropriate payment by insurers. The USPSTF specifically states that "screening should be implemented with adequate systems in place to ensure accurate diagnosis, effective treatment, and appropriate follow up."[21] This requires close partnerships between pediatricians, family physicians, adult primary care physicians, and obstetricians, mental health providers, and other community agencies.

Recent research also has begun to examine the influence of a father's affective state on a child's early development and well-being.[23,24] Available evidence indicates that fathers independently experience higher rates of depression after the birth of a child, which adversely influences parenting and positive interactions.[25] Paternal depression may present differently with substance use (alcohol and drug-related comorbidity), domestic violence, and compulsive behavior, which impairs parenting and can undermine breastfeeding.[26,27] There are virtually no empirical studies on the rates or effects of depression among same-sex partners or nonbiological parents.

This technical report aims to review the definitions of perinatal depression, along with its epidemiology, to discuss the serious consequences for child development and to highlight efforts across the country that have demonstrated effectiveness in increasing early screening and treatment. The technical report reviews the evidence and rationale underlying recommendations in an accompanying policy statement[28] concerning the role of the pediatric provider as a clinician and advocate in ensuring timely identification of perinatal depression and referral to evidence-based treatment programs. With this report, we provide an

update to the 2010 clinical report from the AAP on this subject.[1]

DEFINITIONS

Perinatal depression is characterized by an episode of major depression, including 2 weeks of depressed mood and neurovegetative symptoms (alterations in sleep, appetite, concentration, energy level, etc), as described in the *Diagnostic and Statistical Manual of Mental Disorders, Fifth Edition (DSM-5)*, occurring during pregnancy or after delivery. Although the diagnostic criteria for major depressive disorder (MDD) did not undergo significant change between the fourth edition and the *DSM-5*, the specifier "with perinatal onset" replaced the traditional distinction between antenatal and postpartum onset.[29] The reason for this change is that 50% of MDD identified during the postpartum period actually begins before delivery.[30] With this change, there is emphasis on the utility of early screening, detection, and management throughout pregnancy, not just after delivery. In fact, in 2015, the ACOG released a committee opinion recommending mothers be screened for depression at least once during the perinatal period[3] expanding the window for recommended screening into the antenatal period. Despite changes in nomenclature and disease conceptualization, much of the literature and current guidelines continue to reference only depression after delivery using the term, "postpartum depression."

There is controversy around the time course of perinatal depression, with the *DSM-5* referencing symptom onset occurring any time during pregnancy or within 4 weeks of delivery. However, many professional organizations, including the ACOG, expand the criteria to include onset of symptoms up to 12 months after delivery. Although most of the

biological factors influencing mood may be less relevant at the later stage, there are significant ongoing psychosocial stressors that increase risk, especially with the added responsibilities of caring for an infant.[3]

Perinatal depression is 1 of a few recognized mood disorders that may occur around pregnancy and delivery (Table 1). "Postpartum blues" is a transient state of increased emotional reactivity occurring in approximately 50% to 80% of mothers after labor and delivery. They may cry more easily, be irritable, or demonstrate emotional lability. Peak onset is 3 to 5 days after delivery, often when women begin lactating, and duration is days to weeks. Psychiatric history, environmental stress, cultural context, and breastfeeding do not seem to be related.[2,31] Mothers with postpartum blues do not meet *DSM-5* criteria for a mood disorder, and treatment is generally supportive, because symptoms generally lessen and resolve with time.

"Postpartum psychosis" is a rare event with an estimated incidence of 2 in every 1000 deliveries. Often, the onset is within the first 1 to 4 weeks of delivery, with agitation, irritability, mood lability, delusions, and disorganized behavior. Often, it is conceptualized as on a spectrum with perinatal depression, but the preponderance of data suggests that postpartum psychosis is an overt presentation of bipolar disorder.[33] In the *DSM-5*, such a patient may meet criteria for major depression or bipolar disorder (type I or II) with psychotic features or a brief psychotic episode. Again, the "with peripartum onset" specifier is added if onset is within 4 weeks of delivery.[30] Risk factors include personal and family history of bipolar depression and schizoaffective disorder. Hormonal shifts, sleep deprivation, environmental stress, and stopping mood-stabilizing medications are believed to be

TABLE 1 Characteristics of Postpartum Blues, Perinatal Depression, and Postpartum Psychosis

Type	Course	Prevalence	Symptoms
Postpartum blues	Onset in first few wk after labor, peaks at 3–5 d postpartum (with lactation), and usually resolves in <2 wk.	50%–80% of mothers	Crying, weeping Sadness Irritability Exaggerated sense of empathy Anxiety Mood lability ("ups and downs") Feeling overwhelmed Insomnia Fatigue and/or exhaustion Frustration
Perinatal depression		15%–20% of mothers from conception to 1 y postpartum	Persistent sadness, emptiness, hopelessness, frequent crying, irritability Loss of interest in caring for self and/or child, enjoyable activities, and/or poor bonding with infant (attachment) Changes in appetite or wt
Prenatal depression	Onset during pregnancy, peaks in first trimester, then declines. Symptoms last at least 2 wk.	Up to 13% of mothers (incidence: 2%–7%)	Insomnia or hypersomnia Fatigue and/or exhaustion, decreased motivation Poor concentration or indecisiveness; difficulty remembering
Postpartum depression	After delivery, rates increase and peak at 3 mo postpartum. Symptoms present any time in the first y after delivery and last at least 2 wk.	Up to 10% mothers (incidence: about 7%). Up to 4% of fathers (incidence 4%–25%)[32]	Feelings of worthlessness, guilt, inadequacy Suicidal thoughts Possibly anxiety, including bizarre thoughts, obsessions, and/or fears
Postpartum psychosis	Onset 1–4 wk postpartum.	1–2 cases in every 1000 new mothers	Auditory hallucinations and delusions (including commands and/or beliefs that need to harm the infant) Visual hallucinations Agitation, irritability, anger Insomnia Mood lability or highly elevated mood Disorganized thoughts and behaviors High levels of anxiety Paranoia; distrusting of others Confusion Thoughts of harming or killing self, others, or the infant

Adapted from Santoro K, Peabody H. *Identifying and Treating Maternal Depression: Strategies and Considerations for Health Plans. NIHCM Foundation Issue Brief.* Washington DC: National Institutes of Health Care Management; 2010:3.

contributing factors. Postpartum psychosis is an emergency, because there is risk of infanticide and up to a 70-fold increased risk of suicide.[33]

EPIDEMIOLOGY

Various sources estimate up to 15% to 20% of women experience perinatal depression in the United States, with worldwide prevalence almost double in low-income countries.[3,9,34–36] The Centers for Disease Control and Prevention surveyed 29 reporting areas across the United States in the 2009 Pregnancy Risk Assessment Monitoring System (PRAMS) (most recent published data) and found a prevalence of self-reported depressive symptoms ranging from 7.7% in Illinois to 19.9% in Arkansas.[37] The Agency for Healthcare Research and Quality conducted a systematic review as part of its Evidence-Based Practice Program in 2015, reviewing 30 epidemiological studies of perinatal depression (as confirmed by clinical assessment or structured interview). They estimated that at any given time, 12.7% of women meet criteria for an episode of MDD during pregnancy, with an additional 7.1% meeting criteria in the first 3 months postpartum. The rate of newly diagnosed cases or incidence of MDD during pregnancy was 7.5% during pregnancy and 6.5% in the first 3 months postpartum.[35] Authors of a more recent large epidemiological study found comparable results, with period prevalence rates of 12.4% during pregnancy and 9.6% in the postpartum period; incidence rates were 2.2% and 6.8%, respectively.[38] Studies have suggested that even higher rates of postpartum depression may be seen in low-income or ethnically diverse populations, teenagers, individuals with a previous history of perinatal depression, and those with a personal

TABLE 2 Risk Factors for Perinatal Depression

Risk Factors	Additional Risk Factors Specific for Depression After Delivery
History of depression	Depression before or during pregnancy
History of anxiety	Anxiety before or during pregnancy
Preexisting stressor or relationship issues	Experiencing stressful life events during pregnancy or the early postpartum period
Lack of social support	Traumatic birth experience
Unintended, unwanted pregnancy	Preterm birth and/or infant admission to neonatal intensive care
Medicaid insurance or uninsured	Breastfeeding problems
Domestic and/or family violence	
Lower income or socioeconomic status	
Lower education	
Smoking and substance use	
Single status	
Young parents (<30 y of age)	
Having previous children	

As reviewed in Lancaster et al,[49] Robertson et al,[50] and Underwood et al.[42]

or family history of postpartum depression or major depression.[7,36,39]

The prevalence of depression during pregnancy is highest during the second 2 trimesters.[40] Controlling for antenatal medical complications and past maternal psychiatric history, including depression, in late pregnancy has been shown to be associated with obstetric and pediatric complications, including increased need for epidural analgesia, operative deliveries, preterm birth, and neonatal intensive care admissions.[41] In the postpartum period, peak prevalence is at 3 months after delivery (12.9%) and then remains steady through 7 months at 9.9% to 10.6%.[35] A recent study in New Zealand revealed that even at 9 months postpartum, more than 5% of women endorsed significant depressive symptoms.[42] These figures provide further empirical support for the expanded definition of perinatal depression with a time course of up to 1 year postpartum and the expanded time frame of monitoring for symptoms.

The incidence of paternal postpartum depression ranges from 4% to 25% in community samples,[32] and maternal postpartum depression was identified as the strongest predictor, with 24% to 50% incidence in families in which there was also maternal postpartum depression.[23]

New fathers are 1.38 times more likely to be depressed than age-matched males.[43] In at least 2 prevalence studies, 4% of fathers experienced clinical depression in the first year of the child's life.[44,45] In an 18-city study, 18% of fathers of children enrolled in Early Head Start had symptoms of depression, and fathers with depression had higher rates of substance use.[23] In general, men are more likely to avoid emotional expression, deny vulnerability, and not seek help, which may help explain discrepancies in prevalence rates.[46,47]

RISK FACTORS AND COMORBIDITIES

Multiple conditions are believed to increase the risk for perinatal depression (Table 2), although it is often difficult to clearly distinguish confounding factors and comorbidities. It was identified in PRAMS data from 2004 to 2005 that younger, non-Hispanic African American mothers were most likely to report postpartum depression symptoms.[48] The PRAMS data also revealed that women who had lower educational attainment and who received Medicaid benefits for their deliveries were more likely to report depressive symptoms. In all or nearly all of the 17 states participating in PRAMS, depressive symptoms were significantly associated with

5 possible co-occurring issues or comorbidities: use of tobacco during the last 3 months of pregnancy, physical abuse before or during pregnancy, partner-related stress, traumatic stress, and financial stress during pregnancy.[48] In 14 states, maternal depressive symptoms were significantly correlated with delivery of an infant with low birth weight and experiencing emotional stress during pregnancy. NICU admission was associated with maternal depressive symptoms in 9 states.[48]

It is documented that maternal stress, whether attributable to complications of the pregnancy or the mother's psychosocial situation, may contribute to and result from perinatal depression. Perinatal depression is strongly associated with previous miscarriage, past pregnancy complications, chronic medical disease, and shorter gestation and labor.[51] Psychosocial risk factors for perinatal depression include low socioeconomic status, being a single mother, being a teenager, having low self-esteem, prenatal anxiety, substance use, poverty, history of mood disorder, family history or past medical history of depression, having poor social support, and experiencing general life stress.[49,50,52,53] Having an infant with a difficult temperament is also a risk factor for perinatal depression, but a mother's perception of her inability to soothe her infant has a stronger association with postpartum depression than the actual duration of infant crying or fussing.[54]

Unwanted and unplanned pregnancies and relationship stress, including domestic violence and lack of social support, also have strong associations with perinatal depression.[49,55] Perinatal depression may be comorbid with marital discord, divorce, family violence (verbal and/or physical), and substance use and abuse.[56] The directionality of effect and potential reinforcement between these issues and perinatal depression is complex and warrants more study.

The etiology of perinatal depression is likely multifactorial, but there is evidence for a significant genetic basis. Familial trends in MDD are well established: first-degree relatives of someone with MDD have nearly 3 times the risk of developing it than those without such a family history.[57] Among women with a family history of postpartum depression, 42% experienced depression after their first delivery compared with only 15% of women with no such family history.[58]

Depression and anxiety are common comorbidities in the general population, with almost 60% of individuals with a diagnosis of MDD meeting criteria for an anxiety disorder at some point during their lifetime.[59,60] Depression and anxiety are also comorbidities in the perinatal period; in 1 review, anxiety had the strongest correlation with antepartum depression.[49] Biologically, studies have revealed that women with perinatal depression have abnormal stress hormone levels, particularly increased cortisol secretion, which is believed to be an underlying factor in anxiety symptoms.[61] Maternal anxiety is independently related to obstetric and pediatric

complications, which compound the risk for perinatal depression. Anxiety symptoms in pregnancy are associated with preterm birth, low birth weight infants,[62] increased rate of cesarean delivery, reduced duration of breastfeeding, and increased maternal health care use within 2 weeks of delivery.[63] Maternal anxiety has also been connected to altered infant immune system function,[64] altered patterns of infant gastrointestinal microorganism growth,[65] and some limited research suggests that neural structures are modified that may predispose the child for anxiety disorders.[66] In terms of fathers, a correlation has also been documented between fathers who have preterm infants and higher levels of self-reported depression and anxiety symptoms.[67]

EFFECTS AND CONSEQUENCES

Effect on the Parent-Child Dyadic Relationship

In a classic experiment from the 1970s, researchers manipulated interactions between mothers and infants, illustrating that infants not only attempt to spontaneously initiate social exchanges but also modulate affect and attention around the presence and absence of reciprocal response. In the experiment, mothers first engaged in face-to-face reciprocal interactions (eg, when the child smiled, the mother smiled back, etc) in a laboratory with their 2- to 6-month-old infants. Mothers were then instructed to leave the room and reenter sitting opposite the infant with a "still face" (ie, an unresponsive "poker face"). In response, the infants reacted with fussiness, averting their gazes, slumping in their infant seats, and then reattempting to elicit interaction with a smile before finally giving up.[68] In later replications, exposure to the still face produced physiologic

changes in the infants, such as increase in heart rate and decreased vagal tone.[69] When the mother reentered and again responded reciprocally, the infant's behavior and physiologic changes recover. This paradigm has been repeated with fathers and their infants demonstrating identical results,[70] and limited additional research further support the important role of paternal attachment.[71,72] This study ultimately reveals that the emotional life of an infant is heavily influenced by social interactions, particularly with parents, and the loss of parental engagement and reciprocity can be emotionally, behaviorally, and physiologically distressing, even if just temporarily.

"Attachment" describes the emotional connection between a child and parent that is characterized by a desire for closeness to maintain a sense of security, especially during times of stress and separation.[73–75] From a psychoanalytic perspective, the primary dyadic relationship serves as a prototype for all future social interactions.[74] Furthermore, the model is transactional, so rejection from a parent may cause the child to interpret the parent as rejecting as well as the self as unlovable.[76] From an organizational perspective, children progress through a hierarchy of relevant developmental tasks, each building on each other. Early effects of being raised by a parent who is emotionally absent and depressed, if sustained, can carry forward and adversely influence future adaptation.[77] Research suggests that parent-child relationships or attachment likely influences a child's ability to integrate positive representations of parents and of the self.[78] Therefore, high-quality parent-child dyadic interaction facilitates a secure attachment, which is 1 important factor in promoting early life resiliency, emotional regulation, and cognitive development.[79] Adaptations to the still-face experiment described provide some support for this claim, because infants at 6 months of age who were assessed as "securely attached" with their parents recovered faster with more "positive expression" immediately after the still-face exposure.[80]

Supportive behaviors by mothers that have been identified as especially important for cognitive and socioemotional development include following the child's interests and attention, responding contingently, and stimulating the child's engagement with his or her environment through verbal and practical encouragement. Parents who are depressed speak less, are less responsive (eg, smiling), present with flat affect, and express more negative emotions.[81–83] Mothers and fathers who are depressed are less likely to engage in enrichment activities with their child, including reading, singing, and storytelling.[25] Mothers with perinatal depression also demonstrate less reciprocal interaction; distorted perceptions of the infant's behavior, particularly rejection; less positive attribution, leading the child to irritability; less sensitivity and attunement; apathy; and lower rates of breastfeeding.[84,85]

Ultimately, insecure mother-child attachment is associated with social withdrawal from daily activities and less interaction. As early as 2 months of age, infants look at mothers who are depressed less, and infants of mothers with a history of poorly or untreated perinatal depression tend to demonstrate poor behavioral regulation, less explorative play, and lower activity levels. The infants have poor orientation skills and tracking, lower activity level, and irritable temperament. There is an increased risk of feeding and sleeping problems as well as failure to thrive.[81,86,87] Infants of mothers with untreated perinatal depression cry a lot because of difficulty with both self-comforting and being soothed

by others. They may be apathetic, avoidant, clingy, or indifferent, and they tend not to exhibit any maternal preference or anxiety around strangers. Long-term impact of insecure attachment extends to preschool and older children with anxiety, behavior problems, poor peer relationships, school problems, and depression.[88] Such behaviors may even serve to worsen a parent's sense of worthlessness, rejection, and depression.[89]

Effect on the Child

In the prenatal period, maternal stress and depression negatively affect fetal growth and development.[90] Stress hormones, such as cortisol, are chronically elevated in states of generalized anxiety and depression, and they readily pass through the placenta. Animal and human studies reveal that increased maternal cortisol levels have been associated with decreased placental size, increased rates of fetal growth restriction, and premature delivery.[91–93] Norepinephrine, another stress hormone, does not cross the placenta, but it may influence the placental environment through peripheral effects, including increasing uterine arterial resistance and decreasing blood flow and oxygenation, resulting in fetal growth deprivation. Norepinephrine has also been associated with increased risk of preeclampsia.[94] Consequently, in 1 study, it was found that antenatal maternal depression led to a 34% increase in the odds of a developmental delay using the Denver II Developmental Screen in children at 18 months of age. This effect was statistically significant and independent of any postnatal depression.[95]

In the postpartum period, the still-face experiment revealed that social development starts early. In the experiment, infants demonstrated basic abilities to connect facial expression to emotional states,

to have social and emotional awareness of others in their environment, and to adjust affect and attention in response to their parent. It also revealed that the absence of reciprocal interactions can have emotional consequences, including distress and withdrawal. This basic understanding of early emotional states combined with attachment research has given rise to transactional or social relational models of development. These models suggest that a child's emotional regulation, as well as possibly the child's physical, cognitive, and social well-being, depends heavily on close, intimate parent-infant relationships that begin early in life. Through mutually reinforcing and reciprocal interaction patterns, infants develop building blocks for social exchanges and future relationships, including the skill of turn taking, which is the basis for the pragmatics of language development. The theory suggests that as the child grows, his or her network of relationships becomes complex, which may promote more advanced levels of interactions, such as language and coordinated behaviors.[96–98] It would follow that physical, social, and cognitive development are likely inextricably linked, and disruption of early reciprocal relationships may have long-term adverse effects on overall development and health.

This reasoning has been supported by the body of research investigating adverse childhood experiences (ACEs), such as abuse, neglect, and family dysfunction. In a retrospective 1998 study of a large adult population, it was found that ACEs were common, which may point to high levels of resiliency present in childhood.[99] Those with high levels of risk behaviors and disease as adults (eg, obesity, smoking, depression, suicidality) reported being exposed to multiple ACEs as children. Childhood exposure to household mental illness, such as perinatal depression, was 1 of the more common ACEs reported, and it was often associated with other ACEs, such as exposure to parental substance use or domestic violence. The conclusion has been that accumulation of ACEs throughout childhood as well as their presence during particularly sensitive periods, such as early childhood, may have long-lasting effects on development and overall health into adulthood and may even contribute to an intergenerational cycle of recurring ACEs.[99,100]

Since the original ACEs study was conducted in 1998, there has been growing evidence, including prospective studies, directly associating perinatal depression with increased risk for problematic psychological and socioemotional development in children over time.[101–105] The longer a mother continues to experience depression, the more likely the child's developmental issues are to persist with less response to intervention.[106–108] In 1 study of children with internalizing symptoms (anxiety, depression), a history of maternal depression during the child's first 2 years of life was the best predictor of elevation in baseline cortisol levels at 7 years of age.[109] Prolonged cortisol elevation in preschool children predisposes them to anxiety disorders and social withdrawal.[110–112] Children of mothers with perinatal depression have been documented to have lower standardized scores of mental and motor development, poorer self-control, and social adjustment difficulties up to 5 years of age. Children of mothers with depression also had lower IQ with more attentional problems and difficulty with mathematical reasoning up to 11 years of age.[88,112,113]

In addition to primary associations with poor long-term outcomes for the child, untreated perinatal depression is also strongly tied with other unfavorable states and events that may add to the adverse effect on a child's overall health and development, including the following:

- child abuse and neglect;
- failure to implement the injury-prevention components from anticipatory guidance (eg, car safety seat and electrical plug covers)[114,115];
- failure to implement preventive health practices for the child (eg, Back to Sleep)[114,116–119]; and
- difficulty managing chronic health conditions such as asthma or disabilities in the young child.[117,120]

Families with a parent with depression have been reported to overuse health care and emergency facilities because of somatic complaints[120] and often fall behind on well-child visits and immunizations.[121] Perinatal depression also reduces a mother's chances of continued breastfeeding because of decreased satisfaction, more reported complications, and lower self-efficacy.[84]

The adverse effect of accumulating ACEs on child development may be mediated through the development of toxic stress, or the state of excessive, persistent, repetitive, and/or uncontrollable adversity without the buffering of a safe, stable, nurturing, and responsive parent to promote adaptive coping. Over time, toxic stress has consequences on brain architecture and disrupts multiple organ systems through chronic activation of stress hormone responses, cytokines, and immune modulators. The association between toxic stress states in early childhood and impaired language, cognitive and socioemotional development, and even lifelong disease has been independently validated.[122–124]

There is growing evidence that perinatal depression in parents contributes to elevated stress hormone levels in infants, suggesting that it is likely a contributing factor to toxic stress states. In 1 study, children exposed to mothers with postpartum depression had elevated levels of salivary cortisol levels during infancy[125] and at 3 years of age compared with children in a control group.[126] This effect was also revealed with adolescents at 13 years of age after controlling for current maternal or adolescent depression, experience of undesirable life events by the adolescent, maternal partner conflict, and duration of maternal depression.[127] Therefore, not only is the parent with depression impaired in his or her ability to function as a supportive buffer of adversity, but also, there may be a direct long-term activation of the child's stress responses. Persistent elevation of cortisol can disrupt the developing brain's architecture in the areas of the amygdala, hippocampus, and prefrontal cortex, affecting learning, memory, and behavioral and emotional adaptation.[122–124]

Animal studies with rats reveal compelling evidence for a causal relationship between maternal behaviors and stress reactivity in offspring through individual differences in neuronal gene expression transmitted from mother to pup through parenting behaviors in the first week of life. There is natural variation in maternal rat licking and/or grooming and nursing behaviors, so litters were split between mothers varying in levels of such behaviors. Pups exposed to less maternal care not only went on to provide less care to their own future young but also demonstrated increased gene expression in brain regions regulating behavioral and endocrine responses to stress.[128]

The influence of paternal depression on children and families has only recently been explored.[27,72] A large study from the United Kingdom revealed that paternal postpartum depression, when maternal postpartum depression was controlled for, was associated with adverse emotional and behavioral outcomes in children at 3 to 5 years of age, particularly conduct disorder in sons.[44] Fathers with depression negatively interact not only with their partners but also with their child, including being less likely to play with the child outside.[25] Furthermore, it is well documented that a father's affective state mirrors that of the mother, so there may be a compounded adverse effect on the child's social and emotional development.[23,71]

Fortunately, perinatal depression is identifiable and treatable. Early identification via screening increases access to timely care and significantly reduces the potential negative consequences for the child and family. Even brief psychosocial interventions within primary care settings have shown to be efficacious.[129] Recent studies have revealed that supports to increase maternal engagement and responsiveness can reverse gene expression patterns related to stress via epigenetic pathways and, thereby, buffer initial adverse effects of perinatal depression (DNA methylation and neuroendocrine functioning).[130]

PREVENTION

Antenatal Depression

Prevention of perinatal depression is challenging, given the complex biopsychosocial factors that influence the entire perinatal period. Historically, much of the focus has been exclusively on reducing risk factors, comorbidities, and adverse outcomes related to depression in the postpartum period, particularly on childhood development. There is growing evidence that untreated antenatal depression is 1 of the highest risk factors for meeting criteria for postpartum depression.[51,94,131,132]

Early identification and management of depressive symptoms antenatally are needed to optimize the postpartum environment and prevent such symptoms from persisting.[50,131,133] Recommendations by several professional organizations, such as the Centers for Disease Control and Prevention,[48] the National Center for Children in Poverty,[134] the Center on the Developing Child,[123] the AAFP,[4] and the ACOG[3] have included screening women for depression routinely by antenatal providers, such as obstetricians, family physicians, nurse midwives, behavioral health providers, and other primary care clinicians.

Ideally, pediatric providers can collaborate with obstetric antenatal care providers so that maternal risk factors for perinatal depression are accurately communicated through all transitions of care.[133] Establishing this line of communication can be facilitated through a prenatal visit with the pediatric provider.[135] A prenatal visit with the pediatric provider is the first visit recommended in *Bright Futures: Guidelines for Health Supervision of Infants, Children, and Adolescents, Fourth Edition.*[15] An AAP clinical report defines the prenatal visit as important in building a relationship with the mother and father, coordinating services, and providing key anticipatory guidance and prevention education in the context of the upcoming birth.[135] If there are identified risk factors for perinatal depression, this visit allows the pediatric patient-centered medical home (PPCMH) to coordinate resources for the anticipated primary care and mental health needs of the mother and the mother-child dyad. More research is needed to understand and promote dyadic mother-child and parent-child mental health across the entire perinatal continuum.[131] Advocacy is needed to ensure payment to pediatric providers for prenatal visits and services.[135]

Postpartum Depression

A variety of interventions have revealed some success in preventing postpartum depression. Delivery room companions who provide early support with child-mother interaction combined with home visitation programs with nursing interventions, including cognitive behavioral therapy (CBT), have been shown to be successful, particularly for women at risk for depression, minorities, and underserved populations.[136–138] In another study, midwives were trained to provide individualized emotional support to mothers throughout their pregnancy, which led to improved continuity of care between antenatal and postpartum providers and reductions in symptoms of postpartum maternal depression.[139] In addition, prenatal childbirth classes or weekly parenting classes offered postpartum are potentially effective educational environments in which mothers and fathers can be engaged with messages around postpartum parental depression recognition and prevention.[139]

Finally, Practical Resources for Effective Postpartum Parenting (PREPP)[140] is 1 promising brief mother-infant dyadic intervention. PREPP is aimed at promoting the infant's sleep while reducing fussing and/or crying. This is achieved through integrating evidence-based caregiving techniques, traditional psychotherapy approaches, psychoeducation, and mindfulness meditation through a training program for at-risk women. As a result, mothers reported an increased sense of accomplishment, rest, and effectiveness while the incidence and severity of postpartum depression symptoms declined. PREPP revealed strong effects on reducing depression symptoms at 6 weeks, but the effect was not sustained beyond that period.[140] This suggests a role for pediatric providers in providing ongoing parenting education along with evidence-based strategies for coping with stress.

SCREENING

National and State Integrated Screening Systems

Despite the growing empirical evidence and support for screening for perinatal depression that leads to early identification and referrals for effective treatment, implementation of screening by pediatricians has been slowly increasing from 13% in 2001 to 47% in 2013 in periodic surveys.[9,21] In January 2016, the USPSTF completed its most recent review of the evidence for perinatal depression screening, providing a "grade B recommendation" for implementation. The task force found that there is a moderate net benefit to screening for perinatal depression, particularly when treatment such as psychotherapy or counseling can be made readily available.[20,141,142] Moderate net benefit refers to a situation in which the evidence supporting a prevention practice indicates a determined effect on health outcomes, but assessing the magnitude of effect may be limited by issues with the number, size, quality, consistency, and generalizability of available studies. The report specifically stated that there is "… convincing evidence that screening of pregnant and postpartum women in primary care improves the accurate identification of depression" and "… adequate evidence that programs combining depression screening with adequate support systems in place improve clinical outcomes for pregnant and postpartum women."[143]

In May 2016, CMS sent an informational bulletin (https://www.medicaid.gov/federal-policy-guidance/downloads/cib051116.pdf) to all state Medicaid directors stating, "since maternal depression screening is for the direct benefit of the child,

state Medicaid agencies may allow such screening to be claimed as a service for the child as part of the Early and Periodic Screening, Diagnostic, and Treatment benefit." State programs can train providers to screen and refer mothers with positive screens if necessary, and states are eligible for Medicaid administrative matching funds to help with the cost of training.

The Well-Women Task Force is a collaborative initiative hosted by the ACOG. Existing guidelines were reviewed to develop consensus recommendations on the care of adolescent and adult women. This task force asserted that, in addition to providers offering annual screening for depression in adolescent and adult women using a validated tool, additional screening for depression is specifically recommended in the postpartum period.[144] The 2017 *Bright Futures: Guidelines for Health Supervision of Infants, Children, and Adolescents, Fourth Edition* recommendations from the AAP also now include screening for maternal depression by the 1-, 2-, 4-, and 6-month well-child visits.[15]

On the state level, health care providers, academic centers, Medicaid programs, legislatures, and local professional bodies, including AAP chapters, have been working for decades to incorporate maternal perinatal depression screening with standardized tools into prenatal, postpartum, and periodic well-child visits. Ideally, screening would be conducted within a system of care that also provides access to additional mental health evaluation and treatment when concerns are identified. Although such interdisciplinary integration is not always available or feasible, progress has been made. New Jersey and Illinois (2008) were the first to pass legislative requirements for perinatal depression screening, which resulted in increased awareness, conducted assessments, and referrals for

treatment. In 2010, Massachusetts policymakers led the way by creating a statewide Postpartum Depression Commission to advocate for screening and treatment and to monitor implementation. Several other states have since made efforts to provide training and support even without a formal legislative mandate. In addition, a growing number of state Medicaid programs are now paying for perinatal depression screening. For more information on related state laws and policies, contact AAP State Advocacy at stgov@aap.org. Many states have developed quality improvement programs, community support groups, media campaigns, and other resources to improve both provider and public awareness of the need for early identification and treatment of perinatal depression.[145] Ultimately, such state-level efforts have fostered early identification and treatment of affected parents and have increased public awareness of screening protocols and procedures and appropriate referrals for additional family assessment, support, and treatment. The recent AAP recommendations are for universal screening of infant behavior and development[146] and partnering with mental health care providers to implement evidence-based treatments during early childhood.[147] These recommendations are increasingly being adopted by pediatric providers in all states.[15] An important aspect of screening is to also assess for common perinatal depression comorbidities that adversely affect child development, behavior, and the family environment, including substance use, domestic violence, and food insecurity. Standardized screening tools are now, more than ever, being used to assess for such comorbidities.[148]

State perinatal depression screening efforts were also aided when the National Quality Forum developed a quality measure (National Quality Forum Measure 1401) that assesses whether a maternal perinatal depression screen was administered to a patient's mother at 1 face-to-face visit with her provider during the first 6 months of the child's life.[149] This measure was endorsed by the CMS for the Electronic Health Record Incentive Program in March 2013.[150] The quality measure was anticipated to help with the adoption of perinatal depression screening by providers participating in Meaningful Use Incentive programs, although these programs have since been modified.

Role of the Primary Pediatric Clinician and the PPCMH

Perinatal depression is a pertinent issue for the primary care clinician because of the significant risks to the health and well-being of the infant and the family.[2] Pediatric primary care practices, particularly those identifying as PPCMHs, can build a system to implement postpartum depression screening, to connect affected families to supportive community resources, and to refer parents for additional treatment when indicated.[1]

Early identification and appropriate treatment of perinatal depression can result in more favorable outcomes for the expectant and postpartum mother,[143] her infant, and the entire family.[1] As mentioned, prevention and screening for risk factors and comorbidities of perinatal depression start well before birth in the preconception and antenatal periods where obstetric providers, midwives, and family and adult primary care practitioners are optimally positioned. The ACOG has specific recommendations for antenatal screening as well as collaboration between obstetric providers and their pediatric colleagues to facilitate ongoing assessment, treatment, and support for women with perinatal depression and their families.[3] Ideally, this occurs through handoffs that include important information on antenatal screening, risk factors, and comorbidities of perinatal depression, particularly the existence of any intimate partner violence, substance use, or obstetric complications. The prenatal visit, recommended by the 2017 *Bright Futures: Guidelines for Health Supervision of Infants, Children, and Adolescents, Fourth Edition* recommendations from the AAP, is an opportunity for obtaining such information, assessing existing supports, and providing direct education to potential parents about expectations during the first few days of a child's life and the symptoms of perinatal depression.[15,135,151]

In the postpartum period, the USPSTF and CMS recommend screening of parents by pediatric providers caring for infants with a validated tool at the 1-, 2-, 4-, and 6-month well-child visits. This recommendation is supported by the current understanding of when postpartum depression peaks in prevalence. Repeated screenings are important, because mothers who may not be comfortable disclosing initially may do so at later visits as trust and familiarity builds with the pediatric provider. Perinatal depression is also associated with missed appointments, so having multiple screening times also increases the probability that such families are screened and maximizes opportunities for identification of concerns and engagement in ongoing supports and pediatric health surveillance. Pediatric providers can also screen for and promote healthy social-emotional development in the infant using general developmental and specific social-emotional screening tools when risks factors for or maternal symptoms of postpartum depression are present. In the postpartum period, the parents' primary care and mental health providers are important partners that can communicate with and work with pediatric providers to prevent, buffer, and ameliorate the adverse effects of postpartum depression on the family.[81–83,142]

The PPCMH setting provides an interdisciplinary infrastructure to both implement postpartum depression screening and respond to specific concerns. PPCMHs may have embedded services or expertise from multiple disciplines, including care managers, lactation consultants, social workers, and pediatric mental health providers. Collocating or integrating mental health and pediatric primary care services has been shown to help with access to and compliance with mental health services for infants, children, and their parents. Having these services collocated or integrated also facilitates communication across services, particularly using a shared medical record.[152,153]

Over the well-child visit schedule, the pediatric provider, ideally as a part of a PPCMH, develops a longitudinal relationship with the infant and his or her parents starting at an early age. As trust is built in the provider-patient relationship, it provides opportunities to emphasize the importance of both infant and parental mental health.[16] Well-child visits have an important role in assessing social determinants of health and promoting healthy social-emotional development in young children.[15,16,154] In addition, well visits offer opportunities for screening for psychosocial stressors and concerns, including parental depression, as mentioned previously, as well as intimate partner violence, substance use, poverty, food insecurity, and homelessness.[154] These psychosocial issues can have a compounding effect with perinatal depression and can promote an environment of toxic stress.[155] Recognized in the AAP policy statement, "The Future of Pediatrics:

Mental Health Competencies for Pediatric Primary Care,"[16] is the unique advantage of the primary care clinician, particularly in a PPCMH context, for surveillance, screening, and addressing child and parental mental health outcomes through:

- longitudinal, trusting relationship with the family, including the creation of a safe space for discussion of psychosocial issues;

- family centeredness, including attention to the parents' emotional needs;

- unique opportunities for prevention and anticipatory guidance, including communication and discussion with families in a way that fosters early detection and intervention of emerging social-emotional and mental health concerns and problems;

- understanding of common social-emotional and learning issues in the context of development;

- experience in coordinating with and referring to a broad range of relevant specialists and community-based agencies, particularly those that are focused on the care of children with special health care needs and their families; and

- familiarity with chronic care principles and practice improvement.[156]

Several validated and effective screening instruments for perinatal depression have been developed and are readily available (reviewed in detail below).[1,3] However, despite having access to these screening tools, many physicians do not screen for perinatal depression.[8,21] Many barriers to screening for perinatal depression are reported by providers, including the lack of time to screen and competing demands, inadequate knowledge about the validated tools available and how to appropriately document findings, lack of or insufficient

reimbursement to screen and discuss results, and fears associated with legal implications of screening.[7,10] Studies reveal that providers who rely solely on observational cues and do not use validated tools to screen tend to underdiagnose parental depression.[157,158] As a result, many women may erroneously attribute their changes in mood, fatigue, sleep, eating, body weight, and other symptoms of postpartum depression to their pregnancy and do not seek necessary support.[3]

There is some evidence that screening for perinatal depression can also be conducted effectively in emergency department and pediatric inpatient settings for the mother of an infant in the first year of life.[159,160]

Perinatal Depression Screening Tools

Multiple screening tools exist that can efficiently identify patients at risk for perinatal depression, and most are available free online (Table 3). If there is an interest in reproducing any of these tools, it is important to check with the authors and/or developers of the tools to honor any of the copyright requirements and/or requests for permission for use. Before using any screening tool, it is also important to have detailed policies and protocols about how to address identified depressive symptoms, including follow-up or referral to a licensed mental health provider, if necessary. Knowledge of appropriate emergency mental health resources is important. Immediate action is required at any time during the administration of a screening tool if a parent expresses any concern about the infant's safety or if the parent reports being (or pediatric provider suspects the parent is) suicidal, homicidal, severely depressed, manic, or psychotic.[161] Appropriate documentation of perinatal depression screenings includes the screen used, results, discussion with the parent including

anticipatory guidance, and the plan for follow-up and/or referrals.[6]

The EPDS[163] is a free, widely-used 10-question instrument that is used specifically to screen for perinatal depression. The EPDS was originally developed for screening postpartum women in outpatient, home-visiting settings or at the 6- to 8-week postpartum examination. The tool has been validated with numerous populations and is available in Spanish[164] and for fathers.[165–167] Of note, it includes reverse-scored items that can be used to assess reliability of responses. The most recent 2016 recommendations of the USPSTF clearly conclude that there is sufficient evidence to support the use of the EPDS as an effective screening tool for depression in pregnant and postpartum women.[20] The Survey of Well-being of Young Children (SWYC) (www.theSWYC.org) is a validated developmental and psychosocial screening tool that now includes the EPDS in the 2-, 4-, and 6-month questionnaires (available in English, Spanish, Burmese, Nepali, and Portuguese).[168] The EPDS has some benefit in identifying anxiety disorders as well but is not focused on somatic symptoms or parent-infant relationships.

A total score of 10 or more on the EPDS is a positive screen indicating a concern for depression, which necessitates further discussion in which providers can clarify the findings, determine acuity of concerns, and, if necessary, make appropriate referrals for further assessment and treatment of the parent (as described below).[129,163] It is important to note that similar to all screening tools, the EPDS is not a diagnostic instrument. In situations in which there is any indication of suicidal ideation (on the EPDS question 10 or in discussion), if the parent expresses concern about his or her ability to maintain the infant's safety, or if the pediatric provider suspects that the parent is suicidal or

TABLE 3 Valid Screening Tools for Perinatal Depression

Screening Tool	No. Items	Sensitivity and Specificity[a,b]	Available for Free
EPDS	10	Mothers (score >9–12) Sensitivity 80%–90% Specificity 80%–90% Fathers (score >10) Sensitivity 90% Specificity 78%	Yes[c]
PDSS	35	Sensitivity 80%–90% Specificity 80%–90%	No http://www.wpspublish.com/store/p/2902/postpartum- depression-screening- scale-pdss
PHQ-2	2	Sensitivity 100% Specificity 44.3%–65.7%	Yes[c]
PHQ-9	9	Sensitivity 75%–89% Specificity 83%–91%	Yes[c]
Beck Depression Inventory—II	21	Sensitivity 75%–90% Specificity 80%–90%	No http://www.pearsonclinical.com/psychology/products/ 100000159/beck-depression-inventoryii-bdi-ii.html

All of the above screening tools take <10 min to complete, on average, and are available in Spanish.
[a] Validity specifically for postpartum depression as reviewed in Myers et al.[162]
[b] For EDPS only; as reviewed in Siu et al.[21]
[c] Indicated free screening tools are available on the AAP Web site: https://www.aap.org/en-us/advocacy-and-policy/aap-health-initiatives/Screening/Pages/Screening-Tools.aspx; https://brightfutures.aap.org/materials-and-tools/tool-and-resource-kit/Pages/Developmental-Behavioral-Psychosocial-Screening-and-Assessment-Forms.aspx.

homicidal, it is considered a positive screen that warrants an immediate evaluation for safety of the parent and/or infant, often in an emergency psychiatric setting. Immediate action with a referral to an emergency psychiatric setting has also been recommended with scores greater than 20 or if there is clinical concern that the parent may be severely depressed, manic, or psychotic.[163]

The accuracy of the EPDS as a screening tool in pregnant and postpartum women has been established by a recent USPSTF review of 23 studies (*n* = 5298) comparing the accuracy of the EPDS with a diagnostic interview. Sensitivity of the EPDS using a cutoff of 13 ranged from 0.67 (95% confidence interval [CI], 0.18–0.96) to 0.8 (95% CI, 0.81–1.00) for the detection of MDD. Specificity for detecting MDD was consistently 0.87 or higher.[20,141,143] Two studies in this review were conducted in the United States (1 specifically among African American women) demonstrating an average sensitivity of approximately 0.80. The positive predictive value for detecting MDD would be 47% to 64% in a population with a 10% prevalence of MDD.[143,169,170] The

Agency for Healthcare Research and Quality also reviewed validity statistics for various screening tools among postpartum women specifically and found that the EPDS had a sensitivity of 80% to 90% and specificity of 80% to 90%.[162] Higher cutoff scores for EPDS have been proposed (up to a threshold of 13) to limit false-positive results.[171] Recently, shorter versions of the EPDS have been validated, including a 2-question screen for adolescent mothers.[172]

The EPDS has demonstrated cross-cultural sensitivity,[163] including the Spanish version, which showed acceptable performance characteristics.[143] The EPDS is also available in French, Dutch, Swedish, Spanish, Chinese, Thai, Turkish, and Arabic. Cutoff scores may vary in different populations.[173]

One screen that has been used over the last decade in some primary care settings is the Patient Health Questionnaire-2 (PHQ-2).[174,175] The PHQ-2 is a simple, free general depression screening tool (ie, not limited to use in the postpartum period or with women) with 2 questions about depressed mood and anhedonia that are derived from

the longer 9-question Patient Health Questionnaire-9 (PHQ-9) (discussed in the following paragraph). The PHQ-2 does not include a question about suicidality. The PHQ-2 has been studied in both primary care and obstetric populations.[176] The 2 questions in the PHQ-2 are:

1. Over the past 2 weeks, have you ever felt down, depressed, or hopeless?

2. Over the past 2 weeks, have you felt little interest or pleasure in doing things?

A person is asked to choose 1 of 4 possible choices for each question that comes closest to how he or she has been feeling: not at all (0), several days (1), more than half the days (2), or nearly every day (3). A score of 3 out of a maximum of 6 is the accepted cutoff for a positive screen, with a sensitivity of 83% and a specificity of 92% for MDD.[176] Studies in postpartum populations, specifically, reveal that the sensitivity of the PHQ-2 is 100% and the specificity is 44.3% to 65.7%.[162]

The most recent USPSTF review[143] concluded that no studies of screening in pregnant or postpartum women conducted with the PHQ-2 met methodologic inclusion criteria. As a result, the USPSTF currently has determined that there is not sufficient evidence to support the use of the PHQ-2 at this time as a primary screening tool in pregnant and postpartum women.[20] Yet many practices continue to use it as an initial screen. If a parent screens positive with the PHQ-2, then the recommendation is that it be followed up with a more comprehensive screening tool (eg, PHQ-9, discussed in the following paragraph, or the EPDS).[174,175]

The longer 9-question PHQ-9 has been used as a primary screening instrument for perinatal depression and to monitor for worsening or improvement of perinatal depression symptoms over time.[177] The PHQ-9 has also been widely used to screen nonpregnant adults[178] and adolescents for depression.[179] The diagnostic validity of the PHQ-9 has been established in both primary care and obstetrical clinics,[179,180] although the USPSTF concluded that the data were insufficient for specific use in postpartum depression screening. In addition to the questions from the PHQ-2, the PHQ-9 also asks how often over the past 2 weeks the person has been bothered by different problems related to sleep, lack of energy, feeling bad or letting someone down (feeling like a failure), appetite, concentration, speaking slowly, or being restless. Similar to the PHQ-2, the respondent is asked to choose 1 of 4 responses for symptoms corresponding to how often they are experienced, ranging from not at all to nearly every day. The PHQ-9 specifically asks about suicidal thoughts and how any of the identified symptoms affect the respondent's ability to function at work, at home, or in interacting with other people. Scores of 5, 10, 15, and 20 on the PHQ-9 represent mild, moderate, moderately severe, and severe depression, respectively. PHQ-9 scores ≥10 had a sensitivity

of 88% and specificity of 88% for MDD[180] and among postpartum women had a specificity of 75% to 89% and specificity of 83% to 91%.[162] However, the most recent USPSTF review[143] concluded that no studies of screening in pregnant or postpartum women conducted using the PHQ-9 met methodologic inclusion criteria. Although the USPSTF currently has determined that there is not sufficient evidence to support the use of the PHQ-9 specifically in pregnant and postpartum women,[20] it still continues to be used widely.

Other screens are available with a cost and may be used by adult and mental health providers during the pregnancy or postpartum period and much less often by pediatric primary care clinicians. However, some adult and pediatric providers may choose to use these in partnership with mental health providers who are collocated, integrated, or linked with an obstetric, family medicine, or pediatric practice. The Beck Depression Inventory (BDI-II)[181] is a 21-question scale that is a self-report tool used to provide more feedback on severity of depressive symptoms. This tool is currently endorsed by the USPSTF[141] as an effective screening tool for postpartum depression and also continues to be endorsed by the USPSTF for use in screening all adolescents between 12 and 18 years of age for depression.[182] Two additional tools are the Hamilton Depression Rating Scale (HAM-D)[183] and the Postpartum Depression Screening Scale (PDSS). The Hamilton Depression Rating Scale uses an interview format and is mostly used in research settings. The PDSS is a 35-question screen that identifies patients at high risk for depression but is less commonly used.[184] Among postpartum women, the PDSS has a sensitivity and specificity of 80% to 90%.[162] It should be noted that these screening tools include constitutional symptoms such as insomnia, changes

in appetite, low energy, etc, which may be normative in pregnancy, so their specificity is lower for perinatal depression.[3]

A drawback to these currently less commonly used questionnaires is that they tend to yield higher estimates than clinician-administered interviews, so clinical assessment is recommended but often not conducted. Also, studies differ in their methods in terms of cutoff scores, reporting of cutoff scores, and use of scores as continuous measures in analysis.[61] Just as with the EPDS, these other questionnaires are only screening tools, and they do not diagnose MDD or perinatal depression. Diagnosis requires a face-to-face clinical assessment and, in some circumstances, referral for clinical correlation by an appropriately licensed health care professional.[129]

Infant Assessment

Routine well-child visits allow for pediatric providers to assess and promote healthy early child development, including assessing overall family strengths and supports and the child's social-emotional adjustment.[15,142,146] Identified developmental concerns and delays in an infant may be the only indication of perinatal depression, difficulty with early adjustment as a new family, as well as many other factors. When developmental delays are present in the child, they often increase the stress and decrease the perceived efficacy experienced by the mother.[185] Therefore, several screening tools (some are free online) can be used to assess the child's social-emotional development, family supports, and early family adjustments. These tools can be used whenever there are developmental concerns or delays, particularly if the mother presents with other risk factors identified or has been previously diagnosed with perinatal depression. These tools include the

Ages and Stages Questionnaire Social Emotional-2,[186] the Early Childhood Screening Assessment,[187] the SWYC,[148,168] and the Baby Pediatric Symptom Checklist, which is included in the SWYC,[188,189] among others. Guidance on these and other similar screening tools is available in a policy statement and technical report about early childhood emotional and behavioral problems.[147]

DIAGNOSIS AND TREATMENT

As discussed, screening tools alone are inadequate for diagnosing perinatal depression, but when they indicate concerns, the pediatric provider's role is to discuss results and facilitate referral for appropriate supports and treatment. Some PPCMHs may have mental health, social work, lactation support, and other such services collocated or even integrated directly into a visit, which decreases stigma and improves access.[153,190] In the context of discussing screening results, an opportunity exists to validate parents' experiences and inquire about existing supports available to them and their family in times of transient acute stress. These supports may include extended family, friends, and even therapists or counselors who are providing mental health treatment. It is also a time when careful attention can be given to assessing for any risk of suicide or harm to the infant as well as the presence of other psychosocial stressors or comorbidities in addition to depression.

As was previously discussed, rates of intimate partner violence and substance use are elevated in families in which a parent has perinatal depression symptoms. If there is specific concern for domestic or intimate partner violence or substance use, especially in the perinatal period, then state agencies may require notification. Many national and community agencies are available to support families as well. Information about local organizations available to support victims of intimate partner violence can be accessed through the National Domestic Violence Hotline at http://www.thehotline.org or 1-800-799-SAFE.

A positive screen leads to a discussion with the parent about the specific mental health concerns and symptoms identified in the screening tool and/or during a patient encounter.[142] There is literature showing that, in addition to pediatric providers, such a discussion can be conducted by the parent's primary care provider, obstetric provider, or a licensed mental health provider with perinatal expertise.[129] There may be times when the screening is positive, without suicidal ideation or risk of harm to the infant, and the mother is not interested in a referral for further evaluation and diagnosis. It is important for the pediatric provider and/or other members of the PPCMH to inquire about existing supports and clarify the psychosocial concerns and comorbidities, such as domestic violence and substance use, that may affect the welfare of the infant and to follow-up to monitor the abatement of risk.

When a screen is positive in "low-risk" situations, without suicidal ideation or risk of harm to the infant, a pediatric provider may consider recommending the mother to follow-up with her obstetric or primary care provider for additional discussion and also closely monitoring the infant and mother with a visit or telephone call before the next scheduled well-child visit. The pediatric provider may also recommend adjustments in schedule to provide adequate sleep, additional supports from community agencies such as quality child care, home visiting, mother's morning out programs, or other programs. There are additional office-based interventions that a pediatric provider can implement that will be discussed below.[1] In discussion with the parent and family, it may be determined that referrals to mental health and specialty providers are necessary for diagnostic evaluation, psychotherapy, or even consideration of psychiatric medication management.[142]

In "high-risk" situations in which there are concerns for suicidal ideation, risk of harm to the infant, or severe mental illness, there may be urgent or emergent need for referral to an emergency psychiatric setting for evaluation and treatment.

Regardless of the level of risk or modality of treatment, it is important to explain to parents the assessed need for follow-up or referral, specifically if further evaluation and treatment is necessary by a parent's primary care provider or a mental health specialist. If perinatal depression is ultimately diagnosed, then reassurance can be offered that pediatric providers can work with such adult providers and community organizations to support the parent and his or her ability to best care for the child. Consideration of risk factors, parent's previous psychiatric history, and former treatments, if known by the pediatric provider at the time of referral, is important to communicate through the transition in care to develop an accurate risk profile.[3,191]

Access to Treatment

Although progress is being made in identifying and effectively treating perinatal depression, the cumulative shortfalls in mothers receiving effective treatment are still large. In a recent study, only 49% of women with antenatal depression and 30.8% of women with postpartum depression were screened and identified in practice. In addition, 13.6% of women with antenatal depression and 15.8% of women with postpartum depression received any treatment, and only

8.6% of women with antenatal depression and 6.3% of women with postpartum depression received adequate treatment. Ultimately, 4.8% of women with antenatal depression and 3.2% of women with postpartum depression achieved remission.[192]

Despite the consequences of untreated perinatal depression and the presence of a range of options for effective, evidence-based treatment, most mothers with perinatal depression do not seek therapy and treatment for themselves and their infants.[11,193] Mothers may not seek therapy because of concern about perceptions of others (ie, stigma), cost and a lack of insurance coverage, need for child care during the mental health visit, lack of access to a trained provider and lack of knowledge about perinatal depression, unrealistic beliefs about coping with being a mother, feelings of failure, and fears about using mental health services.[11] These challenges are compounded by the symptoms of depression, especially low energy and motivation, which adversely affect a mother's ability to access help.

Fortunately, data suggest that when providers speak to patients about their depression, they are more likely to become engaged and seek treatment. Use of provider notification systems and motivational interviewing techniques can assist providers in engaging their patients in discussions about their depression.[194] A study from the University of Michigan found that a single motivational interviewing session can increase rates of treatment adherence, particularly through the process of identifying and challenging practical and psychological barriers to care.[195]

In many pediatric clinics and PPCMHs, care coordinators have a significant role in developing and maintaining a referral network of community resources and specialty providers for perinatal depression. They can often follow through to ensure patients are able to access necessary specialty providers in a timely manner.[16,196] An integrated frontline mental health provider, such as a licensed clinical social worker or counselor, can provide immediate triage for a positive screen, conduct additional assessments, offer support, and coordinate follow-up and referrals for the infant, mother, and family. Regardless of whether a clinic has a care coordinator or integrated mental health provider, many sources emphasize the importance of close working relationships and communication between pediatric providers and mental health providers, adult primary care providers, and other agencies in the community with expertise in the evaluation, treatment, and/or support of the mother with perinatal depression and the mother-infant dyad.[1,3]

Emergency and/or Urgent Situations

Many screening tools have critical thresholds above which they recommend that the pediatric provider take immediate action, which usually means referring the parent to an emergency psychiatric setting to ensure safety with timely evaluation and treatment. If question 10 inquiring about suicidality on the EPDS is positive,[161,163] if question 9 inquiring about suicidality on the PHQ-9 is positive, if the parent expresses concern about maintaining the infant's safety during any screening, or if the pediatric provider is concerned at any time with screening that the parent is suicidal, homicidal, severely depressed, manic, or psychotic, immediate evaluation is warranted in an emergency psychiatric setting (ie, calling 911) or by a crisis team that can respond directly to the provider (if available in the community).[161] Although the ultimate goal is to support the mother so she can best care for her child, in a situation in which the mother requires immediate evaluation, it is important that someone is available to specifically maintain care for the infant. An ideal process is that the mother is not left alone at any time, and if sent to an emergency psychiatric setting, the mother is accompanied by a trusted adult or staff member.

If the provider's level of concern is elevated but an emergency intervention is deemed not necessary, precautions are taken to promote safety, including having the mother leave with a support person (not alone), ensuring adequate supervision of the mother and infant at home, composing a specific safety plan (including phone numbers and steps for accessing help urgently), and scheduling close follow-up. Pediatric providers can be prepared by having a current list of contacts for pediatric and adult emergency mental health providers on hand. Fortunately, most positive perinatal depression screens do not necessitate urgent or emergency action by the pediatric provider.[197] Intervention for the mother ranges from support, to therapy, to therapy plus medication, to emergency mental health services and hospitalization.[198,199]

Infant and/or Dyadic Interventions

In promoting evidence-based mental health treatments for infants and their mothers with perinatal depression, most approaches caution against implying any blame or carrying an exclusive focus on challenges faced by the mother. Strengths-based approaches that are focused on the infant-mother dyad are promoted on the basis of some evidence of efficacy in generally addressing attachment issues and developmental concerns in other settings.[147,200,201] Most of these dyadic interventions are focused on infant-mother attachment, but limited evidence is now suggesting the importance of supporting attachment with fathers and nontraditional families.[202] For example, there are specific evidence-based dyadic interventions that have been used with high-risk families, often in the setting of interpersonal violence or abuse, such as Child Parent Dyadic Psychotherapy[203] and Attachment and Biobehavioral Catch-up.[204] Circle of Security[205] has been specifically validated for use specifically with mothers with perinatal depression and their infants.[147,201] Videotaped interactions of mothers and their infants with feedback and coaching has shown efficacy.[94]

Dyadic psychotherapy is an evolving field. These interventions may not be readily available in all areas and require mental health providers to obtain specialized training. Pediatric providers can play an important role in advocating for increased availability of such services, specialized training, and availability of a specialized workforce with experience working with young children, parents, and families.

Office-Based Supportive Management by Pediatric Providers

Pediatric providers can have an important role in partnering with parents, families, and various other involved providers to manage and support parents with perinatal depression. However, considering the demands placed on pediatric providers in most settings, it is essential to evaluate what is feasible and effective for any given practice and in the context of each individual family. It is important that the pediatric provider consider collaborating closely with the mother's adult providers, mental health care providers, and various local agencies to provide optimal support for the mother-child dyad within the entire family structure.

When time and resources allow, pediatric providers can offer parents in low-risk situations office-based interventions. Components of most office-based interventions include:

- explanation and open dialogue with the mother and family to help reduce stigma, normalize the stress faced by new families, and ultimately, foster early identification of those who may need additional resources ("demystification");

- communication about the potential impact on the infant and need for infant screenings and surveillance;

- initial and ongoing support, which includes providing validation and empathy for the mother's experiences and identifying community resources to promote family wellness; and

- reinforcement, when necessary, through referrals to evidence-based treatment programs. Referrals may take the form of a mental health provider for the parent or lactation support for the mother, as will be discussed later.

Demystification is directed at removing the mystery about maternal and paternal depression—that postpartum depression can affect any parent, that it is not the parents' fault, and that it does not imply "bad" parenting. Depression is treatable, and the support facilitated by the pediatric provider for appropriate intervention is an essential ingredient.[1] Having an infant and expanding the family is a transition that can be difficult when there are other stressors involved. However, many parents also experience resiliency factors, such as stable housing, adequate family and/or friend supports, and access to care, which may help attenuate the risk of perinatal depression.

The AAP Task Force on Mental Health promoted the use of a common factors approach to routine mental health assessment[206] to engage families and build an alliance.[16] *Bright Futures: Guidelines for Health Supervision of Infants, Children, and Adolescents, Fourth Edition* provides health promotion themes, including family support, child development, and mental health. Specifically, it includes surveillance for parental socioemotional well-being and for social determinants of health.[15] The common factors theory asserts that therapies can be designed for broad classes of people rather than specific individuals who are deemed "at-risk" or fit a specific diagnostic category.[206] The common factors theory emphasizes that providers can influence behavioral change in patients and families through specific evidence-based interaction approaches, such as motivational interviewing, integrated into routine visits. A mnemonic for a group of common factors that can be routinely assessed and monitored throughout the scheduled well-child visits is "HELLPPP," which stands for hope, empathy, language, loyalty, permission, partnership, and plan.[206] In the absence of an urgent psychiatric crisis, pediatric providers can build alliance and common understanding over time that will foster greater disclosure and recognition of mental health needs and social-emotional concerns. For example, pediatric providers may recognize the need for anticipatory guidance and education on parenting and lifestyle issues (eg, sleep, exercise, diet, rest) that ultimately could mitigate the risk of depression and promote the mental health of parents and children. More details are available on the AAP Mental Health Initiatives site, with a resource in the AAP Mental Health Toolkit at https://www.aap.org/en-us/advocacy-and-policy/aap-health-initiatives/Mental-Health/Pages/Primary-Care-Tools.aspx.

Following is an example of how a brief intervention can be designed by using the common factors approach within the context of a PPCMH to provide support to a parent when there are concerns for perinatal depression:

- Hope: increase the parent's hopefulness by describing realistic expectations and reinforcing the value and strengths of the mother-infant relationship and understanding and responding to the infant's cues;

- Empathy: communicate empathy by listening attentively;

- Language: use the parent's language to reflect your understanding of the concerns for perinatal depression;

- Loyalty: communicate loyalty to the parent by expressing your support and commitment to help;

- Permission: ask for permission to share information;

- Partnership: partner to work together to address common concerns; and

- Plan:
  o encourage infant and parent routines for predictability and security;
  o encourage focus on wellness: sleep, diet, exercise, stress relief;
  o Ask about concerns regarding breastfeeding, and support and/ or encourage if the mother is able to breastfeed. It is important to address specific worries and try to reassure the mother when she is doing well with the breastfeeding and her infant is adequately gaining weight;
  o encourage social connections and supports;
  o depending on the degree of concern from the perinatal depression screening, refer the parent and infant dyad to mental health providers who use evidence-based treatments, and follow-up closely; and
  o make referrals to a variety of agencies and efforts in your local community as available and described below.[206]

Other brief interventions that could take place when there are concerns for postpartum depression could include:

- encourage understanding and response to the infant's cues; emphasize the importance of observing nonverbal behavior;

- encourage routines for predictability and security;

- encourage focus on wellness (sleep, diet, exercise, stress relief);

- acknowledge personal experiences;

- promote realistic expectations and prioritizing important things; and

- encourage social involvement and bolster social networks and supports.

Partnering With Community Agencies

Mental health providers are an important resource, but many community agencies can also provide essential support, such as home-based services or partial hospitalization programs that specialize in addressing stressors of the postpartum period. Part C of the Individuals with Disabilities in Education Act (IDEA) governs how states and community organizations and programs provide services to infants and children from birth to 3 years of age with disabilities or developmental delays, with or without an established condition. This legislation supports early intervention programs that provide family-centered services to help children from birth to age 3 develop skills necessary to promote health and positive development in early life. Early intervention programs can provide education and assessment targeting the infant-parent dyad, often by modeling positive interactions and play.[1,207] However, in many areas, early intervention referrals can be difficult to facilitate because of limitations in state-specific eligibility requirements (emphasizing cognitive, motor, and language delays but not social-emotional delays) and insufficient funding. Inadequate funding may also limit the ability of such services to provide adequate and uniform interventions addressing social-emotional developmental delays for infants and the mother-infant dyad across sites.[207] These challenges to accessing early intervention are concerning given the inextricable connection of social-emotional development to physical health, language acquisition, and cognitive development.

Early Head Start, Head Start, home-visiting programs, and postpartum support groups are additional examples of community resources that are available in many areas. There are opportunities in various regions for public health nurses, lactation specialists, parent educators, and facilitators of family support groups (see http://www.motherwoman.org or www.postpartum.net) to form partnerships with pediatric providers aimed at reducing perinatal depression.

In Massachusetts, the legislature has funded an adjunct to the Massachusetts Child Psychiatry Access Project (MCPAP) called MCPAP for Moms. This statewide project improves access through providing immediate consultation and referral services to pediatric providers and other providers when a positive perinatal depression screen is identified in the community. Furthermore, MCPAP for Moms has created a toolkit for pediatric providers that is available free of charge (www.mcpapformoms.org). The Substance Abuse and Mental Health Services Administration also has a similar toolkit that describes how community service agencies can approach perinatal depression, specifically through forming

Psychotherapy and Psychological Interventions

Several validated individual psychological treatments are offered by mental health professionals to help mothers with perinatal depression.[199] Psychotherapy is often preferred by women over medication during the perinatal period because of perceived adverse effects of medication on pregnancy and with breastfeeding.[209] Many women identified with mild to moderate postpartum depression are optimally treated with psychotherapy and do not require medication.[198]

The USPSTF[143] evaluated the efficacy of psychological treatment with trials in postpartum women, revealing a 28% to 59% reduction in symptoms of depression at follow-up compared with usual care. All 10 trials of a CBT intervention showed an increased likelihood of remission from depressive symptoms with short-term treatment (7–8 months). At the 1-year follow-up, there was a 35% increase in remission rates with CBT compared with usual care (pooled relative risk, 1.34; 95% CI, 1.19–1.50).[20] There is little risk of adverse effects from psychotherapy. In women with antenatal depression, CBT-based interventions have also been shown to be effective in preventing depression recurrence during the perinatal period.[136] The USPSTF has recommended that clinicians consider CBT or other evidence-based counseling, such as interpersonal psychotherapy, when managing depression in pregnant or breastfeeding women.[141,199]

Different methods of delivering interpersonal psychotherapy and CBT are being developed and preliminarily show reduction in depression prevalence. These methods include postpartum telephone-based and telecare sessions using CBT, relaxation techniques, and problem-solving strategies,[210] Internet-based CBT,[211,212] and home-based CBT.[213] A recent Cochrane review evaluated computer or Internet-based interventions to address perinatal depressive symptoms and suggested promising trends, but such interventions are largely still in development.[212] Small studies of additional alternative treatment options, including yoga, massage, light therapy, acupuncture, and omega-3 fatty acids in fish oil, show some limited efficacy, but more research is needed.[4,214] There are no formal recommendations for these treatments at this time.

Psychotropic Medications*

Pharmacologic treatment of depression is often indicated during pregnancy and/or lactation. Review and discussion of the risk of untreated versus treated depression is advised. Consideration of each patient's previous disease and treatment history, along with the risk profile for individual pharmacologic agents, is important when selecting pharmacologic therapy with the greatest likelihood of treatment success. Psychotropic medications, particularly antidepressants such as selective serotonin reuptake inhibitors (SSRIs), may have a role in the management of postpartum depression depending on the presenting symptoms and needs of individual parents. Most often, psychotropic medications are managed through referrals to adult

---

* This section on pharmacological management of perinatal depression is being included to provide context to the pediatric provider; it is not to imply that pediatric providers would or should be instituting psychiatric care for adult parents. It is acknowledged that even when referred to appropriate mental health specialists, parents will often still return to pediatric providers caring for their children with questions or concerns. This section is not meant to be an exhaustive resource, but rather it is used to provide a basic overview of core understandings around perinatal psychopharmacology that may be relevant.

---

primary care, psychiatric, or other qualified mental health professionals. However, pediatric providers can still play a role in dispelling myths, providing education, and responding to specific concerns about medications that a parent may have, particularly as they relate to the health and welfare of the infant. A detailed discussion comparing psychotherapy and psychopharmacology is outside the scope of this article, but a Cochrane review of a few studies consisting of mothers with postpartum depression showed that there is no difference between the effectiveness of antidepressants and psychological or psychosocial treatments.[215]

Despite the availability of effective medications, many mothers prefer not to use psychotropic medications in the perinatal period because of the fear of adverse effects.[216] Discussions about the risks and benefits of using or withholding medications are important for parents to have with their own adult health care providers so they can make informed decisions regarding the role of antidepressant medications used antenatally or in the postpartum period, especially while breastfeeding. Studies about the long-term effects on the infant of maternal antidepressant medication use, such as SSRIs, during pregnancy are mixed, because it is difficult to control for many other cooccurring factors that may influence birth outcomes, including maternal illness or problematic health behaviors.[216] In 1 study, mothers made a list of potential risks and benefits of treatment with medication in the context of their therapeutic goals for a healthy pregnancy and postpartum period. An exercise like this should be conducted in partnership with appropriate providers, including the parent's prescriber, who can provide accurate information.[4,198] The pediatric provider can also play an important role in reinforcing and sharing accurate information about various treatment options.

Untreated and severe perinatal depression poses significant risk for morbidity and occasionally mortality for the mother and fetus during pregnancy. Studies have demonstrated that the risks associated with untreated depression are far more detrimental (including suicide) than the unclearly associated risks of growth effects, neurobehavioral outcomes, preterm birth, low birth weight, structural malformations, and respiratory distress, which vary among studies.[198,217–219] Yet, many mothers choose to stop taking psychotropic medications during pregnancy, although they report significant symptoms of depression, placing them at high risk for the sequela of perinatal depression.[209] In mothers who are suicidal, homicidal, manic, or psychotic, there is often an urgent need for medication in the context of an emergency or inpatient psychiatric setting.[198]

The AAFP,[4] ACOG,[3] Academy of Breastfeeding Medicine (ABM),[191] and American Psychiatric Association[198] endorse the appropriate use of antidepressant medications during the perinatal period. The ABM recommends consideration of each patient's previous disease and treatment history, along with the risk profiles for individual treatments when choosing the treatment with the greatest likelihood of treatment effect.[191] The ABM states that in the "setting of moderate to severe depression, the benefits of [psychotropic medication] treatment likely outweigh the risks of the medication to the mother or infant."[191] Therefore, antidepressant medications can be an important option to consider for parents with perinatal depression symptoms, particularly if their symptoms are not responsive to therapy or they

have previous positive response to medications.

Detailed guidance in regard to specific medications is outside the scope of this article, but SSRIs have become the mainstay of treatment of moderate to severe major perinatal depression because of their favorable profiles of adverse reactions.

Parents often express concerns to and have questions for pediatric providers regarding the use of antidepressant medication while breastfeeding. There is increasing evidence to support the safe use of these medications during lactation. The ABM has developed a clinical protocol on the use of antidepressants in breastfeeding mothers but stipulates, "[There is] no widely accepted algorithm for antidepressant medication treatment of depression in lactating women."[191] In the context of breastfeeding, it has again been asserted that the benefit of effectively treating perinatal depression far outweighs the risks to the infant through breastfeeding.[220,221] Clinical studies in breastfeeding patients who are using sertraline, fluvoxamine, and paroxetine suggest that the transfer of these medications into human milk is low and that there is even lower uptake by the infant. No or minimal adverse effects on infants have been reported after the use of these 3 medications in lactating mothers themselves.[216,220,221] Sertraline was preferred over the other 2 drugs, because many studies have shown that human milk and infant plasma have low to undetectable concentrations of this drug.[216]

Many parents may experience combined or sequential treatment with psychotherapy, such as CBT, and antidepressant medication management. This may implicate multiple providers, which emphasizes the importance of collateral communication. Evidence suggests that combined treatment may lead to even further benefit[198]

and may be preferred for some women with high risk of relapse and co-occurring conditions, such as anxiety disorders.[199] More studies are needed to evaluate the relative efficacy of different psychotherapeutic approaches as well as other psychological and psychosocial treatments, with and without medication.[199]

CODING AND BILLING

Given the 2016 recommendations by the USPSTF and CMS, providers are encouraged to bill for perinatal depression screening at 1-, 2-, 4- and 6-month well-child visits. However, coding may vary by state or payer. The AAP Web site, state AAP chapters, and specific payers can be consulted with any questions. A new *Current Procedural Terminology* code, 96161, for the administration of a mother-focused health risk assessment for the benefit of the patient was approved by the American Medical Association in 2016. Providers can consider the opportunity to bill for time-based counseling and coordination of care with a separate evaluation and management code with a 25 modifier when there are significant concerns for maternal depression.

CONCLUSIONS

There is strong evidence that parental, particularly maternal, depression during pregnancy and the first year after childbirth (perinatal depression) has profound negative consequences on the well-being of women and infants, including family dysfunction, disruption of critical infant brain development, cessation of breastfeeding, and increased health care use, and may place the child at increased risk for future anxiety and depression. A growing body of research shows that fathers are also at increased risk of perinatal depression, which can magnify the adverse effects on an infant's social-emotional development.[23,45,167] Perinatal depression is the most prevalent ACE and can lead to toxic stress and present challenges to essential early attachments between children and their parents.[100]

With a core responsibility to promote the well-being of children and the benefit of longitudinal relationships with families, pediatric providers have a critical role in screening and supporting parents and their infants with concerns for perinatal depression. This responsibility includes supporting parents at risk for or with a diagnosis of perinatal depression and communicating and working with adult obstetric, primary care, and/or mental health providers. If indicated, referrals to community agencies or specialty providers may be necessary for support, diagnostic evaluation, or treatment.

Over the past decade, multiple professional health care and regulatory bodies have recommended routine perinatal depression screening. Most recently, both the USPSTF and CMS have reviewed the evidence and have recommended screening consistent with those asserted by the AAP's *Bright Futures: Guidelines for Health Supervision of Infants, Children, and Adolescents, Fourth Edition*. These recommendations have encouraged, even mandated, many commercial insurers to pay for screening. Medicaid programs are now encouraged to cover and pay for screening for perinatal depression. The recommendation for maternal depression screening is once during pregnancy and then during the infant's well visits at 1, 2, 4, and 6 months of age.[15,20] However, despite the efforts of many state and local AAP and AAFP chapters and other advocacy groups, perinatal depression screening remains far from universal in clinical practice or payment.[140] As more providers are screening and identifying psychosocial risk factors in diverse clinical settings, more emphasis needs to be put on improving collaboration and transitions of care throughout the perinatal period. Finally, there are many models around the country of creative and effective interventions to promote early identification and treatment of perinatal depression. Best practices and evidence-based treatments for parents and the parent-infant dyad need to be identified, advocated for, and brought to scale to allow access to care to promote the best outcomes for women and their infants.

LEAD AUTHORS

Jason Rafferty, MD, MPH, EdM, FAAP
Gerri Mattson, MD, MPH, FAAP
Marian Earls, MD, FAAP
Michael W. Yogman, MD, FAAP

COMMITTEE ON PSYCHOSOCIAL ASPECTS OF CHILD AND FAMILY HEALTH, 2016–2017

Michael W. Yogman, MD, FAAP, Chairperson
Thresia B. Gambon, MD, FAAP
Arthur Lavin, MD, FAAP
Gerri Mattson, MD, FAAP
Jason Richard Rafferty, MD, MPH, EdM
Lawrence Sagin Wissow, MD, MPH, FAAP

LIAISONS

Sharon Berry, PhD, LP – *Society of Pediatric Psychology*
Terry Carmichael, MSW – *National Association of Social Workers*
Edward R. Christophersen, PhD, FAAP – *Society of Pediatric Psychology*
Norah L. Johnson, PhD, RN, CPNP-BC – *National Association of Pediatric Nurse Practitioners*
Leonard Read Sulik, MD, FAAP – *American Academy of Child and Adolescent Psychiatry*

STAFF

Stephanie Domain, MS

ABBREVIATIONS

AAFP: American Academy of Family Physicians
AAP: American Academy of Pediatrics
ABM: Academy of Breastfeeding Medicine
ACE: adverse childhood experience
ACOG: American College of Obstetricians and Gynecologists
CBT: cognitive behavioral therapy
CI: confidence interval
CMS: Centers for Medicare and Medicaid Services

DSM-5: *Diagnostic and Statistical Manual of Mental Disorders, Fifth Edition*
EPDS: Edinburgh Postnatal Depression Scale
MCPAP: Massachusetts Child Psychiatry Access Project
MDD: major depressive disorder
PDSS: Postpartum Depression Screening Scale
PHQ-2: Patient Health Questionnaire-2
PHQ-9: Patient Health Questionnaire-9

PPCMH: pediatric patient-centered medical home
PRAMS: Pregnancy Risk Assessment Monitoring System
PREPP: Practical Resources for Effective Postpartum Parenting
SSRI: selective serotonin reuptake inhibitor
SWYC: Survey of Well-being of Young Children
USPSTF: US Preventive Services Task Force

All technical reports from the American Academy of Pediatrics automatically expire 5 years after publication unless reaffirmed, revised, or retired at or before that time.

DOI: https://doi.org/10.1542/peds.2018-3260

Address correspondence to Jason Rafferty, MD, MPH, EdM, FAAP. Email: Jason_Rafferty@mail.harvard.edu

PEDIATRICS (ISSN Numbers: Print, 0031-4005; Online, 1098-4275).

FINANCIAL DISCLOSURE: The authors have indicated they have no financial relationships relevant to this article to disclose.

FUNDING: No external funding.

POTENTIAL CONFLICT OF INTEREST: The authors have indicated they have no potential conflicts of interest to disclose.

REFERENCES

1. Earls MF; Committee on Psychosocial Aspects of Child and Family Health American Academy of Pediatrics. Incorporating recognition and management of perinatal and postpartum depression into pediatric practice. *Pediatrics.* 2010;126(5):1032–1039

2. Santoro K, Peabody H. *Identifying and Treating Maternal Depression: Strategies & Considerations for Health Plans. NIHCM Foundation Issue Brief.* Washington, DC: National Institutes of Health Care Management; 2010

3. Committee on Obstetric Practice. The American College of Obstetricians and Gynecologists Committee opinion no. 630. Screening for perinatal depression. *Obstet Gynecol.* 2015;125(5):1268–1271

4. Hirst KP, Moutier CY. Postpartum major depression. *Am Fam Physician.* 2010;82(8):926–933

5. Declerq ER, Sakala C, Corry MP, Applebaum S, Risher P. *Listening to Mothers: Report of the First National U.S. Survey of Women's Childbearing Experiences.* New York, NY: Maternity Center Association; 2002

6. Chaudron LH, Szilagyi PG, Tang W, et al. Accuracy of depression screening tools for identifying postpartum depression among urban mothers. *Pediatrics.* 2010;125(3). Available at: www.pediatrics.org/cgi/content/full/125/3/e609

7. Gjerdingen DK, Yawn BP. Postpartum depression screening: importance, methods, barriers, and recommendations for practice. *J Am Board Fam Med.* 2007;20(3):280–288

8. Leiferman JA, Dauber SE, Heisler K, Paulson JF. Primary care physicians' beliefs and practices toward maternal depression. *J Womens Health (Larchmt).* 2008;17(7):1143–1150

9. Kerker BD, Storfer-Isser A, Stein RE, et al. Identifying maternal depression in pediatric primary care: changes over a decade. *J Dev Behav Pediatr.* 2016;37(2):113–120

10. Nutting PA, Rost K, Dickinson M, et al. Barriers to initiating depression treatment in primary care practice. *J Gen Intern Med.* 2002;17(2):103–111

11. Bilszta J, Ericksen J, Buist A, Milgrom J. Women's experiences of postnatal depression – beliefs and attitudes as barriers to care. *Aust J Adv Nurs.* 2010;27(3):44–54

12. US Department of Health and Human Services. *Mental Health: A Report of the Surgeon General.* Washington, DC: US Public Health Service; 1999

13. US Public Health Service. *Report of the Surgeon General's Conference on Children's Mental Health: A National Action Agenda.* Washington, DC: US Department of Health and Human Services; 2000

14. Stewart DE, Vigod S. Postpartum depression. *N Engl J Med.* 2016;375(22):2177–2186

15. Hagan JF, Shaw JS, Duncan PM, eds. *Bright Futures: Guidelines for Health Supervision of Infants, Children, and Adolescents.* 4th ed. Elk Grove Village, IL: American Academy of Pediatrics; 2017

16. Committee on Psychosocial Aspects of Child and Family Health and Task Force on Mental Health. Policy statement—the future of pediatrics: mental health competencies for pediatric primary care. *Pediatrics.* 2009;124(1):410–421

17. Institute of Medicine. *Depression in Parents, Parenting, and Children. Opportunities to Improve Identification, Treatment, and Prevention.* Washington, DC: National Academies Press; 2009

18. Medical Home Initiatives for Children With Special Needs Project Advisory Committee; American Academy of Pediatrics. The medical home. *Pediatrics.* 2002;110(1 pt 1):184–186

19. Office of Disease Prevention and Health Promotion. *Healthy People 2020. ODPHP Publication No. B0132.* Washington, DC: US Department of Health and Human Services, Office of Disease Prevention and Health Promotion; 2010

20. O'Connor E, Rossom RC, Henninger M, Groom HC, Burda BU. Primary care screening for and treatment of depression in pregnant and postpartum women: evidence report and systematic review for the US Preventive Services Task Force. *JAMA.* 2016;315(4):388–406

21. Siu AL, Bibbins-Domingo K, Grossman DC, et al; US Preventive Services Task Force (USPSTF). Screening for depression in adults: US Preventive Services Task Force recommendation statement. *JAMA.* 2016;315(4):380–387

22. Wachino V; Center for Medicaid and CHIP Services. *Maternal Depression Screening: A Critical Role for Medicaid in the Care of Mothers and Children.* Baltimore, MD: Department of Health and Human Services; 2016. Available at: https://www.medicaid.gov/federal-policy-guidance/downloads/cib051116.pdf. Accessed February 5, 2018

23. Goodman JH. Paternal postpartum depression, its relationship to maternal postpartum depression, and

implications for family health. *J Adv Nurs.* 2004;45(1):26–35

24. Yogman M, Garfield CF; Committee on Psychosocial Aspects of Child and Family Health. Fathers' roles in the care and development of their children: the role of pediatricians. *Pediatrics.* 2016;138(1):e20161128

25. Paulson JF, Dauber S, Leiferman JA. Individual and combined effects of postpartum depression in mothers and fathers on parenting behavior. *Pediatrics.* 2006;118(2):659–668

26. Cochran SV. Assessing and treating depression in men. In: Brooks GR, Good GE, eds. *The New Handbook of Psychotherapy and Counseling With Men.* Vol 1. San Francisco, CA: Jossey-Bass; 2001:3–21

27. Edward KL, Castle D, Mills C, Davis L, Casey J. An integrative review of paternal depression. *Am J Men Health.* 2015;9(1):26–34

28. Earls M, Yogman M, Mattson G, Rafferty J; American Academy of Pediatrics, Committee on Psychosocial Aspects of Child and Family Health. Incorporating recognition and management of perinatal and postpartum depression into pediatric practice. *Pediatrics.* 2018;143(1):e20183259

29. Uher R, Payne JL, Pavlova B, Perlis RH. Major depressive disorder in DSM-5: implications for clinical practice and research of changes from DSM-IV. *Depress Anxiety.* 2014;31(6):459–471

30. American Psychiatric Association. *Diagnostic and Statistical Manual of Mental Disorders (DSM-5).* 5th ed. Washington, DC: American Psychiatric Publishing; 2013

31. Miller LJ. Postpartum depression. *JAMA.* 2002;287(6):762–765

32. Stadtlander L. Paternal postpartum depression. *Int J Childbirth Educ.* 2015;30(2):11–13

33. Sit D, Rothschild AJ, Wisner KL. A review of postpartum psychosis. *J Womens Health (Larchmt).* 2006;15(4):352–368

34. O'Hara MW. Postpartum depression: what we know. *J Clin Psychol.* 2009;65(12):1258–1269

35. Gavin NI, Gaynes BN, Lohr KN, Meltzer-Brody S, Gartlehner G, Swinson T. Perinatal depression: a systematic review of prevalence and incidence. *Obstet Gynecol.* 2005;106(5 pt 1):1071–1083

36. Hearn G, Iliff A, Jones I, et al. Postnatal depression in the community. *Br J Gen Pract.* 1998;48(428):1064–1066

37. Robbins CL, Zapata LB, Farr SL, et al; Centers for Disease Control and Prevention (CDC). Core state preconception health indicators - pregnancy risk assessment monitoring system and behavioral risk factor surveillance system, 2009. *MMWR Surveill Summ.* 2014;63(3):1–62

38. Banti S, Mauri M, Oppo A, et al. From the third month of pregnancy to 1 year postpartum. Prevalence, incidence, recurrence, and new onset of depression. Results from the perinatal depression-research & screening unit study. *Compr Psychiatry.* 2011;52(4):343–351

39. Evins GG, Theofrastous JP, Galvin SL. Postpartum depression: a comparison of screening and routine clinical evaluation. *Am J Obstet Gynecol.* 2000;182(5):1080–1082

40. Bennett HA, Einarson A, Taddio A, Koren G, Einarson TR. Prevalence of depression during pregnancy: systematic review. *Obstet Gynecol.* 2004;103(4):698–709

41. Chung TK, Lau TK, Yip AS, Chiu HF, Lee DT. Antepartum depressive symptomatology is associated with adverse obstetric and neonatal outcomes. *Psychosom Med.* 2001;63(5):830–834

42. Underwood L, Waldie K, D'Souza S, Peterson ER, Morton S. A review of longitudinal studies on antenatal and postnatal depression. *Arch Women Ment Health.* 2016;19(5):711–720

43. Giallo R, D'Esposito F, Christensen D, et al. Father mental health during the early parenting period: results of an Australian population based longitudinal study. *Soc Psychiatry Psychiatr Epidemiol.* 2012;47(12):1907–1966

44. Ramchandani P, Stein A, Evans J, O'Connor TG; ALSPAC Study Team. Paternal depression in the postnatal period and child development: a prospective population study. *Lancet.* 2005;365(9478):2201–2205

45. Escribà-Agüir V, Artazcoz L. Gender differences in postpartum depression: a longitudinal cohort study. *J Epidemiol Community Health.* 2011;65(4):320–326

46. Mansfield AK, Addis ME, Mahalik JR. "Why won't he go to the doctor?": the psychology of men's help seeking. *Int J Mens Health.* 2003;2(2):93–109

47. Rochlen AB. Men in (and out of) therapy: central concepts, emerging directions, and remaining challenges. *J Clin Psychol.* 2005;61(6):627–631

48. Centers for Disease Control and Prevention (CDC). Prevalence of self-reported postpartum depressive symptoms—17 states, 2004-2005. *MMWR Morb Mortal Wkly Rep.* 2008;57(14):361–366

49. Lancaster CA, Gold KJ, Flynn HA, Yoo H, Marcus SM, Davis MM. Risk factors for depressive symptoms during pregnancy: a systematic review. *Am J Obstet Gynecol.* 2010;202(1):5–14

50. Robertson E, Grace S, Wallington T, Stewart DE. Antenatal risk factors for postpartum depression: a synthesis of recent literature. *Gen Hosp Psychiatry.* 2004;26(4):289–295

51. Larsson C, Sydsjö G, Josefsson A. Health, sociodemographic data, and pregnancy outcome in women with antepartum depressive symptoms. *Obstet Gynecol.* 2004;104(3):459–466

52. Woods SM, Melville JL, Guo Y, Fan MY, Gavin A. Psychosocial stress during pregnancy. *Am J Obstet Gynecol.* 2010;202(1):61.e1–61.e7

53. Underwood L, Waldie KE, D'Souza S, Peterson ER, Morton SM. A longitudinal study of pre-pregnancy and pregnancy risk factors associated with antenatal and postnatal symptoms of depression: evidence from growing up in New Zealand. *Matern Child Health J.* 2017;21(4):915–931

54. Radesky JS, Zuckerman B, Silverstein M, et al. Inconsolable infant crying and maternal postpartum depressive symptoms. *Pediatrics.* 2013;131(6). Available at: www.pediatrics.org/cgi/content/full/131/6/e1857

55. Lee AM, Lam SK, Sze Mun Lau SM, Chong CS, Chui HW, Fong DY.

Prevalence, course, and risk factors for antenatal anxiety and depression. *Obstet Gynecol.* 2007;110(5):1102–1112

56. Kahn RS, Wise PH, Wilson K. Maternal smoking, drinking and depression: a generational link between socioeconomic status and child behavior problems [abstract]. *Pediatr Res.* 2002;51(pt 2):191A

57. Sullivan PF, Neale MC, Kendler KS. Genetic epidemiology of major depression: review and meta-analysis. *Am J Psychiatry.* 2000;157(10):1552–1562

58. Forty L, Jones L, Macgregor S, et al. Familiality of postpartum depression in unipolar disorder: results of a family study. *Am J Psychiatry.* 2006;163(9):1549–1553

59. Kessler RC, Berglund P, Demler O, et al; National Comorbidity Survey Replication. The epidemiology of major depressive disorder: results from the National Comorbidity Survey Replication (NCS-R). *JAMA.* 2003;289(23):3095–3105

60. Ross LE, McLean LM. Anxiety disorders during pregnancy and the postpartum period: a systematic review. *J Clin Psychiatry.* 2006;67(8):1285–1298

61. Brummelte S, Galea LA. Depression during pregnancy and postpartum: contribution of stress and ovarian hormones. *Prog Neuropsychopharmacol Biol Psychiatry.* 2010;34(5):766–776

62. Ding XX, Wu YL, Xu SJ, et al. Maternal anxiety during pregnancy and adverse birth outcomes: a systematic review and meta-analysis of prospective cohort studies. *J Affect Disord.* 2014;159:103–110

63. Paul IM, Downs DS, Schaefer EW, Beiler JS, Weisman CS. Postpartum anxiety and maternal-infant health outcomes. *Pediatrics.* 2013;131(4). Available at: www.pediatrics.org/cgi/content/full/131/4/e1218

64. O'Connor TG, Winter MA, Hunn J, et al. Prenatal maternal anxiety predicts reduced adaptive immunity in infants. *Brain Behav Immun.* 2013;32:21–28

65. Zijlmans MA, Korpela K, Riksen-Walraven JM, de Vos WM, de Weerth C. Maternal prenatal stress is associated with the infant intestinal microbiota. *Psychoneuroendocrinology.* 2015;53:233–245

66. Rifkin-Graboi A, Meaney MJ, Chen H, et al. Antenatal maternal anxiety predicts variations in neural structures implicated in anxiety disorders in newborns. *J Am Acad Child Adolesc Psychiatry.* 2015;54(4):313–321.e2

67. Pace CC, Spittle AJ, Molesworth CM, et al. Evolution of depression and anxiety symptoms in parents of very preterm infants during the newborn period. *JAMA Pediatr.* 2016;170(9):863–870

68. Tronick E, Als H, Adamson L, Wise S, Brazelton TB. The infant's response to entrapment between contradictory messages in face-to-face interaction. *J Am Acad Child Psychiatry.* 1978;17(1):1–13

69. Tronick EZ. Emotions and emotional communication in infants. *Am Psychol.* 1989;44(2):112–119

70. Braungart-Rieker J, Garwood MM, Powers BP, Notaro PC. Infant affect and affect regulation during the still-face paradigm with mothers and fathers: the role of infant characteristics and parental sensitivity. *Dev Psychol.* 1998;34(6):1428–1437

71. Fuertes M, Faria A, Beeghly M, Lopes-dos-Santos P. The effects of parental sensitivity and involvement in caregiving on mother-infant and father-infant attachment in a Portuguese sample. *J Fam Psychol.* 2016;30(1):147–156

72. Lucassen N, Tharner A, Prinzie P, et al. Paternal history of depression or anxiety disorder and infant-father attachment. *Infant Child Dev.* 2017;27(2):e2070

73. Bowlby J. Attachment and loss. In: *Attachment.* Vol 1. 2nd ed. New York, NY: Basic Books; 1969/1982

74. Ainsworth MS, Bowlby J. An ethological approach to personality development. *Am Psychol.* 1991;46(4):333–341

75. Bretherton I. The origins of attachment theory: John Bowlby and Mary Ainsworth. *Dev Psychol.* 1992;28(5):759–775

76. Bretherton I. Open communication and internal working models: their role in the development of attachment relationships.*Nebr Symp Motiv.* 1988;36:57–113

77. Toth SL, Rogosch FA, Sturge-Apple M, Cicchetti D. Maternal depression, children's attachment security, and representational development: an organizational perspective. *Child Dev.* 2009;80(1):192–208

78. Steele M, Steele H, Johansson M. Maternal predictors of children's social cognition: an attachment perspective. *J Child Psychol Psychiatry.* 2002;43(7):861–872

79. Letourneau NM. Fostering resiliency in infants and young children through parent-infant interaction. *Infants Young Child.* 1997;9(3):36–45

80. Cohn JF, Campbell SB, Ross S. Infant response in the still-face paradigm at 6 months predicts avoidant and secure attachments at 12 months. *Dev Psychopathol.* 1991;3(4):367–376

81. Righetti-Veltema M, Conne-Perréard E, Bousquet A, Manzano J. Postpartum depression and mother-infant relationship at 3 months old. *J Affect Disord.* 2002;70(3):291–306

82. Korja R, Savonlahti E, Ahlqvist-Björkroth S, et al; PIPARI Study Group. Maternal depression is associated with mother-infant interaction in preterm infants. *Acta Paediatr.* 2008;97(6):724–730

83. Flykt M, Kanninen K, Sinkkonen J, Punamaki RL. Maternal depression and dyadic interaction: the role of maternal attachment style. *Infant Child Dev.* 2010;19:530–550

84. Dennis CL, McQueen K. Does maternal postpartum depressive symptomatology influence infant feeding outcomes? *Acta Paediatr.* 2007;96(4):590–594

85. Agency for Healthcare Research and Quality. *Breastfeeding and Maternal and Infant Health Outcomes in Developed Countries. Evidence Report 153.* Rockville, MD: Agency for Healthcare Research and Quality; 2007:130–131

86. Zero to Three. *Diagnostic Classification of Mental Health and Developmental Disorders of Infancy and Early Childhood (DC: 0-3R).* Washington, DC: Zero to Three; 2005

87. Murray L, Cooper PJ. The impact of postpartum depression on child

development. *Int Rev Psychiatry.* 1996;8(1):55–63

88. Beardslee WR, Versage EM, Gladstone TR. Children of affectively ill parents: a review of the past 10 years. *J Am Acad Child Adolesc Psychiatry.* 1998;37(11):1134–1141

89. Weinberg MK, Tronick EZ. Infant affective reactions to the resumption of maternal interaction after the still-face. *Child Dev.* 1996;67(3):905–914

90. Londono Tobon A, Diaz Stransky A, Ross DA, Stevens HE. Effects of maternal prenatal stress: mechanisms, implications, and novel therapeutic interventions. *Biol Psychiatry.* 2016;80(11):e85–e87

91. Rondó PH, Ferreira RF, Nogueira F, Ribeiro MC, Lobert H, Artes R. Maternal psychological stress and distress as predictors of low birth weight, prematurity and intrauterine growth retardation. *Eur J Clin Nutr.* 2003;57(2):266–272

92. French NP, Hagan R, Evans SF, Godfrey M, Newnham JP. Repeated antenatal corticosteroids: size at birth and subsequent development. *Am J Obstet Gynecol.* 1999;180(1 pt 1):114–121

93. Reinisch JM, Simon NG, Karow WG, Gandelman R. Prenatal exposure to prednisone in humans and animals retards intrauterine growth. *Science.* 1978;202(4366):436–438

94. Field T, Diego M, Hernandez-Reif M. Prenatal depression effects on the fetus and newborn: a review. *Infant Behav Dev.* 2006;29(3):445–455

95. Deave T, Heron J, Evans J, Emond A. The impact of maternal depression in pregnancy on early child development. *BJOG.* 2008;115(8):1043–1051

96. Evangelou M. *Early Years Learning and Development: Literature Review.* Washington, DC: Department for Children, Schools and Families; 2009

97. Sameroff AJ, MacKenzie MJ. A quarter-century of the transactional model: how have things changed? *Zero to Three.* 2003;24(1):14–22

98. Sameroff AJ. Transactional models in early social relations. *Hum Dev.* 1975;18(1–2):65–79

99. Felitti VJ, Anda RF, Nordenberg D, et al. Relationship of childhood abuse and household dysfunction to many of the leading causes of death in adults. The Adverse Childhood Experiences (ACE) study. *Am J Prev Med.* 1998;14(4):245–258

100. McDonnell CG, Valentino K. Intergenerational effects of childhood trauma: evaluating pathways among maternal ACEs, perinatal depressive symptoms, and infant outcomes. *Child Maltreat.* 2016;21(4):317–326

101. Verbeek T, Bockting CL, van Pampus MG, et al. Postpartum depression predicts offspring mental health problems in adolescence independently of parental lifetime psychopathology. *J Affect Disord.* 2012;136(3):948–954

102. Avan B, Richter LM, Ramchandani PG, Norris SA, Stein A. Maternal postnatal depression and children's growth and behaviour during the early years of life: exploring the interaction between physical and mental health. *Arch Dis Child.* 2010;95(9):690–695

103. Murray L, Halligan SL, Cooper PJ. Effects of postnatal depression on mother-infant interactions, and child development. In: Bremner G, Wachs T, eds. *The Wiley-Blackwell Handbook of Infant Development.* London, United Kingdom: John Wiley; 2010:192–220

104. Essex MJ, Klein MH, Miech R, Smider NA. Timing of initial exposure to maternal major depression and children's mental health symptoms in kindergarten. *Br J Psychiatry.* 2001;179:151–156

105. Lahti M, Savolainen K, Tuovinen S, et al. Maternal depressive symptoms during and after pregnancy and psychiatric problems in children. *J Am Acad Child Adolesc Psychiatry.* 2017;56(1):30–39. e7

106. Brennan PA, Hammen C, Andersen MJ, Bor W, Najman JM, Williams GM. Chronicity, severity, and timing of maternal depressive symptoms: relationships with child outcomes at age 5. *Dev Psychol.* 2000;36(6):759–766

107. Campbell SB, Cohn JF, Meyers T. Depression in first-time mothers: mother-infant interaction and depression chronicity. *Dev Psychol.* 1995;31(3):349–357

108. Teti DM, Gelfand DM, Messinger DS, Isabella R. Maternal depression and the quality of early attachment: an examination of infants, preschoolers, and their mothers. *Dev Psychol.* 1995;31(3):364–376

109. Ashman SB, Dawson G, Panagiotides H, Yamada E, Wilkinson CW. Stress hormone levels of children of depressed mothers. *Dev Psychopathol.* 2002;14(2):333–349

110. Smider NA, Essex MJ, Kalin NH, et al. Salivary cortisol as a predictor of socioemotional adjustment during kindergarten: a prospective study. *Child Dev.* 2002;73(1):75–92

111. Essex MJ, Klein MH, Cho E, Kalin NH. Maternal stress beginning in infancy may sensitize children to later stress exposure: effects on cortisol and behavior. *Biol Psychiatry.* 2002;52(8):776–784

112. Kersten-Alvarez LE, Hosman CM, Riksen-Walraven JM, van Doesum KT, Smeekens S, Hoefnagels C. Early school outcomes for children of postpartum depressed mothers: comparison with a community sample. *Child Psychiatry Hum Dev.* 2012;43(2):201–218

113. Milgrom J, Westley DT, Gemmill AW. The mediating role of maternal responsiveness in some longer term effects of postnatal depression on infant development. *Infant Behav Dev.* 2004;27(4):443–454

114. McLennan JD, Kotelchuck M. Parental prevention practices for young children in the context of maternal depression. *Pediatrics.* 2000;105(5):1090–1095

115. Moore T, Kotelchuck M. Predictors of urban fathers' involvement in their child's health care. *Pediatrics.* 2004;113(3 pt 1):574–580

116. Santona A, Tagini A, Sarracino D, et al. Maternal depression and attachment: the evaluation of mother-child interactions during feeding practice. *Front Psychol.* 2015;6:1235

117. Chung EK, McCollum KF, Elo IT, Lee HJ, Culhane JF. Maternal depressive symptoms and infant health practices among low-income women. *Pediatrics.* 2004;113(6). Available at: www.pediatrics.org/cgi/content/full/113/6/e523

118. Kavanaugh M, Halterman JS, Montes G, Epstein M, Hightower AD, Weitzman M. Maternal depressive symptoms are adversely associated with prevention practices and parenting behaviors for preschool children. *Ambul Pediatr.* 2006;6(1):32–37

119. Paulson JF, Bazemore SD. Prenatal and postpartum depression in fathers and its association with maternal depression: a meta-analysis. *JAMA.* 2010;303(19):1961–1969

120. Sills MR, Shetterly S, Xu S, Magid D, Kempe A. Association between parental depression and children's health care use. *Pediatrics.* 2007;119(4). Available at: www.pediatrics.org/cgi/content/full/119/4/e829

121. Field T. Postpartum depression effects on early interactions, parenting, and safety practices: a review. *Infant Behav Dev.* 2010;33(1):1–6

122. Shonkoff JP, Boyce WT, Cameron J, et al. *Excessive Stress Disrupts the Architecture of the Developing Brain. Working Paper No. 3.* Cambridge, MA: Centre on the Developing Child, Harvard University; 2009. Available at: http://developingchild.harvard.edu. Accessed February 5, 2018

123. Shonkoff JP, Duncan GJ, Yoshikawa H, Guyer B, Magnuson K, Philips D. *Maternal Depression Can Undermine the Development of Young Children. Working Paper No. 8.* Cambridge, MA: Centre on the Developing Child, Harvard University; 2009. Available at: http://developingchild.harvard.edu. Accessed February 5, 2018

124. Garner AS, Shonkoff JP; Committee on Psychosocial Aspects of Child and Family Health; Committee on Early Childhood, Adoption, and Dependent Care; Section on Developmental and Behavioral Pediatrics. Early childhood adversity, toxic stress, and the role of the pediatrician: translating developmental science into lifelong health. *Pediatrics.* 2012;129(1). Available at: www.pediatrics.org/cgi/content/full/129/1/e224

125. Brennan PA, Pargas R, Walker EF, Green P, Newport DJ, Stowe Z. Maternal depression and infant cortisol: influences of timing, comorbidity and treatment. *J Child Psychol Psychiatry.* 2008;49(10):1099–1107

126. Hessl D, Dawson G, Frey K, et al. A longitudinal study of children of depressed mothers: psychobiological findings related to stress. In: Hann DM, Huffman LC, Lederhendler KK, Minecke D, eds. *Advancing Research on Developmental Plasticity: Integrating the Behavioral Sciences and the Neurosciences of Mental Health.* Bethesda, MD: National Institutes of Mental Health; 1998:256

127. Halligan SL, Herbert J, Goodyer IM, Murray L. Exposure to postnatal depression predicts elevated cortisol in adolescent offspring. *Biol Psychiatry.* 2004;55(4):376–381

128. Francis D, Diorio J, Liu D, Meaney MJ. Nongenomic transmission across generations of maternal behavior and stress responses in the rat. *Science.* 1999;286(5442):1155–1158

129. Olin SC, Kerker B, Stein RE, et al. Can postpartum depression be managed in pediatric primary care? *J Womens Health (Larchmt).* 2016;25(4):381–390

130. Conradt E, Hawes K, Guerin D, et al. The contributions of maternal sensitivity and maternal depressive symptoms to epigenetic processes and neuroendocrine functioning. *Child Dev.* 2016;87(1):73–85

131. Bonari L, Pinto N, Ahn E, Einarson A, Steiner M, Koren G. Perinatal risks of untreated depression during pregnancy. *Can J Psychiatry.* 2004;49(11):726–735

132. Waters CS, Hay DF, Simmonds JR, van Goozen SH. Antenatal depression and children's developmental outcomes: potential mechanisms and treatment options. *Eur Child Adolesc Psychiatry.* 2014;23(10):957–971

133. Stowe ZN, Hostetter AL, Newport DJ. The onset of postpartum depression: implications for clinical screening in obstetrical and primary care. *Am J Obstet Gynecol.* 2005;192(2):522–526

134. Knitzer J, Theberge S, Johnson K. *Reducing maternal depression and its impact on young children: toward a responsive early childhood policy framework. Project Thrive Issue Brief, 2.* New York, NY: National Center for Children in Poverty; 2008

135. Yogman M, Lavin A, Cohen G; Committee on Psychosocial Aspects of Child and Family Health. The prenatal visit. *Pediatrics.* 2018;142(1):e20181218

136. Ogrodniczuk JS, Piper WE. Preventing postnatal depression: a review of research findings. *Harv Rev Psychiatry.* 2003;11(6):291–307

137. Stuart-Parrigon K, Stuart S. Perinatal depression: an update and overview. *Curr Psychiatry Rep.* 2014;16(9):468

138. Sockol LE. A systematic review of the efficacy of cognitive behavioral therapy for treating and preventing perinatal depression. *J Affect Disord.* 2015;177:7–21

139. Zauderer C. Postpartum depression: how childbirth educators can help break the silence. *J Perinat Educ.* 2009;18(2):23–31

140. Werner EA, Gustafsson HC, Lee S, et al. PREPP: postpartum depression prevention through the mother-infant dyad. *Arch Women Ment Health.* 2016;19(2):229–242

141. O'Connor E, Rossom RC, Henninger M. *Screening for Depression in Adults: An Updated Systematic Evidence Review for the US Preventive Services Task Force: Evidence Synthesis No. 128. AHRQ Publication No. 14-05208-EF-1.* Rockville, MD: Agency for Healthcare Research and Quality; 2016

142. Olin SS, McCord M, Stein REK, et al. Beyond screening: a stepped care pathway for managing postpartum depression in pediatric settings. *J Womens Health (Larchmt).* 2017;26(9):966–975

143. Yogman MW. Postpartum depression screening by pediatricians: time to close the gap. *J Dev Behav Pediatr.* 2016;37(2):157–157

144. Conry JA, Brown H. Well-woman task force: components of the well-woman visit. *Obset Gynecol.* 2015;126(4):697–701

145. Rhodes AM, Segre LS. Perinatal depression: a review of US legislation and law. *Arch Women Ment Health.* 2013;16(4):259–270

146. Weitzman C, Wegner L; Section on Developmental and Behavioral Pediatrics; Committee on Psychosocial Aspects of Child and Family Health; Council on Early Childhood; Society for Developmental and Behavioral Pediatrics; American Academy

of Pediatrics. Promoting optimal development: screening for behavioral and emotional problems [published correction appears in *Pediatrics*. 2015;135(5):946]. *Pediatrics*. 2015;135(2):384–395

147. Gleason MM, Goldson E, Yogman MW; Council on Early Childhood; Committee on Psychosocial Aspects of Child and Family Health; Section on Developmental and Behavioral Pediatrics. Addressing early childhood emotional and behavioral problems. *Pediatrics*. 2016;138(6): e20163025

148. Sheldrick RC, Perrin EC. Evidence-based milestones for surveillance of cognitive, language, and motor development. *Acad Pediatr*. 2013;13(6):577–586

149. National Quality Forum. *Perinatal and Reproductive Health Endorsement Maintenance: Technical Report*. Washington, DC: National Quality Forum; 2012:1–92. Available at: www. qualityforum.org/Publications/2012/ 06/Perinatal_and_Reproductive_ Health_Endorsement_Maintenance. aspx. Accessed February 5, 2018

150. Centers for Medicare and Medicaid Services. *An Introduction to EHR Incentive Programs for Eligible Professionals: 2014 Clinical Quality Measure (CQM) Electronic Reporting Guide*. Washington, DC: Department of Health and Human Services; 2015. Available at: www.cms.gov/ Regulations-and-Guidance/Legislation/ EHRIncentivePrograms/Downloads/ CQM2014_GuideEP.pdf. Accessed February 5, 2018

151. Scharf RJ, Scharf GJ, Stroustrup A. Developmental milestones [published correction appears in *Pediatr Rev*. 2016;37(6):266]. *Pediatrics*. 2016;37(1):25–37; quiz 38, 47

152. Kinman CR, Gilchrist EC, Payne-Murphy JC, Miller BF. *Provider- and Practice-Level Competencies for Integrated Behavioral Health in Primary Care: A Literature Review. Contract No. HHSA 290-2009-00023I*. Rockville, MD: Agency for Healthcare Research and Quality; 2015

153. Williams J, Shore SE, Foy JM. Co-location of mental health professionals in primary care settings: three North Carolina models. *Clin Pediatr (Phila)*. 2006;45(6): 537–543

154. Council on Community Pediatrics. Poverty and child health in the United States. *Pediatrics*. 2016;137(4):e20160339

155. Garg A, Dworkin PH. Applying surveillance and screening to family psychosocial issues: implications for the medical home. *J Dev Behav Pediatr*. 2011;32(5):418–426

156. Wagner EH. Chronic disease management: what will it take to improve care for chronic illness? *Eff Clin Pract*. 1998;1(1):2–4

157. Heneghan AM, Morton S, DeLeone NL. Paediatricians' attitudes about discussing maternal depression during a paediatric primary care visit. *Child Care Health Dev*. 2007;33(3):333–339

158. Heneghan AM, Silver EJ, Bauman LJ, Stein RE. Do pediatricians recognize mothers with depressive symptoms? *Pediatrics*. 2000;106(6):1367–1373

159. Emerson BL, Bradley ER, Riera A, Mayes L, Bechtel K. Postpartum depression screening in the pediatric emergency department. *Pediatr Emerg Care*. 2014;30(11):788–792

160. Trost MJ, Molas-Torreblanca K, Man C, Casillas E, Sapir H, Schrager SM. Screening for maternal postpartum depression during infant hospitalizations. *J Hosp Med*. 2016;11(12):840–846

161. Seehusen DA, Baldwin LM, Runkle GP, Clark G. Are family physicians appropriately screening for postpartum depression? *J Am Board Fam Pract*. 2005;18(2):104–112

162. Myers ER, Aubuchon-Endsley N, Bastian LA, et al. *Efficacy and Safety of Screening for Postpartum Depression: Comparative Effectiveness Review, 106. AHRQ Publication No. 13-EHC064-EF*. Rockville, MD: Agency for Healthcare Research and Quality; 2013. Available at: https://effectivehealthcare.ahrq. gov/topics/depression-postpartum-screening/research. Accessed February 5, 2018

163. Cox JL, Holden JM, Sagovsky R. Detection of postnatal depression. Development of the 10-item Edinburgh Postnatal Depression Scale. *Br J Psychiatry*. 1987;150:782–786

164. Alvarado R, Jadresic E, Guajardo V, Rojas G. First validation of a Spanish-translated version of the Edinburgh postnatal depression scale (EPDS) for use in pregnant women. A Chilean study. *Arch Women Ment Health*. 2015;18(4):607–612

165. Massoudi P, Hwang CP, Wickberg B. How well does the Edinburgh Postnatal Depression Scale identify depression and anxiety in fathers? A validation study in a population based Swedish sample. *J Affect Disord*. 2013;149(1–3):67–74

166. Matthey S, Barnett B, Kavanagh DJ, Howie P. Validation of the Edinburgh Postnatal Depression Scale for men, and comparison of item endorsement with their partners. *J Affect Disord*. 2001;64(2–3):175–184

167. Ramchandani PG, Stein A, O'Connor TG, Heron J, Murray L, Evans J. Depression in men in the postnatal period and later child psychopathology: a population cohort study. *J Am Acad Child Adolesc Psychiatry*. 2008;47(4):390–398

168. Perrin E. *The Survey of Wellbeing of Young Children*. Boston, MA: Tufts Medical Center; 2012. Available at: https://www.floatinghospital.org/ The-Survey-of-Wellbeing-of-Young-Children/Age-Specific-Forms. Accessed November 27, 2018

169. Beck CT, Gable RK. Comparative analysis of the performance of the Postpartum Depression Screening Scale with two other depression instruments. *Nurs Res*. 2001;50(4):242–250

170. Tandon SD, Cluxton-Keller F, Leis J, Le HN, Perry DF. A comparison of three screening tools to identify perinatal depression among low-income African American women. *J Affect Disord*. 2012;136(1–2):155–162

171. Buist AE, Barnett BE, Milgrom J, et al. To screen or not to screen—that is the question in perinatal depression. *Med J Aust*. 2002;177(suppl):S101–S105

172. Venkatesh KK, Zlotnick C, Triche EW, Ware C, Phipps MG. Accuracy of brief screening tools for identifying postpartum depression among

adolescent mothers. *Pediatrics.* 2014;133(1). Available at: www. pediatrics.org/cgi/content/full/133/1/e45

173. Montazeri A, Torkan B, Omidvari S. The Edinburgh Postnatal Depression Scale (EPDS): translation and validation study of the Iranian version. *BMC Psychiatry.* 2007;7:11

174. Olson AL, Dietrich AJ, Prazar G, Hurley J. Brief maternal depression screening at well-child visits. *Pediatrics.* 2006;118(1):207–216

175. Olson AL, Dietrich AJ, Prazar G, et al. Two approaches to maternal depression screening during well child visits. *J Dev Behav Pediatr.* 2005;26(3):169–176

176. Kroenke K, Spitzer RL, Williams JB. The Patient Health Questionnaire-2: validity of a two-item depression screener. *Med Care.* 2003;41(11):1284–1292

177. Löwe B, Unützer J, Callahan CM, Perkins AJ, Kroenke K. Monitoring depression treatment outcomes with the patient health questionnaire-9. *Med Care.* 2004;42(12):1194–1201

178. Wittkampf KA, Naeije L, Schene AH, Huyser J, van Weert HC. Diagnostic accuracy of the mood module of the Patient Health Questionnaire: a systematic review. *Gen Hosp Psychiatry.* 2007;29(5):388–395

179. Richardson LP, McCauley E, Grossman DC, et al. Evaluation of the Patient Health Questionnaire-9 Item for detecting major depression among adolescents. *Pediatrics.* 2010;126(6):1117–1123

180. Kroenke K, Spitzer RL, Williams JB. The PHQ-9: validity of a brief depression severity measure. *J Gen Intern Med.* 2001;16(9):606–613

181. Beck AT, Steer RA, Ball R, Ranieri W. Comparison of Beck Depression Inventories -IA and -II in psychiatric outpatients. *J Pers Assess.* 1996;67(3):588–597

182. Forman-Hoffman V, McClure E, McKeeman J, et al. Screening for major depressive disorder in children and adolescents: a systematic review for the U.S. Preventive Services Task Force. *Ann Intern Med.* 2016;164(5):342–349

183. Ji S, Long Q, Newport DJ, et al. Validity of depression rating scales during pregnancy and the postpartum period: impact of trimester and parity. *J Psychiatr Res.* 2011;45(2):213–219

184. Beck CT. A checklist to identify women at risk for developing postpartum depression. *J Obstet Gynecol Neonatal Nurs.* 1998;27(1):39–46

185. Baker BL, McIntyre LL, Blacher J, Crnic K, Edelbrock C, Low C. Pre-school children with and without developmental delay: behaviour problems and parenting stress over time. *J Intellect Disabil Res.* 2003;47(pt 4–5):217–230

186. Squires J, Bricker D, Twombly E. *Ages & Stages Questionnaires: A Parent-Completed Child Monitoring System for Social-Emotional Behaviors.* 2nd ed. Baltimore, MD: Paul Brooks Publishing Co; 2015. Available at: https://agesandstages.com. Accessed February 5, 2018

187. Gleason MM, Zeanah CH, Dickstein S. Recognizing young children in need of mental health assessment: development and preliminary validity of the early childhood screening assessment. *Infant Ment Health J.* 2010;31(3):335–357

188. Sheldrick RC, Henson BS, Merchant S, Neger EN, Murphy JM, Perrin EC. The Preschool Pediatric Symptom Checklist (PPSC): development and initial validation of a new social/emotional screening instrument. *Acad Pediatr.* 2012;12(5):456–467

189. Sheldrick RC, Henson BS, Neger EN, Merchant S, Murphy JM, Perrin EC. The baby pediatric symptom checklist: development and initial validation of a new social/emotional screening instrument for very young children. *Acad Pediatr.* 2013;13(1):72–80

190. Ader J, Stille CJ, Keller D, Miller BF, Barr MS, Perrin JM. The medical home and integrated behavioral health: advancing the policy agenda. *Pediatrics.* 2015;135(5):909–917

191. Sriraman NK, Melvin K, Meltzer-Brody S; Academy of Breastfeeding Medicine Protocol Committee. ABM clinical protocol #18: use of antidepressants in breastfeeding mothers. *Breastfeed Med.* 2015;10(6):290–299

192. Cox EQ, Sowa NA, Meltzer-Brody SE, Gaynes BN. The perinatal depression treatment cascade: baby steps toward improving outcomes. *J Clin Psychiatry.* 2016;77(9):1189–1200

193. Brealey SD, Hewitt C, Green JM, Morrell J, Gilbody S. Screening for postnatal depression: is it acceptable to women and healthcare professionals? A systematic review and meta-synthesis. *J Reprod Infant Psychol.* 2010;28(4):328–344

194. Marcus SM. Depression during pregnancy: rates, risks and consequences—Motherisk Update 2008. *Can J Clin Pharmacol.* 2009;16(1):e15–e22

195. Marcus SM, Barry KL, Flynn HA, Blow FC. *Improving Detection, Prevention and Treatment of Depression and Substance Abuse in Childbearing Women: Critical Variables in Pregnancy and Pre-Pregnancy Planning.* Ann Arbor, MI: University of Michigan Clinical Ventures, Faculty Group Practice; 1998

196. Thota AB, Sipe TA, Byard GJ, et al; Community Preventive Services Task Force. Collaborative care to improve the management of depressive disorders: a community guide systematic review and meta-analysis. *Am J Prev Med.* 2012;42(5):525–538

197. Howard LM, Flach C, Mehay A, Sharp D, Tylee A. The prevalence of suicidal ideation identified by the Edinburgh Postnatal Depression Scale in postpartum women in primary care: findings from the RESPOND trial. *BMC Pregnancy Childbirth.* 2011;11(1):57

198. Yonkers KA, Wisner KL, Stewart DE, et al. The management of depression during pregnancy: a report from the American Psychiatric Association and the American College of Obstetricians and Gynecologists. *Gen Hosp Psychiatry.* 2009;31(5):403–413

199. Stuart S, Koleva H. Psychological treatments for perinatal depression. *Best Pract Res Clin Obstet Gynaecol.* 2014;28(1):61–70

200. Forman DR, O'Hara MW, Stuart S, Gorman LL, Larsen KE, Coy KC. Effective treatment for postpartum depression is not sufficient to improve the developing mother-child relationship. *Dev Psychopathol.* 2007;19(2):585–602

201. Council on Early Childhood; Committee on Psychosocial Aspects of Child and Family Health; Section on Developmental and Behavioral Pediatrics. Addressing early childhood emotional and behavioral problems. *Pediatrics*. 2016;138(6):e20163023

202. Gaskin-Butler VT, McKay K, Gallardo G, Salman-Engin S, Little T, McHale JP. Thinking 3 rather than 2+1: how a coparenting framework can transform infant mental health efforts with unmarried African American parents. *Zero to Three*. 2015;35(5):49–58

203. Willheim E. Dyadic psychotherapy with infants and young children: child-parent psychotherapy. *Child Adolesc Psychiatric Clin N Am*. 2013;22(2):215–239

204. Cassidy J, Woodhouse SS, Sherman LJ, Stupica B, Lejuez CW. Enhancing infant attachment security: an examination of treatment efficacy and differential susceptibility. *J Dev Psychopathol*. 2011;23(1):131–148

205. Marvin R, Cooper G, Hoffman K, Powell B. The Circle of Security project: attachment-based intervention with caregiver-pre-school child dyads. *Attach Hum Dev*. 2002;4(1):107–124

206. Wissow L, Anthony B, Brown J, et al. A common factors approach to improving the mental health capacity of pediatric primary care. *Adm Policy Ment Health*. 2008;35(4):305–318

207. Feinberg E, Donahue S, Bliss R, Silverstein M. Maternal depressive symptoms and participation in early intervention services for young children. *Matern Child Health J*. 2012;16(2):336–345

208. Substance Abuse and Mental Health Services Administration. *Depression in Mothers: More Than the Blues—A Toolkit for Family Service Providers. HHS Publication No. (SMA) 14-4878.* Rockville, MD: Substance Abuse and Mental Health Services Administration; 2014

209. van Schaik DJ, Klijn AF, van Hout HP, et al. Patients' preferences in the treatment of depressive disorder in primary care. *Gen Hosp Psychiatry*. 2004;26(3):184–189

210. Ugarriza DN, Schmidt L. Telecare for women with postpartum depression. *J Psychosoc Nurs Ment Health Serv*. 2006;44(1):37–45

211. Sheeber LB, Seeley JR, Feil EG, et al. Development and pilot evaluation of an Internet-facilitated cognitive-behavioral intervention for maternal depression. *J Consult Clin Psychol*. 2012;80(5):739–749

212. Ashford MT, Olander EK, Ayers S. Computer- or web-based interventions for perinatal mental health: a systematic review. *J Affect Disord*. 2016;197:134–146

213. Ammerman RT, Putnam FW, Altaye M, Stevens J, Teeters AR, Van Ginkel JB. A clinical trial of in-home CBT for depressed mothers in home visitation. *Behav Ther*. 2013;44(3):359–372

214. Freeman MP, Hibbeln JR, Wisner KL, Brumbach BH, Watchman M, Gelenberg AJ. Randomized dose-ranging pilot trial of omega-3 fatty acids for postpartum depression. *Acta Psychiatr Scand*. 2006;113(1):31–35

215. Molyneaux E, Howard LM, McGeown HR, Karia AM, Trevillion K. Antidepressant treatment for postnatal depression. *Cochrane Database Syst Rev*. 2014;(9):CD002018

216. McDonagh MS, Matthews A, Phillipi C, et al. Depression drug treatment outcomes in pregnancy and the postpartum period: a systematic review and meta-analysis. *Obstet Gynecol*. 2014;124(3):526–534

217. Grigoriadis S. The effects of antidepressant medications on mothers and babies. *J Popul Ther Clin Pharmacol*. 2014;21(3):e533–e541

218. Andersen JT, Andersen NL, Horwitz H, Poulsen HE, Jimenez-Solem E. Exposure to selective serotonin reuptake inhibitors in early pregnancy and the risk of miscarriage. *Obstet Gynecol*. 2014;124(4):655–661

219. Meltzer-Brody S. Treating perinatal depression: risks and stigma. *Obstet Gynecol*. 2014;124(4):653–654

220. Rowe H, Baker T, Hale TW. Maternal medication, drug use, and breastfeeding. *Child Adolesc Psychiatr Clin N Am*. 2015;24(1):1–20

221. Hale TW. *Medication and Mother's Milk 2012: A Manual of Lactational Pharmacology*. 15th ed. Amarillo, TX: Hale Publishing LP; 2012

SECTION 4
Mental Health/ Behavioral Problems

POLICY STATEMENT Organizational Principles to Guide and Define the Child Health
Care System and/or Improve the Health of all Children

American Academy
of Pediatrics

DEDICATED TO THE HEALTH OF ALL CHILDREN™

Addressing Early Childhood Emotional and Behavioral Problems

COUNCIL ON EARLY CHILDHOOD, COMMITTEE ON PSYCHOSOCIAL ASPECTS OF CHILD AND
FAMILY HEALTH, SECTION ON DEVELOPMENTAL AND BEHAVIORAL PEDIATRICS

abstract

Emotional, behavioral, and relationship problems can develop in very young children, especially those living in high-risk families or communities. These early problems interfere with the normative activities of young children and their families and predict long-lasting problems across multiple domains. A growing evidence base demonstrates the efficacy of specific family-focused therapies in reducing the symptoms of emotional, behavioral, and relationship symptoms, with effects lasting years after the therapy has ended. Pediatricians are usually the primary health care providers for children with emotional or behavioral difficulties, and awareness of emerging research about evidence-based treatments will enhance this care. In most communities, access to these interventions is insufficient. Pediatricians can improve the care of young children with emotional, behavioral, and relationship problems by calling for the following: increased access to care; increased research identifying alternative approaches, including primary care delivery of treatments; adequate payment for pediatric providers who serve these young children; and improved education for pediatric providers about the principles of evidence-based interventions.

DOI: 10.1542/peds.2016-3023

PEDIATRICS (ISSN Numbers: Print, 0031-4005; Online, 1098-4275).

To cite: AAP COUNCIL ON EARLY CHILDHOOD, AAP COMMITTEE ON PSYCHOSOCIAL ASPECTS OF CHILD AND FAMILY HEALTH, AAP SECTION ON DEVELOPMENTAL AND BEHAVIORAL PEDIATRICS. Addressing Early Childhood Emotional and Behavioral Problems. *Pediatrics.* 2016;138(6):e20163023

INTRODUCTION

Emotional, relationship, and behavioral problems affect nearly as many preschoolers as older children, with prevalence rates of 7% to 10%.[1–3] Emotional, behavioral, and relationship problems, including disorders of attachment, disruptive behavior disorders, attention-deficit/hyperactivity disorder (ADHD), anxiety and mood disorders, and disorders of self-regulation of sleep and feeding in children younger than 6 years, interfere with development across multiple domains, including social interactions, parent–child relationships, physical safety, ability to participate in child care, and school readiness.[4–6] Importantly, if untreated, these problems can persist and have long-lasting effects, including measurable abnormalities in brain functioning and persistent emotional and behavioral problems.[7–10] In short, early emotional, behavioral, and relationship problems in preschool-aged children interfere with their current well-being, jeopardize the foundations of emotional and behavioral health, and have the potential for long-term consequences.[11]

Pediatricians and other child health care providers can reduce the risk of childhood emotional and behavioral problems by reducing exposure to toxic stress, promoting protective factors, and systematically screening for risk factors for emerging clinical problems.[12,13] Existing policy statements address universal approaches, early identification, and strategies for children at risk. The present policy statement focuses on clinical interventions for children with clinical disorders that warrant targeted treatment. Treatment planning is guided by a comprehensive assessment of the clinical presentation with attention to the child, the parent–child relationships, and community stressors. Beyond assessment, effective treatment of clinical disorders requires the following: (1) access to evidence-based treatments; and (2) primary care providers' sufficient familiarity with evidence-based treatments to implement first-line approaches, make informed and effective referrals, and collaborate with specialty providers who have expertise in early childhood emotional and behavioral well-being.[14] Currently, most young children with an emotional, relationship, or behavioral problem receive no interventions for their disorder. This policy statement provides a summary of empirically supported approaches, describes readily identifiable barriers to accessing quality evidence-based interventions, and proposes recommendations to enhance the care of young children. This statement has been endorsed by Zero to Three and the American Academy of Child and Adolescent Psychiatry.

EVIDENCE-BASED TREATMENTS

Awareness of the relative levels of evidence supporting pharmacologic and nonpharmacologic therapies for emotional, behavioral, and relationship problems can guide clinical decisions in the primary care setting. The evidence base related to psychopharmacologic agents in children younger than 6 years is limited and has only addressed ADHD.[15] Only 2 rigorous trials have examined the safety and efficacy of medications in this age group. Both the trial of methylphenidate and the study of atomoxetine for moderate to severe ADHD demonstrated that the trial medication was more effective than placebo but was less effective for younger children than for older children and produced higher rates of adverse effects in younger children.[16,17] Other medications have been less rigorously evaluated in preschool-aged children, although the rates of prescriptions for atypical antipsychotic agents, with their potential for substantial metabolic morbidity, have increased steadily in this age group.[18-20]

Nonpharmacologic treatments have more durable effects than medications, with documented effects lasting for years.[21-23] A first step in reducing the barriers to evidence-based treatments is to ensure that primary care pediatricians are familiar with these approaches, which should be available to young children with emotional, behavioral, or relationship problems.[24]

For infants and toddlers with clinical-level emotional, behavioral, or relationship concerns, dyadic interventions promote attachment security and child emotional regulation and can promote regulation of stress hormones. Examples of these interventions include infant–parent psychotherapy, video feedback to promote positive parenting, and attachment biobehavioral catch-up. These interventions often use real-time infant–parent interactions to support positive interactions, enhance parents' capacity to reflect on their parenting patterns, and promote sensitivity and an understanding of the infant's needs.[25]

For preschool-aged children, parent management training models, including parent–child interaction therapy (PCIT), the Incredible Years series, the New Forest Program, Triple P (Positive Parenting Program), and Helping the Noncompliant Child,[26] are effective in decreasing symptoms of ADHD and disruptive behavior disorders. Parents are actively involved in all of these interventions, sometimes without the child and sometimes in parent–child interactions. All share similar behavioral principles, most consistently engaging parents as partners to: (1) reinforce positive behaviors; (2) ignore low-level provocative behaviors; and (3) provide clear, consistent, safe responses to unacceptable behaviors. Table 1 presents some of the characteristics of the best-supported programs for disruptive behavior disorders and ADHD.[25,27]

Posttraumatic stress disorder can be treated effectively with cognitive behavioral therapy and child–parent psychotherapy in very young children. In cognitive behavioral therapy for posttraumatic stress disorder, preschool-aged children learn relaxation techniques and are gradually exposed to their frightening memories while using these techniques. Child–parent psychotherapy focuses on supporting parents to create a safe, consistent relationship with the child through helping them understand the child's emotional experiences and needs.[33] Cognitive behavioral therapy is also effective for other common anxiety disorders, and recent promising studies report effectiveness of modified PCIT for selective mutism and depression.[34-36] Adaptations for use in primary care, including

TABLE 1 Characteristics of the Best-Supported Programs for Disruptive Behavior Disorders and ADHD

Program	Ages	Formal Psychoeducation for Parents?	Real-Time Observed Parent–Child Interactions?	Special Characteristics	Duration	Evidence Suggesting Effective for ADHD? (Effect Size)	Evidence Suggesting Effective for Disruptive Behavior Disorders? (Effect Size)
New Forest[28]	30–77 mo	Yes	Yes	Parent–child tasks are specifically intended to require attention Occurs in the home Explicit attention to parental depression	5 weekly sessions	Yes (very large, 1.9)	Yes (moderate, 0.7)
Incredible Years Parent Training and Child Training[29,30] (incredibleyearsseries.org)	24 mo–8 y	Yes	No	Separate parent and child groups Parental training uses video vignettes for discussion Child training includes circle time learning and coached free play	20 weekly 2-h sessions	Yes	Yes
Triple P[31] (triplep.org)	Birth–12 y	Yes (primary)	Yes	Multiple levels of intervention Primarily training parents with some opportunities to observe parent–child interactions Handouts and homework supplement the treatment	Primary care, four 15-min sessions Standard treatment is 10 sessions	No	Yes
PCIT[32] (pcit.org)	24 mo–7 y	Yes, minimal	Yes	Through a 1-way mirror, therapist coaches parent during in vivo interactions with child Homework requires parent child interactions Progress through therapy determined by parents' skill development	Duration depends on parental skill development	Modest	Yes
Helping the Noncomplaint Child[26]	3–8 y	Yes	Yes	Involves 2 phases: (1) differential attention; (2) compliance training using demonstration, role plays, and in-office and at home practice	8–10 average (depends on demonstrated progress)	Yes (1.24 parent report; .23 [NS] teacher report)	Yes

Triple P, the Incredible Years series, and PCIT, similarly show positive outcomes, although further research is warranted.[37–39]

Ensuring that parents have access to appropriate support or clinical care is often an important component of clinical intervention for children.

Effective parental treatment (eg, for depression) may reduce child symptoms substantially.[40]

SYSTEMIC BARRIERS

Despite the strong empirical support for these interventions, most young children with emotional, behavioral,

and relationship problems do not receive nonpharmacologic treatments.[41] Physical separation, challenges coordinating across systems, stigma, parental beliefs, and provider beliefs about mental health services may interfere with identification of concerns and success of referrals. New models such as co-located care, in which mental health professionals work together with medical care providers in the same space, improve care coordination and referral success, decrease stigma, and reduce symptoms compared with traditional referrals.[42–44] There are insufficient numbers of skilled providers to meet the emotional, behavioral, and relationship needs of children (and young children in particular) who require developmentally specialized interventions.[45,46] Therefore, when a primary care pediatrician identifies an emotional, relationship, or behavioral problem in a young child, it is often difficult to identify a professional (eg, social worker, psychologist, child and adolescent psychiatrist, developmental-behavioral pediatrician) with expertise in early childhood to accept the referral and provide evidence-based treatments.

Mental health coverage systems may also reduce access to care.[47] Although mental health parity regulations took effect in 2014, there are still "carved out" mental health programs that prohibit payment to primary care pediatricians for care of a child with an emotional, relationship, or behavioral health diagnosis and may limit access to trained specialists.[48] Even when a trained provider of an evidence-based treatment is identified, communication, coordination of care with primary care pediatricians, and adequate payment can be challenges.[14,49] Many health care systems do not pay for, or underpay for, necessary components of early childhood care such as care conferences, school observations, discussions with additional caregivers, same-day services, care coordination, and appointments that do not include face-to-face treatment of the child.

RECOMMENDATIONS

1. In the context of the focus of the American Academy of Pediatrics on early child and brain development, pediatricians have the opportunity to advocate for legislative and research approaches that will increase access to evidence-based treatments for very young children with emotional, behavioral, and relationship problems.

1a. At the legislative level, pediatricians should advocate for: (1) funding programs that increase dissemination and implementation of evidence-based treatments, especially in areas with limited resources; (2) addressing the early childhood mental health workforce shortage by providing incentives for training in these professions; (3) decreasing third-party payer barriers to accessing mental health services to very young children; and (4) promoting accountable care organization regulations that protect early childhood mental health services.

1b. In collaboration with other child-focused organizations, pediatricians should advocate for prioritization of research that will enhance the evidence base for treatment of very young children with emotional, behavioral, and relationship problems. Comparative effectiveness studies between psychopharmacologic and psychotherapeutic interventions and comparison of mental health service delivery approaches (eg, co-located models, community-based consultation, targeted referrals to specialists) are needed to guide management and policy decisions. In addition, studies that examine moderators of treatment effects, including family, social, and biological factors, are warranted. Studies of interventions adapted to treat young children with mild symptoms in the primary care setting could decrease barriers to care.

2. At the community and organizational levels, pediatricians should collaborate with local governmental and private agencies to identify local and national clinical services that can serve young children and explore opportunities for innovative service delivery models such as consultation or co-location.

3. Primary care pediatricians and developmental-behavioral pediatricians, together with early childhood mental health providers, including child and adolescent psychiatrists, and developmental specialists, can create educational materials for trainees and providers to enhance the care young children receive.

4. Without adequate payment for screening and assessment by primary care providers and management by specialty providers with expertise in early childhood mental health, treatment of very young children with emotional and behavioral problems will likely remain inaccessible for many children. Given existing knowledge regarding the importance of early childhood brain development on lifelong health, adequate payment for early childhood preventive services will benefit not only the patients but society as well and should be supported. Mental health carve-outs should be eliminated because they provide a significant barrier to access to mental health care for children. Additional steps toward equal access to mental health and physical health care include efficient prior authorization processes; adequate panels of early childhood mental health providers; payment to all providers, including primary care providers, for mental health

diagnoses; sustainable payment for co-located mental health providers and care coordination; payment for evidence-based approaches focused on parents; and payment for the necessary collection of information from children's many caregivers and for same-day services. Advocacy for true mental health parity must continue.

5. To ensure that all providers caring for children are knowledgeable participants and partners in the care of young children with emotional, behavioral, and relationship problems, graduate medical education and continuing medical education should include opportunities for training that ensure that pediatric providers: (1) are competent to identify young children with emotional, behavioral, and relationship problems as well as risk and protective factors; (2) are aware that common early childhood emotional, behavioral, and relationship problems can be treated with evidence-based treatments; (3) recognize the limitations in the data supporting use of medications in very young children, even for ADHD; (4) are prepared to identify and address parental factors that influence early child development; and (5) can collaborate and refer across disciplines and specialties, including developmental-behavioral pediatrics, child and adolescent psychiatry, psychology, and other mental health services.

LEAD AUTHORS

Mary Margaret Gleason, MD, FAAP
Edward Goldson, MD, FAAP
Michael W. Yogman, MD, FAAP

COUNCIL ON EARLY CHILDHOOD EXECUTIVE COMMITTEE, 2015–2016

Dina Lieser, MD, FAAP, Chairperson
Beth DelConte, MD, FAAP
Elaine Donoghue, MD, FAAP

Marian Earls, MD, FAAP
Danette Glassy, MD, FAAP
Terri McFadden, MD, FAAP
Alan Mendelsohn, MD, FAAP
Seth Scholer, MD, FAAP
Jennifer Takagishi, MD, FAAP
Douglas Vanderbilt, MD, FAAP
Patricia Gail Williams, MD, FAAP

LIAISONS

Lynette M. Fraga, PhD – *Child Care Aware*
Abbey Alkon, RN, PNP, PhD, MPH – *National Association of Pediatric Nurse Practitioners*
Barbara U. Hamilton, MA – *Maternal and Child Health Bureau*
David Willis, MD, FAAP – *Maternal and Child Health Bureau*
Claire Lerner, LCSW – *Zero to Three*

STAFF

Charlotte Zia, MPH, CHES

COMMITTEE ON PSYCHOSOCIAL ASPECTS OF CHILD AND FAMILY HEALTH, 2015–2016

Michael Yogman, MD, FAAP, Chairperson
Nerissa Bauer, MD, MPH, FAAP
Thresia B. Gambon, MD, FAAP
Arthur Lavin, MD, FAAP
Keith M. Lemmon, MD, FAAP
Gerri Mattson, MD, FAAP
Jason Richard Rafferty, MD, MPH, EdM
Lawrence Sagin Wissow, MD, MPH, FAAP

LIAISONS

Sharon Berry, PhD, LP – *Society of Pediatric Psychology*
Terry Carmichael, MSW – *National Association of Social Workers*
Edward Christophersen, PhD, FAAP – *Society of Pediatric Psychology*
Norah Johnson, PhD, RN, CPNP-BC – *National Association of Pediatric Nurse Practitioners*
Leonard Read Sulik, MD, FAAP – *American Academy of Child and Adolescent Psychiatry*

CONSULTANT

George J. Cohen, MD, FAAP

STAFF

Stephanie Domain, MS, CHES

SECTION ON DEVELOPMENTAL AND BEHAVIORAL PEDIATRICS EXECUTIVE COMMITTEE, 2015–2016

Nathan J. Blum, MD, FAAP, Chairperson
Michelle M. Macias, MD, FAAP, Immediate Past Chairperson
Nerissa S. Bauer, MD, MPH, FAAP
Carolyn Bridgemohan, MD, FAAP

Edward Goldson, MD, FAAP
Peter J. Smith, MD, MA, FAAP
Carol Cohen Weitzman, MD, FAAP
Stephen H. Contompasis, MD, FAAP, Web site Editor
Damon R. Korb, MD, FAAP, Discussion Board Moderator
Michael I. Reiff, MD, FAAP, Newsletter Editor
Robert G. Voigt, MD, FAAP, Program Chairperson

LIAISONS

Beth Ellen Davis, MD, MPH, FAAP – *Council on Children with Disabilities*
Pamela C. High, MD, MS, FAAP – *Society for Developmental and Behavioral Pediatrics*

STAFF

Linda Paul, MPH

ABBREVIATIONS

ADHD: attention-deficit/hyperactivity disorder
PCIT: parent–child interaction therapy

REFERENCES

1. Egger HL, Angold A. Common emotional and behavioral disorders in preschool children: presentation, nosology, and epidemiology. *J Child Psychol Psychiatry.* 2006;47(3–4):313–337

2. Wichstrøm L, Berg-Nielsen TS, Angold A, Egger HL, Solheim E, Sveen TH. Prevalence of psychiatric disorders in preschoolers. *J Child Psychol Psychiatry.* 2012;53(6):695–705

3. Gudmundsson OO, Magnusson P, Saemundsen E, et al. Psychiatric disorders in an urban sample of preschool children. *Child Adolesc Ment Health.* 2013;18(4):210–217

4. Schwebel DC, Speltz ML, Jones K, Bardina P. Unintentional injury in preschool boys with and without early onset of disruptive behavior. *J Pediatr Psychol.* 2002;27(8):727–737

5. Pagliaccio D, Luby J, Gaffrey M, et al. Anomalous functional brain activation following negative mood induction in children with pre-school onset major depression. *Dev Cogn Neurosci.* 2012;2(2):256–267

6. Briggs-Gowan MJ, Carter AS. Social-emotional screening status in early childhood predicts elementary

school outcomes. *Pediatrics*. 2008;121(5):957–962

7. Gaffrey MS, Luby JL, Belden AC, Hirshberg JS, Volsch J, Barch DM. Association between depression severity and amygdala reactivity during sad face viewing in depressed preschoolers: an fMRI study. *J Affect Disord*. 2011;129(1–3):364–370

8. Scheeringa MS, Zeanah CH, Myers L, Putnam F. Heart period and variability findings in preschool children with posttraumatic stress symptoms. *Biol Psychiatry*. 2004;55(7):685–691

9. Lahey BB, Pelham WE, Loney J, et al. Three-year predictive validity of DSM-IV attention deficit hyperactivity disorder in children diagnosed at 4-6 years of age. *Am J Psychiatry*. 2004;161(11):2014–2020

10. Barch DM, Gaffrey MS, Botteron KN, Belden AC, Luby JL. Functional brain activation to emotionally valenced faces in school-aged children with a history of preschool-onset major depression. *Biol Psychiatry*. 2012;72(12):1035–1042

11. Garner AS, Shonkoff JP; Committee on Psychosocial Aspects of Child and Family Health; Committee on Early Childhood, Adoption, and Dependent Care; Section on Developmental and Behavioral Pediatrics. Early childhood adversity, toxic stress, and the role of the pediatrician: translating developmental science into lifelong health. *Pediatrics*. 2012;129(1). Available at: www.pediatrics.org/cgi/content/full/129/1/e224

12. Shonkoff JP, Garner AS; Committee on Psychosocial Aspects of Child and Family Health; Committee on Early Childhood, Adoption, and Dependent Care; Section on Developmental and Behavioral Pediatrics. The lifelong effects of early childhood adversity and toxic stress. *Pediatrics*. 2012;129(1). Available at: www.pediatrics.org/cgi/content/full/129/1/e232

13. Weitzman C, Wegner L. American Academy of Pediatrics, Section on Developmental and Behavioral Pediatrics, Committee on Psychosocial Aspects of Child and Family Health, Council on Early Childhood; Society for Developmental and Behavioral Pediatrics. Promoting optimal

development: screening for behavioral and emotional problems. *Pediatrics*. 2015;135(2):384–395

14. Horwitz SM, Kelleher KJ, Stein REK, et al. Barriers to the identification and management of psychosocial issues in children and maternal depression. *Pediatrics*. 2007;119(1). Available at: www.pediatrics.org/cgi/content/full/119/1/e208

15. Zito JM; American Society of Clinical Psychopharmacology. Pharmacoepidemiology: recent findings and challenges for child and adolescent psychopharmacology. *J Clin Psychiatry*. 2007;68(6):966–967

16. Kratochvil CJ, Vaughan BS, Stoner JA, et al. A double-blind, placebo-controlled study of atomoxetine in young children with ADHD. *Pediatrics*. 2011;127(4). Available at: www.pediatrics.org/cgi/content/full/127/4/e862

17. Greenhill L, Kollins S, Abikoff H, et al. Efficacy and safety of immediate-release methylphenidate treatment for preschoolers with ADHD. *J Am Acad Child Adolesc Psychiatry*. 2006;45(11):1284–1293

18. Correll CU, Carlson HE. Endocrine and metabolic adverse effects of psychotropic medications in children and adolescents. *J Am Acad Child Adolesc Psychiatry*. 2006;45(7):771–791

19. Olfson M, Crystal S, Huang C, Gerhard T. Trends in antipsychotic drug use by very young, privately insured children. *J Am Acad Child Adolesc Psychiatry*. 2010;49(1):13–23

20. Zito JM, Safer DJ, Valluri S, Gardner JF, Korelitz JJ, Mattison DR. Psychotherapeutic medication prevalence in Medicaid-insured preschoolers. *J Child Adolesc Psychopharmacol*. 2007;17(2):195–203

21. Pediatric OCD Treatment Study (POTS) Team. Cognitive-behavior therapy, sertraline, and their combination for children and adolescents with obsessive-compulsive disorder: the Pediatric OCD Treatment Study (POTS) randomized controlled trial. *JAMA*. 2004;292(16):1969–1976

22. Webster-Stratton C, Rinaldi J, Jamila MR. Long-term outcomes of Incredible Years parenting program: predictors

of adolescent adjustment. *Child Adolesc Ment Health*. 2011;16(1):38–46

23. Hood KK, Eyberg SM. Outcomes of parent-child interaction therapy: mothers' reports of maintenance three to six years after treatment. *J Clin Child Adolesc Psychol*. 2003;32(3):419–429

24. Foy JM; American Academy of Pediatrics Task Force on Mental Health. Enhancing pediatric mental health care: algorithms for primary care. *Pediatrics*. 2010;125(suppl 3):S109–S125

25. Substance Abuse and Mental Health Services Administration. *National Registry of Evidence-based Programs and Practices*. Washington, DC: Substance Abuse and Mental Health Services Administration; 2013

26. Abikoff HB, Thompson MJ, Laver-Bradbury C, et al. Parent training for preschool ADHD: a randomized controlled trial of specialized and generic programs. *J Child Psychol Psychiatry*. 2015;56(6):618–631

27. Charach A, Dahshti B, Carson P, et al. *Attention Deficit Hyperactivity Disorder: Effectiveness of Treatment in At-Risk Preschoolers; Long-Term Effectiveness in All Ages; and Variability in Prevalence, Diagnosis, and Treatment*. Rockville, MD: Agency for Healthcare Research and Quality; 2012

28. Thompson MJ, Laver-Bradbury C, Ayres M, et al. A small-scale randomized controlled trial of the revised New Forest parenting programme for preschoolers with attention deficit hyperactivity disorder. *Eur Child Adolesc Psychiatry*. 2009;18(10):605–616

29. Webster-Stratton CH, Reid MJ, Beauchaine T. Combining parent and child training for young children with ADHD. *J Clin Child Adolesc Psychol*. 2011;40(2):191–203

30. Webster-Stratton C, Reid J. The Incredible Years parents, teachers, and children training series: a multifaceted treatment approach for young children with conduct disorders. In: Kazdin AE, ed. *Evidence-based Psychotherapies for Children and Adolescents*. 2nd ed. New York, NY: Guilford Press; 2010:194–210

31. Bodenmann G, Cina A, Ledermann T, Sanders MR. The efficacy of the Triple P-Positive Parenting Program in improving parenting and child behavior: a comparison with two other treatment conditions. *Behav Res Ther.* 2008;46(4):411–427

32. Eyberg SM, Funderburk BW, Hembree-Kigin TL, McNeil CB, Querido JG, Hood KK. Parent-child interaction therapy with behavior problem children: one and two year maintenance of treatment effects in the family. *Child Fam Behav Ther.* 2001;23(4):1–20

33. Lieberman AF, Ghosh Ippen C, Van Horn P. Child-parent psychotherapy: 6-month follow-up of a randomized controlled trial. *J Am Acad Child Adolesc Psychiatry.* 2006;45(8):913–918

34. Choate ML, Pincus DB, Eyberg SM. Parent-child interaction therapy for treatment of separation anxiety disorder in young children: a pilot study. *Cogn Behav Ther.* 2005;12(1):136–145

35. Donovan CL, March S. Online CBT for preschool anxiety disorders: a randomised control trial. *Behav Res Ther.* 2014;58:24–35

36. Hirshfeld-Becker DR, Masek B, Henin A, et al. Cognitive behavioral therapy for 4- to 7-year-old children with anxiety disorders: a randomized clinical trial. *J Consult Clin Psychol.* 2010;78(4):498–510

37. Markie-Dadds C, Sanders MR. Self-Directed Triple P (Positive Parenting Program) for mothers with children at-risk of developing conduct problems. *Behav Cogn Psychother.* 2006;34(03):259–275

38. Berkovits MD, O'Brien KA, Carter CG, Eyberg SM. Early identification and intervention for behavior problems in primary care: a comparison of two abbreviated versions of parent-child interaction therapy. *Behav Ther.* 2010;41(3):375–387

39. Perrin EC, Sheldrick RC, McMenamy JM, Henson BS, Carter AS. Improving parenting skills for families of young children in pediatric settings: a randomized clinical trial. *JAMA Pediatr.* 2014;168(1):16–24

40. Gunlicks ML, Weissman MM. Change in child psychopathology with improvement in parental depression: a systematic review. *J Am Acad Child Adolesc Psychiatry.* 2008;47(4):379–389

41. Luby JL, Stalets MM, Belden AC. Psychotropic prescriptions in a sample including both healthy and mood and disruptive disordered preschoolers: relationships to diagnosis, impairment, prescriber type, and assessment methods. *J Child Adolesc Psychopharmacol.* 2007;17(2):205–215

42. Kolko DJ, Campo JV, Kelleher K, Cheng Y. Improving access to care and clinical outcome for pediatric behavioral problems: a randomized trial of a nurse-administered intervention in primary care. *J Dev Behav Pediatr.* 2010;31(5):393–404

43. Sarvet B, Gold J, Bostic JQ, et al. Improving access to mental health care for children: the Massachusetts Child Psychiatry Access Project. *Pediatrics.* 2010;126(6):1191–1200

44. Kolko DJ, Campo JV, Kilbourne AM, Kelleher K. Doctor-office collaborative care for pediatric behavioral problems: a preliminary clinical trial. *Arch Pediatr Adolesc Med.* 2012;166(3):224–231

45. Thomas CR, Holzer CE III. The continuing shortage of child and adolescent psychiatrists. *J Am Acad Child Adolesc Psychiatry.* 2006;45(9):1023–1031

46. Kautz C, Mauch D, Smith SA. *Reimbursement of Mental Health Services in Primary Care Settings.* Rockville, MD: Center for Mental Health Services, Substance Abuse; 2008

47. Committee on Child Health Financing. Scope of health care benefits for children from birth through age 26. *Pediatrics.* 2012;129(1):185–189

48. Kelleher KJ, Campo JV, Gardner WP. Management of pediatric mental disorders in primary care: where are we now and where are we going? *Curr Opin Pediatr.* 2006;18(6):649–653

49. American Academy of Child and Adolescent Psychiatry. Policy Statements: Collaboration with Pediatric Medical Professionals. Washington, DC: American Academy of Child and Adolescent Psychiatry; 2008. Available at: http://www.aacap.org/aacap/policy_statements/2008/Collaboration_with_Pediatric_Medical_Professionals.aspx. Accessed October 17, 2016

TECHNICAL REPORT

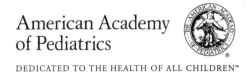

American Academy
of Pediatrics

DEDICATED TO THE HEALTH OF ALL CHILDREN™

Addressing Early Childhood Emotional and Behavioral Problems

Mary Margaret Gleason, MD, FAAP, Edward Goldson, MD, FAAP, Michael W. Yogman, MD, FAAP, COUNCIL ON EARLY CHILDHOOD, COMMITTEE ON PSYCHOSOCIAL ASPECTS OF CHILD AND FAMILY HEALTH, SECTION ON DEVELOPMENTAL AND BEHAVIORAL PEDIATRICS

abstract

More than 10% of young children experience clinically significant mental health problems, with rates of impairment and persistence comparable to those seen in older children. For many of these clinical disorders, effective treatments supported by rigorous data are available. On the other hand, rigorous support for psychopharmacologic interventions is limited to 2 large randomized controlled trials. Access to psychotherapeutic interventions is limited. The pediatrician has a critical role as the leader of the medical home to promote well-being that includes emotional, behavioral, and relationship health. To be effective in this role, pediatricians promote the use of safe and effective treatments and recognize the limitations of psychopharmacologic interventions. This technical report reviews the data supporting treatments for young children with emotional, behavioral, and relationship problems and supports the policy statement of the same name.

All clinical reports from the American Academy of Pediatrics automatically expire 5 years after publication unless reaffirmed, revised, or retired at or before that time.

DOI: 10.1542/peds.2016-3025

PEDIATRICS (ISSN Numbers: Print, 0031-4005; Online, 1098-4275).

FINANCIAL DISCLOSURE: The authors have indicated they have no financial relationships relevant to this article to disclose.

FUNDING: No external funding.

POTENTIAL CONFLICT OF INTEREST: The authors have indicated they have no potential conflicts of interest to disclose.

To cite: Gleason MM, Goldson E, Yogman MW, AAP COUNCIL ON EARLY CHILDHOOD. Addressing Early Childhood Emotional and Behavioral Problems. *Pediatrics.* 2016;138(6):e20163025

At least 8% to 10% of children younger than 5 years experience clinically significant and impairing mental health problems, which include emotional, behavioral, and social relationship problems.[1] An additional 1.5% of children have an autism spectrum disorder, the management of which has been reviewed in a separate report from the American Academy of Pediatrics (AAP).[2] Children with emotional, behavioral, and social relationship problems ("mental health problems"), as well as their families, experience distress and can suffer substantially because of these problems. These children may demonstrate impairment across multiple domains, including social interactions, problematic parent–child relationships, physical safety, inability to participate in child care without expulsion, delayed school readiness, school problems, and physical health problems in adulthood.[3–13] These clinical presentations can be distinguished from the emotional and behavioral patterns of typically developing children by their symptoms, family history, and level of impairment and, in some disorders, physiologic signs.[14–17] Emotional, behavioral, and relationship disorders rarely are transient and often have lasting effects, including measurable differences in brain functioning in school-aged children and a high risk of later mental health problems.[18-24] Exposure to toxic stressors, such as maltreatment or violence, and individual, family, or community stressors can increase the risk of early-onset mental health problems, although such stressors are not necessary for the development of these problems. Early exposure to adversity also has notable effects on the hypothalamic–pituitary–adrenal axis and epigenetic processes, with short-term and long-term consequences in physical and mental health, including adult cardiovascular disease and obesity.[25] In short, young children's early emotional, behavioral, and social relationship problems can cause suffering for young children and families, weaken the developing foundation of emotional and behavioral health, and have the potential for long-term adverse consequences.[26,27] This technical report reviews the data supporting treatment of children with identified clinical disorders, including the efficacy, safety, and accessibility of both pharmacologic and psychotherapeutic approaches.

PREVENTION APPROACHES

Although not the focus of this report, a full system of care includes primary and secondary preventive approaches, which are addressed in separate AAP reports.[28,29] Many family, individual, and community risk factors for adverse emotional, behavioral, and relationship health outcomes, including low-income status, exposure to toxic stressors, and parental mental health problems, can be identified early using systematic surveillance and screening. An extensive review of established prevention programs for the general population and identified children at high risk are described in the Substance

Abuse and Mental Health Services Administration (SAMHSA)'s National Report of Evidence-Based Programs and Practices (http://www.nrepp.samhsa.gov/AdvancedSearch.aspx). Outcomes of these programs highlight the value of early intervention and the potential to improve parenting skills using universal or targeted approaches for children at risk. The programs use a variety of approaches, including home visiting, parent groups, targeted addressing of basic needs, and videos to enhance parental self-reflection skills and have demonstrated a range of outcomes related to positive emotional, behavioral, and relationship development. One model developed specifically for the pediatric primary care setting is the Video Interaction Project, in which parents are paired with a bachelor's-level or master's-level developmental specialist who uses video and educational techniques to support parents' awareness of their child's developmental needs.[30]

Acknowledging that early preventive interventions are an important component of a system of care, the body of this technical report focuses on treatment of identified clinical problems rather than children at risk because of family or community factors.

PSYCHOSOCIAL TREATMENT APPROACHES

The evidence supporting family-focused therapeutic interventions for children with clinical-level concerns is robust, and these are the first-line approaches for young children with significant emotional and behavioral problems in most practice guidelines.[31-35]

Generally, these interventions take an approach that focuses on enhancing emotional and behavioral regulation through specialized parenting tools and approaches. The interventions

are implemented by clinicians with training in the specific treatment modality, following manuals and with fidelity to the treatment model. Primary care providers can be trained in these interventions but more often lead a medical home management approach that includes ongoing primary care management and support and concurrent comanagement with a clinician trained in implementing an evidence-based treatment (EBT).

Effective treatments exist to address early clinical concerns, including relationship disturbances, attention-deficit/hyperactivity disorder (ADHD), disruptive behavior disorders, anxiety, and posttraumatic stress disorder. Measured outcomes include improved attachment relationships, symptom reduction, diagnostic remission, enhanced functioning, and in one study, normalization of diurnal cortisol release patterns, which are known to be related to stress regulation and mood disorders.[31,33-35] Psychotherapies, including treatments that involve cognitive, psychological, and behavioral approaches, have substantially more lasting effects than do medications. Some preschool treatments have been shown to be effective for years after the treatment ended, a finding not matched in longitudinal pharmacologic studies.[36-38] It is for this reason that the recent ADHD treatment guidelines from the AAP emphasize that first-line treatment of preschoolers with well-established ADHD should be family-focused psychotherapy.[39]

EXAMPLES OF EVIDENCE-BASED TREATMENTS FOR EXISTING DIAGNOSES IN YOUNG CHILDREN

Infants and Toddlers

This report focuses on programs that target current diagnoses or clear clinical problems (rather than risk) in infants and toddlers and includes only those with rigorous randomized controlled empirical support. Because the parent–child relationship is a central force in the early emotional and behavioral well-being of children, a number of empirically supported treatments focus on enhancing that relationship to promote child well-being. Each intervention focuses on enhancing parents' ability to identify and respond to the infant's cues and to meet the infant's emotional needs. All interventions use infant–parent interactions in vivo or through video to demonstrate the infant's cues and opportunities to meet them. Some explicitly focus on enhancing parents' self-reflection and increasing awareness of how their own upbringing may influence their parenting approach.

Child Parent Psychotherapy and its partner Infant Parent Psychotherapy are derived from attachment theory and address the parent–child relationship through emotional support for parents, modeling protective behaviors, reflective developmental guidance, and addressing parental traumatic memories as they intrude into parent–child interactions.[40,41] This therapy is flexible in its delivery and can be implemented in the office, at home, or in other locations convenient for the family. On average, child–parent psychotherapy lasts approximately 32 sessions. In infants and toddlers, the empirically supported therapy enhances parent–child relationships, attachment security, child cognitive functioning, and normalization of cortisol regulation.[42-44]

For infants and toddlers who have been adopted internationally, those in foster care, or those thought to be at high risk of maltreatment because of exposure to domestic violence, homelessness, or parental substance abuse, the Attachment and Biobehavioral Catch-Up caregiver training supports

caregivers in developing sensitive, nurturing, nonfrightening parenting behaviors. In 10 sessions, caregivers receive parenting skills training, psychoeducation, and support in understanding the needs of infants and young children. This intervention model is associated with decreased rates of disorganized attachment, the attachment status most closely linked to psychopathology, and is associated with increased caregiver sensitivity and, notably, normalized diurnal cortisol patterns.[45-47]

In the Video Feedback to Promote Positive Parenting program, mothers with low levels of sensitivity to their child's needs review video feedback about their own parent–child interactions, with a focus on supporting sensitive discipline, reading a child's cues, and developing empathy for a child who is frustrated or angry. In the most stressed families, this intervention is associated with decreased infant behavioral difficulties and increased parental sensitivity.[48]

Treatments focused on mother–infant dyads affected by postpartum depression show promising effects on relationships and infant regulation.[49] Data in older children suggest effective treatment of maternal depression may result in reduction of child symptoms or an increase in caregiving quality.[50-52]

Preschoolers (2–6 Years)

ADHD and disruptive behavior disorders (eg, oppositional defiant disorder and conduct disorder) are the most common group of early childhood mental health problems, and a number of parent management training models have been shown to be effective. It should be noted that the criteria for these disorders have been shown to have validity in young children,[22,53] although the validity is dependent on a systematic assessment process that is most easily conducted in specialty settings. All of these parent training

models share similar behavioral principles, most consistently teaching parents: (1) to implement positive reinforcement to promote positive behaviors; (2) to ignore low-level provocative behaviors; and (3) to respond in a clear, consistent, and safe manner to unacceptable behaviors. The specific approaches to sharing these principles with parents vary across interventions. Table 1 presents some of the characteristics of the best-supported programs, all of which are featured on SAMHSA's national registry of evidence-based programs and practices.[34,54] The New Forrest Therapy, Triple P (Positive Parenting Practices), the Incredible Years Series (IYS), Helping the Noncompliant Child, and Parent Child Interaction Therapy (PCIT) all have shown efficacy in reducing clinically significant disruptive behavior symptoms in toddlers, preschoolers, and early school-aged children. The New Forrest Therapy, Helping the Noncompliant Child, and IYS also have proven efficacy in treating ADHD.[35,55-57]

In the New Forrest Therapy, sessions include parent–child activities that require sustained attention, concentration, turn-taking, working memory, and delay of gratification, all followed by positive reinforcement when the child is successful.[32,35] This model has been shown to decrease ADHD symptoms substantially and to decrease parents' negative statements about their children.[35] Triple P is a multilevel intervention that includes targeted treatment of children with disruptive behaviors.[55] The 3 highest levels of care include teaching parents about the causes of disruptive behaviors and effective strategies as well as specific problem solving about the child's individual patterns. The child is included in some sessions to create opportunities to implement the new strategies and for the therapist to model the behaviors. IYS includes a parent-focused treatment approach,

TABLE 1 Evidence-Based Interventions Shown To Reduce Existing Disruptive Problems in Preschoolers

Program	Age Range Supported by Data	Patient Population	No. of Children in Randomized Controlled Trials	Formal Psychoeducation for Parents	Real-Time Observed Parent–Child Interactions	Special Characteristics	Duration	Follow-up Duration (If Applicable)	Evidence Reflecting Efficacy for ADHD (Effect Size)	Evidence Demonstrating Efficacy for ODD and CD (Effect Size)
New Forest[32,35]	30–77 mo	Children with ADHD	202	Yes	Yes	• Parent–child tasks are specifically intended to require attention • Occurs in the home • Explicit attention to parental depression	5 weekly sessions	n/a	Yes (1.9)	Yes (0.7)
IYS parent training, teacher training, and child training[32,53,57–59]	3–8 y	Children with CD, ODD, and ADHD	677	Yes	No	• Separate parent and child groups • Parent training uses video vignettes for discussion • Child training includes circle time learning and coached free play	20 weekly 2-h sessions		Yes (0.8)	Yes (home behavior, 0.4–0.7; school behavior, 0.7–1.25)
Triple P[55,60,61] (levels 3 and 4)	36–48 mo	Children at high risk with parental concerns about behavioral difficulties (level 4)	330	Yes	Yes	• Multiple levels of intervention • Primarily training parents with some opportunities to observe parent–child interactions • Handouts and homework supplement the treatment	• Primary care = 4 sessions of 15 min • Standard treatment is 10 sessions	6 and 12 mo: effect size, 0.66 for children <4 y, 0.65 for children >4 y[62]	No	Yes (level 3: 0.69, level 4: 0.96; lower for children <4 y)[63]
Triple P online[59]	2–9 y	Children with CD and ODD	116	No	No	• Interactive self-directed program delivered via the internet • Instruction in 17 core positive parenting skills	8 modules (45–75 min)	6 mo: effect size from baseline, 0.6–0.7 on ECBI, no effect on SDQ	No effect	Yes (1.0; by parent report)

TABLE 1 Continued

Program	Age Range Supported by Data	Patient Population	No. of Children in Randomized Controlled Trials	Formal Psychoeducation for Parents	Real-Time Observed Parent–Child Interactions	Special Characteristics	Duration	Follow-up Duration (If Applicable)	Evidence Reflecting Efficacy for ADHD (Effect Size)	Evidence Demonstrating Efficacy for ODD and CD (Effect Size)
PCIT[37,64,65]	2–7 y	Children with clinical level disruptive behavior symptoms	358	Yes, minimal	Yes	• Through a 1-way mirror, therapist coaches parent during in vivo interactions with child • Homework requires parent–child interactions • Progress through therapy determined by parents' skill development	Depends on parent skill development	Up to 6 y after treatment, fewer signs of disruptive behavior disorder than baseline	Minimal	Yes (1.45)[58]
Helping the Noncompliant Child[57]	3–8 y	Children with noncompliant behaviors	350	Yes	Yes	Involves two phases 1) Differential Attention 2) Compliance training using demonstration, role plays, and in-office and at home practice	Depends on parent skill development	6.8 mo	Effect size 1.24; inattention 1.09; hyperactivity/impulsivity: 1.21	Yes (but no ES reported)

n/a, not available; ECBI, Eyberg Child Behavior Inventory; SDQ, Strengths and Difficulties Questionnaire; CD, conduct disorder; ODD, oppositional defiant disorder.

in which groups of parents learn effective strategies, practice with each other, and discuss clinical vignettes presented on videos.[56] The child group treatment can occur concurrently with the parent training and focuses on emotional recognition and problem solving. This treatment initially was developed to treat oppositional defiant disorder and conduct disorder, for which a large body of evidence demonstrates its efficacy. Recent studies also have demonstrated effectiveness in treating inattention and hyperactivity.[66] An unintended yet measureable benefit is promoting language.[67] In PCIT, parents are coached in positive interactions and safe discipline with their child by the therapist, who is behind a one-way mirror and communicates to a parent via a small microphone in the parent's ear ("bug in the ear"). This treatment is unique because parents' achievement of specific skills determines the pace of the therapy, allowing movement from the first phase, focused on positive reinforcement, to the second phase, focused on safe, consistent consequences. PCIT has been shown to have large effects on child behavior problems and parent negative behaviors in real time. Importantly, it is also effective in reducing recidivism of maltreating parents.[68] Helping the Noncompliant Child also provides 2 portions of the treatment, with the first focused on differential attention and the second focused on compliance training. Parents move through the therapy based on observed skill acquisition, learning by demonstration, role plays, and practice at home and in the office with their child. Helping the Noncompliant Child has been shown to have similar effectiveness as NFP in treating ADHD in children 3 to 4 years old and those wtih comorbid ODD.[69]

Anxiety disorders also are common in very young children, with nearly

10% of children meeting criteria for at least 1 anxiety disorder. Cognitive behavioral therapy and child–parent psychotherapy, both of which also are listed on the SAMHSA registry of EBTs, are effective in reducing anxiety in very young children. When cognitive behavioral therapy is modified to match young children's developmental levels, children as young as 4 years can learn the necessary skills, including relaxation strategies, naming their feelings, and learning to rate the intensity of the feelings.[31] In cognitive behavioral therapy, children are exposed to the story of their trauma in a systematic, graduated fashion, using the coping strategies and measuring feeling intensity skills that they practice simultaneously throughout the intervention. Two randomized studies have examined cognitive behavioral therapy in trauma-exposed preschoolers, and both have shown that children in the cognitive behavioral therapy treatment arm showed fewer posttraumatic stress symptoms as well as fewer symptoms of disruptive behavior disorders than did children in supportive treatment.[70,71] Effects are sustained for up to a year after treatment.[71,72] Child–parent psychotherapy is similarly effective in treating children exposed to trauma. Child–parent psychotherapy is an attachment-focused treatment that supports the parent in creating a safe, consistent relationship with the child through helping the parent understand the child's emotional experiences and needs as well as parental reactions.[40] Child–parent psychotherapy is more effective in reducing child and parent trauma symptoms than supportive case management and community referral.[73] Importantly, child–parent psychotherapy shows treatment durability with sustained results at least 6 months after treatment.

Other more common anxiety disorders and mood disorders have received less research attention.

CBT has been shown effective in addressing mixed anxiety disorders including selective mutism, generalized anxiety disorders, separation anxiety disorder, and social phobia.[62,63] A randomized controlled trial demonstrated that modified PCIT was effective in helping parents recognize emotions, although not better than parent education in reducing depressive symptoms.[74] Significant controversy and limited data about the validity of diagnostic criteria for bipolar disorder remain, and no rigorous studies of nonpharmacologic interventions in this age group exist.[75]

Although the studies described previously show positive effects of parent management training approaches, limitations are notable. Attrition of up to 30% is not uncommon among these approaches, suggesting that there is a significant proportion of the population for whom these treatments do not seem to be a good fit, whether because of the frequency of appointments, the content, the therapeutic relationship, stigma about mental health care, or other barriers.[60,76,77]

PSYCHOPHARMACOLOGIC TREATMENT APPROACHES

As highlighted in both the professional and lay press, an increasing number of publicly and privately insured preschool and even younger children are receiving prescriptions for psychotropic medications.[78–81] After increasing drastically in the 1990s, claims data indicate that rates of stimulant prescriptions have plateaued in recent years, but the rates of prescriptions of atypical antipsychotic agents continue to increase.[78,81–83] Although prescribing data are limited, it appears that pediatric providers are the primary prescribers for psychopharmacologic treatment in children younger

than 5 years, as they are for older children.[84,85]

The evidence base related to psychopharmacologic medications in young children is limited, and clinical practice has far outpaced the evidence supporting safety or efficacy, especially for children in foster care.[33,81] Specifically, 2 rigorous randomized controlled trials have examined the safety and efficacy of medications in young children. Both studies found that treatment of ADHD in young children with medication, specifically methylphenidate and atomoxetine, was more effective than placebo but less effective than documented in older children.[36,86,87] Both also reported that young children had higher rates of adverse effects, especially negative emotionality and appetite and sleep problems, than did older children.[86,87] Less rigorously studied are the atypical antipsychotic agents, such as risperidone, olanzapine, and aripiprazole, for which prescription rates have increased substantially.[33,88] These agents have known metabolic risks, including obesity, hyperlipidemia, glucose intolerance, and hyperprolactinemia, as well the potential for extrapyramidal effects.[89,90] Long-term safety data regarding use of these medications in humans, including the effects on the brain during its most rapid development, are not available.

ACCESS TO EVIDENCE-BASED TREATMENTS

The balance of risks and benefits of treatment of early childhood emotional, behavioral, or relationship problems strongly favors the safety and established efficacy of the EBTs over the potential for medical risks and lower levels of evidence supporting the medication. Fewer than 50% of young children with emotional, behavioral, or relationship disturbances, even those with severity sufficient to warrant medication trials, receive any treatment, especially nonpharmacologic treatments.[11,78,91,92] A number of barriers limit access to nonpharmacological EBTs.

Residency training and continuing medical education has traditionally provided limited opportunities for collaboration between pediatric and child psychiatry residents and with other mental health providers, including doctoral level and master's level clinicians, although there are calls to increase these opportunities.[93,94] The limited opportunities for collaboration in training and limited supervised opportunities to assess young children with mental health problems likely result in graduating residents having limited experience in early childhood mental health as they enter the primary care workforce. The AAP has worked to address this gap by developing practice transformation approaches, including educational modules and anticipatory guidance approaches that promote emotional, behavioral, and relationship wellness (see the AAP Early Brain and Child Development Web site at http://www.aap.org/en-us/advocacy-and-policy/aap-health-initiatives/EBCD), and around the country, there appears to be an increase in collaborative training opportunities for pediatric residents with developmental–behavioral pediatrics faculty and fellows, triple board residents, child and adolescent psychiatry trainees, and other mental health professionals.

Many of these barriers are not specific to early childhood emotional, behavioral, and relationship health but are quite apparent in this area. Although representative epidemiologic data examining the rates of psychotherapeutic treatment of preschoolers are not available, only 1 in 5 older children with a mental health problem receives treatment,[95] and it seems likely that the rate is lower among preschool-aged children. A major challenge is the workforce shortage among child psychiatrists, child mental health professionals, and pediatric specialists trained to meet the specialized emotional, behavioral, and relationship needs of very young children and their families.[96–99] Anecdotally, it seems that many therapists trained in EBTs remain close to academic centers, further exacerbating the shortage in regions without such a center. Promising statewide initiatives, such as "PCIT of the Carolinas" learning collaborative, which promote organizational readiness and capacity within agencies, clinician competence, and treatment fidelity and consultation with therapists, may begin to foster access to EBTs. Such models are promising approaches to improving access to clinicians trained to evaluate a very young child or to implement EBTs.

Even in communities with early childhood experts who are trained in EBTs, third-party payment systems traditionally have rewarded brief medication-focused visits.[28] When emotional and behavioral health services are "carved out" of health insurance, important barriers to accessing care include limitations on primary care physicians' ability to bill for "mental health" diagnoses, limits on numbers of visits, payer restriction of mental health providers, and low payment rates.[98,100–102] Until 2013, the *Current Procedural Terminology* coding system did not recognize the extended time needed for early childhood emotional and behavioral assessment and treatment (and the payment for the new code tends to be minimal), and many payers will not reimburse for services without the patient present or for phone consultation or case conferences. Lastly, the billing and coding system does not recognize relationship-focused therapy, requiring the individual participants to have an *International Classification of Diseases*–codable diagnosis, and only a few states accept developmentally specific diagnoses, such as the Diagnostic Criteria: 0-5, as reimbursable conditions.[103]

Finally, stigma and parental beliefs may interfere with referrals to EBTs for very young children with emotional, behavioral, and relationship problems.[104–108] Parents' interest in treatment may be influenced by perceived stigma related to the mental health problem or their own experiences with the mental health system.[109] Provider stigma about mental health and concerns about a child being "labeled" may reduce referrals as well. Some parents also may be concerned that involvement with a mental or behavioral health specialist may increase their risk of referral to child protection services.

INNOVATIVE MODELS OF ACCESS THROUGH THE MEDICAL HOME

For children with emotional, behavioral, or relationship problems, the pediatric medical home remains the hub of a child's care, just as it is for other children with special health care needs.[110] Even without a comprehensive diagnostic assessment or knowledge of the details of each EBT, use of specific communication strategies, the "common factors" approach, has been shown to improve outcomes in older children. Specifically, implementation of the common factors approach was associated with reduced impairment from symptoms and reduced parent symptoms in a randomized controlled trial of 58 providers.[111] Subsequently, the mnemonic "HELP" was introduced by the AAP Task Force on Mental Health to prompt clinicians in key elements of the model, including offering **h**ope, demonstrating **e**mpathy, demonstrating **l**oyalty, using the language the family uses about the concerns, and **p**artnering with the family to develop a clearly stated **p**lan, with the parents' **p**ermission.[112] Because of the stigma related to mental health issues, "hope" and "loyalty" are especially powerful first steps.

Innovative and successful adaptations of EBTs have been developed for the primary care setting.[55,64,65] Triple P has been implemented successfully in primary care settings using nurse visits to provide the psychoeducation for parents and also has been studied as a self-directed intervention for parents of children with clinically significant disruptive behavior symptoms, with modest but sustained effects up to 6 months.[61] A pilot PCIT adaptation for primary care showed promising results, although larger studies are needed.[113] Most recently, a randomized controlled trial demonstrated that the Incredible Years Series can be implemented effectively in the pediatric medical home for children with mild to moderate behavior problems. In this study, parent-reported behavioral problems decreased significantly compared with the group on the wait list, as did observed negative parent–child interactions.[114]

The strategy for identifying providers of EBTs varies state to state. However, all but 3 states have an Early Childhood Comprehensive Services grant from the Human Resources and Service Administration (http://mchb.hrsa.gov/programs/earlychildhood/comprehensivesystems/grantees/) and are developing systems of care for young children. EBTs tend to be concentrated around academic settings, so contacting local developmental–behavioral pediatric divisions and child and adolescent psychiatry and psychology divisions often helps, and the originator of the model often knows providers trained in the intervention (eg, www.pcit.

org). Innovative practice models, such as consultation or colocated mental health professionals, can be effective approaches to ensuring children have access to care.[115]

In areas with more trained EBT providers, opportunities for colocated care seem promising. In such models, a clinician, who is often a master's level clinician or psychologist, works in the practice as part of the team to provide short-term mental health interventions, such as skills-training in behavioral management. In older children, such interventions are effective in decreasing ADHD and oppositional defiant disorder, although not conduct disorder or anxiety, and in increasing the likelihood of treatment completion.[116] Models of consultation that support primary care providers in the management of children who have been referred for EBT or who have no access to an EBT are under development, often through federally funded projects, such as SAMHSA's Linking Actions to Unmet Needs in Child Health Project (http://media.samhsa.gov/samhsaNewsletter/Volume_18_Number_3/PromotingWellness.aspx).

COMPREHENSIVE TREATMENT PLAN

Clinical emotional, behavioral, or relationship problems commonly cooccur with other developmental delays, especially speech problems. For example, in one mental health program for toddlers, 77% of children also had a developmental delay.[117] A comprehensive treatment plan includes attention to any comorbid conditions, although such combined or serial treatments have not been studied explicitly. Similarly, family mental health problems, such as maternal depression, can reduce the efficacy of parent management training approaches. In older children, effective treatment of maternal depression is effective in reducing child symptoms and fewer diagnoses.[51]

SUMMARY

Very young children can experience significant and impairing mental health problems at rates comparable to older children. Early adversity, including abuse and neglect, increases the risk of early childhood emotional, behavioral, and relationship problems and is associated with developmental, medical, and mental health problems through the lifespan. EBTs can address early childhood mental health problems effectively, reducing symptoms and impairment and even normalizing biological markers. By contrast, the research base examining safety and efficacy of pharmacologic interventions is sparse and inadequate. Systems issues, including graduate medical education systems, access to trained providers of EBTs for very young children, and coding, billing, and payment structures all interfere with access to effective interventions. Not insignificantly, social stigma related to mental health held by parents, primary care providers, and the greater society likely work against access to care for children.

CONCLUSIONS

The existing data demonstrate strong empirical support for family-focused interventions for young children with emotional, behavioral, and relationship problems, especially disruptive behavior disorders and anxiety or trauma exposure. By contrast, the empirical literature examining psychopharmacologic treatment is limited and highlights risks of adverse effects. A number of workforce and other barriers may contribute to the limited access.

LEAD AUTHORS

Mary Margaret Gleason, MD, FAAP
Edward Goldson, MD, FAAP
Michael W. Yogman, MD, FAAP

ABBREVIATIONS

AAP: American Academy of Pediatrics
ADHD: attention-deficit/hyperactivity disorder
EBT: evidence-based treatment
IYS: Incredible Years Series
PCIT: Parent Child Interaction Therapy
SAMHSA: Substance Abuse and Mental Health Services Administration

---

REFERENCES

1. Egger HL, Angold A. Common emotional and behavioral disorders in preschool children: presentation, nosology, and epidemiology. *J Child Psychol Psychiatry*. 2006;47(3-4):313–337

2. Myers SM, Johnson CP; American Academy of Pediatrics Council on Children With Disabilities. Management of children with autism spectrum disorders. *Pediatrics*. 2007;120(5):1162–1182

3. Kim-Cohen J, Arseneault L, Caspi A, Tomás MP, Taylor A, Moffitt TE. Validity of DSM-IV conduct disorder in 4½-5-year-old children: a longitudinal epidemiological study. *Am J Psychiatry*. 2005;162(6):1108–1117

4. Harvey EA, Youngwirth SD, Thakar DA, Errazuriz PA. Predicting attention-deficit/hyperactivity disorder and oppositional defiant disorder from preschool diagnostic assessments. *J Consult Clin Psychol*. 2009;77(2):349–354

5. Wilens TE, Biederman J, Brown S, et al. Psychiatric comorbidity and functioning in clinically referred preschool children and school-age youths with ADHD. *J Am Acad Child Adolesc Psychiatry*. 2002;41(3):262–268

6. Schwebel DC, Speltz ML, Jones K, Bardina P. Unintentional injury in preschool boys with and without early onset of disruptive behavior. *J Pediatr Psychol*. 2002;27(8):727–737

7. Pagliaccio D, Luby J, Gaffrey M, et al. Anomalous functional brain activation following negative mood induction in children with pre-school onset major depression. *Dev Cogn Neurosci*. 2012;2(2):256–267

8. Luby JL, Si X, Belden AC, Tandon M, Spitznagel E. Preschool depression: homotypic continuity and course over 24 months. *Arch Gen Psychiatry*. 2009;66(8):897–905

9. Briggs-Gowan MJ, Carter AS, Bosson-Heenan J, Guyer AE, Horwitz SM. Are infant-toddler social-emotional and behavioral problems transient? *J Am Acad Child Adolesc Psychiatry*. 2006;45(7):849–858

10. Briggs-Gowan MJ, Carter AS. Social-emotional screening status in early childhood predicts elementary school outcomes. *Pediatrics*. 2008;121(5):957–962

11. Lavigne JV, Arend R, Rosenbaum D, Binns HJ, Christoffel KK, Gibbons RD. Psychiatric disorders with onset in the preschool years: I. Stability of diagnoses. *J Am Acad Child Adolesc Psychiatry*. 1998;37(12):1246–1254

12. Leblanc N, Boivin M, Dionne G, et al. The development of hyperactive-impulsive behaviors during the preschool years: the predictive validity of parental assessments. *J Abnorm Child Psychol*. 2008;36(7):977–987

13. Gaffrey MS, Luby JL, Belden AC, Hirshberg JS, Volsch J, Barch DM. Association between depression severity and amygdala reactivity during sad face viewing in depressed preschoolers: an fMRI study. *J Affect Disord*. 2011;129(1-3):364–370

14. Wakschlag LS, Leventhal BL, Briggs-Gowan MJ, et al. Defining the "disruptive" in preschool behavior: what diagnostic observation can teach us. *Clin Child Fam Psychol Rev.* 2005;8(3):183–201

15. Luby JL, Mrakotsky C, Heffelfinger A, Brown K, Hessler M, Spitznagel E. Modification of DSM-IV criteria for depressed preschool children. *Am J Psychiatry.* 2003;160(6):1169–1172

16. Scheeringa MS, Zeanah CH, Myers L, Putnam F. Heart period and variability findings in preschool children with posttraumatic stress symptoms. *Biol Psychiatry.* 2004;55(7):685–691

17. Lahey BB, Applegate B. Validity of DSM-IV ADHD. *J Am Acad Child Adolesc Psychiatry.* 2001;40(5):502–504

18. Luby JL, Belden AC, Pautsch J, Si X, Spitznagel E. The clinical significance of preschool depression: impairment in functioning and clinical markers of the disorder. *J Affect Disord.* 2009;112(1-3):111–119

19. Tyrka AR, Burgers DE, Philip NS, Price LH, Carpenter LL. The neurobiological correlates of childhood adversity and implications for treatment. *Acta Psychiatr Scand.* 2013;128(6):434–447

20. Luking KR, Repovs G, Belden AC, et al. Functional connectivity of the amygdala in early-childhood-onset depression. *J Am Acad Child Adolesc Psychiatry.* 2011;50(10):1027–41.e3

21. Felitti VJ, Anda RF, Nordenberg D, et al. Relationship of childhood abuse and household dysfunction to many of the leading causes of death in adults. The Adverse Childhood Experiences (ACE) Study. *Am J Prev Med.* 1998;14(4):245–258

22. Lahey BB, Pelham WE, Loney J, et al. Three-year predictive validity of DSM-IV attention deficit hyperactivity disorder in children diagnosed at 4-6 years of age. *Am J Psychiatry.* 2004;161(11):2014–2020

23. Wakschlag LS, Leventhal BL, Thomas J, et al. Disruptive behavior disorders and ADHD in preschool children: Characterizing heterotypic continuities for a developmentally informed nosology for DSM-V. In: Rieger D, First MB, Narrow WE, eds. *Age and gender considerations in psychiatric diagnosis: A research agenda for DSM-V.* Arlington, VA: American Psychiatric Publishing, Inc.; 2007:243–258

24. Scheeringa MS. Post -Traumatic Stress Disorder. In: DelCarmen-Wiggins R, Carter A, eds. *Handbook of Infant, Toddler, and Preschool Mental Health Assessment USA.* Oxford, United Kingdom: Oxford Univeristy Press; 2004:377–397

25. Dong M, Giles WH, Felitti VJ, et al. Insights into causal pathways for ischemic heart disease: adverse childhood experiences study. *Circulation.* 2004;110(13):1761–1766

26. Shonkoff JP, Phillips D. *From neurons to neighborhoods: The science of early childhood development.* Washington, D.C.: National Academy Press; 2000

27. Garner AS, Shonkoff JP; Committee on Psychosocial Aspects of Child and Family Health; Committee on Early Childhood, Adoption, and Dependent Care; Section on Developmental and Behavioral Pediatrics. Early childhood adversity, toxic stress, and the role of the pediatrician: translating developmental science into lifelong health. *Pediatrics.* 2012;129(1). Available at: http://pediatrics. aappublications.org/content/129/1/e224

28. Committee On Child Health Financing. Scope of health care benefits for children from birth through age 26. *Pediatrics.* 2012;129(1):185–189

29. Weitzman C, Wegner L; American Academy of Pediatrics, Section on Developmental and Behavioral Pediatrics; Committee on Psychosocial Aspects of Child and Family Health; Council on Early Childhood; Society for Developmental and Behavioral Pediatrics. Promoting optimal development: screening for behavioral and emotional problems. *Pediatrics.* 2015;135(2):384–395

30. Mendelsohn AL, Valdez PT, Flynn V, et al. Use of videotaped interactions during pediatric well-child care: impact at 33 months on parenting and on child development. *J Dev Behav Pediatr.* 2007;28(3):206–212

31. Scheeringa MS, Salloum A, Arnberger RA, Weems CF, Amaya-Jackson L, Cohen JA. Feasibility and effectiveness of cognitive-behavioral therapy for posttraumatic stress disorder in preschool children: two case reports. *J Trauma Stress.* 2007;20(4):631–636

32. Sonuga-Barke EJ, Daley D, Thompson M, Laver-Bradbury C, Weeks A. Parent-based therapies for preschool attention-deficit/hyperactivity disorder: a randomized, controlled trial with a community sample. *J Am Acad Child Adolesc Psychiatry.* 2001;40(4):402–408

33. Gleason MM, Egger HL, Emslie GJ, et al. Psychopharmacological treatment for very young children: contexts and guidelines. *J Am Acad Child Adolesc Psychiatry.* 2007;46(12):1532–1572

34. Charach A, Dashti B, Carson P, et al; Agency for Healthcare Research and Quality. Attention deficit hyperactivity disorder: effectiveness of treatment in at-risk preschoolers; long-term effectiveness in all ages; and variability in prevalence, diagnosis, and treatment. *Comparitive Effectiveness Review.* 2011;44: AHRQ Publication No. 12-EHC003-EF. Available at: www.effectivehealthcare.ahrq.gov/ehc/products/191/818/CER44-ADHD_20111021.pdf. Accessed October 17, 2016

35. Thompson MJ, Laver-Bradbury C, Ayres M, et al. A small-scale randomized controlled trial of the revised new forest parenting programme for preschoolers with attention deficit hyperactivity disorder. *Eur Child Adolesc Psychiatry.* 2009;18(10):605–616

36. Riddle MA, Yershova K, Lazzaretto D, Paykina N, Yenokyan G, Greenhill L, et al The preschool attention-deficit/hyperactivity disorder treatment study (PATS) 6-year follow-up. *J Am Acad Child Adolesc Psychiatry.* 2013;52(3):264–278.e2

37. Hood KK, Eyberg SM. Outcomes of parent-child interaction therapy: mothers' reports of maintenance three to six years after treatment. *J Clin Child Adolesc Psychol.* 2003;32(3):419–429

38. Pediatric OCD Treatment Study (POTS) Team. Cognitive-behavior therapy, sertraline, and their combination for children and adolescents with obsessive-compulsive disorder: the Pediatric OCD Treatment Study (POTS) randomized controlled trial. *JAMA.* 2004;292(16):1969–1976

39. Wolraich M, Brown L, Brown RT, et al; Subcommittee on Attention-Deficit/ Hyperactivity Disorder; Steering Committee on Quality Improvement and Management. ADHD: clinical practice guideline for the diagnosis, evaluation, and treatment of attention-deficit/hyperactivity disorder in children and adolescents. *Pediatrics*. 2011;128(5):1007–1022

40. Lieberman AF, Van Horn P, Ippen CG. Toward evidence-based treatment: child-parent psychotherapy with preschoolers exposed to marital violence. *J Am Acad Child Adolesc Psychiatry*. 2005;44(12):1241–1248

41. Fraiberg S, Adelson E, Shapiro V. Ghosts in the nursery. A psychoanalytic approach to the problems of impaired infant-mother relationships. *J Am Acad Child Psychiatry*. 1975;14(3):387–421

42. Cicchetti D, Rogosch FA, Toth SL, Sturge-Apple ML. Normalizing the development of cortisol regulation in maltreated infants through preventive interventions. *Dev Psychopathol*. 2011;23(3):789–800

43. Toth SL, Rogosch FA, Manly JT, Cicchetti D. The efficacy of toddler-parent psychotherapy to reorganize attachment in the young offspring of mothers with major depressive disorder: a randomized preventive trial. *J Consult Clin Psychol*. 2006;74(6):1006–1016

44. Lieberman AF, Weston DR, Pawl JH. Preventive intervention and outcome with anxiously attached dyads. *Child Dev*. 1991;62(1):199–209

45. Dozier M, Peloso E, Lewis E, Laurenceau JP, Levine S. Effects of an attachment-based intervention on the cortisol production of infants and toddlers in foster care. *Dev Psychopathol*. 2008;20(3):845–859

46. Bernard K, Dozier M, Bick J, Lewis-Morrarty E, Lindhiem O, Carlson E. Enhancing attachment organization among maltreated children: results of a randomized clinical trial. *Child Dev*. 2012;83(2):623–636

47. Fisher PA, Burraston B, Pears K. The early intervention foster care program: permanent placement outcomes from a randomized trial. *Child Maltreat*. 2005;10(1):61–71

48. Van Zeijl J, Mesman J, Van IJzendoorn MH, et al. Attachment-based intervention for enhancing sensitive discipline in mothers of 1- to 3-year-old children at risk for externalizing behavior problems: a randomized controlled trial. *J Consult Clin Psychol*. 2006;74(6):994–1005

49. Murray L, Cooper PJ, Wilson A, Romaniuk H. Controlled trial of the short- and long-term effect of psychological treatment of post-partum depression: 2. Impact on the mother-child relationship and child outcome. *Br J Psychiatry*. 2003;182(5):420–427

50. Gunlicks ML, Weissman MM. Change in child psychopathology with improvement in parental depression: a systematic review. *J Am Acad Child Adolesc Psychiatry*. 2008;47(4):379–389

51. Weissman MM, Pilowsky DJ, Wickramaratne PJ, et al; STAR*D-Child Team. Remissions in maternal depression and child psychopathology: a STAR*D-child report. *JAMA*. 2006;295(12):1389–1398

52. Beardslee WR, Ayoub C, Avery MW, Watts CL, O'Carroll KL. Family Connections: an approach for strengthening early care systems in facing depression and adversity. *Am J Orthopsychiatry*. 2010;80(4):482–495

53. Keenan K, Wakschlag LS. Can a valid diagnosis of disruptive behavior disorder be made in preschool children? *Am J Psychiatry*. 2002;159(3):351–358

54. SAMHSA. National registry of evidence-based programs and practices. Available at: http://www.samhsa.gov/nrepp. Accessed October 17, 2016

55. Bodenmann G, Cina A, Ledermann T, Sanders MR. The efficacy of the Triple P-Positive Parenting Program in improving parenting and child behavior: a comparison with two other treatment conditions. *Behav Res Ther*. 2008;46(4):411–427

56. Webster-Stratton CH, Reid MJ, Beauchaine T. Combining parent and child training for young children with ADHD. *J Clin Child Adolesc Psychol*. 2011;40(2):191–203

57. Abikoff HB, Thompson MJ, Laver-Bradbury C, et al. Parent training for preschool ADHD: A randomized controlled trial of specialized and generic programs. *J Child Psychol Psychiatry*. 2015;56(6):618–631

58. Thomas R, Zimmer-Gembeck MJ. Behavioral outcomes of Parent-Child Interaction Therapy and Triple P-Positive Parenting Program: a review and meta-analysis. *J Abnorm Child Psychol*. 2007;35(3):475–495

59. Sanders MR, Baker S, Turner KM. A randomized controlled trial evaluating the efficacy of Triple P Online with parents of children with early-onset conduct problems. *Behav Res Ther*. 2012;50(11):675–684

60. Bor W, Sanders MR, Markie-Dadds C. The effects of the Triple P-positive Parenting Program on preschool children with co-occurring disruptive behavior and attentional/hyperactive difficulties. *J Abnorm Child Psychol*.2002;30(6):571–587

61. Markie-Dadds C, Sanders MR. Self-directed Triple P (Positive Parenting Program) for mothers with children at-risk of developing conduct problems. *Behav Cogn Psychother*. 2006;34(3):259–275

62. Comer JS, Puliafico AC, Aschenbrand SG, et al. A pilot feasibility evaluation of the CALM Program for anxiety disorders in early childhood. *J Anxiety Disord*. 2012;26(1):40–49

63. Hirshfeld-Becker DR, Masek B, Henin A, et al. Cognitive behavioral therapy for 4- to 7-year-old children with anxiety disorders: a randomized clinical trial. *J Consult Clin Psychol*. 2010;78:498–510

64. Matos M, Bauermeister JJ, Bernal G. Parent-child interaction therapy for Puerto Rican preschool children with ADHD and behavior problems: a pilot efficacy study. *Fam Process*. 2009;48(2):232–252

65. Fernandez MA, Butler AM, Eyberg SM. Treatment outcome for low socioeconomic status African American families in parent-child interaction therapy: A pilot study. *Child Fam Behav Ther*. 2011;33(1):32–48

66. Webster-Stratton C, Rinaldi J, Jamila MR. Long-term outcomes of Incredible Years parenting program: Predictors of adolescent adjustment. *Child Adolesc Ment Health*. 2011;16(1):38–46

67. Gridley N, Hutchings J, Baker-Henningham H. The Incredible Years Parent-Toddler Programme and parental language: a randomised controlled trial. *Child Care Health Dev.* 2015;41(1):103–111

68. Chaffin M, Funderburk B, Bard D, Valle LA, Gurwitch R. A combined motivation and parent-child interaction therapy package reduces child welfare recidivism in a randomized dismantling field trial. *J Consult Clin Psychol.* 2011;79(1):84–95

69. Forehand R, Parent J, Sonuga-Barke E, Peisch VD, Long N, Abikoff HB. Which type of parent training works best for preschoolers with comorbid ADHD and ODD? A secondary analysis of a randomized controlled trial comparing generic and specialized programs. *J Abnorm Child Psychol.* 2016;44(8):1503–1513

70. Cohen JA, Mannarino AP. A treatment outcome study for sexually abused preschool children: initial findings. *J Am Acad Child Adolesc Psychiatry.* 1996;35(1):42–50

71. Scheeringa MS, Weems CF, Cohen JA, Amaya-Jackson L, Guthrie D. Trauma-focused cognitive-behavioral therapy for posttraumatic stress disorder in three-through six year-old children: a randomized clinical trial. *J Child Psychol Psychiatry.* 2011;52(8): 853–860

72. Cohen JA, Mannarino AP. A treatment study for sexually abused preschool children: outcome during a one-year follow-up. *J Am Acad Child Adolesc Psychiatry.* 1997;36(9):1228–1235

73. Lieberman AF, Ghosh Ippen C, VAN Horn P. Child-parent psychotherapy: 6-month follow-up of a randomized controlled trial. *J Am Acad Child Adolesc Psychiatry.* 2006;45(8):913–918

74. Luby J, Lenze S, Tillman R. A novel early intervention for preschool depression: findings from a pilot randomized controlled trial. *J Child Psychol Psychiatry.* 2012;53(3):313–322

75. Connolly SD, Bernstein GA; Work Group on Quality Issues. Practice parameter for the assessment and treatment of children and adolescents with anxiety disorders. *J Am Acad Child Adolesc Psychiatry.* 2007;46(2): 267–283

76. Shepard SA, Dickstein S. Preventive intervention for early childhood behavioral problems: an ecological perspective. *Child Adolesc Psychiatr Clin N Am.* 2009;18(3):687–706

77. Nock MK, Ferriter C. Parent management of attendance and adherence in child and adolescent therapy: a conceptual and empirical review. *Clin Child Fam Psychol Rev.* 2005;8(2):149–166

78. Olfson M, Crystal S, Huang C, Gerhard T. Trends in antipsychotic drug use by very young, privately insured children. *J Am Acad Child Adolesc Psychiatry.* 2010;49(1):13–23

79. Wilson DO. Child's ordeal shows risks of psychosis drugs for young. *New York Times.* September 2, 2010:A1.

80. Zuvekas SH, Vitiello B, Norquist GS. Recent trends in stimulant medication use among U.S. children. *Am J Psychiatry.* 2006;163(4):579–585

81. Zito JM, Safer DJ, Valluri S, Gardner JF, Korelitz JJ, Mattison DR. Psychotherapeutic medication prevalence in Medicaid-insured preschoolers. *J Child Adolesc Psychopharmacol.* 2007;17(2):195–203

82. Cooper WO, Hickson GB, Fuchs C, Arbogast PG, Ray WA. New users of antipsychotic medications among children enrolled in TennCare. *Arch Pediatr Adolesc Med.* 2004;158(8):753–759

83. Fontanella CA, Hiance DL, Phillips GS, Bridge JA, Campo J. Trends in psychotropic medication utilization for medicaid-enrolled preschool children. *J Child Fam Stud.* 2014;23(4):617–631

84. Rappley MD, Mullan PB, Alvarez FJ, Eneli IU, Wang J, Gardiner JC. Diagnosis of attention-deficit/hyperactivity disorder and use of psychotropic medication in very young children. *Arch Pediatr Adolesc Med.* 1999;153(10):1039–1045

85. Rappley MD, Eneli IU, Mullan PB, et al. Patterns of psychotropic medication use in very young children with attention-deficit hyperactivity disorder. *J Dev Behav Pediatr.* 2002;23(1):23–30

86. Greenhill L, Kollins S, Abikoff H, et al. Efficacy and safety of immediate-release methylphenidate treatment for preschoolers with ADHD. *J Am Acad Child Adolesc Psychiatry.* 2006;45(11):1284–1293

87. Kratochvil CJ, Vaughan BS, Stoner JA, et al. A double-blind, placebo-controlled study of atomoxetine in young children with ADHD. *Pediatrics.* 2011;127(4). Available at: http://pediatrics.aappublications.org/content/127/4/e862

88. Egger H. A perilous disconnect: antipsychotic drug use in very young children. *J Am Acad Child Adolesc Psychiatry.* 2010;49(1):3–6

89. Correll CU, Carlson HE. Endocrine and metabolic adverse effects of psychotropic medications in children and adolescents. *J Am Acad Child Adolesc Psychiatry.* 2006;45(7):771–791

90. Luby J, Mrakotsky C, Stalets MM, et al. Risperidone in preschool children with autistic spectrum disorders: an investigation of safety and efficacy. *J Child Adolesc Psychopharmacol.* 2006;16(5):575–587

91. Horwitz SM, Leaf PJ, Leventhal JM. Identification of psychosocial problems in pediatric primary care: do family attitudes make a difference? *Arch Pediatr Adolesc Med.* 1998;152(4):367–371

92. Horwitz SM, Gary LC, Briggs-Gowan MJ, Carter AS; Do Needs Drive Services Use in Young Children. Do needs drive services use in young children? *Pediatrics.* 2003;112(6 Pt 1):1373–1378

93. Accreditation Council for Graduate Medical Education. ACGME program requirements for graduate medical education in Pediatrics. Available at: www.acgme.org/Portals/0/PFAssets/ProgramRequirements/320_pediatrics_2016.pdf. Accessed October 17, 2016

94. Committee on Psychosocial Aspects of Child and Family Health and Task Force on Mental Health. Policy statement--The future of pediatrics: mental health competencies for pediatric primary care. *Pediatrics.* 2009;124(1):410–421

95. Jensen PS, Goldman E, Offord D, et al. Overlooked and underserved: "action signs" for identifying children with unmet mental health needs. *Pediatrics.* 2011;128(5):970–979

96. Cohen J, Oser C, Quigley K Making it happen: overcoming barriers to

providing infant-early childhood mental health. Available at: www.zerotothree.org/resources/511-making-it-happen-overcoming-barriers-to-providing-infant-early-childhood-mental-health

97. Thomas CR, Holzer CE III. The continuing shortage of child and adolescent psychiatrists. *J Am Acad Child Adolesc Psychiatry.* 2006;45(9):1023–1031

98. Kautz C, Mauch D, Smith SA. *Reimbursement of Mental Health Services in Primary Care Settings.* Rockville, MD: Center for Mental Health Services, Substance Abuse and Mental Health Services Administration; 2008

99. The Lewin Group. *Accessing Children's Mental Health Services in Massachusetts: Workforce Capacity Assessment.* Boston, MA: Blue Cross; 2009

100. Jellinek M, Little M. Supporting child psychiatric services using current managed care approaches: you can't get there from here. *Arch Pediatr Adolesc Med.* 1998;152(4):321–326

101. Kelleher KJ, Campo JV, Gardner WP. Management of pediatric mental disorders in primary care: where are we now and where are we going? *Curr Opin Pediatr.* 2006;18(6):649–653

102. American Academy of Child and Adolescent Psychiatry Committee on Health Care Access and Economics Task Force on Mental Health. Improving mental health services in primary care: reducing administrative and financial barriers to access and collaboration. *Pediatrics.* 2009;123(4):1248–1251

103. Zero to Three. *Diagnostic Classification of Mental Health and Developmental Disorders in Infants and Young*

Children. Washington, DC: Zero to Three; in press

104. dosReis S, Barksdale CL, Sherman A, Maloney K, Charach A. Stigmatizing experiences of parents of children with a new diagnosis of ADHD. *Psychiatric Services.* 2010;61(6):811–816

105. Harwood MD, O'Brien KA, Carter CG, Eyberg SM. Mental health services for preschool children in primary care: a survey of maternal attitudes and beliefs. *J Pediatr Psychol.* 2009;34(7):760–768

106. Pescosolido BA. Culture, children, and mental health treatment: special section on the national stigma study-children. *Psychiatr Serv.* 2007;58(5):611–612

107. Pescosolido BA, Jensen PS, Martin JK, Perry BL, Olafsdottir S, Fettes D. Public knowledge and assessment of child mental health problems: findings from the National Stigma Study-Children. *J Am Acad Child Adolesc Psychiatry.* 2008;47(3):339–349

108. Sayal K, Tischler V, Coope C, et al. Parental help-seeking in primary care for child and adolescent mental health concerns: qualitative study. *Br J Psychiatry.* 2010;197(6):476–481

109. Steele MM, Lochrie AS, Roberts MC. Physician identification and management of psychosocial problems in primary care. *J Clin Psychol Med Settings.* 2010;17(2):103–115

110. American Academy of Pediatrics Council on Children with Disabilities. Care coordination in the medical home: integrating health and related systems of care for children with special health care needs. *Pediatrics.* 2005;116(5):1238–1244

111. Wissow L, Anthony B, Brown J, et al. A common factors approach to improving the mental health capacity of pediatric primary care. *Adm Policy Ment Health.* 2008;35(4):305–318

112. Foy JM, Kelleher KJ, Laraque D; American Academy of Pediatrics Task Force on Mental Health. Enhancing pediatric mental health care: strategies for preparing a primary care practice. *Pediatrics.* 2010;125(suppl 3):S87–S108

113. Berkovits MD, O'Brien KA, Carter CG, Eyberg SM. Early identification and intervention for behavior problems in primary care: a comparison of two abbreviated versions of parent-child interaction therapy. *Behav Ther.* 2010;41(3):375–387

114. Perrin EC, Sheldrick RC, McMenamy JM, Henson BS, Carter AS. Improving parenting skills for families of young children in pediatric settings: a randomized clinical trial. *JAMA Pediatr.* 2014;168(1):16–24

115. Hilt RJ, McDonell MG, Thompson J, et al. Telephone consultation assisting primary care child mental health. In: *55th National Meeting of the American Academy of Child and Adolescent Psychiatry;* October 28–November 2, 2008; Chicago, IL.

116. Kolko DJ, Campo JV, Kilbourne AM, Kelleher K. Doctor-office collaborative care for pediatric behavioral problems: a preliminary clinical trial. *Arch Pediatr Adolesc Med.* 2012;166(3):224–231

117. Fox RA, Keller KM, Grede PL, Bartosz AM. A mental health clinic for toddlers with developmental delays and behavior problems. *Res Dev Disabil.* 2007;28(2):119–129

CLINICAL REPORT   Guidance for the Clinician in Rendering Pediatric Care

American Academy
of Pediatrics

DEDICATED TO THE HEALTH OF ALL CHILDREN™

Evaluation and Management of Children and Adolescents With Acute Mental Health or Behavioral Problems. Part I: Common Clinical Challenges of Patients With Mental Health and/or Behavioral Emergencies

Thomas H. Chun, MD, MPH, FAAP, Sharon E. Mace, MD, FAAP, FACEP, Emily R. Katz, MD, FAAP, AMERICAN ACADEMY OF PEDIATRICS, COMMITTEE ON PEDIATRIC EMERGENCY MEDICINE, AND AMERICAN COLLEGE OF EMERGENCY PHYSICIANS, PEDIATRIC EMERGENCY MEDICINE COMMITTEE

INTRODUCTION

Mental health problems are among the leading contributors to the global burden of disease.[1] Unfortunately, pediatric populations are not spared of mental health problems. In the United States, 21% to 23% of children and adolescents have a diagnosable mental health or substance use disorder.[2,3] Among patients of emergency departments (EDs), 70% screen positive for at least 1 mental health disorder,[4] 23% meet criteria for 2 or more mental health concerns,[5] 45% have a mental health problem resulting in impaired psychosocial functioning,[5] and 10% of adolescents endorse significant levels of psychiatric distress at the time of their ED visit.[6] In pediatric primary care settings, the reported prevalence of mental health and behavioral disorders is between 12% to 22% of children and adolescents.[7]

Although the American Academy of Pediatrics (AAP) has published a policy statement on mental health competencies and a Mental Health Toolkit for pediatric primary care providers, no such guidelines or resources exist for clinicians who care for pediatric mental health emergencies.[8,9] This clinical report supports the 2006 joint policy statement of the AAP and American College of Emergency Physicians (ACEP) on pediatric mental health emergencies, with the goal of addressing the knowledge gaps in this area.[10,11] The report is written primarily from the perspective of ED clinicians, but it is intended for all clinicians who care for children and adolescents with acute mental health and behavioral problems.

Recent epidemiologic studies of mental health visits have revealed a rapid burgeoning of both ED and primary care visits.[12–20] An especially problematic trend is the increase in "boarding" of psychiatric patients in

DOI: 10.1542/peds.2016-1570

PEDIATRICS (ISSN Numbers: Print, 0031-4005; Online, 1098-4275).

Copyright © 2016 by the American Academy of Pediatrics

FINANCIAL DISCLOSURE: The authors have indicated they do not have a financial relationship relevant to this article to disclose.

FUNDING: No external funding.

POTENTIAL CONFLICT OF INTEREST: The authors have indicated they have no potential conflicts of interest to disclose.

To cite: Chun TH, Mace SE, AAP FACEP, Katz ER. Evaluation and Management of Children and Adolescents With Acute Mental Health or Behavioral Problems. Part I: Common Clinical Challenges of Patients With Mental Health and/or Behavioral Emergencies. *Pediatrics.* 2016;138(3):e20161570

the ED and inpatient pediatric beds (ie, extended stays lasting days or even weeks). Although investigation of boarding practices is still in its infancy, the ACEP[21] and the American Medical Association[22] have both expressed concern about it, because it significantly taxes the functioning and efficiency of both the ED and hospital, and mental health services may not be available in the ED.[23-26]

In addition, compared with other pediatric care settings, ED patients are known to be at higher risk of mental health disorders, including depression,[27,28] anxiety,[29] posttraumatic stress disorder,[30] and substance abuse.[31] These mental health conditions may be unrecognized not only by treating clinicians but also by the child/adolescent and his or her parents.[32-36] A similar phenomenon has been described with suicidal patients. Individuals who have committed suicide frequently visited a health care provider in the months preceding their death.[37,38] Although a minority of suicidal patients present with some form of self-harm, many have vague somatic complaints (eg, headache, gastrointestinal tract distress, back pain, concern for a sexually transmitted infection) masking their underlying mental health condition.[34-36]

Despite studies demonstrating moderate agreement between emergency physicians and psychiatrists in the assessment and management of patients with mental health problems,[39,40] ED clinicians frequently cite lack of training and confidence in their abilities as barriers to caring for patients with mental health emergencies.[41-44] Another study of emergency medicine and pediatric emergency medicine training programs found that formal training in psychiatric problems is not required nor offered by most programs.[45] Pediatric primary care providers report similar

barriers to caring for their patients with mental health problems.[46,47]

Part I of this clinical report focuses on the issues relevant to patients presenting to the ED with a mental health chief complaint and covers the following topics:

- Medical clearance of pediatric psychiatric patients

- Suicidal ideation and suicide attempts

- Involuntary hospitalization

- Restraint of the agitated patient

  o Verbal restraint

  o Chemical restraint

  o Physical restraint

- Coordination with the medical home

Part II discusses challenging patients with primarily medical or indeterminate presentations, in which the contribution of an underlying mental health condition may be unclear or a complicating factor, including:

- Somatic symptom and related disorders

- Adverse effects to psychiatric medications

  o Antipsychotic adverse effects

  o Neuroleptic malignant syndrome

  o Serotonin syndrome

- Children with special needs in the ED (autism spectrum and developmental disorders)

- Mental health screening in the ED

An executive summary of this clinical report can be found at www.pediatrics.org/cgi/doi/10.1542/peds.2016-1571.

MEDICAL CLEARANCE OF PEDIATRIC PSYCHIATRIC PATIENTS

Background

Medical clearance can be defined as the process of excluding acute

medical illnesses or injuries in patients presenting with psychiatric complaints. Concern that medical illness may be the underlying cause of a psychiatric problem has led some to suggest "that emergency patients with psychiatric complaints receive a full medical evaluation."[48] Medical clearance originates from the perspective that an ED evaluation of a psychiatric patient may be the only opportunity to diagnose underlying illnesses or injuries that could result in morbidity or mortality because resources for diagnosing and treating medical conditions may not be readily available in some psychiatric facilities. In addition, many psychiatric complaints and disorders can be exacerbated or precipitated by medical illness,[49] and some psychiatric patients may have unmet medical needs.[50-52]

Medical Diseases in ED Psychiatric Patients

Previous studies of medical conditions in ED psychiatric patients have been almost exclusively conducted with adults and have had highly variable findings. Past reports have found underlying medical problems in 19% to 63% of ED psychiatric patients.[53-55] Studies of adults admitted to psychiatric units after an ED medical evaluation have had similarly disparate results. Some have reported missed medical conditions in up to half of patients,[53,56] including diabetes, uremic and hepatic encephalopathy, pneumonia, urinary tract infections, and sepsis,[57] but another found that only 4% (12 of 298) needed treatment of a medical condition within 24 hours of admission to the psychiatric unit.[58] To address these concerns, some have suggested a standardized evaluation and documentation of the ED medical evaluation.[59] Major limitations of these studies are that they are from older literature, and they did not include children. More recent adult and pediatric studies, discussed later, suggest that significant rates of medical morbidity in psychiatric patients may be less likely.

Some authors argue that it is not possible to rule out all potential medical etiologies for psychiatric symptoms and believe that the role of the ED evaluation is to determine whether the patient is "medically stable" rather than "medically cleared."[60] Although the concept of "medical stability," which can be defined as the lack of medical conditions requiring acute evaluation and/or treatment, is gaining traction, for the purposes of this discussion, the term "medical clearance" will be used. A growing body of adult and pediatric studies suggest that an ED patient's history, physical examination, and vital signs provide important data for determining the appropriate medical evaluation for a psychiatric patient. These findings support the 2006 ACEP policy statement, which recommends "focused medical assessment" for ED psychiatric patients, in which laboratory testing is obtained on the basis of history and physical examination rather than a predetermined battery of tests for all patients with psychiatric complaints.[61] When ED resource utilization and the cost of medical screening evaluations for pediatric psychiatric patients are considered, additional questions are raised about such evaluations and whether the ED is the optimal site for them.[62,63]

The Goals of Medical Clearance

Medical clearance of psychiatric patients focuses on determining whether the patient's behavioral or psychiatric signs and symptoms are caused or exacerbated by an underlying medical condition and whether there are medical conditions that would benefit from acute treatment in the ED. Given the vast number of medical illnesses that can masquerade as a behavioral problem or psychiatric disorder,

a comprehensive list of such conditions is beyond the scope of this article. Table 1 focuses on medical conditions that can be evaluated within the context and time frame of an ED visit. Examples of medical conditions requiring ED treatment includes suturing, wound or injury care, and treatment of an overdose. In addition, some psychiatric patients may have comorbidities that are not contributing to their behavioral or psychiatric complaints but would benefit from ED care, such as asthma or diabetes.[58]

Key elements for detecting underlying medical condition(s) include careful assessment of abnormal vital signs, a complete history and physical examination, with particular attention to the neurologic, cardiac, and respiratory systems.[64] Various screening tools have been developed to assist in the medical clearance of psychiatric patients in the ED,[60,65] although these authors also stress the importance of an adequate history and physical examination and do not mandate laboratory or other investigations.[65] After medical clearance has been performed, the AAP and ACEP support the development of transport protocols to definitive psychiatric treatment facilities for EDs that transfer patients with mental health care needs.[10,11]

Diagnostic Laboratory Testing and Medical Clearance

In 1 study of emergency physicians, "routine testing" was performed in 35% of respondents, with 16% of the testing performed because it was ED protocol and 84% of the testing performed at request of the mental health service. Of those with protocol testing, the most frequently ordered tests were urine toxicology screen (86%), serum alcohol (85%), complete blood cell count (56%), electrolytes (56%), blood urea nitrogen (45%), creatinine (40%), serum toxicology screen (31%), and

electrocardiogram (18%).[66] Other commonly obtained laboratory evaluations for medical clearance include testing for pregnancy and sexually transmitted infections.

Recently, the utility of routine medical screening tests has been questioned. In contrast to the older literature, more contemporary studies are finding much lower rates of unsuspected, clinically emergent, or urgent laboratory abnormalities. Two studies of adult ED patients with psychiatric complaints found low rates of clinically significant abnormalities on routine laboratory testing,[55,67] the majority (94%) of which were clinically suspected on the basis of the patient's history and physical examination.[55] Similar results have been reported in admitted adult psychiatric patients after an ED evaluation. One study of 250 psychiatric inpatients found a mean of 27.7 tests were ordered per patient, with only 4% (11 of 250) having "important" medical problems discovered and less than 1 test in 50 resulting in any clinically useful information.[10] Another study identified only 1 patient of 519 (0.2%) with an abnormal laboratory test result that would have changed ED management or patient disposition.[68]

Similar results have emerged for ED pediatric psychiatric patients. Several studies have found little to no utility for routine urine drug testing. Shihabuddin et al evaluated such testing in 547 patients presenting with a psychiatric complaint. A positive result was found in 20.8% of patients, half of which were suspected on the basis of the patients' reported substance use history. Urine drug testing resulted in no changes in patient management, and all were medically cleared.[69] Fortu et al examined 652 (385 routine and 267 medically indicated) urine toxicology screens.[70] For the routine toxicology screens, only 5% were positive, and there were no changes

TABLE 1 Medical Disorders That Can Present as a Psychiatric Disorder or Behavioral Problem[a]

Neurologic (CNS) Diseases
   Stroke/transient ischemic attacks
   Hemorrhage: intracerebral, subdural, subarachnoid, epidural
   CNS vascular: aneurysms, venous thrombosis, ischemia, vertebrobasilar insufficiency
   CNS malignancy/tumors
   CNS trauma: primary injury, secondary injury or sequelae of head trauma
   CNS infections: meningitis, encephalitis, abscess (brain, epidural, spinal), HIV, syphilis
   Congenital malformations
   Hydrocephalus
   Seizures
   Headaches including migraines
   Neurodegenerative disorders: multiple sclerosis, Huntington chorea
   Tuberous sclerosis
   Delirium ("ICU psychosis")
Metabolic, Endocrine, and Electrolyte Disturbances
   Hyponatremia
   Hypocalcemia
   Hypoglycemia
   Hyperglycemia
   Ketoacidosis
   Uremia
   Hyperammonemia
   Inborn errors of metabolism: lipid storage diseases, Gaucher disease, Niemann-Pick disease
   Thyroid disease: hyperthyroidism, thyroid storm, hypothyroidism
   Adrenal disease: Addison disease, Cushing disease
   Pituitary: hypopituitarism
   Parathyroid disease: hypoparathyroidism, hyperparathyroidism
   Pheochromocytoma
Respiratory
   Hypoxia
   Hypercarbia/hypercapnia
   Respiratory failure
Medications
   Drug withdrawal: alcohol, amphetamines, barbiturates, benzodiazepines, cocaine, psychiatric
      medications
   Drug overdose:
      Drugs of abuse: phencyclidine, heroin, cocaine, marijuana, MDMA (3,4-methylenedioxy-
         methamphetamine), LSD (lysergic acid diethylamide), alcohol, amphetamines, "bath salts"
      Prescription drugs: steroids, birth control, antihypertensives, statins, anticonvulsants,
         barbiturates, benzodiazepines, opioids, anticholinergics, antibiotics, antifungal agents, antiviral
         agents, asthmatic medications, muscle relaxants, gastrointestinal tract drugs, anesthetics,
         anticholinergics, cardiac medications (such as digoxin), decongestants, antiarrhythmics,
         immunosuppressives
      Drugs for psychiatric patients: antidepressants, antipsychotics, lithium
Hematologic/Oncologic
   Malignancies
   Tumors
   Paraneoplastic syndromes
Inflammatory/Rheumatologic
   Sarcoidosis
   Systemic lupus erythematosus
Toxins
   Carbon monoxide
   Lead poisoning
   Organophosphates
   Volatile substances
Other
   Fever
   Child maltreatment

[a] This is not an exhaustive inclusive list but one that provides examples of the many diseases/conditions and drugs/medications that can masquerade as a psychiatric/behavioral disorder.

in management and no significant differences in disposition between those with positive and negative toxicology screens. Tenenbein reviewed 3 retrospective case studies of urine drug testing in children and concluded, "The emergency drug screen is unlikely to impact significantly upon the management of the patient in the emergency department."[71]

Santiago et al prospectively studied 208 children and adolescents presenting to the ED with psychiatric conditions.[62] Half of the patients underwent medical testing, 26% (55 patients) were medically indicated (ie, because of clinical suspicions based on the elicited history and physical examination), and 24% (54 patients) were obtained at the request of the mental health consultant. Only 3 patients had laboratory abnormalities that required further medical intervention, all of which were suspected on the basis of patient's presenting history and physical examination. Among patients for whom "routine testing" was performed, 9% (5 patients) had unsuspected abnormalities, none of which altered ED patient management.

Two recent studies of ED pediatric psychiatric patients have raised similar questions about the utility of routine medical testing and of "medical clearance" evaluations. Donofrio et al investigated the utility of extensive laboratory testing of these patients.[72] Of 1082 eligible patients, more than 68% had multiple laboratory testing, including urine toxicology, urinalysis, and blood tests for complete blood cell count, electrolytes, hepatic transferases, thyroid stimulating hormone, and syphilis. Of these tested patients, only 7 had a laboratory abnormality that resulted in a disposition change. Not only was the number of disposition changing laboratory abnormalities low, only 1 of these abnormalities·

was not suspected from the patient's history and physical examination. Santillanes et al studied all patients referred to their ED for medical screening clearance by a mobile psychiatric crisis team.[63] All patients had been placed on an involuntary psychiatric hold. Among 789 patients, 9.1% met criteria for a medical screening examination (ie, altered mental status, ingestion, hanging, traumatic injury, sexual assault, or medical complaints), and only 1.2% (9 patients) were admitted for medical reasons. Of these 9 patients, only 2 did not meet criteria for a medical screening evaluation, although both patients' conditions (possible disorientation and urinary tract infection in an HIV-positive patient) were suspected on the basis of a basic history and physical examination.

Diagnostic Radiology Testing and Medical Clearance

All studies of radiographic evaluation of psychiatric patients have been conducted with adults. Although central nervous system (CNS) abnormalities such as oligodendroglioma, glioblastoma, meningioma, intracerebral cysts, and hydrocephalus can present with primarily psychiatric symptoms,[73] other studies have found low rates of clinically significant findings on computed tomography (CT) scan. In 1 study of 127 young military recruits with new-onset psychosis, none had clinically significant findings on brain CT scans.[74] In another analysis of new-onset acute psychosis in patients admitted to a psychiatric unit, only 1.2% had clinically significant findings.[75] A larger study of 397 patients with a psychiatric presentation and no focal neurologic findings detected specific abnormalities in 5%, all of which had no relevance to the patient's condition. The pretest probability of a space occupying lesion or any relevant abnormality was no greater than finding one

in the general population.[76] These findings have led some authors to question the utility of routine brain CT scans.[64] Given the concerns about the long-term effects of radiation exposure on pediatric patients,[77-79] the utility of routine brain CT in children and adolescents is, at best, unclear.

Summary

The current body of literature supports focused medical assessments for ED psychiatric patients, in which laboratory and radiographic testing is obtained on the basis of a patient's history and physical examination. Routine diagnostic testing generally is low yield, costly, and unlikely to be of value or affect the disposition or management of ED psychiatric patients. When patients are clinically stable (ie, alert, cooperative, normal vital signs, with noncontributory history and physical examination and psychiatric symptoms), the ACEP states that routine laboratory testing need not be performed as part of the ED assessment.[61] If a discrepancy occurs between the ED and psychiatry clinicians regarding the appropriate ED medical evaluation of a psychiatric patient, direct communication between the ED and psychiatry attending physicians may be helpful. For patients with concerning findings on history and/or physical examination (eg, altered mental status or unexplained vital signs abnormalities) or with new-onset or acute changes in psychiatric symptoms, a careful evaluation for possible underlying medical conditions may be important.

SUICIDAL IDEATION AND SUICIDE ATTEMPTS

For an extended discussion on the assessment and management of suicidal adolescents, please refer to the AAP clinical report on suicide.[80]

Epidemiology and Risk Factors

Suicide is the third leading cause of death among people 10 to 24 years of age, accounting for more than 4000 deaths per year.[81] Although only a small percentage of suicide attempts lead to medical attention,[82] they nonetheless account for a significant number of ED visits.[83] Suicidal ideation in the absence of a suicide attempt is also a common chief complaint in pediatric EDs.

Approximately 16% of teenagers report having seriously considered suicide in the past year, 12.8% report having planned a suicide attempt, and 7.8% report having attempted suicide in the past year. Females are more likely to consider and attempt suicide, but males are more than 5 times more likely to die by suicide. The higher fatality rate among males is primarily accounted for by their use of more lethal means: males are more likely to attempt suicide via firearms and hanging, whereas females are more likely to attempt via overdose.[82]

American Indian/Alaska Native males have the highest suicide rates among ethnic groups. Non-Hispanic white males are also at increased risk.[81] Adolescents who have previous suicide attempts,[84] impulsivity, a mood or disruptive behavior disorder,[85] recent psychiatric hospitalization,[86,87] substance abuse,[88] a family history of suicide,[89] or a history of sexual or physical abuse[90]; are homeless/runaway[91]; or who identify as lesbian, gay, bisexual, or transgender[92] are also at higher risk for attempting and/or completing suicide. Suicide and suicide attempts are often precipitated by significant psychosocial stressors. These can include family conflict, the breakup of a romantic relationship, bullying, academic difficulties, or disciplinary actions/legal troubles. Younger patients tend to be triggered more often by family conflict, whereas older adolescents are more likely to cite peer or romantic conflicts as a precipitant.[93]

Evaluation

For patients reporting current or recent suicidal ideation and those who present after clear or suspected intentional self-injury, best practices include an evaluation by a clinician experienced in evaluating pediatric mental health conditions. Whenever concern for suicidal ideation or attempt is present, having the patient undergo a personal and belongings search, change into hospital attire, and be placed in as safe a setting as possible (eg, a room without easy access to medical equipment) with close staff supervision may be important.

Interviewing patients and caregivers both together and separately may be beneficial. Obtaining collateral information from caregivers or other individuals who may have knowledge about the patient's state of mind or the details of the event in question often has significant clinical utility, as patients frequently minimize the severity of their symptoms or the intention behind their acts. When interviewing adolescents alone, a discussion about the limits of patient confidentiality may facilitate an open and honest conversation. If there are significant concerns that the patient may be at high risk of harm to himself or herself or others (see "Determination of Level of Care"), the physician may decide to break doctor-patient confidentiality.

A thorough medical examination with careful evaluation for signs of self-injury or toxidromes and a mental status examination may be helpful. The mental status examination typically includes assessment of the patient's appearance, behavior, thought process, thought content (including presence or absence of hallucinations or delusions), mood and affect, and insight and judgment. An evaluation for delirium may also be indicated. When suspicion of delirium is high, a number of screening tools (eg, the Folstein Mini-Mental Status Examination)[94] may be useful.

Determination of Level of Care

No validated criteria exist for assessing level of risk for subsequent suicide or determining level of care. However, most experts agree that patients who continue to endorse a desire to die, remain agitated or severely hopeless, cannot engage in a discussion around safety planning, do not have an adequate support system, cannot be adequately monitored or receive follow-up care, or had a high-lethality suicide attempt or an attempt with clear expectation of death may be at high risk of suicide, and consideration should be given to admission to an inpatient psychiatric facility once medically cleared.[80] Additional risk factors, such as gender, comorbid substance abuse, and high levels of anger or impulsivity, may also be considered.

Patients who do not meet criteria for inpatient psychiatric hospitalization may be candidates for outpatient mental health treatment and intervention. Where available, partial hospital programs, intensive outpatient services, or in-home treatment/ crisis stabilization interventions may be considered, especially when ED clinicians believe that a patient may benefit from more intensive or urgent treatment. Experts suggest that even patients who are deemed to be at relatively low risk of future suicidal or self-injurious acts benefit from outpatient follow-up. Whenever possible, a follow-up appointment with the medical home provider and an outpatient mental health clinician may be helpful. When outpatient mental health services are not readily accessible or wait times for intake appointments are considerable, the medical home providers can play an important bridging role. These providers may also continue to work with patients and families to promote engagement in and adherence to mental health treatment. Consensus expert opinion suggests direct contact with these outpatient providers, either by the mental health consultant or the ED clinician, documentation of this contact, and documentation of the discharge treatment plan.[95,96]

Discharge Planning

Some patients evaluated in the ED for suicidal ideation or a suicide attempt struggle to obtain follow-up care.[97,98] The ED visit may, therefore, be a valuable link in obtaining care for these patients. ED physicians may stress the importance of follow-up to both the patient and the family and attempt to identify and address barriers to subsequent treatment. Counseling and educating families about suicide risk and treatment may be beneficial. The greatest risk of reattempting suicide is in the months after an initial attempt. In addition, given that counseling takes time to work, emphasizing the importance of consistent follow-up may help patients and families.[99–101]

Although having a patient sign a no-suicide contract has not been shown to prevent subsequent suicides,[95] a safety-planning discussion is still an important element of ED care. A safety plan typically includes steps such as identification of (1) warning signs and potential triggers for recurrence of suicidal ideation; (2) coping strategies the patient may use if suicidal ideation returns; (3) healthy activities that could provide distraction or suppression of suicidal thoughts; (4) responsible social supports to which the patient could turn if suicidal urges recur; (5) contact information for professional supports, including instructions on how and when to reaccess emergency services; and (6) means restriction.[102]

Studies suggest that means restriction counseling may be a key component of discharge planning discussions. A large percentage of suicide attempts are impulsive. One study of patients 13 to 34 years of age who had near-lethal suicide attempts found that 24% of patients went from deciding to attempt suicide to implementing their plan within 0 to 5 minutes, 24% took 5 to 19 minutes, and 23% took 20 minutes to 1 hour.[103] Several studies have demonstrated that patients usually misjudge the lethality of their suicide attempts.[104–106] There is also a wide variation in the case-fatality rates of common methods of suicide attempt, ranging from 85% for gunshot wounds to 2% for ingestions and 1% for cutting.[107] It follows that interventions that decrease access to more lethal means and/or increase the amount of time and effort it takes for someone to carry out their suicidal plan and, as a result, increase the amount of time they have to reconsider or for someone to intervene may have a positive effect.

It may be helpful to ask and counsel patients and families about restricting access to potentially lethal means, including access to such means in the homes of friends or family. Means restriction counseling includes suggestions for securing knives, locking up medicines, and removing firearms. It is important to note that parents often underestimate their children's abilities to locate and access firearms and that simply having a gun in the home has been shown to double the risk of youth suicide.[108,][109] Families who are reluctant to permanently remove firearms from the home may be open to temporarily relocating them (eg, for safe keeping with a relative, friend, or local law enforcement) until the child is in a better emotional state. If families insist on keeping firearms in the home, counseling them on how to store them as safely as possible (eg,

by locking all firearms unloaded in a specialized or tamper-proof safe, separately locking or temporarily removing ammunition, and restricting access to keys or lock combinations) may be helpful. Given the high rates of drug and alcohol intoxication among individuals who attempt and complete suicide, physicians may also want to suggest alcohol access restriction and, where indicated, referral for substance abuse counseling and treatment.

INVOLUNTARY HOSPITALIZATION

Under certain circumstances, physicians may insist on admission to a psychiatric inpatient unit over the objections of patients and/or their guardians. This type of admission is often referred to as a "psychiatric hold." Every state has laws governing involuntary admission for inpatient psychiatric hospitalization. Specific details of such laws vary from state to state, as do laws regarding confidentiality and an adolescent's right to seek mental health or substance abuse treatment without parental consent. As such, ED clinicians may benefit from familiarizing themselves with the relevant laws, statutes, and involuntary commitment procedures in the states in which they practice. In general, physicians are able to admit a patient against his or her will for a brief period of time, typically up to 72 hours, but ranging from 1 to 30 days. After that initial period, the psychiatric facility works to obtain a court order for civil commitment for ongoing treatment, if the patient and/or his or her guardian still object to the hospitalization. Criteria for involuntary hospitalization typically include the patient having a mental disorder and being at immediate risk of harm to self or others. Some states also allow for involuntary hospitalization if the patient is "gravely disabled." The criteria for being gravely disabled may include

the inability to meet basic physical needs including nourishment, shelter, safety, and/or basic medical care.[110] State laws differ over whether and, if so, at what age, assent for psychiatric admission must be obtained from minors. For more information on related state laws, contact the AAP Division of State Government Affairs at stgov@aap.org.

RESTRAINT OF THE AGITATED PATIENT

Restraint typically refers to methods of restricting an individual's freedom of movement, physical activity, or normal access to his or her body because of concerns about the person harming himself or herself or others. Some experts believe that interventions to help control a person's activity and behavior span a wide gamut, including verbal and behavioral strategies and favor the term "de-escalation interventions." Restraints may be used for either "medical" or "psychiatric" patients[111] and have been subdivided into verbal, chemical, and physical restraints. Chemical restraint, sometimes called "rapid tranquilization," is the use of pharmacologic means for the acute management of an agitated patient.[112]

Four guiding principles for working with agitated patients are as follows: (1) maximizing the safety of the patient and treating staff; (2) assisting the patient in managing his or her emotions and maintaining or regaining control of his or her behavior; (3) using the least restrictive, age-appropriate methods of restraint possible; and (4) minimizing coercive interventions that may exacerbate agitation.[113]

Verbal Restraint

The general principles of verbal restraint can be found across a wide variety of disciplines, including various psychotherapeutic approaches (eg, anger management, stress reduction), linguistic science, law enforcement, martial arts, and nursing.[113–116] Although consensus is that verbal restraint is preferable to chemical or physical restraint,[117] reviews of the literature find primarily case studies, with a paucity of rigorous studies of verbal restraint, and little on specific strategies or efficacy.[113,118] For example, although a study by Jonikas et al found a decrease in restraint use, it was not clear whether the decrease was attributable to staff training in de-escalation techniques or to crisis intervention training, which occurred at the same time.[119] Other protocols emphasize the importance of prevention in behavior management protocols.[115,120]

Detailed in Table 2 are Fishkind's "Ten Commandments of De-escalation," which incorporate practical, commonly used verbal restraint strategies.[112–114,121–123] Other strategies that may improve the chances of successful de-escalation include a calming physical environment with decreased sensory stimulation, rooms that have been "safety-proofed" (ie, removal or securing of objects that could be used as weapons) or close monitoring if this is not possible,[113] modifying or eliminating triggers of agitation (eg, an argumentative acquaintance, friend, or family or staff member, a long ED wait time),[117,124,125] and staff training in behavioral emergencies.[126,127] A child life specialist may also be an excellent resource to help calm an agitated child. To minimize risk to themselves, health care providers may take precautions, such as removing neck ties, stethoscopes, or securing long hair.

Chemical Restraint

All controlled trials of medications for acute agitation in the ED or inpatient psychiatric setting have been conducted with adults. In the literature, different terms have been used to describe the use of medications to treat agitation, violent or aggressive behavior, or excessive psychomotor activity (eg, psychosis or mania), including pharmacologic or chemical restraint[128] and rapid tranquilization.[112] The 3 most commonly used classes of drugs for this purpose are the typical antipsychotics, atypical antipsychotics, and benzodiazepines.[124,125,129]

Antipsychotics

Antipsychotics exert their effect primarily as CNS dopamine receptor antagonists.[130,131] "Low-potency" agents (eg, chlorpromazine and thioridazine) are more sedating, with fewer extrapyramidal symptoms than "high-potency" agents (eg, haloperidol and droperidol), which are less sedating but more likely to cause extrapyramidal symptoms.[132] The second-generation "atypical" antipsychotics are both serotonin-dopamine receptor antagonists.[130] Some consider aripiprazole the first "third-generation" antipsychotic, because it has partial dopamine receptor agonist activity, distinguishing it from other antipsychotics.[130,132,133] Antipsychotics also have varying ability to block other CNS neurotransmitters, which, combined with their disparate affinity for the postsynaptic D_2 receptors, account for the side effect profiles of each medication, which are discussed in greater detail below and in part II of this clinical report.[130,132]

Benzodiazepines

Benzodiazepines exert their CNS depressant effect by binding to presynaptic γ-aminobutyric acid (GABA) receptors. GABA, the primary CNS inhibitory neurotransmitter, decreases neuronal excitability. Benzodiazepines that have been commonly used to treat agitation are lorazepam, midazolam, and diazepam. Some experts prefer lorazepam for the management of acute agitation because it has fast onset of action, rapid and complete absorption, and no active metabolites. Midazolam may have a more rapid onset of action, but it also has a shorter duration of action. Diazepam has a longer half-life and erratic absorption when given intramuscularly (IM).[134,135]

Less Commonly Used Drugs

Other drugs also used for management of the agitated patient include the antihistamines diphenhydramine, and hydroxyzine and the α-adrenergic agent clonidine.[117,134,136,137] Diphenhydramine and hydroxyzine have sedative effects and are commonly used as nighttime sleep aids for insomnia. Clonidine is a presynaptic α_2-agonist, often used off-label for attention-deficit/hyperactivity disorder and opiate withdrawal. Doses are typically given at night because a significant effect of the medication is somnolence. Although there have been some controlled trials of diphenhydramine as a sedative,[138,139] clonidine has been less well studied.[140]

Drug Selection for Chemical Restraint

Drug selection for chemical restraint will depend largely on the specific details of the clinical scenario (Table 3) and collaboration among ED, psychiatric, and pharmacy colleagues. The combination of a benzodiazepine and an antipsychotic is a regimen frequently suggested by experts for acutely agitated patients, including children and adolescents[124,134,141–147] (Table 4). The route of administration, orally or IM, will depend on the patient's condition. The choice of medication(s) also depend(s) on the patient's current medications. If a patient is already on an antipsychotic, an additional or increased dose of that medication may be preferred.[61,145,147]

TABLE 2 Verbal Restraint Strategies

	Guiding Principle	Strategies, Suggestions, and Examples
1. Respect personal space	• Physical environment can make a patient feel threatened and/or vulnerable	• Two arms' length distance from patient • Unobstructed path out of room for both patient and ED staff
2. Minimize provocative behavior	• Posture and behavior can make a patient feel threatened and/or vulnerable • Concealed hands might imply a hidden weapon	• Calm demeanor and facial expressions • Visible, unclenched hands • Minimize defensive and/or confrontational body language, eg, hands on hips, arms crossed, aggressive posture, directly facing patient (instead, stand at an angle to the patient)
3. Establish verbal contact	• Multiple messages and "messengers" may confuse and agitate the patient	• Ideally, designate 1 or limited staff members to interact with the patient • Introduce self and staff to patient • Orient patient to ED and what to expect • Reassure patient that you will help him or her
4. Be concise	• Agitated patients may be impaired in verbally processing information • Repeating the message may be helpful	• Simple language, concise sentences • May be helpful to frequently repeat/reinforce message • Allow the patient adequate time to process information and respond
5. Identify patient's goals and expectations	• Use body language and verbal acknowledgment to convey	• "I'd like to know what you hoped or expected would happen here." • "What helps you at times like this?" • "Even if I can't provide it, I'd like to know so we can work on it."
6. Use active listening	• Convey to the patient that what he or she said is heard, understood, and valued	• "Tell me if I have this right …" • "What I heard is that …"
7. Agree <u>OR</u> agree to disagree	• Builds empathy for patient's situation • Minimize arguing	• (Agree) "What you're (specific example) going through/experiencing is difficult." • (Agree) "I think everyone would want (the same as you)." • (Agree) "That (what patient is complaining about) would upset other people too." • (Agree to disagree) "People have a lot of different views on (the focus of disagreement)."
8. Clear limits and expectations	• Reasonable and respectful limit setting • Set expectations of mutual respect and dignity, as well as consequences of unacceptable behaviors • Minimize "bargaining" • Coach patient on how to maintain control	• "We're here to help, but it's also important that we're safe with each other and respect each other." • "Safety comes first. If you're having a hard time staying safe or controlling your behavior, we will … (clear, nonpunitive consequence)." • "It'll help me if you (sit, calm yourself, etc). I can better understand you if you calmly tell me your concerns."
9. Offer choices and optimism	• Realistic choice helps empower the patient, regain control of himself/herself, and feel like a partner in the process • Link patient's goals to his or her action • Minimize deception and/or bargaining	• "Instead of (violence/agitation), what else could you do? Would (offer choice) help?" • Acts of kindness (eg, food, blanket, magazine, access to a phone or family member) may help • "You'd like (desired outcome). How can we work together to accomplish (their goal)?"
10. Debrief patient and staff	• If an involuntary intervention is indicated, debriefing may help restore working relationship with the patient and help staff plan for possible future interventions	• Explain why the intervention was necessary • Ask patient to explain his or her perspective • Review options/alternative strategies if the situation arises again

TABLE 3 Acute Agitation Medication Considerations

Suspected Etiology of Agitation	Symptom Severity	
	Mild/Moderate	Severe
Medical/intoxication	Benzodiazepine	Benzodiazepine first, consider adding antipsychotic
Psychiatric	Benzodiazepine or antipsychotic	Antipsychotic
Unknown	Dose of benzodiazepine or antipsychotic; consider a dose of the other medication if the first dose is not effective	

In situations in which the cause of agitation is unclear, many clinicians prefer a stepwise rather than combination approach, administering either a benzodiazepine or first-generation antipsychotic. When treating an agitated patient with a known psychiatric disorder, either a first- or second-generation antipsychotic is generally preferred.

TABLE 4 Medications for the Acutely Agitated Pediatric Patient[a]

Drug: How Supplied	Dose: Route of Administration	Time: Course/Onset Peak/Duration	Side Effects	Advantages	Comments
Benzodiazepines	See individual drugs	See individual drugs	• Sedation	• No EPS	• Contraindicated for intoxication due to other GABAergic drugs (eg, barbiturates, benzodiazepine abuse) • Use with caution in patients with respiratory compromise
			• Respiratory depression	• Preferred agent for many intoxications (eg, cocaine can cause seizures), withdrawal (eg, alcohol)	• Pregnancy class D
			• Hypotension • Paradoxical disinhibition (especially younger children and those with developmental disabilities)		
Lorazepam PO, IM, IV	0.05–0.1 mg/kg PO/IM/IV Usual dose: Adult: 2 mg PO/IM May repeat every 30–60 min	Onset: 5–10 min IV 15 min IM 20–30 min PO Peak: 30 min IV 1 h IM 2 h PO Duration: 2 h IV 6–8 h PO/IM			• Most commonly used drug for acute pediatric agitation
Midazolam PO, IM, IV	0.1 mg/kg PO/IM/IV Usual dose: Adult: 2 mg/PO/IM May repeat every 30–60 min	Onset: 5–10 min IV 10–15 min IM 20 min PO Peak: 5–15 min IV 15–30 min IM 1 h PO Duration: 3–4 h			
Antipsychotics First-generation, "typical antipsychotics"[b]			• Prolonged QT_c • Torsades de pointes • Dysrhythmias • Hypotension • Dystonia/EPS[c] • NMS		• Pregnancy class C
Haloperidol PO, IM	0.025–0.075 mg/kg IM/PO	Onset:		• Most commonly used drug in adults for acute agitation	• Lowers seizure threshold in animals

TABLE 4 Continued

Drug: How Supplied	Dose: Route of Administration	Time: Course/Onset Peak/Duration	Side Effects	Advantages	Comments
	Usual dose:	20–30 min IM		• Second most commonly used drug in pediatric patients	
	Child: 0.5–2 mg			• Low addiction potential	
	Adolescent: 2–5 mg	45–60 min PO		• High therapeutic index	
	Adult: 5–10 mg	Peak:		• Lack of tolerance	
	May repeat IM every 20–30 min, PO every 60 min	60 min IM			
		3 h PO			
	Usual total dose for tranquilization: 10–20 mg (adults)	Duration:			
		4–8 h			
Second-generation, "atypical antipsychotics"			• Same as first-generation drugs	• May be better tolerated and may cause fewer EPS than first-generation drugs	• Pregnancy class C
			• Hyperglycemia	• May have higher risk of dystonia, especially with higher doses and in male and/or young patients	
			• Hyperprolactinemia		
Risperidone PO (liquid, tablet, ODT), IM	0.025–0.050 mg/kg PO/IM	Onset:			
	Usual dose:	30–60 min PO			
	Child: 0.25–0.50 mg	Peak:			
	Adolescent: 0.5–1 mg	1–2 h PO			
	May repeat PO every 60 min				
Olanzepine PO (tablet, ODT) IM	0.1 mg/kg PO/IM	Onset:	• Postinjection delirium/sedation		• FDA investigating 2 unexplained deaths 3–4 d after appropriate IM dose
	Usual dose:	10–20 min IM			• Consider monitoring for at least 3 h after IM injection
	Child: 2.5 mg	20–30 min PO			
	Adolescent: 5–10 mg	Peak:			
	Adult: 10 mg	15–45 min IM			
	Maximum: 30 mg daily	6 h PO			
	May repeat IM every 20–30 min, PO every 30–45 min	Duration:			
		24 h			
Ziprasidone PO, IM	Usual dose:	Onset:			
	Younger adolescent (12–16 y): 10 mg	60 min IM			
	Older adolescent (>16 y): 10–20 mg	4–5 h PO			
		Peak:			
	Maximum: 40 mg daily	IM ≤60 min			
	May repeat every 2 h	PO 6–8 h PO			
Combinations[d]					
Antipsychotic (typical) + benzodiazepine	Haloperidol + lorazepam or midazolam				

TABLE 4 Continued

Drug: How Supplied	Dose: Route of Administration	Time: Course/Onset Peak/Duration	Side Effects	Advantages	Comments
Antipsychotic (typical) + antihistamine	Haloperidol + diphenhydramine				
Antipsychotic (atypical) + benzodiazepine	Risperidone + lorazepam or midazolam				
Antipsychotic (atypical) + antihistamine	Risperidone + diphenhydramine				

Side effects for all drugs in the class are given in the row for the drug class. Side effects for a specific drug in the class are given in the row for the drug class. Pregnancy class is based on limited data, but according to Lexicomp (http://www.wolterskluwercdi.com/lexicomp-online/community-pharmacy/), the benzodiazepines are class D and the first- and second-generation antipsychotics listed in the table are class C (last accessed December 2, 2013). EPS, extrapyramidal symptom; FDA, US Food and Drug Administration; IV, intravenous; NMS, neuroleptic malignant syndrome; ODT, oral disintegrating tablet; PO, oral administration.

a This table provides suggestions for some of the most commonly used drugs for management of the agitated pediatric patient. Child (prepubertal) ages 6–12 y; adolescent 13 y or older. Adult doses have been used in adolescents with high BMI.[125,129,135,143,148,149]

b Chlorpromazine, a phenothiazine that can be used to treat nausea/vomiting and intractable hiccups, has also been used with agitated patients[118,126,150] but has many of the same adverse effects as the other drugs (extrapyramidal/dystonic symptoms, neuroleptic malignant syndrome) as well as anticholinergic side effects and a decrease in the seizure threshold, without having any major advantages over the other drugs.

c EPSs include dystonia and akathisia, which may be treated with diphenhydramine (1.0 mg/kg/dose IV or PO, maximum 50 mg, usual dose in adults is 25 mg or 50 mg) and/or benztropine (1–2 mg in adults).

d Studies of the coadministration of these drugs have been reported. There may be research with other combinations studied in the future. Combinations of a butyrophenone (eg, haloperidol) and a benzodiazepine (eg, lorazepam) may be given together for an additive effect and may be administered in the same syringe. Data in some adult studies suggest that coadministration of a butyrophenone with a benzodiazepine may be more effective than either medication alone.

In other clinical situations, benzodiazepines alone may be the drug of choice. A common scenario is when the agitation is attributable to drug withdrawal or drug intoxication, especially drugs that decrease seizure threshold (eg, cocaine).[117,123,143,145,151] Because of their anticholinergic properties, antipsychotics may worsen the condition of patients who present with intoxication from drugs with anticholinergic properties (eg, hallucinogens) or with an anticholinergic delirium.[123,124,143]

Adverse Effects of and Clinical Monitoring During Chemical Restraint

Monitoring of patients who have received chemical restraint is similar to patients under physical restraint, which are discussed in detail in the subsequent section on physical restraint.[152–154] Medications used for chemical restraint may result in myriad adverse effects that benefit from close medical monitoring, including respiratory depression; hypotension; paradoxical behavioral disinhibition from benzodiazepines, especially in younger children and those with developmental disabilities[134,148,155]; dystonic reactions; orthostatic hypotension; sinus tachycardia; and other dysrhythmias attributable to antipsychotics.[61,130,132–134,149] Given these concerns, monitoring patients who receive antipsychotics may include close clinical observation, cardiorespiratory monitoring, pulse oximetry,[156] and/or an electrocardiogram, when and if the patient will tolerate them.

The most feared cardiac adverse effect of antipsychotics is a quinidine-like QT_c prolongation, resulting in dysrhythmias such as torsades de pointes. QT_c prolongation has been noted to occur with therapeutic dosing of antipsychotics and is possible with any antipsychotic medication. Potential risk factors for QT_c prolongation and dysrhythmia include coadministration with

TABLE 5 QT-Interval-Prolonging Medications in Pediatrics

Antiemetics	Cardiac	Antidepressants
• Ondansetron	• Adenosine	• Fluoxetine
• Dolasetron	• Dopamine	• Sertraline
Macrolides	• Epinephrine	• Paroxetine
• Azithromycin	• Dobutamine	• Venlafaxine
• Clarithromycin	• Quinidine	• Amitriptyline
• Erythromycin	• Procainamide	• Desipramine
Fluoroquinolones	• Flecainide	• Imipramine
• Ciprofloxacin	• Amiodarone	Mood-stabilizing agents
• Levofloxacin	• Bretylium	• Lithium
• Moxifloxacin	• Nicardipine	Antipsychotics
Other Antibiotics	• Sotalol	• Please see Table 4 at www.pediatrics.org/cgi/doi/10.1542/peds.2016-1573
• Amantadine	Antihistamines	Other medications
• Trimethoprim-sulfamethoxazole	• Diphenhydramine	• Cisapride
Antimalarials	• Hydroxyzine	• Octreotide
• Quinine	• Loratadine	• Pentamidine
• Chloroquine	• Astemizole	• Tacrolimus
Neurologic	• Terfenadine	• Vasopressin
• fos-Phenytoin	Respiratory tract	
• Sumatriptan	• Albuterol	
• Zolmitriptan	• Terbutaline	
• Chloral hydrate	• Phenylephrine	
	• Pseudoephedrine	

This is an incomplete list of QT-interval-prolonging medications, limited to those that are commonly used in pediatrics. For a more comprehensive list, please refer to the cited references Haddad et al, Olsen et al, and Yap et al.[159–161]

other drugs that prolong the QT_c; administration of high doses of haloperidol[157,158]; and underlying medical illness (eg, electrolyte abnormalities, hepatic or renal impairment, heart failure, elderly, congenital long QT syndromes). Among the typical and atypical antipsychotics, thioridazine and ziprasidone, respectively, are associated with the greatest degrees of QTc prolongation.[130,134,145,159] Many other commonly used pediatric medications may prolong the QT_c, including antiemetics (eg, ondansetron), antibiotics such as macrolides, fluoroquinolones, and antifungal agents (eg, ketoconazole), antiarrhythmics, and other psychiatric medications (Table 5).[160–162] US Food and Drug Administration "black box" warnings have been issued for both droperidol and thioridazine because of this risk, although the actual clinical risk of and dangers from antipsychotic-induced cardiac dysrhythmias is unclear and is being vigorously debated.[61,134,149,163–168] However, since the black box

warning, the use of droperidol has declined exponentially.[114,117,125,157]

Acute dystonia usually presents as involuntary motor tics or spasms usually involving the face, neck, back, and limb muscles and may occur after antipsychotic administration. Oculogyric crisis is a specific form of acute dystonia, characterized by continuous rotatory eye movements. A rare, life-threatening form of dystonia is laryngeal dystonia, which presents as a choking sensation, difficulty breathing, or stridor. Acute dystonia is commonly treated with diphenhydramine or benztropine administered intravenously or IM. Additional doses of these medications may be indicated, given that their half-life is shorter than antipsychotics.

Among the less commonly used chemical restraint medications, antihistamines, such as diphenhydramine and hydroxyzine, can cause anticholinergic adverse effects including dry mouth, dry skin, urinary retention, constipation, flushing, dizziness,

mydriasis, delirium, and conduction abnormalities. Clonidine can result in hypotension and sedation.[136,137]

Physical Restraint

Physical restraint involves the use of mechanical restrictive devices to limit physical activity. Some differentiate physical restraint from "therapeutic holding," a method in which health care providers or caregivers hold the individual to contain the agitated behavior. Therapeutic holding is most often used in patients of younger ages as a method to help patients regain control of their behavior.[169] In 1 study, restraint was achieved with a mean of 3.5 people per patient, with patients held for an average of 21 minutes.[170] Another technique is seclusion, which refers to the placement of an individual in isolation in an enclosed space.[171]

The prevalence of the use of physical restraints among ED adult psychiatric patients varies widely, ranging from 8% to 59%.[172–177] There are much fewer data on the use of restraint among pediatric patients.[62,144]

Complications of Physical Restraints

Over the past 2 decades, there has been increasing concern regarding adverse events, including deaths, associated with the use of physical restraints in psychiatric facilities.[111] The New York State Commission on Quality of Care in 1994 reported 111 deaths over a 10-year period in New York facilities that were linked to the use of physical restraints.[178] Four years later, the *Hartford Courant* detailed 142 mortalities nationwide attributed to physical restraint use, with children disproportionately represented among the deaths.[179] Among child and adolescent psychiatric facilities, between 1993 and 2003, 45 deaths were ascribed to the use of restraints.[180]

There is also significant morbidity associated with the use of physical restraints. The most common complication is skin breakdown at the site of the restraint, with the possibility of neurovascular damage also occurring.[123] Rhabdomyolysis may occur, especially in patients who continue to struggle, which can lead to kidney failure. Other reported complications include accidental strangulation from vest restraints, brachial plexus injuries, electrolyte abnormalities, hyperthermia, deep vein thrombosis, pulmonary injury/diseases, and asphyxia.[171]

Physical Restraint Policies and Regulations

Because of increasing awareness of the potential complications and dangers of physical restraint, federal agencies and hospital accreditation organizations have developed formal regulations regarding physical restraint. In 2006, the Centers for Medicare and Medicaid Services published its most recent guidelines on patients' rights regarding the use of restraints and seclusion.[152] The US General Accounting Office and The Joint Commission (formerly, The Joint Commission for the Accreditation of Health Care Organizations) have published similar policies and regulations.[153,181] Medical professional organizations, including the AAP,[182] the ACEP,[183] the American Academy of Child and Adolescent Psychiatry,[115] and the American Medical Association,[184] all have policies supporting these regulations, the principles of the humane and least restrictive possible use of restraint, and the need for further research in this area.

The use of restraints remains controversial. Although restraints can be a component of patient treatment in certain situations,[61,182,185] the use of restraints and seclusion has been questioned by some. According to the National Association of State Mental Health Program Directors, "Seclusion and restraint should be considered a security measure, not a form of

'medical treatment' that should only be used as 'last resort measure.'"[186] Adding to the complexity of this issue, it is important to keep in mind the potential liability for failure to restrain a patient who loses control and injures someone and/or destroys property, which may be greater than the liability for appropriately restraining an aggressive/violent patient.[114]

Indications for the Use of Physical Restraints

There are specific indications for the use of restraints: when the patient is an acute danger to harm himself/herself or others,[111,123,124,176,187] to prevent significant disruption of the treatment plan including considerable disruption of property, and when other less restrictive measures have failed or are not possible options.[61,129,182,185] It is unethical to use restraints for convenience or punishment and when prohibited by law or regulation or by untrained personnel.[185]

Techniques for Application of Physical Restraints

If other less restrictive measures have failed, nursing staff may initiate restraint use in extenuating circumstances, with a physician or other licensed independent practitioner performing a face-to-face evaluation and reviewing and approving the order within 1 hour.[123] Sometimes, the mere show of force by a cohort of trained professionals may induce the agitated/violent individual to deescalate, rendering restraint unnecessary. When possible, 5 or more individuals may be included in the application of physical restraints. One person supports the head, and 4 other individuals secure each limb. Experts suggest applying restraints securely to each extremity, then to the bed frame rather than the side rails. Maximizing patient safety includes allowing the patient's head to rotate freely, elevating the head of the bed, if possible, to decrease the risk of

aspiration. If a female patient is being restrained, having at least 1 female on the restraint team may be helpful. In some cases, a "sandwiching" technique between 2 mattresses has been used, with careful monitoring for risk for asphyxia.[122]

Although definitive studies evaluating the best and safest restraint practices are lacking, experts suggest the use of age-appropriate or leather restraints. Restraints made of softer, makeshift, or other materials may be less effective and more likely to result in patient injury. After their review of deaths of patients who were being physically restrained, The Joint Commission made the following suggestions[188]:

- Proper staff training on alternatives to and proper application of physical restraints
- Continuous monitoring of restrained patients
- Supine positioning, with
    o the head of the bed elevated, and
    o free cervical range of motion, to decrease aspiration risk
- Prone positioning may be used if other measures have failed or are not possible. Deaths have been associated with its use. If used, helpful strategies include the following:
    o monitoring for airway obstruction,
    o minimizing or eliminating pressure on the neck and back, and
    o discontinuing as soon as possible
- Minimize covering of the patient's face or head
- Minimize the use of high vests, waist restraints, and beds with unprotected, split side rails
- Remove smoking materials from the patient
- Minimize restraint of medically compromised or unstable patients
- In cases of agitation because of suspected illicit stimulant

use, chemical restraint may be preferable, as a rapid increase in serum potassium secondary to rhabdomyolysis may result in cardiac arrest.

The Joint Commission guidelines also include a schedule for the evaluation of the need for and ordering of restraints, as well as patient monitoring and assistance, by a licensed independent practitioner (licensed independent practitioner; eg, physician, nurse practitioner, physician assistant) and the staff members who apply or monitor the restrained patient (Table 6).[153]

Techniques for Removal of Restraints

Before removal of restraints, it may be helpful to inform the patient of what behavior is expected to minimize the chance that restraints will be reapplied. The same number of staff members that was used to apply the restraints may be present when the restraints are removed. A common strategy is removing 1 restraint at a time, usually starting with 1 lower extremity, next the other leg, then 1 of the upper extremities, and then the other arm, to monitor the patient's response. If the patient becomes violent or disruptive, then the limb restraint(s) may be reapplied; if the patient is cooperative, the restraint removal process may continue.

COORDINATION WITH THE MEDICAL HOME

Experts strongly endorse the benefits of a "medical home"—patient-centered care that is coordinated and integrated by the patient's personal physician, especially for high-risk and/or high-utilization patients.[189,190] The AAP also supports the integration of mental health treatment within the medical home so that youth can "benefit from the strength and skills of the primary care clinician in establishing rapport with the child and family, using the primary care clinicians' unique

TABLE 6 The Joint Commission Requirements for Evaluating and Ordering Restraint

	Age		
	<9 y	9–17 y	>18 y
LIP in-person evaluation to order restraint	Within 1 h of placement of restraints	Within 1 h of placement of restraints	Within 1 h of placement of restraints
Renew restraint order by qualified staff	Every 1 h	Every 2 h	Every 4 h
LIP in-person evaluation to renew restraint order	Every 4 h	Every 4 h	Every 8 h
Assessments every 15 min (all ages)	• Vital signs • Signs of injury due to restraint or seclusion • Nutrition/hydration • Extremities circulation and range of motion • Hygiene and elimination (bowel/bladder) • Physical and psychological status/comfort • Readiness to discontinue restraint		

LIP, licensed independent practitioner.

opportunities to engage children and families in mental health care without stigma."[191] Unfortunately, nearly half of adolescents lack a medical home, with those with mental health problems being even less likely to have the benefit of a medical home.[192] Whenever possible, best practices include consulting primary care pediatricians regarding level-of-care determination, follow-up planning, and referrals. When referral to an outpatient mental health specialist is indicated, providers who are either colocated within or have established collaborations with the medical home may be strongly considered. The medical home provider can follow up with the family to help facilitate and encourage adequate aftercare. In circumstances when a referral to a mental health specialist or higher level of psychiatric care is either not indicated or unavailable, encouraging patients to seek follow-up treatment through their medical home may be beneficial.

There are likely additional health benefits to involving a child's medical home in the aftercare plan. Although data in children are limited, there is a body of data demonstrating that access to primary care may be problematic and morbidity and

mortality are increased in adults with psychiatric illness. In fact, studies suggest that the life expectancy of adults with severe psychiatric illness is between 13 and 35 years lower than their peers without psychiatric illness.[193] Pediatric studies have demonstrated increased rates of obesity and worse self-reported health in adolescents with mental illness.[194] Youth with attention-deficit/hyperactivity disorder and developmental disabilities, such as autism spectrum disorders, have been found to have elevated rates of medical conditions including asthma, frequent ear infections, severe headaches or migraines, and seizures. They also have increased utilization of specialists and higher unmet health needs, including delays in care and inability to afford prescriptions.[150] Therefore, emergency physicians may have a significant effect on children presenting with mental health concerns by referring and encouraging them to participate in coordinated care through a suitable medical home.

LEAD AUTHORS

Thomas H. Chun, MD, MPH, FAAP
Sharon E. Mace, MD, FAAP, FACEP
Emily R. Katz, MD, FAAP

AMERICAN ACADEMY OF PEDIATRICS, COMMITTEE ON PEDIATRIC EMERGENCY MEDICINE, 2015-2016

Joan E. Shook, MD, MBA, FAAP, Chairperson
James M. Callahan, MD, FAAP
Thomas H. Chun, MD, MPH, FAAP
Gregory P. Conners, MD, MPH, MBA, FAAP
Edward E. Conway Jr, MD, MS, FAAP
Nanette C. Dudley, MD, FAAP
Toni K. Gross, MD, MPH, FAAP
Natalie E. Lane, MD, FAAP
Charles G. Macias, MD, MPH, FAAP
Nathan L. Timm, MD, FAAP

LIAISONS

Kim Bullock, MD – *American Academy of Family Physicians*
Elizabeth Edgerton, MD, MPH, FAAP – *Maternal and Child Health Bureau*
Tamar Magarik Haro – *AAP Department of Federal Affairs*
Madeline Joseph, MD, FACEP, FAAP – *American College of Emergency Physicians*
Angela Mickalide, PhD, MCHES – *EMSC National Resource Center*
Brian R. Moore, MD, FAAP – *Natonal Association of EMS Physicians*
Katherine E. Remick, MD, FAAP – *National Association of Emergency Medical Technicians*
Sally K. Snow, RN, BSN, CPEN, FAEN – *Emergency Nurses Association*
David W. Tuggle, MD, FAAP – *American College of Surgeons*
Cynthia Wright-Johnson, MSN, RNC – *National Association of State EMS Officials*

FORMER MEMBERS AND LIAISONS, 2013–2015

Alice D. Ackerman, MD, MBA, FAAP
Lee Benjamin, MD, FACEP, FAAP - *American College of Physicians*
Susan M. Fuchs, MD, FAAP
Marc H. Gorelick, MD, MSCE, FAAP
Paul Sirbaugh, DO, MBA, FAAP - *National Association of Emergency Medical Technicians*
Joseph L. Wright, MD, MPH, FAAP

STAFF

Sue Tellez

AMERICAN COLLEGE OF EMERGENCY PHYSICIANS, PEDIATRIC EMERGENCY MEDICINE COMMITTEE, 2013–2014

Lee S. Benjamin, MD, FACEP, Chairperson
Isabel A. Barata, MD, FACEP, FAAP
Kiyetta Alade, MD
Joseph Arms, MD
Jahn T. Avarello, MD, FACEP
Steven Baldwin, MD
Kathleen Brown, MD, FACEP
Richard M. Cantor, MD, FACEP
Ariel Cohen, MD

Ann Marie Dietrich, MD, FACEP
Paul J. Eakin, MD
Marianne Gausche-Hill, MD, FACEP, FAAP
Michael Gerardi, MD, FACEP, FAAP
Charles J. Graham, MD, FACEP
Doug K. Holtzman, MD, FACEP
Jeffrey Hom, MD, FACEP
Paul Ishimine, MD, FACEP
Hasmig Jinivizian, MD
Madeline Joseph, MD, FACEP
Sanjay Mehta, MD, Med, FACEP
Aderonke Ojo, MD, MBBS
Audrey Z. Paul, MD, PhD
Denis R. Pauze, MD, FACEP
Nadia M. Pearson, DO
Brett Rosen, MD
W. Scott Russell, MD, FACEP
Mohsen Saidinejad, MD
Harold A. Sloas, DO
Gerald R. Schwartz, MD, FACEP
Orel Swenson, MD
Jonathan H. Valente, MD, FACEP
Muhammad Waseem, MD, MS
Paula J. Whiteman, MD, FACEP
Dale Woolridge, MD, PhD, FACEP

FORMER COMMITTEE MEMBERS

Carrie DeMoor, MD
James M. Dy, MD
Sean Fox, MD
Robert J. Hoffman, MD, FACEP
Mark Hostetler, MD, FACEP
David Markenson, MD, MBA, FACEP
Annalise Sorrentino, MD, FACEP
Michael Witt, MD, MPH, FACEP

STAFF

Dan Sullivan
Stephanie Wauson

ABBREVIATIONS

AAP:　American Academy of Pediatrics
ACEP:　American College of Emergency Physicians
CNS:　central nervous system
CT:　computed tomography
ED:　emergency department
GABA:　γ-aminobutyric acid
IM:　intramuscularly

REFERENCES

1. World Health Organization. *The Global Burden of Disease: 2004 Update.* Geneva, Switzerland: World Health Organization Press; 2008

2. Merikangas KR, He JP, Burstein M, et al. Lifetime prevalence of mental disorders in U.S. adolescents: results from the National Comorbidity Survey Replication—Adolescent Supplement (NCS-A). *J Am Acad Child Adolesc Psychiatry.* 2010;49(10):980–989

3. National Institute of Mental Health, Substance Abuse and Mental Health Services Administration, Department of Health and Human Services. *Mental Health: A Report of the Surgeon General. Executive Summary.* Rockville, MD: US Department of Health and Human Services; 1999

4. Grupp-Phelan J, Delgado SV, Kelleher KJ. Failure of psychiatric referrals from the pediatric emergency department. *BMC Emerg Med.* 2007;7:12

5. Grupp-Phelan J, Wade TJ, Pickup T, et al. Mental health problems in children and caregivers in the emergency department setting. *J Dev Behav Pediatr.* 2007;28(1):16–21

6. Fein JA, Pailler ME, Barg FK, et al. Feasibility and effects of a Web-based adolescent psychiatric assessment administered by clinical staff in the pediatric emergency department. *Arch Pediatr Adolesc Med.* 2010;164(12):1112–1117

7. Sheldrick RC, Merchant S, Perrin EC. Identification of developmental-behavioral problems in primary care: a systematic review. *Pediatrics.* 2011;128(2):356–363

8. Committee on Psychosocial Aspects of Child and Family Health and Task Force on Mental Health. Policy statement—The future of pediatrics: mental health competencies for pediatric primary care. *Pediatrics.* 2009;124(1):410–421

9. Foy JM, Kelleher KJ, Laraque D; American Academy of Pediatrics Task Force on Mental Health. Enhancing pediatric mental health care: strategies for preparing a primary care practice. *Pediatrics.* 2010;125(suppl 3):S87–S108

10. Dolan MA, Mace SE; American Academy of Pediatrics, Committee on Pediatric Emergency Medicine; American College of Emergency Physicians and Pediatric Emergency Medicine Committee. Pediatric mental health emergencies in the emergency medical services system. *Pediatrics.* 2006;118(4):1764–1767

11. American College of Emergency Physicians, Pediatric Emergency Medicine Committee. American Academy of Pediatrics, Committee on Pediatric Emergency Medicine. Pediatric mental health emergencies in the emergency medical services system. *Ann Emerg Med.* 2006;48(4):484–486

12. Sills MR, Bland SD. Summary statistics for pediatric psychiatric visits to US emergency departments, 1993–1999. *Pediatrics.* 2002;110(4). Available at: www.pediatrics.org/cgi/content/full/110/4/e40

13. Goldstein AB, Silverman MA, Phillips S, Lichenstein R. Mental health visits in a pediatric emergency department and their relationship to the school calendar. *Pediatr Emerg Care.* 2005;21(10):653–657

14. Larkin GL, Claassen CA, Emond JA, Pelletier AJ, Camargo CA. Trends in U.S. emergency department visits for mental health conditions, 1992 to 2001. *Psychiatr Serv.* 2005;56(6):671–677

15. Grupp-Phelan J, Harman JS, Kelleher KJ. Trends in mental health and chronic condition visits by children presenting for care at U.S. emergency departments. *Public Health Rep.* 2007;122(1):55–61

16. Mahajan P, Alpern ER, Grupp-Phelan J, et al; Pediatric Emergency Care Applied Research Network (PECARN). Epidemiology of psychiatric-related visits to emergency departments in a multicenter collaborative research pediatric network. *Pediatr Emerg Care.* 2009;25(11):715–720

17. Newton AS, Ali S, Johnson DW, et al. A 4-year review of pediatric mental health emergencies in Alberta. *CJEM.* 2009;11(5):447–454

18. Pittsenbarger ZE, Mannix R. Trends in pediatric visits to the emergency department for psychiatric illnesses. *Acad Emerg Med.* 2014;21(1):25–30

19. Anderson LE, Chen ML, Perrin JM, Van Cleave J. Outpatient visits and medication prescribing for us children with mental health conditions. *Pediatrics.* 2015;136(5). Available at: www.pediatrics.org/cgi/content/full/136/5/e1178

20. Olfson M, Blanco C, Wang S, Laje G, Correll CU. National trends in the mental health care of children, adolescents, and adults by office-based physicians. *JAMA Psychiatry.* 2014;71(1):81–90

21. American College of Emergency Physicians. *ACEP Psychiatric and Substance Abuse Survey 2008.* Irving, TX: American College of Emergency Physicians; 2008

22. American Medical Association. *Report of the Council on Medical Service: Access to Psychiatric Beds and Impact on Emergency Medicine.* Chicago, IL: American Medical Association; 2007

23. Claudius I, Donofrio JJ, Lam CN, Santillanes G. Impact of boarding pediatric psychiatric patients on a medical ward. *Hosp Pediatr.* 2014;4(3):125–132

24. Kutscher B. Bedding, not boarding. Psychiatric patients boarded in hospital EDs create crisis for patient care and hospital finances. *Mod Healthc.* 2013;43(46):15–17

25. Nicks BA, Manthey DM. The impact of psychiatric patient boarding in emergency departments. *Emerg Med Int.* 2012;2012:360308

26. Wharff EA, Ginnis KB, Ross AM, Blood EA. Predictors of psychiatric boarding in the pediatric emergency department: implications for emergency care. *Pediatr Emerg Care.* 2011;27(6):483–489

27. Biros MH, Hick K, Cen YY, et al. Occult depressive symptoms in adolescent emergency department patients. *Arch Pediatr Adolesc Med.* 2008;162(8):769–773

28. Scott EG, Luxmore B, Alexander H, Fenn RL, Christopher NC. Screening for adolescent depression in a pediatric emergency department. *Acad Emerg Med.* 2006;13(5):537–542

29. Ramsawh HJ, Chavira DA, Kanegaye JT, Ancoli-Israel S, Madati PJ, Stein MB. Screening for adolescent anxiety disorders in a pediatric emergency department. *Pediatr Emerg Care.* 2012;28(10):1041–1047

30. Winston FK, Kassam-Adams N, Garcia-España F, Ittenbach R, Cnaan A. Screening for risk of persistent posttraumatic stress in injured children and their parents. *JAMA.* 2003;290(5):643–649

31. Rhodes KV, Gordon JA, Lowe RA; Society for Academic Emergency Medicine Public Health and Education Task Force Preventive Services Work Group. Preventive care in the emergency department, Part I: Clinical preventive services—are they relevant to emergency medicine? Society for Academic Emergency Medicine Public Health and Education Task Force Preventive Services Work Group. *Acad Emerg Med.* 2000;7(9):1036–1041

32. Downey LV, Zun LS, Burke T. Undiagnosed mental illness in the emergency department. *J Emerg Med.* 2012;43(5):876–882

33. Pan YJ, Lee MB, Chiang HC, Liao SC. The recognition of diagnosable psychiatric disorders in suicide cases' last medical contacts. *Gen Hosp Psychiatry.* 2009;31(2):181–184

34. Porter SC, Fein JA, Ginsburg KR. Depression screening in adolescents with somatic complaints presenting to the emergency department. *Ann Emerg Med.* 1997;29(1):141–145

35. Slap GB, Vorters DF, Chaudhuri S, Centor RM. Risk factors for attempted suicide during adolescence. *Pediatrics.* 1989;84(5):762–772

36. Slap GB, Vorters DF, Khalid N, Margulies SR, Forke CM. Adolescent suicide attempters: do physicians recognize them? *J Adolesc Health.* 1992;13(4):286–292

37. Luoma JB, Martin CE, Pearson JL. Contact with mental health and primary care providers before suicide: a review of the evidence. *Am J Psychiatry.* 2002;159(6):909–916

38. Gairin I, House A, Owens D. Attendance at the accident and emergency department in the year before suicide: retrospective study. *Br J Psychiatry.* 2003;183:28–33

39. Garbrick L, Levitt MA, Barrett M, Graham L. Agreement between emergency physicians and psychiatrists regarding admission decisions. *Acad Emerg Med.* 1996;3(11):1027–1030

40. Tse SK, Wong TW, Lau CC, Yeung WS, Tang WN. How good are accident and emergency doctors in the evaluation of psychiatric patients? *Eur J Emerg Med.* 1999;6(4):297–300

41. Cronholm PF, Barg FK, Pailler ME, Wintersteen MB, Diamond GS, Fein JA. Adolescent depression: views of health care providers in a pediatric emergency department. *Pediatr Emerg Care*. 2010;26(2):111–117

42. Habis A, Tall L, Smith J, Guenther E. Pediatric emergency medicine physicians' current practices and beliefs regarding mental health screening. *Pediatr Emerg Care*. 2007;23(6):387–393

43. Hoyle JD Jr, White LJ; Emergency Medical Services for Children. Health Resources Services Administration. Maternal and Child Health Bureau. National Association of EMS Physicians. Treatment of pediatric and adolescent mental health emergencies in the United States: current practices, models, barriers, and potential solutions. *Prehosp Emerg Care*. 2003;7(1):66–73

44. Hoyle JD Jr, White LJ. Pediatric mental health emergencies: summary of a multidisciplinary panel. *Prehosp Emerg Care*. 2003;7(1):60–65

45. Santucci KA, Sather J, Baker MD. Emergency medicine training programs' educational requirements in the management of psychiatric emergencies: current perspective. *Pediatr Emerg Care*. 2003;19(3):154–156

46. Horwitz SM, Storfer-Isser A, Kerker BD, et al. Barriers to the identification and management of psychosocial problems: changes from 2004 to 2013. *Acad Pediatr*. 2015;15(6):613–620

47. Al-Osaimi FD, Al-Haidar FA. Assessment of pediatricians' need for training in child psychiatry. *J Family Community Med*. 2008;15(2):71–75

48. Riba M, Hale M. Medical clearance: fact or fiction in the hospital emergency room. *Psychosomatics*. 1990;31(4):400–404

49. Glauser JG. Functional versus organic illness: identifying medical illness in patients with psychiatric symptoms. *Crit Decis Emerg Med*. 2005;19(6):12–21

50. Newcomer JW. Metabolic considerations in the use of antipsychotic medications: a review of recent evidence. *J Clin Psychiatry*. 2007;68(suppl 1):20–27

51. Allen MH, Currier GW. Medical assessment in the psychiatric emergency service. *New Dir Ment Health Serv*. 1999;82(82):21–28

52. Krummel S, Kathol RG. What you should know about physical evaluations in psychiatric patients. Results of a survey. *Gen Hosp Psychiatry*. 1987;9(4):275–279

53. Hall RC, Gardner ER, Stickney SK, LeCann AF, Popkin MK. Physical illness manifesting as psychiatric disease. II. Analysis of a state hospital inpatient population. *Arch Gen Psychiatry*. 1980;37(9):989–995

54. Henneman PL, Mendoza R, Lewis RJ. Prospective evaluation of emergency department medical clearance. *Ann Emerg Med*. 1994;24(4):672–677

55. Olshaker JS, Browne B, Jerrard DA, Prendergast H, Stair TO. Medical clearance and screening of psychiatric patients in the emergency department. *Acad Emerg Med*. 1997;4(2):124–128

56. Herridge CF. Physical disorders in psychiatric illness. A study of 209 consecutive admissions. *Lancet*. 1960;2(7157):949–951

57. Worster A, Elliott L, Bose TJ, Chemeris E. Reliability of vital signs measured at triage. *Eur J Emerg Med*. 2003;10(2):108–110

58. Tintinalli JE, Peacock FW IV, Wright MA. Emergency medical evaluation of psychiatric patients. *Ann Emerg Med*. 1994;23(4):859–862

59. Pinto T, Poynter B, Durbin J. Medical clearance in the psychiatric emergency setting: a call for more standardization. *Healthc Q*. 2010;13(2):77–82

60. Zun LS. Evidence-based evaluation of psychiatric patients. *J Emerg Med*. 2005;28(1):35–39

61. Lukens TW, Wolf SJ, Edlow JA, et al; American College of Emergency Physicians Clinical Policies Subcommittee (Writing Committee) on Critical Issues in the Diagnosis and Management of the Adult Psychiatric Patient in the Emergency Department. Clinical policy: critical issues in the diagnosis and management of the adult psychiatric patient in the emergency department. *Ann Emerg Med*. 2006;47(1):79–99

62. Santiago LI, Tunik MG, Foltin GL, Mojica MA. Children requiring psychiatric consultation in the pediatric emergency department: epidemiology, resource utilization, and complications. *Pediatr Emerg Care*. 2006;22(2):85–89

63. Santillanes G, Donofrio JJ, Lam CN, Claudius I. Is medical clearance necessary for pediatric psychiatric patients? *J Emerg Med*. 2014;46(6):800–807

64. Glauser J, Marshall M. Medical clearance of psychiatric patients. *Emerg Med Rep*. 2011;32(23):273–283

65. Shah SJ, Fiorito M, McNamara RM. A screening tool to medically clear psychiatric patients in the emergency department. *J Emerg Med*. 2012;43(5):871–875

66. Broderick KB, Lerner EB, McCourt JD, Fraser E, Salerno K. Emergency physician practices and requirements regarding the medical screening examination of psychiatric patients. *Acad Emerg Med*. 2002;9(1):88–92

67. Korn CS, Currier GW, Henderson SO. "Medical clearance" of psychiatric patients without medical complaints in the emergency department. *J Emerg Med*. 2000;18(2):173–176

68. Janiak BD, Atteberry S. Medical clearance of the psychiatric patient in the emergency department. *J Emerg Med*. 2012;43(5):866–870

69. Shihabuddin BS, Hack CM, Sivitz AB. Role of urine drug screening in the medical clearance of pediatric psychiatric patients: is there one? *Pediatr Emerg Care*. 2013;29(8):903–906

70. Fortu JM, Kim IK, Cooper A, Condra C, Lorenz DJ, Pierce MC. Psychiatric patients in the pediatric emergency department undergoing routine urine toxicology screens for medical clearance: results and use. *Pediatr Emerg Care*. 2009;25(6):387–392

71. Tenenbein M. Do you really need that emergency drug screen? *Clin Toxicol (Phila)*. 2009;47(4):286–291

72. Donofrio JJ, Santillanes G, McCammack BD, et al. Clinical utility of screening laboratory tests in pediatric psychiatric patients presenting to the

emergency department for medical clearance. *Ann Emerg Med.* 2013

73. Bunevicius A, Deltuva VP, Deltuviene D, Tamasauskas A, Bunevicius R. Brain lesions manifesting as psychiatric disorders: eight cases. *CNS Spectr.* 2008;13(11):950–958

74. Bain BK. CT scans of first-break psychotic patients in good general health. *Psychiatr Serv.* 1998;49(2):234–235

75. Gewirtz G, Squires-Wheeler E, Sharif Z, Honer WG. Results of computerised tomography during first admission for psychosis. *Br J Psychiatry.* 1994;164(6):789–795

76. Agzarian MJ, Chryssidis S, Davies RP, Pozza CH. Use of routine computed tomography brain scanning of psychiatry patients. *Australas Radiol.* 2006;50(1):27–28

77. Brody AS, Frush DP, Huda W, Brent RL; American Academy of Pediatrics Section on Radiology. Radiation risk to children from computed tomography. *Pediatrics.* 2007;120(3):677–682

78. Newman B, Callahan MJ. ALARA (as low as reasonably achievable) CT 2011--executive summary. *Pediatr Radiol.* 2011;41(Suppl 2):453–455

79. Mathews JD, Forsythe AV, Brady Z, et al. Cancer risk in 680,000 people exposed to computed tomography scans in childhood or adolescence: data linkage study of 11 million Australians. *BMJ.* 2013;346:f2360

80. Shain BN; American Academy of Pediatrics Committee on Adolescence. Suicide and suicide attempts in adolescents. *Pediatrics.* 2016;138(1):e20161420

81. Centers for Disease Control and Prevention. Leading Causes of Death 1999–2010. Web-Based Injury Statistics Query and Reporting System (WISQARS) [database]. Available at: https://www.cdc.gov/injury/wisqars/. Accessed April 14, 2012

82. Eaton DK, Kann L, Kinchen S, et al; Centers for Disease Control and Prevention (CDC). Youth risk behavior surveillance—United States, 2011. *MMWR Surveill Summ.* 2012;61(4):1–162

83. Ting SA, Sullivan AF, Boudreaux ED, Miller I, Camargo CA Jr. Trends in

US emergency department visits for attempted suicide and self-inflicted injury, 1993–2008. *Gen Hosp Psychiatry.* 2012;34(5):557–565

84. Shaffer D, Craft L. Methods of adolescent suicide prevention. *J Clin Psychiatry.* 1999;60(suppl 2):70–74, discussion 75–76, 113–116

85. Foley DL, Goldston DB, Costello EJ, Angold A. Proximal psychiatric risk factors for suicidality in youth: the Great Smoky Mountains Study. *Arch Gen Psychiatry.* 2006;63(9):1017–1024

86. Lewinsohn PM, Rohde P, Seeley JR. Psychosocial risk factors for future adolescent suicide attempts. *J Consult Clin Psychol.* 1994;62(2):297–305

87. Shaffer D, Gould MS, Fisher P, et al. Psychiatric diagnosis in child and adolescent suicide. *Arch Gen Psychiatry.* 1996;53(4):339–348

88. Esposito-Smythers C, Spirito A. Adolescent substance use and suicidal behavior: a review with implications for treatment research. *Alcohol Clin Exp Res.* 2004;28(suppl 5):77S–88S

89. McKeown RE, Garrison CZ, Cuffe SP, Waller JL, Jackson KL, Addy CL. Incidence and predictors of suicidal behaviors in a longitudinal sample of young adolescents. *J Am Acad Child Adolesc Psychiatry.* 1998;37(6):612–619

90. Brown J, Cohen P, Johnson JG, Smailes EM. Childhood abuse and neglect: specificity of effects on adolescent and young adult depression and suicidality. *J Am Acad Child Adolesc Psychiatry.* 1999;38(12):1490–1496

91. Smart RG, Walsh GW. Predictors of depression in street youth. *Adolescence.* 1993;28(109):41–53

92. McDaniel JS, Purcell D, D'Augelli AR. The relationship between sexual orientation and risk for suicide: research findings and future directions for research and prevention. *Suicide Life Threat Behav.* 2001;31(Suppl):84–105

93. Olverholser J. Predisposing factors in suicide attempts: life stressors. In: Spirito A, Overholser JC, eds. *Evaluating and Treating Adolescent Suicide Attempters: From Research to Practice.* New York, NY: Academic Press; 2002:42–54

94. Folstein MF, Folstein SE, McHugh PR. "Mini-Mental State." A practical method for grading the cognitive state of patients for the clinician. *J Psychiatr Res.* 1975;12(3):189–198

95. American Academy of Child and Adolescent Psychiatry. Practice parameter for the assessment and treatment of children and adolescents with suicidal behavior. *J Am Acad Child Adolesc Psychiatry.* 2001;40(suppl 7):24S–51S

96. Fontanella CA, Bridge JA, Campo JV. Psychotropic medication changes, polypharmacy, and the risk of early readmission in suicidal adolescent inpatients. *Ann Pharmacother.* 2009;43(12):1939–1947

97. Spirito A, Lewander WJ, Levy S, Kurkjian J, Fritz G. Emergency department assessment of adolescent suicide attempters: factors related to short-term follow-up outcome. *Pediatr Emerg Care.* 1994;10(1):6–12

98. Trautman PD, Stewart N, Morishima A. Are adolescent suicide attempters noncompliant with outpatient care? *J Am Acad Child Adolesc Psychiatry.* 1993;32(1):89–94

99. Prinstein MJ, Nock MK, Simon V, Aikins JW, Cheah CS, Spirito A. Longitudinal trajectories and predictors of adolescent suicidal ideation and attempts following inpatient hospitalization. *J Consult Clin Psychol.* 2008;76(1):92–103

100. Spirito A, Plummer B, Gispert M, et al. Adolescent suicide attempts: outcomes at follow-up. *Am J Orthopsychiatry.* 1992;62(3):464–468

101. Yen S, Weinstock LM, Andover MS, Sheets ES, Selby EA, Spirito A. Prospective predictors of adolescent suicidality: 6-month post-hospitalization follow-up. *Psychol Med.* 2013;43(5):983–993

102. Sher L, LaBode V. Teaching health care professionals about suicide safety planning. *Psychiatr Danub.* 2011;23(4):396–397

103. Simon OR, Swann AC, Powell KE, Potter LB, Kresnow MJ, O'Carroll PW. Characteristics of impulsive suicide attempts and attempters. *Suicide Life Threat Behav.* 2001;32(suppl 1):49–59

104. Brown GK, Henriques GR, Sosdjan D, Beck AT. Suicide intent and accurate expectations of lethality: predictors of medical lethality of suicide attempts. *J Consult Clin Psychol.* 2004;72(6):1170–1174

105. Swahn MH, Potter LB. Factors associated with the medical severity of suicide attempts in youths and young adults. *Suicide Life Threat Behav.* 2001;32(suppl 1):21–29

106. Plutchik R, van Praag HM, Picard S, Conte HR, Korn M. Is there a relation between the seriousness of suicidal intent and the lethality of the suicide attempt? *Psychiatry Res.* 1989;27(1):71–79

107. Vyrostek SB, Annest JL, Ryan GW. Surveillance for fatal and nonfatal injuries—United States, 2001. *MMWR Surveill Summ.* 2004;53(7):1–57

108. Baxley F, Miller M. Parental misperceptions about children and firearms. *Arch Pediatr Adolesc Med.* 2006;160(5):542–547

109. Brent DA, Perper JA, Allman CJ, Moritz GM, Wartella ME, Zelenak JP. The presence and accessibility of firearms in the homes of adolescent suicides. A case-control study. *JAMA.* 1991;266(21):2989–2995

110. Treatment Advocacy Center. State Standards Charts for Assisted Treatment. Civil Commitment Criteria and Initiation Procedures by State. Available at: www.treatmentadvocacy center.org/storage/documents/State_ Standards_Charts_for_Assisted_ Treatment_-_Civil_Commitment_ Criteria_and_Initiation_Procedures. pdf. Accessed July 9, 2015

111. Glezer A, Brendel RW. Beyond emergencies: the use of physical restraints in medical and psychiatric settings. *Harv Rev Psychiatry.* 2010;18(6):353–358

112. Hockberger RS. Richards J. Thought disorders. In: Marx JA, Hockberger R, Walls RM, eds. *Rosen's Emergency Medicine: Concepts and Clinical Practice.* Philadelphia, PA: Saunders; 2014:1460–1465

113. Richmond JS, Berlin JS, Fishkind AB, et al. Verbal de-escalation of the agitated patient: consensus statement of the American Association for Emergency Psychiatry Project BETA De-escalation Workgroup. *West J Emerg Med.* 2012;13(1):17–25

114. Heiner JD, Moore GP. The combatative patient. In: Marx JA, Hockberger R, Walls RM, eds. *Rosen's Emergency Medicine: Concepts and Clinical Practice.* Philadelphia, PA: Saunders; 2014:2414–2421

115. Masters KJ, Bellonci C, Bernet W, et al; American Academy of Child and Adolescent Psychiatry. Practice parameter for the prevention and management of aggressive behavior in child and adolescent psychiatric institutions, with special reference to seclusion and restraint. *J Am Acad Child Adolesc Psychiatry.* 2002;41(suppl 2):4S–25S

116. Stevenson S. Heading off violence with verbal de-escalation. *J Psychosoc Nurs Ment Health Serv.* 1991;29(9):6–10

117. Adimando AJ, Poncin YB, Baum CR. Pharmacological management of the agitated pediatric patient. *Pediatr Emerg Care.* 2010;26(11):856–860, quiz 861–863

118. Delaney KR. Evidence base for practice: reduction of restraint and seclusion use during child and adolescent psychiatric inpatient treatment. *Worldviews Evid Based Nurs.* 2006;3(1):19–30

119. Jonikas JA, Cook JA, Rosen C, Laris A, Kim JB. A program to reduce use of physical restraint in psychiatric inpatient facilities. *Psychiatr Serv.* 2004;55(7):818–820

120. dosReis S, Barnett S, Love RC, Riddle MA; Maryland Youth Practice Improvement Committee. A guide for managing acute aggressive behavior of youths in residential and inpatient treatment facilities. *Psychiatr Serv.* 2003;54(10):1357–1363

121. Fishkind A. Calming agitation with words, not drugs: 10 commandments for safety. *Curr Psychiatr.* 2002;1(4):32–39

122. Larkin GL, Beautrais AL. Behavioral disorders: emergency assessment. In: Tintinalli JE, Stapczynski S, Ma OJ, Cline DM, Cydulka RK, Mecklereds GD, eds. *Tintinalli's Emergency Medicine: A Comprehensive Study Guide.* New York, NY: McGraw-Hill Education; 2011:1939–1946

123. Rossi J, Swan MC, Isaacs ED. The violent or agitated patient. *Emerg Med Clin North Am.* 2010;28(1):235–256, x

124. Marder SR. A review of agitation in mental illness: treatment guidelines and current therapies. *J Clin Psychiatry.* 2006;67(suppl 10):13–21

125. Mace SE. Behavioral and psychiatric disorders in children and infants. In: Tintinalli JE, Stapczynski S, Ma OJ, Cline DM, Cydulka RK, Mecklereds GD, eds. *Tintinalli's Emergency Medicine: A Comprehensive Study Guide.* New York, NY: McGraw-Hill Education; 2011:967–971

126. Allen MH, Forster P, Zealberg J, Currier G; American Psychiatric Association, Task Force on Psychiatric Emergency Services. *Report and Recommendations Regarding Psychiatric Emergency and Crisis Services: A Review and Model Program Descriptions.* Bloomfield, CT: American Association for Emergency Psychiatry; 2002

127. Cowin L, Davies R, Estall G, Berlin T, Fitzgerald M, Hoot S. De-escalating aggression and violence in the mental health setting. *Int J Ment Health Nurs.* 2003;12(1):64–73

128. Tan D. Medications for psychiatric emergencies. In: Khouzam HR, Tan DT, Gill TS, eds. *Handbook of Emergency Psychiatry.* Philadelphia, PA: Mosby-Elsevier; 2007:22–31

129. Downes MA, Healy P, Page CB, Bryant JL, Isbister GK. Structured team approach to the agitated patient in the emergency department. *Emerg Med Australas.* 2009;21(3):196–202

130. Miyamoto S, Lieberman JA, Fleischacker WW, Marder SR. Antipsychotic drugs. In: Tasman A, Kay J, Lieberman A, First MB, Maj M, eds. *Psychiatry.* 3rd ed. West Sussex, England: John Wiley & Sons; 2008:2161–2201

131. Smith T, Horwath E, Cournos F. Schizophrenia and other psychotic disorders. In: Cutler JL, Marcus E, eds. *Psychiatry.* New York, NY: Oxford University Press; 2010:101–131

132. Levine M, LoVecchio F. Antipsychotics. In: Tintinalli JE, Stapczynski S, Ma OJ, Cline DM, Cydulka RK, Mecklereds GD,

eds. *Tintinalli's Emergency Medicine: A Comprehensive Study Guide.* New York, NY: McGraw-Hill Education; 2011:1207–1211

133. Minns AB, Clark RF. Toxicology and overdose of atypical antipsychotics. *J Emerg Med.* 2012;43(5):906–913

134. Sonnier L, Barzman D. Pharmacologic management of acutely agitated pediatric patients. *Paediatr Drugs.* 2011;13(1):1–10

135. Nobay F, Simon BC, Levitt MA, Dresden GM. A prospective, double-blind, randomized trial of midazolam versus haloperidol versus lorazepam in the chemical restraint of violent and severely agitated patients. *Acad Emerg Med.* 2004;11(7):744–749

136. May DE, Kratochvil CJ. Attention-deficit hyperactivity disorder: recent advances in paediatric pharmacotherapy. *Drugs.* 2010;70(1):15–40

137. Yoon EY, Cohn L, Rocchini A, Kershaw D, Clark SJ. Clonidine utilization trends for Medicaid children. *Clin Pediatr (Phila).* 2012;51(10):950–955

138. Cengiz M, Baysal Z, Ganidagli S. Oral sedation with midazolam and diphenhydramine compared with midazolam alone in children undergoing magnetic resonance imaging. *Paediatr Anaesth.* 2006;16(6):621–626

139. Roach CL, Husain N, Zabinsky J, Welch E, Garg R. Moderate sedation for echocardiography of preschoolers. *Pediatr Cardiol.* 2010;31(4):469–473

140. Lustig SL, Botelho C, Lynch L, Nelson SV, Eichelberger WJ, Vaughan BL. Implementing a randomized clinical trial on a pediatric psychiatric inpatient unit at a children's hospital: the case of clonidine for post-traumatic stress. *Gen Hosp Psychiatry.* 2002;24(6):422–429

141. Battaglia J, Moss S, Rush J, et al. Haloperidol, lorazepam, or both for psychotic agitation? A multicenter, prospective, double-blind, emergency department study. *Am J Emerg Med.* 1997;15(4):335–340

142. Chan EW, Taylor DM, Knott JC, Phillips GA, Castle DJ, Kong DC. Intravenous droperidol or olanzapine as an adjunct to midazolam for the acutely agitated

patient: a multicenter, randomized, double-blind, placebo-controlled clinical trial. *Ann Emerg Med.* 2013;61(1):72–81

143. Allen MH. Managing the agitated psychotic patient: a reappraisal of the evidence. *J Clin Psychiatry.* 2000;61(suppl 14):11–20

144. Dorfman DH, Mehta SD. Restraint use for psychiatric patients in the pediatric emergency department. *Pediatr Emerg Care.* 2006;22(1):7–12

145. Isaacs E. The violent patient. In: Marx JA, Hockberger R, Walls RM, eds. *Rosen's Emergency Medicine: Concepts and Clinical Practice.* Philadelphia, PA: Saunders; 2014:1460–1465

146. Bieniek SA, Ownby RL, Penalver A, Dominguez RA. A double-blind study of lorazepam versus the combination of haloperidol and lorazepam in managing agitation. *Pharmacotherapy.* 1998;18(1):57–62

147. Currier GW, Medori R. Orally versus intramuscularly administered antipsychotic drugs in psychiatric emergencies. *J Psychiatr Pract.* 2006;12(1):30–40

148. Garris S, Hughes C. Management of acute agitation. In: Tintinalli JE, Stapczynski S, Ma OJ, Cline DM, Cydulka RK, Mecklereds GD, eds. *Tintinalli's Emergency Medicine: A Comprehensive Study Guide.* New York, NY: McGraw-Hill Education; 2011

149. Whittler MA, Lavonas EJ. Antipsychotics. In: Marx JA, Hockberger RS, Walls RM, et al, eds. *Rosen's Emergency Medicine: Concepts and Clinical Practice.* Philadelphia, PA: Saunders; 2014:2042–2046

150. Schieve LA, Gonzalez V, Boulet SL, et al. Concurrent medical conditions and health care use and needs among children with learning and behavioral developmental disabilities, National Health Interview Survey, 2006–2010. *Res Dev Disabil.* 2012;33(2):467–476

151. Sorrentino A. Chemical restraints for the agitated, violent, or psychotic pediatric patient in the emergency department: controversies and recommendations. *Curr Opin Pediatr.* 2004;16(2):201–205

152. Centers for Medicare & Medicaid Services (CMS), DHHS. Medicare and Medicaid programs; hospital conditions of participation: patients' rights. Final rule. *Fed Regist.* 2006;71(236):71377–71428

153. The Joint Commission. *Standards on Restraint and Seclusion.* Oakbrook Terrace, IL: The Joint Commission; 2009

154. Health Care Finance Administration. Medicare and Medicaid Programs; Hospital Conditions of Participation: Patients' Rights; Interim Final Rule. *Fed Regist.* 1999;64(127):36088–36089

155. Baren JM, Mace SE, Hendry PL, Dietrich AM, Goldman RD, Warden CR. Children's mental health emergencies—part 2: emergency department evaluation and treatment of children with mental health disorders. *Pediatr Emerg Care.* 2008;24(7):485–498

156. Masters KJ. Pulse oximetry use during physical and mechanical restraints. *J Emerg Med.* 2007;33(3):289–291

157. Walters H, Killius K. *Guidelines for the Acute Psychotropic Medication Management of Agitation in Children and Adolescents.* Boston, MA: Boston Medical Center Emergency Department Policy and Procedure Guidelines; 2012

158. Meyer-Massetti C, Cheng CM, Sharpe BA, Meier CR, Guglielmo BJ. The FDA extended warning for intravenous haloperidol and torsades de pointes: how should institutions respond? *J Hosp Med.* 2010;5(4):E8–E16

159. Haddad PM, Anderson IM. Antipsychotic-related QTc prolongation, torsade de pointes and sudden death. *Drugs.* 2002;62(11):1649–1671

160. Olsen KM. Pharmacologic agents associated with QT interval prolongation. *J Fam Pract.* 2005;(suppl):S8–S14

161. Yap YG, Camm AJ. Drug induced QT prolongation and torsades de pointes. *Heart.* 2003;89(11):1363–1372

162. Labellarte MJ, Crosson JE, Riddle MA. The relevance of prolonged QTc measurement to pediatric psychopharmacology. *J Am Acad Child Adolesc Psychiatry.* 2003;42(6):642–650

163. Bailey P, Norton R, Karan S. The FDA droperidol warning: is it justified? *Anesthesiology.* 2002;97(1):288–289

164. Chase PB, Biros MH. A retrospective review of the use and safety of droperidol in a large, high-risk, inner-city emergency department patient population. *Acad Emerg Med.* 2002;9(12):1402–1410

165. Dershwitz M. Droperidol: should the black box be light gray? *J Clin Anesth.* 2002;14(8):598–603

166. Gan TJ, White PF, Scuderi PE, Watcha MF, Kovac A. FDA "black box" warning regarding use of droperidol for postoperative nausea and vomiting: is it justified? *Anesthesiology.* 2002;97(1):287

167. Hilt RJ, Woodward TA. Agitation treatment for pediatric emergency patients. *J Am Acad Child Adolesc Psychiatry.* 2008;47(2):132–138

168. Horowitz BZ, Bizovi K, Moreno R. Droperidol—behind the black box warning. *Acad Emerg Med.* 2002;9(6):615–618

169. Baren JM, Mace SE, Hendry PL, Dietrich AM, Grupp-Phelan J, Mullin J. Children's mental health emergencies—part 1: challenges in care: definition of the problem, barriers to care, screening, advocacy, and resources. *Pediatr Emerg Care.* 2008;24(6):399–408

170. Miller D, Walker MC, Friedman D. Use of a holding technique to control the violent behavior of seriously disturbed adolescents. *Hosp Community Psychiatry.* 1989;40(5):520–524

171. Di Lorenzo R, Baraldi S, Ferrara M, Mimmi S, Rigatelli M. Physical restraints in an Italian psychiatric ward: clinical reasons and staff organization problems. *Perspect Psychiatr Care.* 2012;48(2):95–107

172. Allen MH, Currier GW. Use of restraints and pharmacotherapy in academic psychiatric emergency services. *Gen Hosp Psychiatry.* 2004;26(1):42–49

173. Beck JC, White KA, Gage B. Emergency psychiatric assessment of violence. *Am J Psychiatry.* 1991;148(11):1562–1565

174. Bell CC, Palmer JM. Security procedures in a psychiatric emergency service. *J Natl Med Assoc.* 1981;73(9):835–842

175. Currier GW, Allen MH. Emergency psychiatry: physical and chemical restraint in the psychiatric emergency service. *Psychiatr Serv.* 2000;51(6):717–719

176. Currier GW, Walsh P, Lawrence D. Physical restraints in the emergency department and attendance at subsequent outpatient psychiatric treatment. *J Psychiatr Pract.* 2011;17(6):387–393

177. Lavoie FW. Consent, involuntary treatment, and the use of force in an urban emergency department. *Ann Emerg Med.* 1992;21(1):25–32

178. Sundram CJ, Stack EW, Benjamin WP. *Restraint and Seclusion Practices in New York State Psychiatric Facilities.* Albany, NY: New York State Commission on Quality of Care for the Mentally Disabled; 1994

179. Weiss EM, Altamira D, Blinded DF, et al. Deadly restraint: a Hartford Courant investigative report. *Hartford Courant.* October 11-15, 1998:A10

180. Nunno MA, Holden MJ, Tollar A. Learning from tragedy: a survey of child and adolescent restraint fatalities. *Child Abuse Negl.* 2006;30(12):1333–1342

181. US General Accounting Office. *Report to Congressional Requestors: Mental Health: Improper Restraint or Seclusion Places People at Risk. US Department of Health and Human Services.* Washington, DC: US General Accounting Office; 1999

182. American Academy of Pediatrics Committee on Pediatric Emergency Medicine. The use of physical restraint interventions for children and adolescents in the acute care setting. *Pediatrics.* 1997;99(3):497–498

183. American College of Emergency Physicians. Emergency physicians' patient care responsibilities outside the emergency department. *Ann Emerg Med.* 2006;47(3):304

184. Brown RL, Genel M, Riggs JA; American Medical Association, Council on Scientific Affairs. Use of seclusion and restraint in children and adolescents. Council on Scientific Affairs, American Medical Association. *Arch Pediatr Adolesc Med.* 2000;154(7):653–656

185. American Psychiatric Association, Task Force on the Psychiatric Uses of Seclusion and Restraint. *Seclusion and Restraint: The Psychiatric Uses (Task Force Report 22).* Washington, DC: American Psychiatric Association; 1985

186. Medical Directors Council of the National Association of State Mental Health Program Directors. *Reducing the Use of Seclusion and Restraints: Findings, Strategies and Recommendations.* Alexandria, VA: National Association of State Mental Health Program Directors; 1999

187. Fisher WA. Restraint and seclusion: a review of the literature. *Am J Psychiatry.* 1994;151(11):1584–1591

188. The Joint Commission. Preventing Restraint Deaths. In: *Sentinel Event Alert.* Oakbrook Terrace, IL: The Joint Commission; 1998:2

189. Higgins S, Chawla R, Colombo C, Snyder R, Nigam S. Medical homes and cost and utilization among high-risk patients. *Am J Manag Care.* 2014;20(3):e61–e71

190. Schwenk TL. The patient-centered medical home: one size does not fit all. *JAMA.* 2014;311(8):802–803

191. American Academy of Child and Adolescent Psychiatry Committee on Health Care Access and Economics Task Force on Mental Health. Improving mental health services in primary care: reducing administrative and financial barriers to access and collaboration. *Pediatrics.* 2009;123(4):1248–1251

192. Adams SH, Newacheck PW, Park MJ, Brindis CD, Irwin CE Jr. Medical home for adolescents: low attainment rates for those with mental health problems and other vulnerable groups. *Acad Pediatr.* 2013;13(2):113–121

193. DE Hert M, Correll CU, Bobes J, et al. Physical illness in patients with severe mental disorders. I. Prevalence, impact of medications and disparities in health care. *World Psychiatry.* 2011;10(1):52–77

194. Burnett-Zeigler I, Walton MA, Ilgen M, et al. Prevalence and correlates of mental health problems and treatment among adolescents seen in primary care. *J Adolesc Health.* 2012;50(6):559–564

CLINICAL REPORT Guidance for the Clinician in Rendering Pediatric Care

American Academy
of Pediatrics

DEDICATED TO THE HEALTH OF ALL CHILDREN™

Evaluation and Management of Children With Acute Mental Health or Behavioral Problems. Part II: Recognition of Clinically Challenging Mental Health Related Conditions Presenting With Medical or Uncertain Symptoms

Thomas H. Chun, MD, MPH, FAAP, Sharon E. Mace, MD, FAAP, FACEP, Emily R. Katz, MD, FAAP,
AMERICAN ACADEMY OF PEDIATRICS Committee on Pediatric Emergency Medicine, AMERICAN
COLLEGE OF EMERGENCY PHYSICIANS Pediatric Emergency Medicine Committee

INTRODUCTION

Part I of this clinical report (http://www.pediatrics.org/cgi/doi/10. 1542/peds.2016-1570) discusses the common clinical issues that may be encountered in caring for children and adolescents presenting to the emergency department (ED) or primary care setting with a mental health condition or emergency and includes the following:

- Medical clearance of pediatric psychiatric patients

- Suicidal ideation and suicide attempts

- Involuntary hospitalization

- Restraint of the agitated patient

  o Verbal restraint

  o Chemical restraint

  o Physical restraint

- Coordination with the medical home

Part II discusses the challenges a pediatric clinician may face when evaluating patients with a mental health condition, which may be contributing to or a complicating factor for a medical or indeterminate clinical presentation. Topics covered include the following:

- Somatic symptom and related disorders

- Adverse effects of psychiatric medications

DOI: 10.1542/peds.2016-1573

PEDIATRICS (ISSN Numbers: Print, 0031-4005; Online, 1098-4275).

To cite: Chun TH, Mace SE, Katz ER, AAP AMERICAN ACADEMY OF PEDIATRICS Committee on Pediatric Emergency Medicine. Evaluation and Management of Children With Acute Mental Health or Behavioral Problems. Part II: Recognition of Clinically Challenging Mental Health Related Conditions Presenting With Medical or Uncertain Symptoms. *Pediatrics.* 2016;138(3):e20161573

TABLE 1 Common Symptoms of Somatic Symptom and Related Disorders[14]

Pseudoneurologic	Gastrointestinal symptoms
Amnesia	Abdominal pain
Difficulty with swallowing or voice	Nausea
Vision or hearing impairment	Vomiting
Syncope	Bloating
Seizure	Diarrhea
Paralysis or paresis	Multiple food intolerances
Pain symptoms	Cardiopulmonary symptoms
Headache	Chest pain
Back pain	Dyspnea
Extremity pain	Palpitations
Dysuria	Dizziness

o Antipsychotic adverse effects

o Neuroleptic malignant syndrome

o Serotonin syndrome

• Children with special needs (autism spectrum disorders [ASDs] and developmental disorders [DDs])

• Mental health screening

The report is written primarily from the perspective of ED clinicians, but it is intended for all clinicians who care for children and adolescents with acute mental health and behavioral problems. An executive summary of this clinical report can be found at http://www.pediatrics.org/cgi/doi/ 10.1542/peds.2016-1574.

SOMATIC SYMPTOM AND RELATED DISORDERS

Overview

The *Diagnostic and Statistical Manual of Mental Disorders, Fifth Edition* recognizes 7 distinct somatic symptom and related disorders, including somatic symptom disorder, illness anxiety disorder, conversion disorder (functional neurologic symptom disorder), psychological factors affecting other medical conditions, factitious disorder, other specified somatic symptom and related disorder, and unspecified somatic symptom and related disorder.[1] Each disorder has specific diagnostic criteria, which apply to both adults and children and which are not adjusted for children. All these disorders

refer to an individual's subjective experience of physical symptoms. These diagnoses can also be applied to situations in which the level of distress or disability is thought to be disproportionate to what is typically associated with the physical findings. For example, when a medical condition is present, if the physical problems do not fully explain the reported symptoms or severity, a somatic symptom and related disorder may apply.[2]

Additional criteria for somatic symptom disorders include the requirement that the complaints or fixations are not associated with material gain, nor are they intentionally produced.[3] Symptoms that are intentionally created are classified as factitious disorders; those that result in material gain are categorized as malingering. Lastly, the symptoms result in significant impairment in psychosocial functioning (eg, relationships with family or friends, academic or occupational difficulties).[1]

Epidemiologic studies have found that somatic symptom and related disorders are both common and a significant contributor to health care usage and costs. In adult primary care populations, between 10% and 15% of patients have a diagnosis of 1 of these disorders.[4] Among children and adolescents, recurrent abdominal pain and headaches account for 5% and between 20% and 55% of pediatric office visits, respectively; 10% of adolescents report frequent

headaches, chest pain, nausea, and fatigue.[5] Patients with somatic symptom and related disorders use all types of medical services (eg, primary, specialty, ED, and mental health care) more frequently,[4,6–8] are more likely to "doctor shop,"[4] and in 2005, were estimated to have incrementally added $265 billion to the cost of health care in the United States.[9]

Clinical Features and Studies of Pediatric Somatic Symptom and Related Disorders

The clinical presentations of somatic symptom and related disorders are myriad, most often involving neurologic, pain, autonomic, or gastrointestinal tract symptoms (Table 1). Children and adolescents often report such symptoms[10,11] and often have multiple visits for these symptoms in primary care and other settings.[3,5,12,13] Vague, poorly described complaints, recent or current stressful events, symptoms that fluctuate with activity or stress, and lack of physical findings and laboratory abnormalities are common.[3]

Symptoms of pediatric somatic symptom and related disorders often do not meet strict *Diagnostic and Statistical Manual of Mental Disorders, Fifth Edition* diagnostic criteria and defy categorization. Other difficulties in caring for patients with these disorders in the ED are that few patients will have received a formal diagnosis, and ED clinicians rarely have access to sufficient clinical information to confirm the diagnosis.[15–17] In addition, the diagnosis of a "psychosomatic" illness can be stigmatizing to patients and families, resulting in them feeling unheard, disrespected, and defensive about their symptoms.[5] For these and other reasons, some prefer the term "medically unexplained symptoms".[2,6,18,19]

Several studies, including 1 performed jointly in the Pediatric

Research in Office Settings and Ambulatory Sentinel Practice Network collaboratives, have identified demographic and risk factors associated with pediatric somatic symptom and related disorders.[2,8,20,21] Patients who are adolescents, female, from minority ethnicities, from nonintact families, or from urban dwellings; who have past histories of psychological trauma; whose parents have lower education levels; and who have other family members with somatic symptom and related disorders are more likely to present with unexplained medical symptoms. Such patients are also at much higher risk of comorbid psychiatric problems.[8]

Other studies have approached this topic by investigating the prevalence of and relationships between psychiatric conditions in patients with unexplained medical symptoms. Emiroğlu et al[22] studied 31 patients referred to a pediatric neurology clinic for headache, vertigo, and syncope. When comprehensive testing did not reveal an identifiable medical cause for their symptoms, the patients were interviewed by a child psychiatrist. A large majority (93.5%) were found to have a diagnosable disorder according to *Diagnostic and Statistical Manual of Mental Disorders, Fourth Edition* criteria, the most common being mood and somatic symptom and related disorders. Other pediatric headache studies have found similar results.[23,24] Guidetti et al[25] followed patients for 8 years after referral to a pediatric neurology headache clinic. At follow-up, persistence or worsening of headaches was highly associated with the presence of comorbid psychiatric conditions, and resolution of headaches strongly correlated with the absence of mental health conditions. In this study, the most common mental health conditions were anxiety disorders and depression.

Other studies in other settings echo these findings. In a pediatric cardiology clinic study, Tunaoglu et al[26] reported a prevalence of 74% for psychiatric disorders, primarily depression, anxiety, and somatic symptom and related disorders, in patients referred for chest pain with normal medical workups. Campo et al[27] recruited patients from a pediatric primary care office. Using standardized psychiatric interviews, they found that patients with recurrent abdominal pain were significantly more likely to be diagnosed with anxiety (79%) and depressive disorders (43%) than controls. In a study from a pediatric rheumatology clinic, Kashikar-Zuck et al[28] also conducted standardized psychiatric interviews among patients with juvenile fibromyalgia. A high prevalence of current and lifetime anxiety and mood disorders was detected in this population.

Somatic Symptom and Related Disorders and the ED

Somatic symptom and related disorders are a particularly vexing problem in the ED because of the potential harm to patients that may result from diagnostic uncertainty. It is understandable that a patient with 1 of these disorders might undergo extensive, invasive testing such as a lumbar puncture, be exposed to radiographic studies with ionizing radiation, or be given potent medications to treat their symptoms, which in turn could result in significant respiratory, cardiac, central nervous system (CNS), or hematologic adverse effects, potentially necessitating additional medications or procedures such as endotracheal intubation and mechanical ventilation to treat these adverse effects.

Psychogenic nonepileptic seizures (PNES, previously called "pseudoseizures") in pediatric ED patients are an illustrative example of this conundrum. In their review

of identified PNES patients (the authors recognize that PNES is often unrecognized and underdiagnosed in the ED), Selbst and Clancy[29] found that all had multiple previous ED visits, 8 of 10 patients had been prescribed anticonvulsants in the past, 6 received anticonvulsants either in the ED or before arrival in the ED by prehospital personnel, all but 1 had invasive procedures and testing, and 8 were admitted to the hospital. Other studies have found similar rates of extensive medical testing in children with PNES.[30] Accurate diagnosis and appropriate referrals for these patients may be important, as Wyllie et al[31] found that on follow-up, 72% of patients' PNES had resolved after psychiatric treatment. A particularly challenging problem when treating potential PNES in the ED is that some of these patients will have both a true seizure disorder and PNES, making airway management and the decision to give anticonvulsants for apparent seizure activity difficult and complex for ED physicians.

Several studies have investigated the impact of somatic symptom and related disorders on emergency department patients. Knockaert et al[32] prospectively enrolled 578 adult patients presenting to a Belgian ED with chest pain. Although the majority of these patients were found to have a cardiac or pulmonary disease as the etiology of their chest pain, the authors classified "somatization disorder" as the third leading cause (9.2%) of these ED visits. Another interesting finding from this study was that somatization disorder was more common among patients who were self-referred to the ED and those brought by ambulance. Although formal psychiatric evaluation was not performed on all patients, and classification as somatization disorder was based on the available clinical information and the final discharge diagnoses, the authors believe that their methods underestimated the true prevalence. Other studies have found a higher prevalence of mental health disorders among adult ED patients with chest pain.[17]

Lipsitz et al[33] studied 32 pediatric ED patients who presented with chest pain and for whom no medical cause was found. Using a semistructured *Diagnostic and Statistical Manual of Mental Disorders, Fourth Edition* interview to detect anxiety disorders, they found that 81% met diagnostic criteria for an anxiety disorder, with 28% meeting full criteria for panic disorder. Other pain symptoms such as headaches, abdominal pain, and back pain were common in these children, as were impaired quality of life and multiple domains of daily functioning. In a secondary analysis of a larger study on maternal and pediatric mental health problems, Dang et al[34] explored the relationship between mothers' somatic symptoms and subsequent pediatric ED use for their child. Maternal somatic symptoms were assessed with the Patient Health Questionnaire 15, a validated measure for inquiring about common somatic problems in outpatient settings. After covariates were adjusted for, mothers with high somatic symptom scores reported higher rates of depression symptoms, difficulty caring for themselves and their child, and a greater use of the ED for their child (odds ratio, 1.8; 95% confidence interval [CI], 0.99–3.38; $P = .055$).

Although there are no known studies of interventions for pediatric ED patients, Abbass et al[35] performed an intriguing prospective study of adult ED patients with suspected somatic symptom and related disorders. If the treating ED physician made a provisional diagnosis of somatization after completing the medical evaluation of the patient, a referral was made for an outpatient mental health evaluation and intensive, short-term psychotherapy.

The mental health evaluation and treatment typically took place a few weeks after the ED visit, with patients receiving a mean of 3.8 psychotherapy sessions (range: 1–25 sessions). After the psychotherapy intervention, at 1-year follow-up, they found a mean reduction of 3.2 ED (69%) visits per patient (SD, 6.4; 95% CI, 1.3–5.0; $P < .001$), compared with the year before the index ED visit. In addition, at follow-up patients reported significant improvement in their somatic symptoms and high satisfaction with the psychotherapeutic referral and intervention. Although this was not a randomized controlled trial, patients who were referred to psychotherapy but did not attend treatment did not show any changes in their ED use at 1 year follow-up.

Treatment Strategies

Medically unexplained symptoms are extremely frustrating for patients, families, and medical providers. Parents and children often think that they are not being listened to and that physicians have misdiagnosed the problem, or potential causes of the symptoms have not been adequately evaluated.[2,10] These feelings can be intense and may be rooted in a fear that a medical illness is being missed, frustration over the lack of success in resolving the symptoms, the stigma of being labeled or perceived as "psychosomatic," or difficulty in acknowledging that psychological and physical symptoms may be related.[18]

Prognosis often is unpredictable. In some cases, the episode can be brief and resolve. In other cases, the course is chronic and difficult to treat. The chronicity of the symptoms and previous response to treatment may be informative about the likely treatment course. Most experts agree that an empathetic, consistent, multidisciplinary, long-term treatment plan is helpful for chronic

cases.[2,5,10,18] This may include various psychotherapies (eg, cognitive–behavioral, rehabilitative, operant interventions, self-management strategies, and family or group therapy), consistent communication between all treating providers, and comprehensive treatment of comorbid psychiatric conditions.[2]

Although these treatment modalities are not practical or possible for the ED setting, there are some strategies that are applicable and may be helpful. Experts suggest the following[2,5,18]:

- *Provide reassurance*: First and foremost, it is important to convey to the patient and family that the patient's symptoms are being heard and taken seriously. Taking time to obtain a detailed history and comprehensive physical examination can help accomplish this goal. Some children and families may be reassured by the knowledge that their symptoms are not life or limb threatening. In addition, eliciting and addressing the child's and family's anxiety and fears about the patient's symptoms may be both clinically illuminating for the ED provider and comforting to the patient and family. It may also be important to reaffirm that their ED and outpatient providers are working and will continue to work with them to continue to evaluate and treat their symptoms.

- *Communicate*: Strategies to improve communication include emphasizing collaboration between the patient, family, and all caregivers; identifying common goals and outcomes; and introducing the idea of working on improving functioning in addition to working toward symptom resolution. In addition, educating the patient and family about the limitations of the ED setting, as well as the benefits of other settings for evaluation and treatment, may be helpful. Lastly, exploring the patient and family's openness to the possibility that the symptoms may be psychologically related may be an important first step. Determining and using terms such as stress, temperament, anxiety, "nerves," and other terms that are acceptable to the patient and family may assist in this goal.

- *Coordinate care*: Contacting and communicating with all involved care providers may be time consuming but is important in implementing a cohesive, comprehensive evaluation and treatment plan and may have the added benefit of providing reassurance to the patient and family as well as decreasing frustration and improving satisfaction.

ADVERSE EFFECTS OF PSYCHIATRIC MEDICATIONS

The use of all psychotropic medications in pediatric populations over the last 2 decades has markedly increased.[36,37] Antipsychotic use, in particular, has shown large increases.[38] Especially notable is their burgeoning off-label use,[39–41] including in preschool-aged children.[42–44] Given the frequency and multiple medication regimens with which psychotropic agents are being prescribed,[36] ED clinicians are likely to encounter children and adolescents taking 1 or many of these medications. This section focuses on the clinical problems and diagnostic and treatment dilemmas one may encounter in the ED when caring for pediatric patients on antipsychotics and antidepressants.

An additional important consideration for ED clinicians is that many commonly used medications not typically thought of as psychotropic agents have dopaminergic and serotonergic properties similar to those of antipsychotics and antidepressants. For example, drugs used as antiemetics and for

TABLE 2 Antipsychotic Adverse Symptoms

Neurotransmitter	Symptoms	Antipsychotics Commonly Associated With Symptom
Dopamine		
Nigrostriatal tract	Extrapyramidal symptoms (eg, dystonia, dyskinesia, akathisia, Parkinsonism)	High-potency "typical" antipsychotics (haloperidol)
Tuberoinfundibular tract	Hyperprolactinemia	All "typical" antipsychotics, risperidone
Preoptic tract	Hypothermia	Rare, possibly more common with atypical antipsychotics
Acetylcholine (muscarinic)	Sinus tachycardia, dry mucous membranes, mydriasis, urinary retention	Low-potency "typical" antipsychotics (chlorpromazine)
α-Adrenergic	Orthostatic hypotension, reflex tachycardia	Atypical antipsychotics
Histamine	Sedation	"Typical" antipsychotics
Mechanism unknown		
Potential etiology: Pancreatic versus CNS adrenergic α_1, α_2, dopamine D_2, muscarinic, histamine H_1, serotonin$_1$, serotonin$_2$, or serotonin$_6$	Wt gain, obesity, hyperlipidemia, metabolic syndrome, impaired glucose tolerance, hyperglycemia, type 2 diabetes	Atypical antipsychotics Highest risk: clozapine, olanzapine Lower risk: quetiapine, risperidone Lowest risk: ziprasidone, aripiprazole

migraines (ie, prochlorperazine, metoclopramide, promethazine, and trimethobenzamide) are phenothiazines, the same type of medications as first-generation, "typical" antipsychotics. Droperidol, which has been used as an antiemetic and for agitation, is a butyrophenone, the same class as the antipsychotic haloperidol.[45] The number and scope of medications with serotonergic effects are surprising and are detailed in this section. Either alone or in combination with psychotropic serotonergic drugs, these medications can result in serotonin toxicity. Given how frequently these medications are used in clinical practice, familiarizing oneself with them and their potential adverse effects may be beneficial to ED clinicians.

Antipsychotic Adverse Effects

Antipsychotics are prescribed for various childhood disorders, including oppositional–defiant disorder, conduct disorder, attention-deficit/hyperactivity disorder, and ASDs.[46–49] These medications have

also been used as antiemetics and antipruritics and to treat headaches, hiccups, and various neurologic disorders such as Parkinson disease, hemiballismus, ballismus, Tourette syndrome, and Huntington chorea.[50,51]

The common adverse effects of antipsychotics can be conceptualized and organized around the CNS neurotransmitters on which they act.[45,50–54] Table 2 lists the common adverse effects of antipsychotics and the medications with which they are most commonly associated.

It is important to note that antipsychotics have other clinically significant effects, including "black box" warnings from the US Food and Drug Administration (FDA) for thioridazine and droperidol because of their potential to cause dysrhythmias. Almost all antipsychotics cause some degree of QT_c prolongation because of a quinidinelike effect. For most of the medications, however, the degree of QT_c prolongation is small, which has given rise to a debate about the actual risk of dysrhythmias and torsades de pointes with antipsychotics administered in their usual doses and routes of administration.[45,47,48,55-60] Of note, intravenous (IV) haloperidol has been studied[61] but carries an FDA non–black box warning because of deaths associated with high doses and IV administration.[62] Therefore, experts suggest that intramuscular dosing of antipsychotics in the ED is the parental preferred route of administration. Table 3 details the factors that are thought to increase the risk of QT_c prolongation and sudden death.[48,51,63,64] Table 4 lists the degree of QT_c prolongation for common antipsychotics.[65]

Cardiac: Black Box Warning

Both thioridazine and droperidol have been issued FDA black box warnings for a potential association with prolonged QT interval, torsades de pointes, and sudden death. Since then, several studies have disputed this risk with droperidol.[55-60] A large retrospective review of 2468 patients given droperidol in the ED found that no cardiovascular event occurred that did not have an alternative explanation, and only 6 serious adverse events occurred, with 1 cardiac arrest in a patient with a normal QT interval out of 2468 patients (0.2% = 6/2468).[56] A pediatric study also suggested the safety and efficacy of droperidol when used to treat agitation, nausea and vomiting, headache, and pain.[66] Thus, "although droperidol can be associated with prolongation of the QT interval, there is not convincing evidence that the drug causes severe cardiac events."[60] Despite these and other studies, since the black box warning was issued, use of droperidol has declined exponentially.[67,68]

Neurologic

Acute extrapyramidal syndromes associated with antipsychotic medications include acute dystonia, akathisia, and a Parkinsonian syndrome. Acute dystonia is characterized by involuntary motor

TABLE 3 Risk Factors for QT_c Prolongation or Dysrhythmias With Antipsychotic Use

Coadministration with other QT_c-prolonging medications
IV administration or high doses
Medically ill patients
Electrolyte abnormalities
Hepatic, renal, or cardiac impairment
Congenital long QT syndromes

tics or spasms usually involving the face, the extraocular muscles (oculogyric crisis), and the neck, back, and limb muscles and tends to occur after the first few doses of medication or after an increase in dosage. Laryngeal dystonia is a rare, potentially life-threatening adverse event that presents as a choking sensation, difficulty breathing, or stridor.[45,48]

Akathisia is a subjective feeling of restlessness, which generally occurs within the first few days of antipsychotic medication administration. Akathisia is found in up to 25% of patients[51] and has also been reported in patients receiving a single, standard dose (10 mg) of prochlorperazine. Both acute dystonia and acute akathisia tend to occur early in the course of treatment (ie, days to weeks after beginning an antipsychotic) and are easily reversed. To minimize these adverse effects, some advocate coadministering 25 to 50 mg of diphenhydramine or 1 to 2 mg of benztropine when giving an antipsychotic.[69] Others prefer to treat with anticholinergic agents (ie, diphenhydramine or benztropine) only if acute symptoms occur, followed by 2 days of oral therapy, given the prolonged half-life of antipsychotics.

The delayed-onset neurologic syndromes are Parkinsonism and tardive dyskinesia. The hallmarks of Parkinsonism are shuffling gait, cogwheel muscle rigidity, mask facies, bradykinesia or akinesia, pill-rolling tremors, and cognitive impairment. These symptoms are found in up to 13% of patients and

TABLE 4 QT_c Prolongation Associated With Antipsychotics

Medication	Mean QT_c Prolongation, ms
Thioridazine	25–30
Ziprasidone	5–22
Pimozide	13
Clozapine	8–10
Haloperidol	7
Quetiapine	6
Risperidone	0–5
Olanzapine	2
Aripiprazole	0

generally occur weeks to months after the patient starts antipsychotic therapy.[51] Drug-induced Parkinsonism syndrome is often treated by adding an anticholinergic agent, adding a dopaminergic agonist (eg, amantadine), or decreasing the dosage of a typical antipsychotic or switching to an atypical antipsychotic. Considering the diagnosis of drug-induced Parkinsonism may be important, because early diagnosis and rapid withdrawal of the antipsychotic drug may improve the possibility of complete recovery.[50] Tardive dyskinesia is characterized by rapid involuntary facial movements (eg, blinking, grimacing, chewing, or tongue movements) and extremity or truncal movements. Respiratory dyskinesia is often undiagnosed, can lead to recurrent aspiration pneumonia, and includes orofacial dyskinesia, dysphonia, dyspnea, and respiratory alkalosis.[45] Tardive dyskinesia occurs in 5% of young patients per year and is more common with older, "typical" antipsychotics.[50]

Although antipsychotic medications have been noted to lower the seizure threshold in a dose-dependent manner, antipsychotic medication–induced seizures are rare (usually <1%) when therapeutic doses are used, except for clozapine, which has a 5% incidence of seizures at high dosages.[45,51]

Metabolic

Adverse effects, such as weight gain, hyperglycemia, and

hyperlipidemia, are common, especially with second-generation, "atypical" antipsychotics.[45,50,51,70] Antipsychotics vary in their metabolic adverse effects, with the highest risk associated with clozapine and olanzapine, an intermediate risk with quetiapine, risperidone, and chlorpromazine, and the lowest risk with haloperidol, ziprasidone, and aripiprazole.[53]

Other

Agranulocytosis is a potential adverse effect of the atypical antipsychotic drug clozapine. Patients on clozapine regularly have complete blood cell counts performed, usually weekly or monthly, to monitor for this adverse effect. Other adverse effects of various atypical antipsychotics include somnolence, anxiety, agitation, oral hypoesthesia, headache, nausea, vomiting, insomnia, and tremor.[51]

Neuroleptic Malignant Syndrome

Neuroleptic malignant syndrome (NMS) is a potentially lethal syndrome consisting of the tetrad of mental status changes, fever, hypertonicity or rigidity, and autonomic dysfunction. It is presumed to be attributable to a lack of dopaminergic activity in the CNS, although hyperactivity of the sympathetic nervous system may also be involved. The deficiency of central dopaminergic activity can be attributable to dopamine antagonists or dopamine receptor blockade, dysfunction of the dopamine receptors, or withdrawal of dopamine agonists.[50,71,72]

With the increasing use of antipsychotic medications in the pediatric population, clinicians caring for children and adolescents may encounter this syndrome.[73] Given that NMS can be difficult to recognize and attenuated or incomplete presentations are possible, NMS is challenging to diagnose.[71,74] The incidence of NMS has been difficult

to determine, with estimates ranging from 0.02% to 3%.[45,71,75] Fortunately, mortality from NMS has decreased from 76% in the 1960s to <10% to 15% more recently.[72,76-78] Experts suggest considering NMS in the differential diagnosis of patients presenting with fever and altered mental status who are taking or may have taken an antipsychotic.[74]

NMS affects patients of all ages, with an apparent predominance in young adults and male patients (2:1).[73,79-81] It is unclear whether these are truly risk factors or reflect the patient population with the greatest use of antipsychotic medications.[75] Coadministration of psychotropic agents seems to be an especially high risk factor for precipitating NMS; in 1 study, more than half of people with reported NMS cases were taking concomitant psychotropic agents.[77] Other risk factors include dehydration, physical exhaustion, preexisting organic brain disease, and the use of long-acting depot antipsychotics. Neither duration of exposure to the drug nor toxic overdoses of antipsychotics appear to be associated with NMS. In addition, reintroducing the original precipitating drug may not lead to a reoccurrence of NMS, although patients with a history of NMS are at increased risk of recurrence.[76,77] The onset of NMS generally occurs within 7 days of starting or increasing antipsychotics and may last for 5 to 10 days even after the initiating agent is stopped. With depot forms of antipsychotics, however, onset of NMS symptoms may be more insidious and may last longer, up to 15 to 30 days.[71,76,82]

It was initially thought that newer atypical antipsychotics, which have both serotonin and dopamine-blocking properties, would not cause NMS because of their lower activity at dopamine receptors and their greater antiserotoninergic activity. This has not turned out to

be the case. Both second-generation atypical antipsychotics and the third-generation aripiprazole, which has partial dopamine agonist activity, have all been implicated in causing NMS.[76,79,83-87]

Despite its name, NMS can also be triggered by the administration or withdrawal of other, nonantipsychotic medications. Administration of tricyclic antidepressants, selective serotonin reuptake inhibitors (SSRIs), and lithium have been associated with NMS.[75] NMS also has been associated with the abrupt withdrawal of medications (eg, dopaminergic drugs used to treat Parkinson disease, such as levodopa, as well as baclofen, amantadine, some antipsychotics, and some antidepressants).[74] Lastly, the introduction to this section enumerates some of the medications commonly thought to be antiemetics or antimigraine therapies. They are, in fact, phenothiazines (ie, the same class of medications as first-generation, typical antipsychotics), but because of the clinical conditions for which they are used, they may not be suspected for being at risk for triggering NMS.

Pathophysiology

The cause of NMS is postulated to be a lack of dopaminergic activity in the CNS, principally affecting the D_2 receptors. Dopamine D_2 receptor antagonism leads to the manifestations of the NMS. Blockade of D_2 receptors in the hypothalamus produces an increased set point and loss of heat-dissipating mechanisms. Antagonism of the D_2 receptors in the nigrostriatal pathways and spinal cord via extrapyramidal pathways produces muscle rigidity and tremor. In the periphery, the increased release of calcium from the sarcoplasmic reticulum causes increased contractility, leading to muscle rigidity, increased heat production (with worsening of hyperthermia), and muscle cell

TABLE 5 Differential Diagnosis of NMS[72,89]

Toxicologic	Psychiatric
Serotonin syndrome	Delirium
Anticholinergic poisoning	Lethal catatonia
Sympathomimetics	Factitious fever
Malignant hyperthermia	Munchausen syndrome
Monoamine oxidase inhibitor	CNS
Monoamine oxidase inhibitor interaction with drugs	Intracranial tumors
or foods	
Central anticholinergic syndrome	Vasculitis
Lithium	Stroke
Phencyclidine	Seizure
Infectious disease	Other
Encephalitis	Heatstroke
Meningitis	Rheumatologic (eg, systemic lupus
	erythematosus, lupus cerebritis)
Tetanus	Malignancies
Endocrine	HIV/AIDS
Pheochromocytoma	Porphyria
Thyroid disease	Familial Mediterranean fever
Adrenal disease	

breakdown with elevated creatine kinase and rhabdomyolysis. In addition, D_2 receptor antagonism by eliminating tonic inhibition of the sympathetic nervous system leads to sympathoadrenal hyperactivity and autonomic instability.[72,75]

Clinical Presentation

The hallmarks of NMS are hyperthermia, altered mental status, muscle rigidity, and autonomic instability. Manifestations of autonomic dysfunction, which may occur before other symptoms, include fever up to 41°C or higher, tachycardia, blood pressure instability, diaphoresis, pallor, cardiac dysrhythmia, diaphoresis, sialorrhea, and dysphagia.[71,88]

The most common neurologic finding is lead pipe rigidity, although akinesia, dyskinesia, or waxy flexibility may be present.[45,77] The alteration in mental status often takes the form of delirium but varies from alert mutism to agitation to stupor to coma.[50,76] Motor abnormalities may include rigidity, akinesia, intermittent tremors, and involuntary movements. Other less common neurologic or neuromuscular signs include a positive Babinski, chorea, seizures, opisthotonos, trismus, and oculogyric crisis.[76,86]

Complications include renal failure from rhabdomyolysis, thromboemboli, dysrhythmias, cardiovascular collapse, and respiratory failure from aspiration pneumonia or tachypneic hypoventilation caused by diminished chest wall compliance from muscle rigidity, which may result in endotracheal intubation and ventilatory support.[50,71]

Diagnosis

Because there are no pathognomonic clinical or laboratory criteria, NMS is a clinical diagnosis. The differential diagnosis for NMS is broad and is outlined in Table 5. An important component of the diagnosis is a history of antipsychotic use or withdrawal of a dopaminergic agent.[45,86] Numerous diagnostic criteria have been proposed, which have included the classic clinical symptoms and other supplemental criteria.[1,79,81,88] Additional proposed criteria include elevated creatine kinase,[81] leukocytosis, incontinence, dysphagia, mutism, and metabolic acidosis.[1,79,81]

Recently, a Delphi panel of international NMS experts convened to discuss NMS diagnostic criteria.[90] Although its purpose was not to create a new set of criteria, the

results reflect consensus on the relative importance of individual clinical and diagnostic features for making a diagnosis of NMS. On a 100-point scoring system (ie, the total number of points sum up to 100), each clinical feature of NMS was assigned a number of "priority points." The point system is not meant to be used as a method for making the diagnosis of NMS; that is, there is no threshold number of points that indicate the presence or absence of NMS. Rather, it is meant to help clinicians determine which features of NMS are more important in making the diagnosis. The greater the number of points assigned, the greater the significance of the feature in making the diagnosis of NMS. The Delphi panel made the following assignments: exposure to dopamine antagonist or withdrawal of dopamine agonist within 3 days (20 points), hyperthermia (>100.4°F oral on ≥2 occasions [18 points]), rigidity (17 points), mental status alteration (13 points), creatine kinase elevation (≥4 times upper limit of normal [10 points]), sympathetic nervous system lability (10 points), hypermetabolism (5 points), and negative workup for infectious, toxic, metabolic, or neurologic causes (7 points). Sympathetic nervous system lability was defined as 2 or more of the following: elevated (systolic or diastolic ≥25% of baseline) or fluctuations (≥20 mm Hg diastolic or ≥25 mm Hg systolic change within 24 hours) in blood pressure, diaphoresis, or urinary incontinence. Hypermetabolism was defined as a heart rate increase ≥25% above baseline and respiratory rate ≥50% above baseline.

Leukocytosis, generally in the range of 15 000 to 30 000 cells per cubic millimeter, and electrolyte findings consistent with dehydration may be present. The etiology of elevated alkaline phosphatase, lactic dehydrogenase, and transaminases indicating impaired liver function is unknown but may be secondary to acute fatty liver changes from the hyperpyrexia. An elevated serum aldolase and creatine kinase, often greater than 16 000 IU/L, may be attributable to severe, sustained muscle contractions. The elevated creatine kinase may lead to rhabdomyolysis, acute myoglobinuria, and renal failure. A nonspecific common finding is the presence of a low serum iron concentration in patients with NMS.[77,86,91] If a lumbar puncture is performed, the cerebrospinal fluid results may be normal or have nonspecific findings. Findings on an EEG, if obtained, are variable. The EEG results may be normal or demonstrate findings of a nonspecific encephalopathy, such as diffuse slowing.[71,76] There are no specific findings on postmortem histopathology of the brain.[71]

Differentiating NMS from serotonin syndrome and other toxidromes can be challenging. Clinical features that may help are detailed in Table 7 and the section on serotonin syndrome.

Treatment

Management of NMS involves primarily supportive care and removal of the initiating agent. If NMS is triggered by the abrupt withdrawal of an anti-Parkinsonism drug, reintroduction of the drug may be considered.[72] Cardiorespiratory compromise may be managed with standard, supportive measures. Dehydration or elevated creatine kinase and rhabdomyolysis may be treated with IV fluids. If renal failure occurs, hemodialysis may be necessary (however, dialysis does not remove antipsychotics that are protein bound). For agitation, experts suggest benzodiazepines as the first-line agent. Fever can be treated with external cooling measures, such as cooling blankets.[72,75]

Suggestions for NMS treatment are based on case reports and clinical experience, not rigorous clinical

trials, limiting the strength of the evidence base. The most frequently administered drugs have been dantrolene, bromocriptine, and amantadine. Dantrolene decreases muscle rigidity, and thermogenesis caused by the tonic contraction of muscles. It blocks the release of calcium from smooth muscle cells' sarcoplasmic reticulum, uncoupling actin and myosin chains, resulting in muscle relaxation. Commonly used dosages in NMS are 1 mg/kg by IV push followed by 0.25 to 0.75 mg/kg every 6 hours. The drug may be continued until symptoms resolve or a maximum of 10 mg/kg is reached.[72,77]

The utility of CNS dopaminergic agents is unclear and controversial. Therefore, consultation with a toxicologist or poison control center may be helpful. Bromocriptine is a centrally acting dopamine agonist. Experts suggest an initial dosage of 1.25 to 2.5 mg twice a day, which may be increased to 10 mg 3 times a day. Muscle rigidity usually responds quickly to bromocriptine, but fever, blood pressure, and creatine kinase levels may take several days to normalize. Amantadine has dopaminergic and anticholinergic effects. A common starting dosage is 100 mg orally, with a maximum dosage of 200 mg twice a day.[72,77,86] Benzodiazepines are often used for agitation and rigidity. Electroconvulsive therapy has been used in some pharmacotherapy-resistant cases.[72,77]

ED clinicians may not have seen or treated many cases of NMS. Potential resources for caring for these patients include toxicologists, a poison control center, and the NMS Information Service, which can be accessed through its Web site (http://www.nmsis.org/index.asp). Staffed by NMS experts, the NMS Information Service provides information, education, and phone consultation regarding the diagnosis and treatment of NMS.

Serotonin Syndrome

Serotonin syndrome occurs in all ages, from infants and children to older adults. It has even been reported in newborn infants as a result of in utero exposure.[92] The incidence of and mortality from serotonin syndrome have been increasing and may escalate in the future[93,94] because of the growing number and use of proserotonergic medications, such as SSRIs, other classes of psychiatric medications (eg, other antidepressants and anxiolytics), antibiotics, opiate analgesics, antiemetics, anticonvulsants, antimigraine drugs, anti-Parkinsonism drugs, muscle relaxants, and weight-reduction or bariatric medications (Table 6). In addition to prescription medications, a wide variety of over-the-counter medications, herbal and dietary supplements, and drugs of abuse have all been associated with serotonin syndrome.[95]

Serotonin syndrome occurs in approximately 16% to 18% of patients who overdose with an SSRI.[93] The true incidence of serotonin syndrome is difficult to estimate, given that many instances are probably undiagnosed or misdiagnosed.[96,97] Variable clinical manifestations (eg, lack of the classic triad of symptoms), wide spectrum of disease from mild to life-threatening, symptoms that are easily misattributed to the patient's underlying mental condition (eg, anxiety and akathisia), lack of awareness of the disorder, and the vast number of medications, other agents, and combinations of medicines or agents that can cause serotonin syndrome all may contribute to missed diagnoses.[93,97,98]

Pathophysiology

In the CNS, serotonin (5-hydroxytryptamine) regulates temperature, attention, and behavior. Peripherally, serotonin

TABLE 6 Medications and Other Agents Associated With Serotonin Syndrome

Psychiatric drugs
  Antianxiety drugs: direct serotonin antagonists
    Buspirone
  Antimanic drugs: increased postsynaptic receptor sensitivity
    Lithium
    Antidepressants
  Antidepressants: tricyclic antidepressants
    Amitriptyline
    Clomipramine
    Nortriptyline
  Antidepressants: monoamine oxidase inhibitors
    Phenelzine
  Antidepressants: SSRIs
    Citalopram
    Fluoxetine
    Paroxetine
    Sertraline
  Antidepressants: $5HT_{2A}$ receptor blockers
    Nefazodone
    Trazodone
  Antidepressants: serotonin-norepinephrine reuptake inhibitors
    Venlafaxine
    Duloxetine
Nonpsychiatric drugs
  Skeletal muscle relaxants
    Cyclobenzaprine
  Opioid analgesics
    Fentanyl
    Meperidine
    Oxycodone
    Pentazocine
    Tramadol
    Hydrocodone
  Antibiotics
    Linezolid
  Antiretroviral (protease inhibitor)
    Ritonavir
  Anticonvulsants
    Carbamazepine
    Valproic acid
  Antiemetics
    Metoclopramide (Reglan)
    $5HT_3$ receptor antagonists
    Ondansetron
  Antimigraine drugs
    Ergot alkaloids: ergotamines
    Triptans ($5 HT_{1B}$ and $5HT_{1B}$ receptor agonists; eg, sumatriptan)
    Antiparkinsonian drugs
    Carbidopa/levodopa
  Bariatric medications (weight reduction)
    Sibutramine
Over-the-counter medications
  Dextromethorphan (cough suppressants and cold remedies)
Drugs of abuse
  3,4–Methylenedioxymethamphetamine (Ecstasy)
  Cocaine
  Lysergic acid diethylamide
  Methamphetamine
Herbals
  Hypericum perforatum (St John's wort)
Dietary supplements
  Panax ginseng (ginseng)
  L-tryptophan
  5-hydroxytryptophan

This is not an all-inclusive list but gives an overview of the wide range of agents that can trigger the serotonin syndrome. Drugs are listed by their therapeutic category. This list is not intended to endorse any given drug or product.

modulates gastrointestinal tract motility, vasoconstriction, bronchoconstriction, and platelet aggregation. Seven families of serotonin receptors have been identified, with serotonin syndrome resulting from excess CNS serotonin,[98,99] primarily caused by overstimulation of serotonin$_{2A}$ receptors.[100,101]

Excessive serotonin activity may result from myriad mechanisms, including increased release of serotonin (eg, cocaine, amphetamines), increased production of serotonin (eg, L-tryptophan in stimulant products), inhibiting reuptake of synaptic serotonin (eg, tricyclic antidepressants, SSRIs), decreased neuronal metabolism of serotonin via inhibition of monoamine oxidase inhibitors, direct stimulation of serotonin receptors (eg, lysergic acid diethylamide, migraine drugs such as sumatriptan, buspirone), and increased postsynaptic receptor responsivity (eg, lithium).[93,95]

A single dose of a single proserotonergic agent may precipitate serotonin syndrome. However, many cases occur after exposure to 2 or more drugs that increase the serotonin activity. Examples of combinations of proserotonergic medications causing serotonin syndrome include reports of SSRIs and fentanyl (given during procedural sedation),[102] erythromycin,[96] and St John's wort (an over-the-counter herbal supplement).[95] In addition, serotonin syndrome has also been reported in a patient withdrawing from a serotonergic agent.[100]

Clinical Presentation

The clinical triad of the serotonin syndrome consists of mental status changes, autonomic hyperactivity, and neuromuscular abnormalities. One of the greatest challenges of this diagnosis is its extremely variable presentation. Many patients do not exhibit all these clinical characteristics.[103] Some patients will have severe symptoms, such as high fever (up to 41.1°C), severe hypertension, and tachycardia that may deteriorate into hypotension, shock, agitated delirium, muscular rigidity, and hypertonicity. Mild cases may range from tremor and diarrhea to tachycardia and hypertension but no fever. Symptom onset is generally rapid, often within minutes of exposure to the precipitating agent, with most patients presenting within 6 to 24 hours.[100]

Agitated delirium is the most common form of mental status change, although this too has a wide spectrum of severity, including mild agitation, hypervigilance, slightly pressured speech, and easy startle. Diaphoresis, shivering, mydriasis, increased bowel sounds, and diarrhea are common signs of autonomic dysfunction.[95,100] Myoclonus is the most common neuromuscular finding,[98] but other abnormalities are possible, including muscular rigidity, hypertonicity (which may in turn contribute to hyperthermia), hyperreflexia and clonus (which are more pronounced in the lower than the upper extremities), horizontal ocular clonus, tremor, and akathisia. In some cases, muscle hypertonicity may be so severe that it overpowers and obscures tremor and hyperreflexia.

Significant morbidity and mortality are associated with serotonin syndrome. Severe cases are characterized by rhabdomyolysis with an elevated creatine kinase, metabolic acidosis, elevated serum aminotransferase, renal failure with an elevated serum creatinine, seizures, and disseminated intravascular coagulopathy. Approximately one-quarter of patients are treated with intubation, mechanical ventilation, and admission to an ICU. The mortality rate is approximately 11%, with the most common cause of death being inadequate management of hyperthermia.[98]

Diagnosis

The differential diagnosis of serotonin syndrome includes other disorders precipitated by medications or drug toxicity reactions (eg, NMS and malignant hyperthermia, anticholinergic syndrome, and withdrawal syndromes including delirium tremens); CNS disorders spanning infection (meningitis, encephalitis), tumors, and seizures; and psychiatric disorders such as acute catatonia.

Differentiating between serotonin syndrome and other medication-induced syndromes can be challenging and may be important, given that treatment may differ depending on the underlying etiology. Table 7 details both the similar and differentiating features of these syndromes. The most common clinical finding of serotonin syndrome is myoclonus, which occurs in slightly more than half (57%) of cases.[98] Some experts believe that clonus and hyperreflexia are "highly diagnostic for the serotonin syndrome and their occurrence in the setting of serotonergic drug use establishes the diagnosis."[100]

As with NMS, there are no pathognomonic laboratory or radiographic findings of serotonin syndrome. Testing may be obtained on the basis of clinical suspicion and may include a complete blood cell count, electrolytes, serum urea nitrogen, creatinine, arterial blood gas (checking respiratory status and for metabolic acidosis), hepatic transaminases, creatine kinase, urinalysis, toxicology screens, coagulation studies, electrocardiography, EEG, and brain imaging studies.

Clinical diagnostic criteria for serotonin syndrome have been proposed.[104,105] Hunter criteria[104] have a higher sensitivity (84% vs 75%) and specificity (97% vs 96%) than Sternbach criteria.[105] In addition, the use of the Sternbach criteria may exclude mild, early, or subacute serotonin syndrome. Others prefer modified Dunkley criteria.[100,104] According to the modified Dunkley criteria, the diagnosis can be made if the patient has taken a serotonergic drug within the last 5 weeks and has any of the following: tremor and hyperreflexia; spontaneous clonus; muscle rigidity, temperature >38°C, and either ocular clonus or inducible clonus; ocular clonus and either agitation or diaphoresis; or inducible clonus and either agitation or diaphoresis.[100] Other variations of these diagnostic criteria have been proposed. They all include a serotonergic drug having been started or the dosage increased and other possible etiologies (eg, NMS, substance abuse, withdrawal, infection, other toxidromes) having been ruled out, plus the presence of specific signs and symptoms.[95,106,107]

Treatment

Treatment often involves discontinuing the precipitating agent and providing supportive care. Supportive care may include treatment of agitation (eg, benzodiazepines), amelioration of hyperthermia, and management of the autonomic instability (eg, IV fluids and other agents to address abnormal vital signs). In addition, for those with severe serotonin syndrome (eg, temperature >41.1°C), emergency sedation, neuromuscular paralysis, and intubation may be considered. Physical restraints may be detrimental, because they may exacerbate isometric contractions, thereby worsening hyperthermia and lactic acidosis and increasing mortality.[98]

In severe cases, serotonin$_{2A}$ antagonists may be considered, with cyproheptadine being most commonly used. The adult dosage of

TABLE 7 Differentiation of the Drug Toxicity Syndromes

	Serotonin Syndrome	NMS	Malignant Hyperthermia	Anticholinergic Poisoning
Etiology	Excessive serotonin	Decreased dopamine	Calcium release from sarcoplasmic reticulum	Inhibit acetylcholine binding to muscarinic receptors
Precipitant	Proserotonergic drugs	Dopamine antagonist or withdrawal of dopaminergic drug	Inhalational anesthetic with or without succinylcholine	Anticholinergic drugs or antimuscarinic drugs
History	Nonidiosyncratic, add new drug, ↑ dosage of drug, or add second drug	Idiosyncratic, exposure to dopamine antagonist drug or withdrawal from dopaminergic drug	Inherited (+ family history) or new genetic mutation	Anticholinergic drug exposure antihistamines, tricyclic antidepressants, sleep aids, cold preparations, diphenhydramine, atropine
Onset	Minutes to hours Usual: 6–24 h	Days Usual: 1–7 d	Hours Usual: <12 h	Minutes to hours Usual: 0.5–24 h
Vital signs				
Temperature	Elevated (≤41.1°C)	Elevated (≤41.1°C)	Elevated (≤46°C)	Mild elevation (<38.8°C)
Heart rate	Tachycardia	Tachycardia	Tachycardia	Tachycardia
Respirations	Tachypnea	Tachypnea	Tachypnea	Tachypnea
Blood pressure	Hypertension (may deteriorate to hypotension)	Hypertension	Hypertension	Hypertension (mild)
Mental status	Agitated delirium	Variable: alert, mutism, stupor, coma	Agitation	Agitated delirium
Neuromuscular abnormalities				
Muscle tone	Increased, lower extremities greater than upper extremities	"Lead pipe" rigidity	Rigor mortis–like rigidity (masseters or generalized)	Normal
Muscle reflexes	Hyperreflexic, clonus; may be masked by hypertonicity	Slowed, bradyreflexic	Hyporeflexic	Normal
Physical examination				
Skin	Diaphoretic	Diaphoretic	Diaphoretic, mottled	Hot, dry, erythema[a]
Pupils	Mydriasis	Normal	Normal	Mydriasis
Mucous membranes	Sialorrhea	Sialorrhea	Normal	Dry[a]
Gastrointestinal motility	Hyperactive bowel sounds, may have diarrhea	Normal or hypoactive bowel sounds	Hypoactive bowel sounds	Hypoactive or absent bowel sounds
Treatment considerations				
General	Discontinue precipitant drug, supportive care, benzodiazepine for agitation			
Specific	If severe: serotonin$_{2A}$ antagonists (eg, cyproheptadine)	If severe: smooth muscle relaxant (eg, dantrolene), dopamine agonists (eg, bromocriptine, amantadine)	If severe: dantrolene	Sodium bicarbonate for prolonged QRS or dysrhythmias, treat hyperthermia, physostigmine

All of these drug toxicity syndromes can present with altered mental status, autonomic dysfunction, and neuromuscular abnormalities as manifested by abnormal vital signs including fever, hypertension, and tachycardia. Treatment in all 4 syndromes may include removing the precipitating agent and providing supportive care. Other specific therapy may differ depending on the disorder. Not all patients will have all the classic signs and symptoms. For example, a patient with mild serotonin syndrome may be afebrile but have tachycardia and hypertension. Typical findings are listed in this table.

[a] Anticholinergic syndrome described as "Red as a beet, dry as a bone, hot as a hare, blind as a bat, mad as a hatter, full as a flask."

cyproheptadine is usually 12 to 24 mg over 24 hours, typically starting with 12 mg, followed by 2 mg every 2 hours for continuing symptoms, and a maintenance dose of 8 mg every 6 hours, given orally. There is no parenteral form, but tablets have been crushed and administered via a nasogastric tube. The pediatric dosage is usually 0.25 mg/kg per day, divided into 2 or 3 doses daily, up to a maximum of 12 mg. Chlorpromazine, an antagonist of serotonin$_{2A}$ receptors as well, is available in a parenteral form but has the disadvantage that it can cause hypotension and may increase muscle rigidity, decrease the seizure threshold, and worsen NMS.[98] Both drugs may be effective,[108] but cyproheptadine is preferred by most experts.[99,100]

Low dosages of direct-acting sympathomimetic amines (eg, phenylephrine, norepinephrine, and epinephrine) or short-acting drugs such as esmolol or nitroprusside have been used to manage fluctuating blood pressure and heart rate. Use of indirect agents (eg, dopamine) may not be efficacious, because the mechanism of action of these drugs includes intracellular metabolism via catecholamine-O-methyl transferase to metabolize the dopamine to epinephrine and norepinephrine, which may result in overshooting the desired effect.

Management of hyperthermia often involves terminating the extreme muscle activity. In addition to treating agitation, benzodiazepines may be useful in controlling muscular activity in moderate cases. In severe cases, paralysis with nondepolarizing drugs (eg, vecuronium or rocuronium) and intubation may be considered. Some experts suggest that succinylcholine may be risky with these patients, secondary to hyperkalemia and rhabdomyolysis, which may be present and ultimately result in dysrhythmias. Because the fever of NMS is secondary to muscular hyperactivity and not effects on the hypothalamic thermoregulation set point, antipyretics typically are not efficacious.[96,99,108]

Patients with serotonin syndrome can deteriorate rapidly; therefore, close observation and preparation for rapid intervention may be considered. In milder cases, evaluation, observation, and discharge with close, additional outpatient management may be considered. As mentioned previously, discussing these patients' care with a toxicologist or poison control center may be helpful.

CHILDREN WITH SPECIAL NEEDS

Autism Spectrum and Developmental Disorders

In recent years, there has been a sharp increase in the incidence of ASDs and DDs,[109] with corresponding interest and growth in treatment strategies. Investigated therapeutic modalities include psychobehavioral therapies,[110-115] psychopharmacology,[116-118] occupational and language therapies,[119-121] and complementary and alternative medicines.[122] Unfortunately, many studies have had methodologic limitations (eg, small sample sizes, variability in study populations, methods or interventions used, and outcomes measures) and are not applicable to the medical setting.[123-125] Three evidence-based reviews of this topic conclude that there is adequate evidence for only a limited number of therapies (eg, pharmacotherapy), although several other strategies show promise (eg, early and intensive behavioral therapy, social skills training, and visual communication systems).[125-128] Given these limitations, the strategies discussed below are based primarily on expert, consensus opinion.

ASD-DD–Sensitive Care Resources

A wide range of ED health professionals can champion, organize, design, and coordinate ASD-sensitive ED care, including physicians, nurses, nursing assistants, nurse practitioners and physician assistants, social workers, and child life specialists. Non-ED professionals who may be helpful include developmental–behavioral pediatricians, child psychologists and psychiatrists, special education teachers, speech–language therapists, and occupational therapists.

Often, the most important ASD-DD "experts" to consult are the child's parents. Parents of children with ASDs or DDs know what strategies work with their children (eg, which words, actions, or stimuli calm and help their child and which have the opposite effect). Parents can also be "interpreters" for ED clinicians, deciphering the significance of their child's actions and behaviors and facilitating communication with their child. Spending some time asking parents about their child is likely to be a productive, efficient method for tailoring effective ED care for these patients.

Strategies for ASD-DD–Sensitive ED Care

Typical strategies for caring for children with ASD-DD are listed in Table 8.[128] Children with ASD-DD are often hypersensitive to environmental stimuli (eg, light, sound, and activity). Simple solutions include using a quiet office or counseling room (if available) instead of a loud, stimulating examination room. If this type of patient space is not available, an alternative solution may be to use a quiet examination room, away from the busy, noisy areas of the ED, with dimmed lighting (eg, turning off some lights or using a single lamp).

Studies have demonstrated that visual communication systems (VCSs) can improve communication with children with language disabilities.[129-132] VCS products are the most commonly used communication adjuncts and are widely available. There are numerous commercial or free and print and electronic products (eg, Web sites, "apps," devices). A visual schedule (Fig 1) exemplifies how a VCS can be used to prepare a child with ASD-DD for an upcoming event or activity. Visual schedules help children organize themselves, understand what will happen next, highlight or introduce activities that are unfamiliar to them, and create smoother transitions, all of which may decrease children's anxiety.

If a child has his or her own personal VCS, it may be advantageous to use

TABLE 8 Nonpharmacologic Strategies for Caring for Children With ASD-DD

Environmental modification (light, noise, other stimuli)
Visual communication systems
Transition planning
Occupational or physical therapy techniques

the VCS, because the child will be familiar with pictures. A potential disadvantage of a personal VCS is that the set of images may not have the necessary medical pictures. A simple and inexpensive solution to this problem is to create a custom set of images of the ED setting. This can easily be done with clip art or digital photography images, which are then printed and laminated. If digital photography is used, taking pictures of the ED staff, equipment, and commonly performed procedures is a simple method for creating a customized VCS for your setting (Fig 2).

Transitions are often problematic for children with ASD-DD, including changing from 1 activity to the next, moving from 1 setting to another (especially new settings), and breaks or deviations from their usual routines. For these reasons, a medical visit may be upsetting or unsettling to these children. Fortunately, many parents are familiar with anticipating and planning for these types of transitions. For example, these parents talk to their children before a new experience, describe what will happen and the sequence of events, and explain what might be upsetting to the children and how they will handle these stressful situations. Preparing children with ASD-DD for a medical visit ideally begins before or while en route to the visit and is an ongoing process once they arrive.

Anticipating and building breaks in a schedule may be helpful. Many children with ASD-DD are able to remain on task for only short periods of time. Regular, brief breaks in the schedule may be helpful to these children. As time consuming as it may be, in the total calculus of planning

Triage Schedule

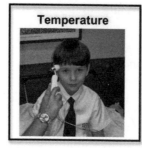 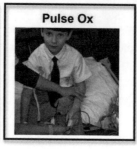 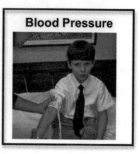

FIGURE 1
Digital photograph visual schedule. Photo credit: Thomas H. Chun, MD, MPH, FAAP.

Triage Schedule

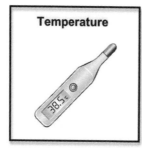 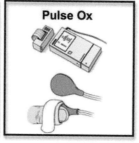 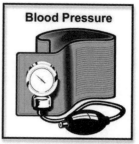

FIGURE 2
Clip art visual schedule.

the ED visit this may still be a time-neutral strategy relative to the time consumed by unsuccessful strategies. At the least, this strategy is likely to be more satisfactory to children, their parents, and ED clinicians.

Desensitization strategies that are used with all children (eg, gradually approaching and engaging with children, bending down to interact at children's level, allowing children to play with medical instruments or to use them on you or their parent first, distracting them with a toy or game, and having children held or comforted by parents while they are examined) also may help with children with ASD-DD. For some, however, the same strategies may benefit from significant augmentation, literally breaking each step down into several incremental, smaller steps. It may take several visits and interactions and multiple attempts before children will allow you to approach and examine them.

Other children with ASD-DD are very sensitive about their personal space. Starting at the periphery (ie, toes and fingers) and slowly moving centrally may help relax children and facilitate the examination. These types of desensitization strategies have been successfully used for phlebotomy attempts in children with ASD-DD.[133]

Many children with ASD-DD find value in occupational therapy (OT). OT techniques that are directly applicable to medical settings involve sensory integration and tasks that can be used as distraction techniques. Children with ASD-DD have variable responses to touch, with some finding it soothing and others becoming distressed by touch. Some find "deep pressure" (ie, the feeling of weight on their bodies) relaxing, but others respond to light touch. Devices such as weighted blankets or shawls for deep pressure and gentle massaging devices for light touch frequently are used. These products can be purchased through OT supply vendors, but simple substitutes can be found easily in medical settings. For example, a radiology lead vest or apron is an easy facsimile of a weighted blanket. Gently stroking the child with gauze or cast underpadding provides an excellent light touch massage.

Distraction may be a useful adjunct in children with ASD-DD. Occupying a child's hands or body with "fidget toys" is a typical strategy. OT devices (eg, grip strengthening and manual dexterity devices, devices to improve balance) also may serve this function. With appropriate supervision, simple substitutes for these devices are also easily made (eg, a loosely wound roll of gauze or cast underpadding can be a substitute for a squeeze toy). Rocking in a rocking chair or nylon folding sports stadium seat also can calm children (Fig 3).

Psychopharmacology and ASD-DD

There are no rigorous evidence-based guidelines regarding psychotropic medications for children with ASD-DD. Although there is strong evidence for the use of psychotropic medications in ASD-DD,[116,117,125] there are no controlled trials of these medications for acute agitation or sedation. Currently, there are no known contraindications to using common sedating medications for children with ASD-DD, although some experts believe that atypical medication responses may be more common (eg, idiosyncratic, disinhibition, or paradoxical reactions). Inquiring about the previous reaction to medications often is helpful, as may be beginning with lower medication dosages to observe and determine the child's response to the medication.[134]

MENTAL HEALTH SCREENING

For a discussion of mental health screening strategies in primary care settings, please refer to the American Academy of Pediatrics clinical report on screening for behavioral and emotional problems.[135]

The Advantages of the ED Setting

The ED may be an ideal setting for screening and identifying high-risk, difficult-to-reach pediatric populations with mental health problems. Many teenagers either do not have a primary care provider or face significant barriers to accessing such health care. For these adolescents, the ED often is their main or only source of medical care.[136,137] Other high-risk groups for mental health and substance use problems are homeless adolescents and school dropouts,[138-143] both of whom disproportionately seek medical care in the ED.

Finally, male adolescents may preferentially seek care in EDs because they are less likely to participate in primary or mental health care.[144,145]

Feasibility and Acceptability of ED Mental Health Screening

Several rapid, efficient, and accurate ED mental health screening tools have been developed and show promising results. As few as 2 screening questions have been found to be helpful in detecting depression in both adult and pediatric ED settings as well as problematic adolescent alcohol use.[146-148] A 4-question adolescent suicide screen has been shown to have good sensitivity, specificity, and predictive value across a range of teenagers seeking care in the ED and can be accurately administered by non–mental health professionals.[149-151] Similarly, an 8-question screen was shown to have excellent predictive characteristics for detecting posttraumatic stress symptoms in children who sustained traffic-related injuries.[152]

Given the clinical and time pressures of the ED setting, it is important that mental health screening be

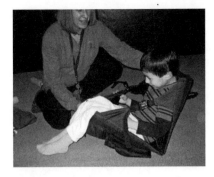

FIGURE 3
Example of rocking in a sports chair. Photo credit: Thomas H. Chun, MD, MPH, FAAP.

acceptable to adolescents, their parents, and ED clinicians. Numerous studies have shown the acceptability of such screening. Teenagers and parents both report favorable attitudes toward mental health screening during an ED visit.[153,154] In this study, suicide and drug and alcohol screening rated as more important than other mental health problems. Female adolescents and their parents, more than male adolescents, expressed positive views on screening. In another study, both teenagers and their caregivers perceived ED depression screening as a sign of caring and concern for the adolescent.[155] Suicide screening has been found to be acceptable to 60% to 66% of patients and parents, with 96% of participants agreeing that suicide screening is appropriate in the ED.[149,150,156]

What do ED clinicians think about mental health screening in the ED? Is such screening acceptable to them? Perceived and real barriers to such screening exist, including lack of training, time constraints, and increasing ED patients' length of stay. Williams et al[154] investigated this question and found that 99% of physicians and 97% of nurses stated that a brief, validated screening tool did not interfere with patient care. In addition, research staff endorsed "no difficulty" in administering the screen to 73% of participants. Lastly, a significant and important finding of the study by Horowitz et al[149] was that real-time evaluation of positive suicide screens did not increase ED patients' length of stay.

ED Mental Health Screens

Many mental health screening tools have been developed or tested in the ED setting. Although not validated in general ED populations, they have the potential to increase ED mental health screening. One example is an abbreviated version of the Home, Education/School, Activities, Drugs, Depression, Sexuality, Suicide, Safety (HEADDSSS) mnemonic for adolescent psychosocial assessment, which was adapted for and tested in an ED.[157] The Home, Education, Activities and Peers, Drugs and Alcohol, Suicidality, Emotions and Behaviors, Discharge Resources (HEADS-ED) was found to be reliable and accurate, with good concurrent and predictive validity for future psychiatric evaluation and hospitalization.[158]

Horowitz et al[149,151,159] have performed several studies on ED suicide screening, most recently by using multiple logistic regression modeling to determine which suicide screening questions best screen for and identify occult suicidal youth.[150] A 4-question model was found to optimize sensitivity (97%; 95% CI, 91%–99%), specificity (88%; 95% CI, 84%–91%), and negative predictive value (99%, 95% CI, 98%–99%) for ED patients presenting with both psychiatric and nonpsychiatric conditions. The 4 domains of suicidal ideation are current suicidal ideation, past suicide attempts, current wish to die, and current thoughts of being better off dead. Given the prevalence of suicidal ideation and attempts and the morbidity and mortality associated with attempts, screening patients with unclear or high risk of suicide (eg, those presenting with ingestions, acute intoxication, single-car motor vehicle crashes, and significant falls) also may be important.

Both depression and alcohol abuse may be screened for with 2 questions. Rutman et al[147] found that the 2 questions "During the past month, have you often been bothered by feeling down, depressed, or hopeless?" and "During the past month, have you often been bothered by little interest or pleasure in doing things?" were 78% sensitive (95% CI, 73%–84%) and 82% specific (95% CI, 77%–87%) for adolescent depression. These 2 questions have similar screening properties in adult ED patients as well.[146] Both Newton et al and the National Institute of Alcohol Abuse and Alcoholism (NIAAA) have developed 2-question screens for problematic teenage alcohol use.[148,160] Newton et al also believe that a single question may efficiently screen for marijuana use. They used the following questions: "In the past year, have you sometimes been under the influence of alcohol in situations where you could have caused an accident or gotten hurt?", "Have there often been times when you have a lot more to drink than you intended to have?", and "In the past year, how often have your used cannabis: 0 to 1 time, or greater than 2 times?" Teenagers who answer "yes" to 1 alcohol question or to the marijuana question have an eightfold and sevenfold increased risk of having a substance use disorder, respectively. The 2 NIAAA questions vary according to the patient's age and explore the patient's and their friends' experience with alcohol. The NIAAA currently is investigating the reliability as well as the concurrent, convergent, discriminant, and predictive validity of this screen.[161]

Computerized screening may add advantages and efficiency to ED mental health screening. They can be administered with little ED clinician time or effort and have been used successfully in both pediatric and general ED settings for general health and mental health screening, alcohol use,[162-164] interpersonal and intimate

partner violence,[165,166] weapons,[167] injury prevention,[168] and HIV risk behaviors.[169] Adolescents not only rated these screens as highly acceptable but also may prefer such health interventions.[170-172] Fein and Pailler[140,173] have developed and implemented an electronic tool for universal screening of ED adolescent physical and mental health risks. The screen was presented to patients by a nurse or medical technician. After the screen was scored, the adolescent's results were printed out and reviewed by the treating physicians. This method resulted in a 68% increase in identification of psychiatric illnesses and subsequently a 47% increase in mental health assessments.

LEAD AUTHORS

Thomas H. Chun, MD, MPH, FAAP
Sharon E. Mace, MD, FAAP, FACEP
Emily R. Katz, MD, FAAP

AMERICAN ACADEMY OF PEDIATRICS COMMITTEE ON PEDIATRIC EMERGENCY MEDICINE, 2014–2015

Joan E. Shook, MD, MBA, FAAP, Chairperson
James M. Callahan, MD, FAAP
Thomas H. Chun, MD, MPH, FAAP
Gregory P. Conners, MD, MPH, MBA, FAAP
Edward E. Conway Jr, MD, MS, FAAP
Nanette C. Dudley, MD, FAAP
Toni K. Gross, MD, MPH, FAAP
Natalie E. Lane, MD, FAAP
Charles G. Macias, MD, MPH, FAAP
Nathan L. Timm, MD, FAAP

LIAISONS

Kim Bullock, MD – *American Academy of Family Physicians*
Elizabeth Edgerton, MD, MPH, FAAP – *Maternal and Child Health Bureau*
Tamar Magarik Haro – *AAP Department of Federal Affairs*
Madeline Joseph, MD, FACEP, FAAP – *American College of Emergency Physicians*
Angela Mickalide, PhD, MCHES – *EMSC National Resource Center*
Brian R. Moore, MD, FAAP – *National Association of EMS Physicians*
Katherine E. Remick, MD, FAAP – *National Association of Emergency Medical Technicians*
Sally K. Snow, RN, BSN, CPEN, FAEN – *Emergency Nurses Association*
David W. Tuggle, MD, FAAP – *American College of Surgeons*

ABBREVIATIONS

ASD: autism spectrum disorder
CI: confidence interval
CNS: central nervous system
DD: developmental disorder
ED: emergency department
FDA: US Food and Drug Administration
IV: intravenous
NIAAA: National Institute of Alcohol Abuse and Alcoholism
NMS: neuroleptic malignant syndrome
OT: occupational therapy
PNES: psychogenic nonepileptic seizures
SSRI: selective serotonin reuptake inhibitor
VCS: visual communication system

Copyright © 2016 by the American Academy of Pediatrics

FINANCIAL DISCLOSURE: The authors have indicated they have no financial relationships relevant to this article to disclose.

FUNDING: No external funding.

POTENTIAL CONFLICT OF INTEREST: The authors have indicated they have no potential conflicts of interest to disclose.

REFERENCES

1. American Psychiatric Association. *Diagnostic and Statistical Manual of Mental Disorders.* 5th ed (DSM-5). Washington, DC: American Psychiatric Association Press; 2013

2. Dell ML, Campo JV. Somatoform disorders in children and adolescents. *Psychiatr Clin North Am.* 2011;34(3):643–660

3. Sater N, Constantino JN. Pediatric emergencies in children with psychiatric conditions. *Pediatr Emerg Care.* 1998;14(1):42–50

4. Barsky AJ, Orav EJ, Bates DW. Distinctive patterns of medical care utilization in patients who somatize. *Med Care.* 2006;44(9):803–811

5. Silber TJ. Somatization disorders: diagnosis, treatment, and prognosis. *Pediatr Rev.* 2011;32(2):56–63, quiz 63–64

6. Reid S, Wessely S, Crayford T, Hotopf M. Medically unexplained symptoms in frequent attenders of secondary health care: retrospective cohort study. *BMJ.* 2001;322(7289):767

7. Livingston R, Witt A, Smith GR. Families who somatize. *J Dev Behav Pediatr.* 1995;16(1):42–46

8. Campo JV, Jansen-McWilliams L, Comer DM, Kelleher KJ. Somatization in pediatric primary care: association with psychopathology, functional impairment, and use of services. *J Am Acad Child Adolesc Psychiatry.* 1999;38(9):1093–1101

9. Barsky AJ, Orav EJ, Bates DW. Somatization increases medical utilization and costs independent of psychiatric and medical comorbidity. *Arch Gen Psychiatry.* 2005;62(8):903–910

10. Campo JV, Fritsch SL. Somatization in children and adolescents. *J Am Acad Child Adolesc Psychiatry.* 1994;33(9):1223–1235

11. Garralda ME. Somatisation in children. *J Child Psychol Psychiatry.* 1996;37(1):13–33

12. Garralda ME, Bailey D. Children with psychiatric disorders in primary care. *J Child Psychol Psychiatry.* 1986;27(5):611–624

13. Garralda ME, Bailey D. Psychosomatic aspects of children's consultations in primary care. *Eur Arch Psychiatry Neurol Sci.* 1987;236(5):319–322

14. Schecker N. Childhood conversion reactions in the emergency department: Part II--general and specific features. *Pediatr Emerg Care.* 1990;6(1):46–51

15. Lee J, Dade LA. The buck stops where? What is the role of the emergency physician in managing panic disorder in chest pain patients? *CJEM.* 2003;5(4):237–238

16. Pollard CA, Lewis LM. Managing panic attacks in emergency patients. *J Emerg Med.* 1989;7(5):547–552

17. Fleet RP, Dupuis G, Marchand A, Burelle D, Arsenault A, Beitman BD. Panic disorder in emergency department chest pain patients: prevalence, comorbidity, suicidal ideation, and physician recognition. *Am J Med.* 1996;101(4):371–380

18. Garralda ME. Unexplained physical complaints. *Pediatr Clin North Am.* 2011;58(4):803–813, ix

19. Stephenson DT, Price JR. Medically unexplained physical symptoms in emergency medicine. *Emerg Med J.* 2006;23(8):595–600

20. Alfvén G. The covariation of common psychosomatic symptoms among children from socio-economically differing residential areas. An epidemiological study. *Acta Paediatr.* 1993;82(5):484–487

21. Haugland S, Wold B, Stevenson J, Aaroe LE, Woynarowska B. Subjective health complaints in adolescence. A cross-national comparison of prevalence and dimensionality. *Eur J Public Health.* 2001;11(1):4–10

22. Emiroğlu FN, Kurul S, Akay A, Miral S, Dirik E. Assessment of child neurology outpatients with headache, dizziness, and fainting. *J Child Neurol.* 2004;19(5):332–336

23. Egger HL, Angold A, Costello EJ. Headaches and psychopathology in children and adolescents. *J Am Acad Child Adolesc Psychiatry.* 1998;37(9):951–958

24. Galli F, Patron L, Russo PM, Bruni O, Ferini-Strambi L, Guidetti V. Chronic daily headache in childhood and adolescence: clinical aspects and a 4-year follow-up [published correction appears in *Cephalalgia.* 2004;24(11):1011]. *Cephalalgia.* 2004;24(10):850–858

25. Guidetti V, Galli F, Fabrizi P, et al. Headache and psychiatric comorbidity: clinical aspects and outcome in an 8-year follow-up study. *Cephalalgia.* 1998;18(7):455–462

26. Tunaoglu FS, Olguntürk R, Akcabay S, Oguz D, Gücüyener K, Demirsoy S. Chest pain in children referred to a cardiology clinic. *Pediatr Cardiol.* 1995;16(2):69–72

27. Campo JV, Bridge J, Ehmann M, et al. Recurrent abdominal pain, anxiety, and depression in primary care. *Pediatrics.* 2004;113(4):817–824

28. Kashikar-Zuck S, Parkins IS, Graham TB, et al. Anxiety, mood, and behavioral disorders among pediatric patients with juvenile fibromyalgia syndrome. *Clin J Pain.* 2008;24(7):620–626

29. Selbst SM, Clancy R. Pseudoseizures in the pediatric emergency department. *Pediatr Emerg Care.* 1996;12(3):185–188

30. Bhatia MS, Sapra S. Pseudoseizures in children: a profile of 50 cases. *Clin Pediatr (Phila).* 2005;44(7):617–621

31. Wyllie E, Glazer JP, Benbadis S, Kotagal P, Wolgamuth B. Psychiatric features of children and adolescents with pseudoseizures. *Arch Pediatr Adolesc Med.* 1999;153(3):244–248

32. Knockaert DC, Buntinx F, Stoens N, Bruyninckx R, Delooz H. Chest pain in the emergency department: the broad spectrum of causes. *Eur J Emerg Med.* 2002;9(1):25–30

33. Lipsitz JD, Gur M, Sonnet FM, et al. Psychopathology and disability in children with unexplained chest pain presenting to the pediatric emergency department. *Pediatr Emerg Care.* 2010;26(11):830–836

34. Dang AT, Ho M, Kroenke K, Grupp-Phelan J. Maternal somatic symptoms, psychosocial correlates, and subsequent pediatric emergency department use. *Pediatr Emerg Care.* 2013;29(2):170–174

35. Abbass A, Campbell S, Magee K, Tarzwell R. Intensive short-term dynamic psychotherapy to reduce rates of emergency department return visits for patients with medically unexplained symptoms: preliminary evidence from a pre–post intervention study. *CJEM.* 2009;11(6):529–534

36. Comer JS, Olfson M, Mojtabai R. National trends in child and adolescent psychotropic polypharmacy in office-based practice, 1996–2007. *J Am Acad Child Adolesc Psychiatry.* 2010;49(10):1001–1010

37. Olfson M, Blanco C, Wang S, Laje G, Correll CU. National trends in the mental health care of children, adolescents, and adults by office-based physicians. *JAMA Psychiatry.* 2014;71(1):81–90

38. Pringsheim T, Lam D, Patten SB. The pharmacoepidemiology of antipsychotic medications for Canadian children and adolescents: 2005–2009. *J Child Adolesc Psychopharmacol.* 2011;21(6): 537–543

39. Alexander GC, Gallagher SA, Mascola A, Moloney RM, Stafford RS. Increasing off-label use of antipsychotic medications in the United States, 1995–2008. *Pharmacoepidemiol Drug Saf.* 2011;20(2):177–184

40. Matone M, Localio R, Huang YS, dosReis S, Feudtner C, Rubin D. The relationship between mental health diagnosis and treatment with second-generation antipsychotics over time: a national study of US Medicaid-enrolled children. *Health Serv Res.* 2012;47(5):1836–1860

41. Pathak P, West D, Martin BC, Helm ME, Henderson C. Evidence-based use of second-generation antipsychotics in a state Medicaid pediatric population, 2001–2005. *Psychiatr Serv.* 2010;61(2):123–129

42. Harrison JN, Cluxton-Keller F, Gross D. Antipsychotic medication prescribing trends in children and adolescents. *J Pediatr Health Care.* 2012;26(2):139–145

43. Cooper WO, Arbogast PG, Ding H, Hickson GB, Fuchs DC, Ray WA. Trends in prescribing of antipsychotic medications for US children. *Ambul Pediatr.* 2006;6(2):79–83

44. Olfson M, Crystal S, Huang C, Gerhard T. Trends in antipsychotic drug use by very young, privately insured children.

J Am Acad Child Adolesc Psychiatry. 2010;49(1):13–23

45. Whittler MA, Lavonas EJ. Antipsychotics. In: Marx JA, Hockberger R, Walls RM, eds. *Rosen's Emergency Medicine: Concepts and Clinical Practice.* Philadelphia, PA: Saunders; 2014:2042–2046

46. Amaral DG, Rubenstein JLR, Rogers SJ. Neuroscience of autism. In: Tasman A, Kay J, Lieberman A, First MB, Maj M, eds. *Psychiatry.* 3rd ed. West Sussex, England: John Wiley & Sons; 2008:386–392

47. Hilt RJ, Woodward TA. Agitation treatment for pediatric emergency patients. *J Am Acad Child Adolesc Psychiatry.* 2008;47(2):132–138

48. Sonnier L, Barzman D. Pharmacologic management of acutely agitated pediatric patients. *Paediatr Drugs.* 2011;13(1):1–10

49. Newcorn JH, Ivanov I, Sharma V. Childhood disorders: attention-deficit and disruptive behavior disorders. In: Tasman A, Kay J, Lieberman A, First MB, Maj M, eds. *Psychiatry.* 3rd ed. West Sussex, England: John Wiley & Sons; 2008:816–831

50. Levine M, LoVecchio F. Antipsychotics. In: Tintinalli JE, Stapczynski S, Ma OJ, Cline DM, Cydulka RK, Mecklereds GD, eds. *Tintinalli's Emergency Medicine: A Comprehensive Study Guide.* New York, NY: McGraw-Hill Education; 2011:1207–1211

51. Miyamoto S, Merrill DB, Lieberman JA, Fleischacker WW, Marder SR. Antipsychotic drugs. In: Tasman A, Kay J, Lieberman A, First MB, Maj M, eds. *Psychiatry.* 3rd ed. West Sussex, England: John Wiley & Sons; 2008:2161–2201

52. Guenette MD, Giacca A, Hahn M, et al. Atypical antipsychotics and effects of adrenergic and serotonergic receptor binding on insulin secretion in-vivo: an animal model. *Schizophr Res.* 2013;146(1–3):162–169

53. Reynolds GP, Kirk SL. Metabolic side effects of antipsychotic drug treatment: pharmacological mechanisms. *Pharmacol Ther.* 2010;125(1):169–179

54. Starrenburg FC, Bogers JP. How can antipsychotics cause diabetes mellitus? Insights based on receptor-binding profiles, humoral factors and transporter proteins. *Eur Psychiatry.* 2009;24(3):164–170

55. Bailey P, Norton R, Karan S. The FDA droperidol warning: is it justified? *Anesthesiology.* 2002;97(1):288–289

56. Chase PB, Biros MH. A retrospective review of the use and safety of droperidol in a large, high-risk, inner-city emergency department patient population. *Acad Emerg Med.* 2002;9(12):1402–1410

57. Dershwitz M. Droperidol: should the black box be light gray? *J Clin Anesth.* 2002;14(8):598–603

58. Gan TJ, White PF, Scuderi PE, Watcha MF, Kovac A. FDA "black box" warning regarding use of droperidol for postoperative nausea and vomiting: is it justified? *Anesthesiology.* 2002;97(1):287

59. Horowitz BZ, Bizovi K, Moreno R. Droperidol: behind the black box warning. *Acad Emerg Med.* 2002;9(6):615–618

60. Lukens TW, Wolf SJ, Edlow JA, et al; American College of Emergency Physicians Clinical Policies Subcommittee (Writing Committee) on Critical Issues in the Diagnosis and Management of the Adult Psychiatric Patient in the Emergency Department. Clinical policy: critical issues in the diagnosis and management of the adult psychiatric patient in the emergency department. *Ann Emerg Med.* 2006;47(1):79–99

61. Walters H, Killius K. *Guidelines for the Acute Psychotropic Medication Management of Agitation in Children and Adolescents.* Boston, MA: Boston Medical Center Emergency Department Policy and Procedure Guidelines; 2012

62. Meyer-Massetti C, Cheng CM, Sharpe BA, Meier CR, Guglielmo BJ. The FDA extended warning for intravenous haloperidol and torsades de pointes: how should institutions respond? *J Hosp Med.* 2010;5(4):E8–E16

63. Haddad PM, Anderson IM. Antipsychotic-related QTc prolongation, torsade de pointes and sudden death. *Drugs.* 2002;62(11):1649–1671

64. Isaacs E. The violent patient. In: Marx JA, Hockberger R, Walls RM, eds. *Rosen's Emergency Medicine: Concepts and Clinical Practice.* Philadelphia, PA: Saunders; 2014:1460–1465

65. Gören JL, Dinh TA. Psychotropics and sudden cardiac death. *R I Med J (2013).* 2013;96(3):38–41

66. Szwak K, Sacchetti A. Droperidol use in pediatric emergency department patients. *Pediatr Emerg Care.* 2010;26(4):248–250

67. Baren JM, Mace SE, Hendry PL, Dietrich AM, Goldman RD, Warden CR. Children's mental health emergencies--part 2: emergency department evaluation and treatment of children with mental health disorders [published correction appears in *Pediatr Emerg Care.* 2008;24(11):748]. *Pediatr Emerg Care.* 2008;24(7):485–498

68. Hockberger R, Walls R. Thought disorders. In: Marx JA, Hockberger R, Walls RM, eds. *Rosen's Emergency Medicine: Concepts and Clinical Practice.* Philadelphia, PA: Saunders; 2014:1430–1436

69. Pringsheim T, Doja A, Belanger S, Patten S; Canadian Alliance for Monitoring Effectiveness and Safety of Antipsychotics in Children (CAMESA) guideline group. Treatment recommendations for extrapyramidal side effects associated with second-generation antipsychotic use in children and youth. *Paediatr Child Health.* 2011;16(9):590–598

70. Minns AB, Clark RF. Toxicology and overdose of atypical antipsychotics. *J Emerg Med.* 2012;43(5):906–913

71. Guzé BH, Baxter LR Jr. Current concepts. Neuroleptic malignant syndrome. *N Engl J Med.* 1985;313(3):163–166

72. Meeks TW, Jeste DV. Medication-induced movement disorders. In: Tasman A, Kay J, Lieberman A, First MB, Maj M, eds. *Psychiatry.* 3rd ed. West Sussex, England: John Wiley & Sons; 2008:2142

73. Silva RR, Munoz DM, Alpert M, Perlmutter IR, Diaz J. Neuroleptic malignant syndrome in children and adolescents. *J Am Acad Child Adolesc Psychiatry.* 1999;38(2):187–194

74. Young MC, Miller AD, Clark RF. Antipsychotic agents. In: Wolfson AB, Hendey GW, Ling LJ, Rosen CL, Schaider

JJ, Sharieff GQ, eds. *Harwood-Nuss Clinical Practice of Emergency Medicine*. Philadelphia, PA: Wolters-Kluwer/Lippincott Williams & Wilkins; 2010:1493–1497

75. Margetić B, Aukst-Margetić B. Neuroleptic malignant syndrome and its controversies. *Pharmacoepidemiol Drug Saf*. 2010;19(5):429–435

76. Jacobson JL. Neuroleptic malignant syndrome. In: Jacobson JL, ed. *Psychiatric Secrets*. Philadelphia, PA: Hanley & Belfus; 2000:447–451

77. Perry PJ, Wilborn CA. Serotonin syndrome vs neuroleptic malignant syndrome: a contrast of causes, diagnoses, and management. *Ann Clin Psychiatry*. 2012;24(2):155–162

78. Shalev A, Hermesh H, Munitz H. Mortality from neuroleptic malignant syndrome. *J Clin Psychiatry*. 1989;50(1):18–25

79. Caroff SN, Mann SC. Neuroleptic malignant syndrome. *Med Clin North Am*. 1993;77(1):185–202

80. Chung T, Smith GT, Donovan JE, et al. Drinking frequency as a brief screen for adolescent alcohol problems. *Pediatrics*. 2012;129(2):205–212

81. Levenson JL. Neuroleptic malignant syndrome. *Am J Psychiatry*. 1985;142(10):1137–1145

82. Agar L. Recognizing neuroleptic malignant syndrome in the emergency department: a case study. *Perspect Psychiatr Care*. 2010;46(2):143–151

83. Bajjoka I, Patel T, O'Sullivan T. Risperidone-induced neuroleptic malignant syndrome. *Ann Emerg Med*. 1997;30(5):698–700

84. Kogoj A, Velikonja I. Olanzapine induced neuroleptic malignant syndrome: a case review. *Hum Psychopharmacol*. 2003;18(4):301–309

85. Trollor JN, Chen X, Chitty K, Sachdev PS. Comparison of neuroleptic malignant syndrome induced by first- and second-generation antipsychotics. *Br J Psychiatry*. 2012;201(1):52–56

86. Wijdicks EFM. Neuroleptic malignant syndrome. In: Aminoff MJ, ed. *UpToDate*. Updated May 30, 2014. Available at: www.uptodate.com/contents/neuroleptic-malignant-syndrome. Accessed July 7, 2015

87. Hammerman S, Lam C, Caroff SN. Neuroleptic malignant syndrome and aripiprazole. *J Am Acad Child Adolesc Psychiatry*. 2006;45(6):639–641

88. Martel ML, Biros MH. Psychotropic medications and rapid tranquilization. In: Tintinalli JE, Stapczynski S, Ma OJ, Cline DM, Cydulka RK, Mecklereds GD, eds. *Tintinalli's Emergency Medicine: A Comprehensive Study Guide*. New York, NY: McGraw-Hill Education; 2011:1952–1955

89. Hatfield-Keller E, Thomas HA. Fever. In: Wolfson AB, Hendey GW, Ling LJ, Rosen CL, Schaider JJ, Sharieff GQ, eds. *Harwood-Nuss Clinical Practice of Emergency Medicine*. Philadelphia, PA: Wolters-Kluwer/Lippincott Williams & Wilkins; 2010:99–101

90. Gurrera RJ, Caroff SN, Cohen A, et al. An international consensus study of neuroleptic malignant syndrome diagnostic criteria using the Delphi method. *J Clin Psychiatry*. 2011;72(9):1222–1228

91. Anglin RE, Rosebush PI, Mazurek MF. Neuroleptic malignant syndrome: a neuroimmunologic hypothesis. *CMAJ*. 2010;182(18):E834–E838

92. Isbister GK, Dawson A, Whyte IM, Prior FH, Clancy C, Smith AJ. Neonatal paroxetine withdrawal syndrome or actually serotonin syndrome? *Arch Dis Child Fetal Neonatal Ed*. 2001;85(2):F147–F148

93. Kant S, Liebelt E. Recognizing serotonin toxicity in the pediatric emergency department. *Pediatr Emerg Care*. 2012;28(8):817–821, quiz 822–824

94. Spirko BA, Wiley JF II. Serotonin syndrome: a new pediatric intoxication. *Pediatr Emerg Care*. 1999;15(6):440–443

95. Birmes P, Coppin D, Schmitt L, Lauque D. Serotonin syndrome: a brief review. *CMAJ*. 2003;168(11):1439–1442

96. Ables AZ, Nagubilli R. Prevention, recognition, and management of serotonin syndrome. *Am Fam Physician*. 2010;81(9):1139–1142

97. Christensen RC. Identifying serotonin syndrome in the emergency department. *Am J Emerg Med*. 2005;23(3):406–408

98. Mills KC, Bora KM. Atypical antidepressants, serotonin reuptake inhibitors, and serotonin syndrome. In: Tintinalli JE, Stapczynski S, Ma OJ, Cline DM, Cydulka RK, Mecklereds GD, eds. *Tintinalli's Emergency Medicine: A Comprehensive Study Guide*. New York, NY: McGraw-Hill Education; 2011:1198–1203

99. Isbister GK, Buckley NA, Whyte IM. Serotonin toxicity: a practical approach to diagnosis and treatment. *Med J Aust*. 2007;187(6):361–365

100. Boyer EW, Shannon M. The serotonin syndrome. *N Engl J Med*. 2005;352(11):1112–1120

101. Isbister GK, Buckley NA. The pathophysiology of serotonin toxicity in animals and humans: implications for diagnosis and treatment. *Clin Neuropharmacol*. 2005;28(5):205–214

102. Kirschner R, Donovan JW. Serotonin syndrome precipitated by fentanyl during procedural sedation. *J Emerg Med*. 2010;38(4):477–480

103. Barthold CL, Graudins A. Serotonin re-uptake inhibitors and the serotonin syndrome. In: Wolfson AB, Hendey GW, Ling LJ, Rosen CL, Schaider JJ, Sharieff GQ, eds. *Harwood-Nuss Clinical Practice of Emergency Medicine*. Philadelphia, PA: Wolters-Kluwer/Lippincott Williams & Wilkins; 2010:1510–1513

104. Dunkley EJ, Isbister GK, Sibbritt D, Dawson AH, Whyte IM. The Hunter Serotonin Toxicity Criteria: simple and accurate diagnostic decision rules for serotonin toxicity. *QJM*. 2003;96(9):635–642

105. Sternbach H. The serotonin syndrome. *Am J Psychiatry*. 1991;148(6):705–713

106. Boland RJ, Keller MB. Antidepressants. In: Tasman A, Kay J, Lieberman A, First MB, Maj M, eds. *Psychiatry*. 3rd ed. West Sussex, England: John Wiley & Sons; 2008:2142

107. Radomski JW, Dursun SM, Reveley MA, Kutcher SP. An exploratory approach to the serotonin syndrome: an update of clinical phenomenology and revised diagnostic criteria. *Med Hypotheses*. 2000;55(3):218–224

108. Gillman PK. The serotonin syndrome and its treatment. *J Psychopharmacol*. 1999;13(1):100–109

109. Autism and Developmental Disabilities Monitoring Network Surveillance Year

2008 Principal Investigators; Centers for Disease Control and Prevention. Prevalence of autism spectrum disorders: Autism and Developmental Disabilities Monitoring Network, 14 sites, United States, 2008. *MMWR Surveill Summ.* 2012;61(3):1–19

110. Foxx RM. Applied behavior analysis treatment of autism: the state of the art. *Child Adolesc Psychiatr Clin N Am.* 2008;17(4):821–834, ix

111. Hodgetts S, Hodgetts W. Somatosensory stimulation interventions for children with autism: literature review and clinical considerations. *Can J Occup Ther.* 2007;74(5):393–400

112. Karkhaneh M, Clark B, Ospina MB, Seida JC, Smith V, Hartling L. Social Stories to improve social skills in children with autism spectrum disorder: a systematic review. *Autism.* 2010;14(6):641–662

113. LeBlanc LA, Gillis JM. Behavioral interventions for children with autism spectrum disorders. *Pediatr Clin North Am.* 2012;59(1):147–164, xi–xii

114. Meindl JN, Cannella-Malone HI. Initiating and responding to joint attention bids in children with autism: a review of the literature. *Res Dev Disabil.* 2011;32(5):1441–1454

115. Virués-Ortega J. Applied behavior analytic intervention for autism in early childhood: meta-analysis, meta-regression and dose–response meta-analysis of multiple outcomes. *Clin Psychol Rev.* 2010;30(4):387–399

116. McPheeters ML, Warren Z, Sathe N, et al. A systematic review of medical treatments for children with autism spectrum disorders. *Pediatrics.* 2011;127(5). Available at: www.pediatrics.org/cgi/content/full/127/5/e1312

117. Siegel M, Beaulieu AA. Psychotropic medications in children with autism spectrum disorders: a systematic review and synthesis for evidence-based practice. *J Autism Dev Disord.* 2012;42(8):1592–1605

118. Sung M, Fung DS, Cai Y, Ooi YP. Pharmacological management in children and adolescents with pervasive developmental disorder. *Aust N Z J Psychiatry.* 2010;44(5):410–428

119. Case-Smith J, Arbesman M. Evidence-based review of interventions for autism used in or of relevance to occupational therapy. *Am J Occup Ther.* 2008;62(4):416–429

120. Oriel KN, George CL, Peckus R, Semon A. The effects of aerobic exercise on academic engagement in young children with autism spectrum disorder. *Pediatr Phys Ther.* 2011;23(2):187–193

121. Polatajko HJ, Cantin N. Exploring the effectiveness of occupational therapy interventions, other than the sensory integration approach, with children and adolescents experiencing difficulty processing and integrating sensory information. *Am J Occup Ther.* 2010;64(3):415–429

122. Rossignol DA. Novel and emerging treatments for autism spectrum disorders: a systematic review. *Ann Clin Psychiatry.* 2009;21(4):213–236

123. Mesibov GB, Shea V. Evidence-based practices and autism. *Autism.* 2011;15(1):114–133

124. Reichow B, Volkmar FR, Cicchetti DV. Development of the evaluative method for evaluating and determining evidence-based practices in autism. *J Autism Dev Disord.* 2008;38(7):1311–1319

125. Warren Z, Veenstra-VanderWeele J, Stone W, et al. *Therapies for Children With Autism Spectrum Disorders.* Comparative Effectiveness Review no. 26. (Prepared by the Vanderbilt Evidence-Based Practice Center under contract no. 290-02-HHSA-290-2007-10065-I.) AHRQ publication no. 11-EHC029-EF. Rockville, MD: Agency for Healthcare Research and Quality; 2011

126. Maglione MA, Gans D, Das L, Timbie J, Kasari C; Technical Expert Panel; HRSA Autism Intervention Research—Behavioral (AIR-B) Network. Nonmedical interventions for children with ASD: recommended guidelines and further research needs. *Pediatrics.* 2012;130(suppl 2):S169–S178

127. Wong C, Odom SL, Hume K, et al. *Evidence Based Practices for Children, Youth, and Young Adults With Autism Spectrum Disorder.* Chapel Hill, NC: University of North Carolina; 2013

128. Chun TH, Berrios-Candelaria R. Caring for children with autism in emergencies: What can we learn from . . . Broadway? *Contemp Pediatr.* 2012;29(9):56–65

129. Ganz JB, Davis JL, Lund EM, Goodwyn FD, Simpson RL. Meta-analysis of PECS with individuals with ASD: investigation of targeted versus non-targeted outcomes, participant characteristics, and implementation phase. *Res Dev Disabil.* 2012;33(2):406–418

130. Gordon K, Pasco G, McElduff F, Wade A, Howlin P, Charman T. A communication-based intervention for nonverbal children with autism: what changes? Who benefits? *J Consult Clin Psychol.* 2011;79(4):447–457

131. Howlin P, Gordon RK, Pasco G, Wade A, Charman T. The effectiveness of Picture Exchange Communication System (PECS) training for teachers of children with autism: a pragmatic, group randomised controlled trial. *J Child Psychol Psychiatry.* 2007;48(5):473–481

132. Yoder PJ, Lieberman RG. Brief report: randomized test of the efficacy of picture exchange communication system on highly generalized picture exchanges in children with ASD. *J Autism Dev Disord.* 2010;40(5):629–632

133. Autism Treatment Network. Blood draw tool kit (for parents and medical providers). Available at: www.autismspeaks.org/science/resources-programs/autism-treatment-network/tools-you-can-use/blood-draw-toolkits. Accessed July 5, 2015

134. Sullivan M. Autism demands attention in the emergency department. *ACEP News.* April 17, 2012

135. Weitzman C, Wegner L; Section on Developmental and Behavioral Pediatrics; Committee on Psychosocial Aspects of Child and Family Health; Council on Early Childhood; Society for Developmental and Behavioral Pediatrics; American Academy of Pediatrics. Promoting optimal development: screening for behavioral and emotional problems. *Pediatrics.* 2015;135(2):384–395

136. Oster A, Bindman AB. Emergency department visits for ambulatory care sensitive conditions: insights

into preventable hospitalizations. *Med Care*. 2003;41(2):198–207

137. Wilson KM, Klein JD. Adolescents who use the emergency department as their usual source of care. *Arch Pediatr Adolesc Med*. 2000;154(4):361–365

138. Klein JD, Woods AH, Wilson KM, Prospero M, Greene J, Ringwalt C. Homeless and runaway youths' access to health care. *J Adolesc Health*. 2000;27(5):331–339

139. Chen CM, Yi HY, Faden VB. *Trends in Underage Drinking in the United States, 1991–2009. National Institute on Alcohol Abuse and Alcoholism. Surveillance Report #91*. Bethesda, MD: US Department of Health and Human Services; 2011

140. Fein JA, Pailler ME, Barg FK, et al. Feasibility and effects of a Web-based adolescent psychiatric assessment administered by clinical staff in the pediatric emergency department. *Arch Pediatr Adolesc Med*. 2010;164(12):1112–1117

141. Grupp-Phelan J, Delgado SV, Kelleher KJ. Failure of psychiatric referrals from the pediatric emergency department. *BMC Emerg Med*. 2007;7:12

142. Grupp-Phelan J, Wade TJ, Pickup T, et al. Mental health problems in children and caregivers in the emergency department setting. *J Dev Behav Pediatr*. 2007;28(1):16–21

143. Monti PM, Colby SM, Barnett NP, et al. Brief intervention for harm reduction with alcohol-positive older adolescents in a hospital emergency department. *J Consult Clin Psychol*. 1999;67(6):989–994

144. Marcell AV, Klein JD, Fischer I, Allan MJ, Kokotailo PK. Male adolescent use of health care services: where are the boys? *J Adolesc Health*. 2002;30(1):35–43

145. Chandra A, Minkovitz CS. Stigma starts early: gender differences in teen willingness to use mental health services. *J Adolesc Health*. 2006;38(6):754.e1–754.e8

146. Haughey MT, Calderon Y, Torres S, Nazario S, Bijur P. Identification of depression in an inner-city population using a simple screen. *Acad Emerg Med*. 2005;12(12):1221–1226

147. Rutman MS, Shenassa E, Becker BM. Brief screening for adolescent depressive symptoms in the emergency department. *Acad Emerg Med*. 2008;15(1):17–22

148. Newton AS, Gokiert R, Mabood N, et al. Instruments to detect alcohol and other drug misuse in the emergency department: a systematic review. *Pediatrics*. 2011;128(1). Available at: www.pediatrics.org/cgi/content/full/128/1/e180

149. Horowitz L, Ballard E, Teach SJ, et al. Feasibility of screening patients with nonpsychiatric complaints for suicide risk in a pediatric emergency department: a good time to talk? *Pediatr Emerg Care*. 2010;26(11):787–792

150. Horowitz LM, Bridge JA, Teach SJ, et al. Ask Suicide-Screening Questions (ASQ): a brief instrument for the pediatric emergency department. *Arch Pediatr Adolesc Med*. 2012;166(12):1170–1176

151. Horowitz LM, Wang PS, Koocher GP, et al. Detecting suicide risk in a pediatric emergency department: development of a brief screening tool. *Pediatrics*. 2001;107(5):1133–1137

152. Winston FK, Kassam-Adams N, Garcia-España F, Ittenbach R, Cnaan A. Screening for risk of persistent posttraumatic stress in injured children and their parents. *JAMA*. 2003;290(5):643–649

153. O'Mara RM, Hill RM, Cunningham RM, King CA. Adolescent and parent attitudes toward screening for suicide risk and mental health problems in the pediatric emergency department. *Pediatr Emerg Care*. 2012;28(7):626–632

154. Williams JR, Ho ML, Grupp-Phelan J. The acceptability of mental health screening in a pediatric emergency department. *Pediatr Emerg Care*. 2011;27(7):611–615

155. Pailler ME, Cronholm PF, Barg FK, Wintersteen MB, Diamond GS, Fein JA. Patients' and caregivers' beliefs about depression screening and referral in the emergency department. *Pediatr Emerg Care*. 2009;25(11):721–727

156. King CA, O'Mara RM, Hayward CN, Cunningham RM. Adolescent suicide risk screening in the emergency department. *Acad Emerg Med*. 2009;16(11):1234–1241

157. Goldenring JM, Rosen DS. Getting into adolescent heads: an essential update. *Contemp Pediatr*. 2004;21(1):64–90

158. Cappelli M, Gray C, Zemek R, et al. The HEADS-ED: a rapid mental health screening tool for pediatric patients in the emergency department. *Pediatrics*. 2012;130(2). Available at: www.pediatrics.org/cgi/content/full/130/2/e321

159. Horowitz LM, Ballard ED, Pao M. Suicide screening in schools, primary care and emergency departments. *Curr Opin Pediatr*. 2009;21(5):620–627

160. National Institute of Alcohol Abuse and Alcoholism. *Alcohol Screening and Brief Intervention for Youth: A Practitioner's Guide*. Bethesda, MD: National Institutes of Health; 2011

161. National Institute of Alcohol Abuse and Alcoholism. Evaluation of NIAAA's Alcohol Screening Guide for Children and Adolescents. Bethesda, MD: National Institute of Alcohol Abuse and Alcoholism; 2011. Available at: http://grants.nih.gov/grants/guide/rfa-files/RFA-AA-12-008.html. Accessed July 5, 2015

162. Maio RF, Shope JT, Blow FC, et al. A randomized controlled trial of an emergency department-based interactive computer program to prevent alcohol misuse among injured adolescents. *Ann Emerg Med*. 2005;45(4):420–429

163. Suffoletto B, Callaway C, Kristan J, Kraemer K, Clark DB. Text-message–based drinking assessments and brief interventions for young adults discharged from the emergency department. *Alcohol Clin Exp Res*. 2012;36(3):552–560

164. Walton MA, Chermack ST, Shope JT, et al. Effects of a brief intervention for reducing violence and alcohol misuse among adolescents: a randomized controlled trial. *JAMA*. 2010;304(5):527–535

165. Walton MA, Cunningham RM, Goldstein AL, et al. Rates and correlates of violent behaviors among adolescents treated in an urban emergency department. *J Adolesc Health*. 2009;45(1):77–83

166. Whiteside LK, Walton MA, Stanley R, et al. Dating aggression and risk behaviors among teenage girls seeking gynecologic care. *Acad Emerg Med.* 2009;16(7):632–638

167. Cunningham RM, Resko SM, Harrison SR, et al. Screening adolescents in the emergency department for weapon carriage. *Acad Emerg Med.* 2010;17(2): 168–176

168. Gielen AC, McKenzie LB, McDonald EM, et al. Using a computer kiosk to promote child safety: results of a randomized, controlled trial in an urban pediatric emergency department. *Pediatrics.* 2007;120(2):330–339

169. Choo EK, Ranney ML, Aggarwal N, Boudreaux ED. A systematic review of emergency department technology-based behavioral health interventions. *Acad Emerg Med.* 2012;19(3): 318–328

170. Heron KE, Smyth JM. Ecological momentary interventions: incorporating mobile technology into psychosocial and health behaviour treatments. *Br J Health Psychol.* 2010;15(pt 1):1–39

171. Kit Delgado M, Ginde AA, Pallin DJ, Camargo CA Jr. Multicenter study of preferences for health education in the emergency department population. *Acad Emerg Med.* 2010;17(6):652–658

172. Ranney ML, Choo EK, Wang Y, Baum A, Clark MA, Mello MJ. Emergency department patients' preferences for technology-based behavioral interventions. *Ann Emerg Med.* 2012;60(2):218–27.e48

173. Pailler ME, Fein JA. Computerized behavioral health screening in the emergency department. *Pediatr Ann.* 2009;38(3):156–160

CLINICAL REPORT   Guidance for the Clinician in Rendering Pediatric Care

**American Academy
of Pediatrics**

DEDICATED TO THE HEALTH OF ALL CHILDREN™

Executive Summary: Evaluation and Management of Children and Adolescents With Acute Mental Health or Behavioral Problems. Part I: Common Clinical Challenges of Patients With Mental Health and/or Behavioral Emergencies

Thomas H. Chun, MD, MPH, FAAP, Sharon E. Mace, MD, FAAP, FACEP, Emily R. Katz, MD, FAAP,
AMERICAN ACADEMY OF PEDIATRICS, COMMITTEE ON PEDIATRIC EMERGENCY MEDICINE, AMERICAN
COLLEGE OF EMERGENCY PHYSICIANS, PEDIATRIC EMERGENCY MEDICINE COMMITTEE

FREE

EXECUTIVE SUMMARY

The number of children and adolescents seen in emergency departments (EDs) and primary care settings for mental health problems has skyrocketed in recent years, with up to 23% of patients in both settings having diagnosable mental health conditions.[1-4] Even when a mental health problem is not the focus of an ED or primary care visit, mental health conditions, both known and occult, may challenge the treating clinician and complicate the patient's care.[4]

Although the American Academy of Pediatrics has published a policy statement on mental health competencies and a Mental Health Toolkit for pediatric primary care providers, no such guidelines or resources exist for clinicians who care for pediatric mental health emergencies.[5,6] Many ED and primary care physicians report a paucity of training and lack of confidence in caring for pediatric psychiatry patients. The 2 clinical reports (www.pediatrics.org/cgi/doi/10.1542/peds.2016-1570 and www.pediatrics.org/cgi/doi/10.1542/peds.2016-1573) support the 2006 joint policy statement of the American Academy of Pediatrics and the American College of Emergency Physicians on pediatric mental health emergencies,[7] with the goal of addressing the knowledge gaps in this area. Although written primarily from the perspective of ED clinicians, they are intended for all clinicians who care for children and adolescents with acute mental health and behavioral problems.

The clinical reports are organized around the common clinical challenges pediatric caregivers face, both when a child or adolescent presents with a psychiatric chief complaint or emergency (part I) and also when a mental

This document is copyrighted and is property of the American Academy of Pediatrics and its Board of Directors. All authors have filed conflict of interest statements with the American Academy of Pediatrics. Any conflicts have been resolved through a process approved by the Board of Directors. The American Academy of Pediatrics has neither solicited nor accepted any commercial involvement in the development of the content of this publication.

Clinical reports from the American Academy of Pediatrics benefit from expertise and resources of liaisons and internal (AAP) and external reviewers. However, clinical reports from the American Academy of Pediatrics may not reflect the views of the liaisons or the organizations or government agencies that they represent.

The guidance in this report does not indicate an exclusive course of treatment or serve as a standard of medical care. Variations, taking into account individual circumstances, may be appropriate.

All clinical reports from the American Academy of Pediatrics automatically expire 5 years after publication unless reaffirmed, revised, or retired at or before that time.

DOI: 10.1542/peds.2016-1571

PEDIATRICS (ISSN Numbers: Print, 0031-4005; Online, 1098-4275).

To cite: Chun TH, Mace SE, Katz ER, AMERICAN ACADEMY OF PEDIATRICS. Executive Summary: Evaluation and Management of Children and Adolescents With Acute Mental Health or Behavioral Problems. Part I: Common Clinical Challenges of Patients With Mental Health and/or Behavioral Emergencies. Pediatrics. 2016;138(3):e20161571 health condition may be an unclear or complicating factor in a non–mental health clinical presentation (part II). Part II of the clinical reports (www.pediatrics.org/cgi/doi/10.1542/peds.2016-1573) includes discussions of somatic symptom and related disorders, adverse effects of psychiatric medications including neuroleptic malignant syndrome and serotonin syndrome, caring for children with special needs such as autism and developmental disorders, and mental health screening. This executive summary is an overview of part I of the clinical reports. The full text of the below topics can be accessed online at (www.pediatrics.org/cgi/doi/10.1542/peds.2016-1570). Key considerations are shown in the following sections.

1. ED Medical Clearance of Pediatric Psychiatric Patients

- Definition

  1. Medical clearance is the process of excluding potential medical conditions causing or exacerbating the patient's psychiatric symptoms as well as evaluating the patient for medical diseases or injuries for which acute diagnostic or therapeutic interventions in the ED may be indicated.[8,9]

  2. Some favor the term "medically stable," because the goal of the ED visit is not to exclude all possible medical etiologies but rather to rule out acute medical conditions.[10]

  3. For patients with unexplained vital sign abnormalities, a concerning history, or physical examination findings or with new onset or acute changes in their neurologic or psychiatric symptoms, a careful evaluation for potential underlying medical conditions may be important.[11]

- Laboratory Testing

  1. Despite the large number of medical conditions (see Table 1 at [www.pediatrics.org/cgi/doi/10.1542/peds.2016-1570]) that can present with mental health symptoms, there is a growing body of both pediatric and adult literature that casts doubt on the utility of routinely obtaining laboratory or radiologic testing for these patients.[12-19] This literature supports the position of the American College of Emergency Physicians for focused medical assessments and judicious testing of these ED patients.[11]

  2. Mental health consultants often request pregnancy (females), toxicology, and sexually transmitted infection testing for adolescent patients. Whether to obtain these or other medical tests or evaluations can usually be decided with a direct conversation between the ED and mental health clinicians.

2. Suicidal Ideation and Suicide Attempts

- Epidemiology

  1. Suicide is one of the leading causes of death in adolescents,[20] and suicide attempts are one of the most common ED mental health presentations.[21,22] Epidemiologic studies in teenagers have found that 16% reported seriously considering suicide and 7.8% have attempted suicide in the past year.[23]

  2. More females consider and attempt suicide, although males are far more likely to die of suicide because of their frequent use of more lethal means (eg, firearms, hanging).[23] Native Americans have the highest suicide rates among ethnic groups.[21]

- Risk factors: previous suicide attempt(s); mood (eg, depression, bipolar disorder, mood swings, irritable mood, etc), impulsivity, or disruptive behavior disorders; substance abuse; recent psychiatric hospitalization; family history of suicide; interpersonal violence (eg, physical or sexual abuse, bullying, antisocial behavior); homelessness or runaway behavior; self-identification as lesbian, gay, bisexual, or transgender; hopelessness; history of aggressive or impulsive behavior; cultural/religious beliefs; recent loss or stress (eg, relational, social, work, financial, etc) of the patient or family; physical illness; recent high-profile suicides; access to lethal methods; social isolation; and barriers or unwillingness to seek mental health care.[24-29]

- Assessment

  1. Suicidal ideation and attempts are often precipitated by psychosocial stressors.[29] As such, evaluating the pediatric patient for suicide risk includes inquiring about his or her current psychosocial situation, interviewing both the patient and his or her caregivers (eg, family members, school or mental health personnel), and assessing for the aforementioned suicide risk factors.

  2. The ED management of patients with suicidal ideation and attempts includes an evaluation of their current mental health state. Children and adolescents frequently misjudge the lethality of their actions. A potential pitfall is to equate the lethality of a suicide attempt with the patient's suicide intent. A patient whose suicide attempt had low medical lethality may, in fact, have a significant wish to harm himself or herself or to die.[30-32]

  3. The ED workup of patients presenting for suicidal ideation or attempt includes evaluation for signs of self-injury (which

can be concealed under clothing) or occult toxidromes as well as questions about suicidal intent, suicide plans, and other self-injurious behaviors.

- Disposition: The decision for inpatient versus outpatient management depends on many factors, including a careful assessment of suicide risk, and may include consultation with a mental health clinician. Outpatient management may be considered for low-risk patients (those with a low risk of future self-harm, adequate supervision, mental health follow-up, and safety planning; eg, the patient can identify his or her warning signs or triggers for recurrent suicidal ideation and have appropriate coping strategies if he or she becomes suicidal again, such as healthy activities and social support, and means restrictions, that is, limiting access to mechanisms for self-harm, such as firearms, other weapons, medications, etc).[33] "Contracting for safety"/suicide prevention agreements are controversial and remain unproven.[34]

- Involuntary hospitalization: Under certain circumstances, physicians may insist on admission to a psychiatric unit over the objections of patients and/or their parents/guardians, when clinically indicated. Every state has laws governing involuntary admission for inpatient psychiatric hospitalization. These laws vary from state to state, as do laws regarding confidentiality and an adolescent's right to seek mental health or substance abuse treatment without parental consent. As such, it may be beneficial for ED clinicians to familiarize themselves with their state's relevant laws, statutes, and involuntary commitment procedures. For more information

on related state laws, contact the American Academy of Pediatrics' Division of State Government Affairs at stgov@aap.org.

3. Restraint of the Agitated Patient

- Agitated behavior is the final common pathway for a wide number of medical and psychiatric conditions and, in some cases, a combination of the two. Determining the underlying cause of the agitation often guides treatment choices.

- The 4 guiding principles of working with agitated patients are as follows[35]:

  1. prioritizing the safety of the patient and the treating staff;

  2. assisting the patient in managing his or her emotions and regaining control of his or her behavior;

  3. utilizing age-appropriate and the least-restrictive methods possible; and

  4. recognizing that coercive interventions may exacerbate the agitation.

- Monitoring and evaluation of restrained patients (see Table 6 at [www.pediatrics.org/cgi/doi/ 10.1542/peds.2016-1570]) may include the following[36–38]:

  1. in-person evaluation by a licensed independent practitioner within 1 hour of placement of restraints;

  2. review and renewal of restraint orders on a frequent basis (1–8 hours, depending the patient's age); and

  3. frequent assessment of vital signs, injury attributable to restraint, nutrition and hydration status, peripheral circulation, hygiene and elimination status, physical and psychological status, and readiness to discontinue restraint.

- Verbal restraint/de-escalation

  1. A calming (eg, quiet room, soft/ decreased lighting, elimination of triggers of agitation) and safe (eg, removal or securing of objects that can be used as weapons, padded walls) physical environment may help de-escalate a patient.[35,39,40]

  2. Common verbal restraint (see Table 2 at [www.pediatrics. org/cgi/doi/10.1542/peds. 2016-1570]) strategies include the following[41]:

     a. respecting personal space;

     b. minimizing behavior and/ or interventions the patient may find provocative;

     c. using clear, concise language and expectations;

     d. active listening, especially regarding the patient's goals; and

     e. offering clear, realistic choices without "bargaining."

- Chemical restraint

  1. The most commonly used medications for agitation are antihistamines, benzodiazepines, and antipsychotics.[42,43]

  2. Choice of medication(s) usually depends on many factors, including the severity and underlying cause of the agitated behavior; collaboration between ED, psychiatric, and pharmacy colleagues; and which medication(s), if any, the patient is currently taking (see Tables 3 and 4 at [www. pediatrics.org/cgi/doi/10. 1542/peds.2016-1570]).[42,43]

     a. Diphenhydramine may be used for mild agitation.

     b. Benzodiazepines are common first-line drugs for medical causes of agitation.

     c. Either benzodiazepines or antipsychotics may be used

for psychiatric causes of agitation.

d. Some experts favor a combination of an antipsychotic with either a benzodiazepine or an antihistamine for severe agitation.[43,44]

3. Monitoring and precautions

a. For patients receiving chemical restraint, consider the same monitoring and reassessment precautions as for physical restraint.[37,38]

b. Antipsychotics may cause QT_c prolongation and dysrhythmias, especially in patients with underlying cardiac conditions and/or who are taking other QT_c-prolonging medication.[45–47] Many medications commonly used in pediatrics (see Table 5 at [www.pediatrics.org/cgi/doi/10.1542/peds.2016-1570]) can affect QT_c duration. If there are significant concerns for dysrhythmia, cardiac monitoring may be considered for patients receiving antipsychotics.

c. Antipsychotics can exacerbate symptoms in patients with anticholinergic or sympathomimetic toxidromes or delirium.

- Physical restraint

1. Physical restraints have resulted in the death of psychiatric patients and have disproportionately affected children.[48,49]

2. Federal, regulatory, and accreditation agencies all have guidelines and regulations regarding physical restraint.[37,38]

3. Guidelines for when physical restraint may be indicated include the following[11,50–54]:

a. an imminent risk of harm to self or others;

b. significant risk of disrupting treatment; and

c. less restrictive means have failed.

4. For the application of restraints, when possible:

a. apply restraints with ≥5 providers, one for each extremity and one for the patient's head;

b. use leather or other age-appropriate restraints; and

c. secure restraints to the bed frame.

5. To maximize safety during physical restraint, experts suggest, when possible[38]:

a. staff training of alternatives to and proper application of restraints;

b. continuous patient monitoring;

c. utilize the supine position, with free cervical range of motion and elevation of the head of the bed, to reduce aspiration risk;

d. utilize the prone position only if other measures have failed or are not possible; if the prone position is used, monitoring for airway obstruction and excessive pressure on the back and neck of the patient may be helpful, because death has been associated with these factors and prone restraint; experts suggest discontinuing prone positioning as soon as possible[38];

e. minimize covering of the patient's face or head, to reduce aspiration risk;

f. minimize use of high vests, waist restraints, or beds with unprotected side rails to

reduce the risk of respiratory compromise and falls;

g. minimize restraint of medically compromised or unstable patients; and

h. in cases of agitation attributable to suspected illicit stimulant use, chemical restraint may be preferable, because a rapid increase in serum potassium secondary to rhabdomyolysis may result in cardiac arrest.

4. Coordination With the Medical Home

- Coordinating mental health care with the medical home (ie, patient-centered care, coordinated and integrated by the patient's personal physician) offers several benefits.[55,56]

1. Coordinating with the medical home decreases redundant care for high-risk or high-utilization patients.

2. The medical home may be a unique opportunity to address mental health care without stigma.[55]

3. For patients without a medical home, identifying and promptly referring them to a personal physician may be beneficial.

4. Children and adolescents with mental health problems and those taking psychiatric medications are at increased risk of medical problems, including asthma, ear infections, headaches or migraines, seizures, and obesity/metabolic syndrome.

LEAD AUTHORS

Thomas H. Chun, MD, MPH, FAAP
Sharon E. Mace, MD, FAAP, FACEP
Emily R. Katz, MD, FAAP

AMERICAN ACADEMY OF PEDIATRICS, COMMITTEE ON PEDIATRIC EMERGENCY MEDICINE, 2015-2016

Joan E. Shook, MD, MBA, FAAP, Chairperson
James M. Callahan, MD, FAAP
Thomas H. Chun, MD, MPH, FAAP
Gregory P. Conners, MD, MPH, MBA, FAAP
Edward E. Conway Jr, MD, MS, FAAP
Nanette C. Dudley, MD, FAAP
Toni K. Gross, MD, MPH, FAAP
Natalie E. Lane, MD, FAAP
Charles G. Macias, MD, MPH, FAAP
Nathan L. Timm, MD, FAAP

LIAISONS

Kim Bullock, MD – *American Academy of Family Physicians*
Elizabeth Edgerton, MD, MPH, FAAP – *Maternal and Child Health Bureau*
Tamar Magarik Haro – *AAP Department of Federal Affairs*
Madeline Joseph, MD, FACEP, FAAP – *American College of Emergency Physicians*
Angela Mickalide, PhD, MCHES – *EMSC National Resource Center*
Brian R. Moore, MD, FAAP – *National Association of EMS Physicians*
Katherine E. Remick, MD, FAAP – *National Association of Emergency Medical Technicians*
Sally K. Snow, RN, BSN, CPEN, FAEN – *Emergency Nurses Association*
David W. Tuggle, MD, FAAP – *American College of Surgeons*
Cynthia Wright-Johnson, MSN, RNC – *National Association of State EMS Officials*

FORMER MEMBERS AND LIAISONS, 2013-2015

Alice D. Ackerman, MD, MBA, FAAP
Lee Benjamin, MD, FACEP, FAAP - *American College of Physicians*
Susan M. Fuchs, MD, FAAP
Marc H. Gorelick, MD, MSCE, FAAP
Paul Sirbaugh, DO, MBA, FAAP - *National Association of Emergency Medical Technicians*
Joseph L. Wright, MD, MPH, FAAP

STAFF

Sue Tellez

AMERICAN COLLEGE OF EMERGENCY PHYSICIANS, PEDIATRIC EMERGENCY MEDICINE COMMITTEE, 2013–2014

Lee S. Benjamin, MD, FACEP, Chairperson
Isabel A. Barata, MD, FACEP, FAAP
Kiyetta Alade, MD
Joseph Arms, MD
Jahn T. Avarello, MD, FACEP
Steven Baldwin, MD
Kathleen Brown, MD, FACEP
Richard M. Cantor, MD, FACEP
Ariel Cohen, MD
Ann Marie Dietrich, MD, FACEP
Paul J. Eakin, MD
Marianne Gausche-Hill, MD, FACEP, FAAP
Michael Gerardi, MD, FACEP, FAAP
Charles J. Graham, MD, FACEP
Doug K. Holtzman, MD, FACEP
Jeffrey Hom, MD, FACEP
Paul Ishimine, MD, FACEP
Hasmig Jinivizian, MD
Madeline Joseph, MD, FACEP

Sanjay Mehta, MD, Med, FACEP
Aderonke Ojo, MD, MBBS
Audrey Z. Paul, MD, PhD
Denis R. Pauze, MD, FACEP
Nadia M. Pearson, DO
Brett Rosen, MD
W. Scott Russell, MD, FACEP
Mohsen Saidinejad, MD
Harold A. Sloas, DO
Gerald R. Schwartz, MD, FACEP
Orel Swenson, MD
Jonathan H. Valente, MD, FACEP
Muhammad Waseem, MD, MS
Paula J. Whiteman, MD, FACEP
Dale Woolridge, MD, PhD, FACEP

FORMER COMMITTEE MEMBERS

Carrie DeMoor, MD
James M. Dy, MD
Sean Fox, MD
Robert J. Hoffman, MD, FACEP
Mark Hostetler, MD, FACEP
David Markenson, MD, MBA, FACEP
Annalise Sorrentino, MD, FACEP
Michael Witt, MD, MPH, FACEP

STAFF

Dan Sullivan

Stephanie Wauson

> **ABBREVIATION**
>
> ED: emergency department

FINANCIAL DISCLOSURE: The authors have indicated they do not have a financial relationship relevant to this article to disclose.

FUNDING: No external funding.

POTENTIAL CONFLICT OF INTEREST: The authors have indicated they have no potential conflicts of interest to disclose.

REFERENCES

1. Mahajan P, Alpern ER, Grupp-Phelan J, et al; Pediatric Emergency Care Applied Research Network (PECARN). Epidemiology of psychiatric-related visits to emergency departments in a multicenter collaborative research pediatric network. *Pediatr Emerg Care.* 2009;25(11):715–720

2. Pittsenbarger ZE, Mannix R. Trends in pediatric visits to the emergency department for psychiatric illnesses. *Acad Emerg Med.* 2014;21(1):25–30

3. Sheldrick RC, Merchant S, Perrin EC. Identification of developmental-behavioral problems in primary care: a systematic review. *Pediatrics.* 2011;128(2):356–363

4. Grupp-Phelan J, Wade TJ, Pickup T, et al. Mental health problems in children and caregivers in the emergency department setting. *J Dev Behav Pediatr.* 2007;28(1):16–21

5. Committee on Psychosocial Aspects of Child and Family Health; Task Force on Mental Health. The future of pediatrics: mental health competencies for pediatric primary care [policy statement]. *Pediatrics.* 2009;124(1):410–421

6. Foy JM, Kelleher KJ, Laraque D; American Academy of Pediatrics Task Force on Mental Health. Enhancing pediatric mental health care: strategies for preparing a

primary care practice. *Pediatrics.* 2010;125(suppl 3):S87–S108

7. Dolan MA, Mace SE; American Academy of Pediatrics, Committee on Pediatric Emergency Medicine; American College of Emergency Physicians and Pediatric Emergency Medicine Committee. Pediatric mental health emergencies in the emergency medical services system. *Pediatrics.* 2006;118(4):1764–1767

8. Glauser J, Marshall M. Medical clearance of psychiatric patients. *Emerg Med Rep.* 2011;32(23): 273–286

9. Riba M, Hale M. Medical clearance: fact or fiction in the hospital

emergency room. *Psychosomatics.* 1990;31(4):400–404

10. Zun LS. Evidence-based evaluation of psychiatric patients. *J Emerg Med.* 2005;28(1):35–39

11. Lukens TW, Wolf SJ, Edlow JA, et al; American College of Emergency Physicians Clinical Policies Subcommittee (Writing Committee) on Critical Issues in the Diagnosis and Management of the Adult Psychiatric Patient in the Emergency Department. Clinical policy: critical issues in the diagnosis and management of the adult psychiatric patient in the emergency department. *Ann Emerg Med.* 2006;47(1):79–99

12. Agzarian MJ, Chryssidis S, Davies RP, Pozza CH. Use of routine computed tomography brain scanning of psychiatry patients. *Australas Radiol.* 2006;50(1):27–28

13. Donofrio JJ, Santillanes G, McCammack BD, et al. Clinical utility of screening laboratory tests in pediatric psychiatric patients presenting to the emergency department for medical clearance. *Ann Emerg Med.* 2014;63(6):666–75.e3

14. Fortu JM, Kim IK, Cooper A, Condra C, Lorenz DJ, Pierce MC. Psychiatric patients in the pediatric emergency department undergoing routine urine toxicology screens for medical clearance: results and use. *Pediatr Emerg Care.* 2009;25(6):387–392

15. Janiak BD, Atteberry S. Medical clearance of the psychiatric patient in the emergency department. *J Emerg Med.* 2012;43(5):866–870

16. Santiago LI, Tunik MG, Foltin GL, Mojica MA. Children requiring psychiatric consultation in the pediatric emergency department: epidemiology, resource utilization, and complications. *Pediatr Emerg Care.* 2006;22(2):85–89

17. Santillanes G, Donofrio JJ, Lam CN, Claudius I. Is medical clearance necessary for pediatric psychiatric patients? *J Emerg Med.* 2014;46(6):800–807

18. Shihabuddin BS, Hack CM, Sivitz AB. Role of urine drug screening in the medical clearance of pediatric psychiatric patients: is there one? *Pediatr Emerg Care.* 2013;29(8):903–906

19. Tenenbein M. Do you really need that emergency drug screen? *Clin Toxicol (Phila).* 2009;47(4):286–291

20. Shain BN; American Academy of Pediatrics, Committee on Adolescence. Suicide and suicide attempts in adolescents. *Pediatrics.* 2016;138(1):e20161420

21. Centers for Disease Control and Prevention, National Center for Injury Prevention and Control. Web-based Injury Statistics Query and Reporting System (WISQARS) [database]. Available at: www.cdc.gov/injury/wisqars/. Accessed July 7, 2015

22. Ting SA, Sullivan AF, Boudreaux ED, Miller I, Camargo CA Jr. Trends in US emergency department visits for attempted suicide and self-inflicted injury, 1993-2008. *Gen Hosp Psychiatry.* 2012;34(5):557–565

23. Eaton DK, Kann L, Kinchen S, et al; Centers for Disease Control and Prevention. Youth risk behavior surveillance—United States, 2011. *MMWR Surveill Summ.* 2012;61(4 SS-4):1–162

24. Brown J, Cohen P, Johnson JG, Smailes EM. Childhood abuse and neglect: specificity of effects on adolescent and young adult depression and suicidality. *J Am Acad Child Adolesc Psychiatry.* 1999;38(12):1490–1496

25. Esposito-Smythers C, Spirito A. Adolescent substance use and suicidal behavior: a review with implications for treatment research. *Alcohol Clin Exp Res.* 2004;28(5 suppl):77S–88S

26. Foley DL, Goldston DB, Costello EJ, Angold A. Proximal psychiatric risk factors for suicidality in youth: the Great Smoky Mountains Study. *Arch Gen Psychiatry.* 2006;63(9):1017–1024

27. McDaniel JS, Purcell D, D'Augelli AR. The relationship between sexual orientation and risk for suicide: research findings and future directions for research and prevention. *Suicide Life Threat Behav.* 2001;31(suppl):84–105

28. McKeown RE, Garrison CZ, Cuffe SP, Waller JL, Jackson KL, Addy CL. Incidence and predictors of suicidal behaviors in a longitudinal sample of young adolescents. *J Am Acad Child Adolesc Psychiatry.* 1998;37(6):612–619

29. Overholser J. Predisposing factors in suicide attempts: life stressors. In: Spirito A, Overholser JC, Overholser J, eds. *Evaluating and Treating Adolescent Suicide Attempters: From Research to Practice.* New York, NY: Academic Press; 2002:42–54

30. Brown GK, Henriques GR, Sosdjan D, Beck AT. Suicide intent and accurate expectations of lethality: predictors of medical lethality of suicide attempts. *J Consult Clin Psychol.* 2004;72(6):1170–1174

31. Plutchik R, van Praag HM, Picard S, Conte HR, Korn M. Is there a relation between the seriousness of suicidal intent and the lethality of the suicide attempt? *Psychiatry Res.* 1989;27(1):71–79

32. Swahn MH, Potter LB. Factors associated with the medical severity of suicide attempts in youths and young adults. *Suicide Life Threat Behav.* 2001;32(1 suppl):21–29

33. Sher L, LaBode V. Teaching health care professionals about suicide safety planning. *Psychiatr Danub.* 2011;23(4):396–397

34. American Academy of Child and Adolescent Psychiatry. Practice parameter for the assessment and treatment of children and adolescents with suicidal behavior. *J Am Acad Child Adolesc Psychiatry.* 2001;40(7 suppl):24S–51S

35. Richmond JS, Berlin JS, Fishkind AB, et al. Verbal de-escalation of the agitated patient: consensus statement of the American Association for Emergency Psychiatry Project BETA De-escalation Workgroup. *West J Emerg Med.* 2012;13(1):17–25

36. Health and Human Services Division, US General Accounting Office, ed. Report to Congressional Requestors: Mental Health: Improper Restraint or Seclusion Places People at Risk. Washington, DC: US General Accounting Office; 1999

37. Centers for Medicare and Medicaid Services; Department of Health and Human Services. Medicare and Medicaid programs; hospital conditions of participation: patients' rights. Final rule. *Fed Regist.* 2006;71(236):71377–71428

38. The Joint Commission. *Standards on Restraint and Seclusion*. Oakbrook Terrace, IL: The Joint Commission; 2009

39. Cowin L, Davies R, Estall G, Berlin T, Fitzgerald M, Hoot S. De-escalating aggression and violence in the mental health setting. *Int J Ment Health Nurs*. 2003;12(1):64–73

40. American Psychiatric Association, Task Force on the Psychiatric Use of Seclusion and Restraint. *Seclusion and Restraint: The Psychiatric Uses*. Washington, DC: American Psychiatric Association; 1985. Task Force Report 22.

41. Fishkind A. Calming agitation with words, not drugs: 10 commandments for safety. *Curr Psychiatr*. 2002;1(4):32–39

42. Adimando AJ, Poncin YB, Baum CR. Pharmacological management of the agitated pediatric patient. *Pediatr Emerg Care*. 2010;26(11):856–860; quiz: 861–863

43. Sonnier L, Barzman D. Pharmacologic management of acutely agitated pediatric patients. *Paediatr Drugs*. 2011;13(1):1–10

44. Marder SR. A review of agitation in mental illness: treatment guidelines and current therapies. *J Clin Psychiatry*. 2006;67(suppl 10):13–21

45. Labellarte MJ, Crosson JE, Riddle MA. The relevance of prolonged QTc measurement to pediatric psychopharmacology. *J Am Acad Child Adolesc Psychiatry*. 2003;42(6):642–650

46. Olsen KM. Pharmacologic agents associated with QT interval prolongation. *J Fam Pract*. 2005;(suppl):S8–S14

47. Yap YG, Camm AJ. Drug induced QT prolongation and torsades de pointes. *Heart*. 2003;89(11):1363–1372

48. Nunno MA, Holden MJ, Tollar A. Learning from tragedy: a survey of child and adolescent restraint fatalities. *Child Abuse Negl*. 2006;30(12):1333–1342

49. Weiss EM, Altamira D, Blinded DF, et al. Deadly restraint: a Hartford Courant investigative report. *Hartford Courant*. October 11–15, 1998:A10

50. American Academy of Pediatrics Committee on Pediatric Emergency Medicine. The use of physical restraint interventions for children and adolescents in the acute care setting. *Pediatrics*. 1997;99(3):497–498

51. Currier GW, Walsh P, Lawrence D. Physical restraints in the emergency department and attendance at subsequent outpatient psychiatric treatment. *J Psychiatr Pract*. 2011;17(6):387–393

52. Downes MA, Healy P, Page CB, Bryant JL, Isbister GK. Structured team approach to the agitated patient in the emergency department. *Emerg Med Australas*. 2009;21(3):196–202

53. Glezer A, Brendel RW. Beyond emergencies: the use of physical restraints in medical and psychiatric settings. *Harv Rev Psychiatry*. 2010;18(6):353–358

54. Rossi J, Swan MC, Isaacs ED. The violent or agitated patient. *Emerg Med Clin North Am*. 2010;28(1):235–256

55. American Academy of Child and Adolescent Psychiatry Committee on Health Care Access and Economics Task Force on Mental Health. Improving mental health services in primary care: reducing administrative and financial barriers to access and collaboration. *Pediatrics*. 2009;123(4):1248–1251

56. Schwenk TL. The patient-centered medical home: one size does not fit all. *JAMA*. 2014;311(8):802–803

CLINICAL REPORT   Guidance for the Clinician in Rendering Pediatric Care

American Academy
of Pediatrics

DEDICATED TO THE HEALTH OF ALL CHILDREN™

Executive Summary: Evaluation and Management of Children With Acute Mental Health or Behavioral Problems. Part II: Recognition of Clinically Challenging Mental Health Related Conditions Presenting With Medical or Uncertain Symptoms

Thomas H. Chun, MD, MPH, FAAP, Sharon E. Mace, MD, FAAP, FACEP, Emily R. Katz, MD, FAAP, AMERICAN ACADEMY OF PEDIATRICS, COMMITTEE ON PEDIATRIC EMERGENCY MEDICINE, AMERICAN COLLEGE OF EMERGENCY PHYSICIANS, PEDIATRIC EMERGENCY MEDICINE COMMITTEE

FREE

EXECUTIVE SUMMARY

The number of children and adolescents seen in emergency departments (EDs) and primary care settings for mental health problems has skyrocketed in recent years, with up to 23% of patients in both settings having diagnosable mental health conditions.[1-4] Even when a mental health problem is not the focus of an ED or primary care visit, mental health conditions, both known and occult, may challenge the treating clinician and complicate the patient's care.[4]

Although the American Academy of Pediatrics (AAP) has published a policy statement on mental health competencies and a Mental Health Toolkit for pediatric primary care providers, no such guidelines or resources exist for clinicians who care for pediatric mental health emergencies.[5,6] Many ED and primary care physicians report paucity of training and lack of confidence in caring for pediatric psychiatry patients. The 2 clinical reports support the 2006 joint policy statement of the AAP and the American College of Emergency Physicians on pediatric mental health emergencies,[7] with the goal of addressing the knowledge gaps in this area. Although written primarily from the perspective of ED clinicians, it is intended for all clinicians who care for children and adolescents with acute mental health and behavioral problems. They are organized around the common clinical challenges pediatric caregivers face, both when a child or adolescent presents with a psychiatric chief complaint or emergency (part I) and when a mental health condition may be an unclear or complicating factor in a non–mental health ED presentation (part II). Part I of the clinical reports

DOI: 10.1542/peds.2016-1574

Accepted for publication May 12, 2016

PEDIATRICS (ISSN Numbers: Print, 0031-4005; Online, 1098-4275).

To cite: Chun TH, Mace SE, AAP FACEP, Katz ER. Executive Summary: Evaluation and Management of Children With Acute Mental Health or Behavioral Problems. Part II: Recognition of Clinically Challenging Mental Health Related Conditions Presenting With Medical or Uncertain Symptoms. *Pediatrics.* 2016;138(2):e20161574 includes discussions of Medical Clearance of Pediatric Psychiatric Patients, Suicide and Suicidal Ideation, Restraint of the Agitated Patient Including Verbal, Chemical, and Physical Restraint, and Coordination of Care With the Medical Home, and it can be accessed online at www.pediatrics.org/cgi/doi/10.1542/peds.2016-1570. This executive summary is an overview of part II of the clinical reports. Full text of the following topics can be accessed online at www.pediatrics.org/cgi/doi/10.1542/peds.2016-1573.

Key considerations include the following:

Somatic Symptom and Related Disorders

- Somatic symptom and related disorders encompass conditions in which physical symptoms are not intentionally produced or associated with material gain.[8] These disorders are common and are significant contributors to health care usage and costs, because they cause significant functional impairment.[9–11]

- Symptoms of pediatric somatic symptom and related disorders often do not meet strict diagnostic criteria and defy categorization.[12,13] Clinical presentations are myriad, most often involving neurologic, pain, autonomic, or gastrointestinal tract symptoms.[14,15] Patients often have vague, poorly described complaints, recent or current stressful events, and symptoms that fluctuate with activity or stress and often have multiple medical visits for these symptoms.[16]

- *Risk factors:* Studies have found higher rates of somatic symptom and related disorders in patients who are adolescent, female, or of minority ethnicities; patients who live in urban areas; patients from nonintact families; patients whose parents have lower education level; patients whose family members

have somatic symptom and related disorders; and patients who have histories of psychological trauma. Comorbid depression and anxiety disorders are common.[8,17]

- *Somatic symptom and related disorders and the ED:* Caring for such patients in the ED can be particularly vexing, because few patients will have received a formal diagnosis, and ED clinicians often do not have access to sufficient clinical information to confirm the diagnosis.[12,13] In addition, diagnosing a "psychosomatic" illness may be stigmatizing to patients and families and may result in them feeling unheard, disrespected, and defensive about their symptoms.[18] Because of diagnostic uncertainty, patients with somatic symptom and related disorders are at risk for extensive, invasive, or potentially harmful testing and interventions in the ED.[19,20]

- *ED management strategies*[8,18,21]: ED clinicians may consider doing the following:

  i. Reassure the patient and family that the patient's symptoms are being heard and taken seriously and that testing and treatment that are medically indicated will be performed.

  ii. Emphasize collaboration between the patient, family, and all caregivers; make referrals as needed; and identify common goals and outcomes. Educating the patient and family about the limitations of the ED setting and what are alternative settings for evaluation and treatment may be beneficial.

  iii. Introduce the concept of working on improving functioning while also working on symptom resolution.

  iv. Coordinate the patient's care with the medical home and other involved care providers to help the ED clinician avoid unnecessary testing or intervention and reassure the patient and family.

Adverse Effects of Psychiatric Medications

- In recent years, the use of medications for mental health conditions, especially antipsychotics, is burgeoning among children and adolescents.[22–25]

- Many medications commonly used as antiemetics or for migraines (eg, prochlorperazine, metoclopramide, and promethazine) are phenothiazines, the same class of medications as first-generation "typical" antipsychotics.[26] In addition, other medications commonly used in pediatrics have serotonergic properties. Therefore, a working knowledge of the adverse effects of these medications may be helpful to ED clinicians.

- Antipsychotics:

  i. Although antipsychotics exert their effect primarily through the brain's dopaminergic system, they also affect numerous other neurotransmitter systems. Table 2 in the clinical report (see Table 2 at www.pediatrics.org/cgi/doi/10.1542/peds.2016-1573) lists the common adverse effects, which neurotransmitter system is involved, and which adverse effects are most commonly seen with which antipsychotics.

  ii. QT_c prolongation: Almost all antipsychotics cause some degree of QT_c prolongation because of a quinidinelike effect (see Table 4 at www.

pediatrics.org/cgi/doi/10.1542/peds.2016-1573). Risk factors (see Table 3 at www.pediatrics.org/cgi/doi/10.1542/peds.2016-1573) for QT_c prolongation and sudden death include coadministration of other QT_c-prolonging medications (see Table 5 at www.pediatrics.org/cgi/doi/10.1542/peds.2016-1570); intravenous administration or high dosage; medically ill patients; electrolyte abnormalities; hepatic, renal, or cardiac impairment; and congenital long QT syndromes.[27–29]

iii. *Black box warning:* Because of this risk, thioridazine and, more controversially, droperidol carry Food and Drug Administration "black box" warnings.

iv. *Extrapyramidal symptoms:* Dystonia, akathisia, Parkinsonism, and tardive dyskinesia are typical extrapyramidal symptoms. Acute dystonic reactions, the most commonly encountered extrapyramidal symptoms, often respond to diphenhydramine or benztropine. Laryngeal dystonia is rare but potentially life threatening.[26,28]

v. *Metabolic syndrome:* Hyperglycemia, hyperlipidemia, and obesity are often associated with atypical antipsychotic use, with variable severity between medications (see Table 2 at www.pediatrics.org/cgi/doi/10.1542/peds.2016-1573).[30]

vi. *Agranulocytosis:* This rare adverse effect is most commonly associated with clozapine and less commonly with risperidone and olanzapine.[31]

vii. *Neuroleptic malignant syndrome (NMS):* NMS is a potentially lethal condition consisting of the tetrad of mental status changes, fever, muscular hypertonicity or rigidity, and autonomic dysfunction caused by central dopamine deficiency and can occur with any antipsychotic.[32,33]

1. NMS occurs idiosyncratically but is most common within 7 days of starting or increasing antipsychotic doses and later (15–30 days) if depot medications have been used.[32,34]

2. In addition to the classic tetrad, symptoms can include tachycardia, blood pressure instability, diaphoresis, pallor, cardiac dysrhythmia, diaphoresis, sialorrhea, dysphagia, rhabdomyolysis, renal failure, thromboembolic events, hypoventilation, and respiratory failure.[32,35]

3. NMS is a clinical diagnosis, because there are no pathognomonic clinical or laboratory criteria. Leukocytosis and elevated serum creatine phosphokinase and aldose are commonly observed.[36]

4. Treatment may include supportive measures, such as removal of the initiating agent, and when indicated may also include intravenous fluids for dehydration and rhabdomyolysis, benzodiazepines for agitation, external cooling measures, and cardiorespiratory support. The smooth muscle relaxant dantrolene may be used to directly treat the abnormal muscle contractions of NMS.[37,38] The utility of central nervous system dopaminergic agents, such as bromocriptine and amantadine, is less clear and controversial.

5. Potential resources for caring for patients with NMS include toxicologists, a poison control center, and the NMS Information Service, which can be accessed through its Web site (http://www.nmsis.org/index.asp).[37,38]

• Serotonin syndrome:

i. Given the large number of non–mental health medications with serotonergic properties (see Table 6 at www.pediatrics.org/cgi/doi/10.1542/peds.2016-1573) in addition to antidepressants and some antipsychotics, it is not surprising that the incidence of serotonin syndrome is increasing. It can occur in cases of overdose but also in the course of standard use.[39,40] The classic clinical triad consists of mental status changes, autonomic hyperactivity, and neuromuscular abnormalities, although many patients do not exhibit all these clinical characteristics. Given the wide variability in the severity of symptoms and the lack of pathognomonic clinical and laboratory findings, diagnosing serotonin syndrome can be particularly challenging.[40,41]

ii. *Signs and symptoms:* Agitated delirium is the most common form of mental status change, although it also has a wide spectrum of severity, including mild agitation, hypervigilance, slightly pressured speech, and easy startle. Diaphoresis, shivering, mydriasis, increased bowel sounds, and diarrhea are common signs of autonomic dysfunction. Myoclonus is the most common neuromuscular finding, but other abnormalities are possible, including, muscular rigidity, hypertonicity, hyperreflexia, clonus, horizontal ocular clonus, tremor, akathisia, and seizures.[39,42] Laboratory findings can include elevated CPK and hepatic transaminases, metabolic acidosis, renal failure, and disseminated intravascular coagulopathy.

iii. *Diagnosis:* Differentiating serotonin syndrome from other medication-induced syndromes can be challenging. Table 7 in the clinical report (www. pediatrics.org/cgi/doi/10. 1542/peds.2016-1573) details both the similar and differentiating features of these syndromes. In addition to the aforementioned laboratory abnormalities, other diagnostic testing may include a complete blood cell count, serum electrolytes, arterial blood gas, urinalysis, toxicology screens, electrocardiogram, electroencephalogram, and brain imaging studies.

iv. *Treatment:* Similar to NMS, treatment of serotonin syndrome most often includes supportive measures. For severe cases, centrally acting serotonin agents may be considered, including cyproheptadine

and chlorpromazine. Some experts prefer cyproheptadine, because chlorpromazine may cause hypotension and increase muscle rigidity, decrease seizure threshold, and worsen NMS (eg, in diagnostically challenging cases when the diagnosis is unclear and the patient has NMS, not serotonin syndrome).[42,43] Toxicologists, poison control centers, and the NMS Information Service, as mentioned previously in the NMS section, may be helpful resources in caring for these patients. Evaluation and observation in the ED and additional outpatient management may be considered in mild cases.

Children With Special Needs: Caring for Patients With Autism Spectrum Disorders and Developmental Disorders

- In recent years, there has been a sharp increase in the incidence of autism spectrum disorders, with corresponding interest and growth in treatment strategies. Most studies have methodological or generalizability limitations. Therefore, the following strategies are based primarily on expert, consensus opinion.

- *Resources:* Often, the most important autism spectrum disorder or developmental delay (ASD-DD) "expert" to consult is the child's parent. Parents of children with ASD-DD often know what strategies work with their child (eg, which words, actions, stimuli, calm and help their child) and which have the opposite effect. They can also be an "interpreter" for ED clinicians, deciphering the significance of their child's actions and behaviors and facilitating communication with their child. Spending some time asking the parents about their child can be

a very productive, efficient method for tailoring effective ED care for patients with ASD-DD. A wide range of ED professionals can assist with or champion ASD-DD–sensitive care, including physicians, nurses, nursing assistants, nurse practitioners or physician assistants, social workers, and child life specialists. Non-ED resources that may be helpful include developmental–behavioral pediatricians, child psychologist and psychiatrists, special education teachers, speech–language therapists, and occupational therapists.

- *Strategies:* A variety of environmental modifications, communication adjuncts, and distraction techniques may assist in caring for children with ASD-DD (see Table 8 at www. pediatrics.org/cgi/doi/10. 1542/peds.2016-1573). A quiet, darkened room may be soothing to a child with an ASD-DD. These children often communicate with a visual communication system (VCS).[44] If they do not have their usual VCS, a wide variety of free and commercial products are available. Digital photography is an alternative, inexpensive method of creating a custom VCS for the ED. Transition planning and desensitization strategies may help children with ASD-DD acclimate to the ED and the care they will receive. Distraction techniques that may be useful include physical activity, electronic games, and tactile stimulation.

- *Medications:* There are no rigorous, evidence-based recommendations for which medications to use for children with ASD-DD. Although there are no known contraindications, other than the patient's past response to medications, atypical, idiosyncratic responses to medications may be common with these patients. Consultation with an ASD-DD expert before starting medication may be helpful. Many suggest starting with lower medication dosages and closely monitoring the patient's response.[45]

Mental Health Screening

- *Advantages of the ED:* Many children and adolescents who visit EDs are at high risk of mental health problems that may not be addressed in other settings.[46,47] For example, they may not attend school or have a medical home, effectively making the ED the sole safety net for these patients.[48,49]

- *Feasibility and acceptability of ED mental health screening:* Many rapid and efficient mental health screening tools have been tested in the ED, including for depression, suicide, anxiety, and posttraumatic stress.[50–53] Studies have found these screening tools to have high feasibility (eg, they can be completed in a few seconds to a few minutes) and acceptability by patients, their families, and ED clinicians.[54–58] Electronic screening tools have been developed, are being tested, and may be advantageous to the ED setting.[59–61]

LEAD AUTHORS

Thomas H. Chun, MD, MPH, FAAP
Sharon E. Mace, MD, FAAP, FACEP
Emily R. Katz, MD, FAAP

AMERICAN ACADEMY OF PEDIATRICS, COMMITTEE ON PEDIATRIC EMERGENCY MEDICINE, 2015-2016

Joan E. Shook, MD, MBA, FAAP, Chairperson
James M. Callahan, MD, FAAP
Thomas H. Chun, MD, MPH, FAAP
Gregory P. Conners, MD, MPH, MBA, FAAP
Edward E. Conway Jr, MD, MS, FAAP
Nanette C. Dudley, MD, FAAP

Toni K. Gross, MD, MPH, FAAP
Natalie E. Lane, MD, FAAP
Charles G. Macias, MD, MPH, FAAP
Nathan L. Timm, MD, FAAP

LIAISONS

Kim Bullock, MD — *American Academy of Family Physicians*
Elizabeth Edgerton, MD, MPH, FAAP — *Maternal and Child Health Bureau*
Brian R. Moore, MD, FAAP — *National Association of EMS Physicians*
Tamar Magarik Haro — *AAP Department of Federal Affairs*
Madeline Joseph, MD, FACEP, FAAP — *American College of Emergency Physicians*
Angela Mickalide, PhD, MCHES — EMSC National Resource Center
Katherine E. Remick, MD, FAAP — National Association of Emergency Medical Technicians
Sally K. Snow, RN, BSN, CPEN, FAEN — Emergency Nurses Association
David W. Tuggle, MD, FAAP — American College of Surgeons
Cynthia Wright-Johnson, MSN, RNC — National Association of State EMS Officials

FORMER MEMBERS AND LIAISONS, 2013-2015

Alice D. Ackerman, MD, MBA, FAAP
Lee Benjamin, MD, FACEP, FAAP - *American College of Physicians*
Susan M. Fuchs, MD, FAAP
Marc H. Gorelick, MD, MSCE, FAAP
Paul Sirbaugh, DO, MBA, FAAP - *National Association of Emergency Medical Technicians*
Joseph L. Wright, MD, MPH, FAAP

STAFF

Sue Tellez

AMERICAN COLLEGE OF EMERGENCY PHYSICIANS, PEDIATRIC EMERGENCY MEDICINE COMMITTEE, 2013–2014

Lee S. Benjamin, MD, FACEP, Chairperson
Isabel A. Barata, MD, FACEP, FAAP
Kiyetta Alade, MD
Joseph Arms, MD
Jahn T. Avarello, MD, FACEP
Steven Baldwin, MD
Kathleen Brown, MD, FACEP
Richard M. Cantor, MD, FACEP
Ariel Cohen, MD
Ann Marie Dietrich, MD, FACEP
Paul J. Eakin, MD

Marianne Gausche-Hill, MD, FACEP, FAAP
Michael Gerardi, MD, FACEP, FAAP
Charles J. Graham, MD, FACEP
Doug K. Holtzman, MD, FACEP
Jeffrey Hom, MD, FACEP
Paul Ishimine, MD, FACEP
Hasmig Jinivizian, MD
Madeline Joseph, MD, FACEP
Sanjay Mehta, MD, MEd, FACEP
Aderonke Ojo, MD, MBBS
Audrey Z. Paul, MD, PhD
Denis R. Pauze, MD, FACEP
Nadia M. Pearson, DO
Brett Rosen, MD
W. Scott Russell, MD, FACEP
Mohsen Saidinejad, MD
Harold A. Sloas, DO
Gerald R. Schwartz, MD, FACEP
Orel Swenson, MD
Jonathan H. Valente, MD, FACEP
Muhammad Waseem, MD, MS
Paula J. Whiteman, MD, FACEP
Dale Woolridge, MD, PhD, FACEP

FORMER COMMITTEE MEMBERS

Carrie DeMoor, MD
James M. Dy, MD
Sean Fox, MD
Robert J. Hoffman, MD, FACEP
Mark Hostetler, MD, FACEP
David Markenson, MD, MBA, FACEP
Annalise Sorrentino, MD, FACEP
Michael Witt, MD, MPH, FACEP

STAFF

Dan Sullivan
Stephanie Wauson

ABBREVIATIONS

AAP: American Academy of Pediatrics
ASD-DD: autism spectrum disorder or developmental delay
ED: emergency department
NMS: neuroleptic malignant syndrome
VCS: visual communication system

FINANCIAL DISCLOSURE: The authors have indicated they do not have a financial relationship relevant to this article to disclose.

FUNDING: No external funding.

POTENTIAL CONFLICT OF INTEREST: The authors have indicated they have no potential conflicts of interest to disclose.

REFERENCES

1. Mahajan P, Alpern ER, Grupp-Phelan J, et al; Pediatric Emergency Care Applied Research Network (PECARN). Epidemiology of psychiatric-related visits to emergency departments in a multicenter collaborative research pediatric network. *Pediatr Emerg Care*. 2009;25(11):715–720

2. Pittsenbarger ZE, Mannix R. Trends in pediatric visits to the emergency department for psychiatric illnesses. *Acad Emerg Med*. 2014;21(1):25–30

3. Sheldrick RC, Merchant S, Perrin EC. Identification of developmental–behavioral problems in primary care: a systematic review. *Pediatrics*. 2011;128(2):356–363

4. Grupp-Phelan J, Wade TJ, Pickup T, et al. Mental health problems in children and caregivers in the emergency department setting. *J Dev Behav Pediatr*. 2007;28(1):16–21

5. Committee on Psychosocial Aspects of Child and Family Health and Task Force on Mental Health. Policy statement-- The future of pediatrics: mental health competencies for pediatric primary care. *Pediatrics*. 2009;124(1):410–421

6. Foy JM, Kelleher KJ, Laraque D; American Academy of Pediatrics Task Force on Mental Health. Enhancing pediatric mental health care: strategies for preparing a primary care practice. *Pediatrics*. 2010;125(suppl 3):S87–S108

7. Dolan MA, Mace SE; American Academy of Pediatrics, Committee on Pediatric Emergency Medicine; American College of Emergency Physicians and Pediatric Emergency Medicine Committee. Pediatric mental health emergencies in the emergency medical services system. *Pediatrics*. 2006;118(4):1764–1767

8. Dell ML, Campo JV. Somatoform disorders in children and adolescents. *Psychiatr Clin North Am*. 2011;34(3):643–660

9. Barsky AJ, Orav EJ, Bates DW. Somatization increases medical utilization and costs independent of psychiatric and medical comorbidity. *Arch Gen Psychiatry*. 2005;62(8):903–910

10. Campo JV, Jansen-McWilliams L, Comer DM, Kelleher KJ. Somatization in pediatric primary care: association with psychopathology, functional impairment, and use of services. *J Am Acad Child Adolesc Psychiatry*. 1999;38(9):1093–1101

11. Reid S, Wessely S, Crayford T, Hotopf M. Medically unexplained symptoms in frequent attenders of secondary health care: retrospective cohort study. *BMJ*. 2001;322(7289):767

12. Fleet RP, Dupuis G, Marchand A, Burelle D, Arsenault A, Beitman BD. Panic disorder in emergency department chest pain patients: prevalence, comorbidity, suicidal ideation, and physician recognition. *Am J Med*. 1996;101(4):371–380

13. Pollard CA, Lewis LM. Managing panic attacks in emergency patients. *J Emerg Med*. 1989;7(5):547–552

14. Campo JV, Fritsch SL. Somatization in children and adolescents. *J Am Acad Child Adolesc Psychiatry*. 1994;33(9):1223–1235

15. Garralda ME. Somatisation in children. *J Child Psychol Psychiatry*. 1996;37(1):13–33

16. Sater N, Constantino JN. Pediatric emergencies in children with psychiatric conditions. *Pediatr Emerg Care*. 1998;14(1):42–50

17. Haugland S, Wold B, Stevenson J, Aaroe LE, Woynarowska B. Subjective health complaints in adolescence. A cross-national comparison of prevalence and dimensionality. *Eur J Public Health*. 2001;11(1):4–10

18. Silber TJ. Somatization disorders: diagnosis, treatment, and prognosis. *Pediatr Rev*. 2011;32(2):56–63, quiz 63–64

19. Bhatia MS, Sapra S. Pseudoseizures in children: a profile of 50 cases. *Clin Pediatr (Phila)*. 2005;44(7):617–621

20. Selbst SM, Clancy R. Pseudoseizures in the pediatric emergency department. *Pediatr Emerg Care*. 1996;12(3):185–188

21. Garralda ME. Unexplained physical complaints. *Pediatr Clin North Am*. 2011;58(4):803–813, ix

22. Alexander GC, Gallagher SA, Mascola A, Moloney RM, Stafford RS. Increasing off-label use of antipsychotic medications in the United States, 1995–2008. *Pharmacoepidemiol Drug Saf*. 2011;20(2):177–184

23. Harrison JN, Cluxton-Keller F, Gross D. Antipsychotic medication prescribing trends in children and adolescents. *J Pediatr Health Care*. 2012;26(2):139–145

24. Matone M, Localio R, Huang YS, dosReis S, Feudtner C, Rubin D. The relationship between mental health diagnosis and treatment with second-generation antipsychotics over time: a national study of US Medicaid-enrolled children. *Health Serv Res*. 2012;47(5):1836–1860

25. Pringsheim T, Doja A, Belanger S, Patten S; Canadian Alliance for Monitoring Effectiveness and Safety of Antipsychotics in Children (CAMESA) guideline group. Treatment recommendations for extrapyramidal side effects associated with second-generation antipsychotic use in children and youth. *Paediatr Child Health*. 2011;16(9):590–598

26. Whittler MA, Lavonas EJ. Antipsychotics. In: Marx JA, Hockberger RS, Walls RM, et al, eds. *Rosen's Emergency Medicine: Concepts and Clinical Practice*. Philadelphia, PA: Saunders; 2014:2042–2046

27. Lukens TW, Wolf SJ, Edlow JA, et al; American College of Emergency Physicians Clinical Policies Subcommittee (Writing Committee) on Critical Issues in the Diagnosis and Management of the Adult Psychiatric Patient in the Emergency Department. Clinical policy: critical issues in the diagnosis and management of the adult psychiatric patient in the emergency department. *Ann Emerg Med*. 2006;47(1):79–99

28. Sonnier L, Barzman D. Pharmacologic management of acutely agitated pediatric patients. *Paediatr Drugs*. 2011;13(1):1–10

29. Hilt RJ, Woodward TA. Agitation treatment for pediatric emergency patients. *J Am Acad Child Adolesc Psychiatry*. 2008;47(2):132–138

30. Reynolds GP, Kirk SL. Metabolic side effects of antipsychotic drug treatment: pharmacological mechanisms. *Pharmacol Ther*. 2010;125(1):169–179

31. Miyamoto S, Lieberman JA, Fleischacker WW, Marder SR. Antipsychotic drugs. In: Tasman A, Kay J, Lieberman A, First MB, Maj M, eds. *Psychiatry*. 3rd ed. West Sussex, England: John Wiley & Sons; 2008:2161–2201

32. Guzé BH, Baxter LR Jr. Current concepts. Neuroleptic malignant syndrome. *N Engl J Med*. 1985;313(3):163–166

33. Levine M, LoVecchio F. Antipsychotics. In: Tintinalli JE, Stapczynski S, Ma OJ, Cline DM, Cydulka RK, Mecklereds GD, eds. *Tintinalli's Emergency Medicine: A Comprehensive Study Guide*. New York, NY: McGraw-Hill Education; 2011:1207–1211

34. Agar L. Recognizing neuroleptic malignant syndrome in the emergency department: a case study. *Perspect Psychiatr Care*. 2010;46(2):143–151

35. Martel ML, Biros MH. Psychotropic medications and rapid tranquilization. In: Tintinalli JE, Stapczynski S, Ma OJ, Cline DM, Cydulka RK, Mecklereds GD, eds. *Tintinalli's Emergency Medicine: A Comprehensive Study Guide*. New York, NY: McGraw-Hill Education; 2011:1952–1955

36. Wijdicks EFM. Neuroleptic malignant syndrome. In: Aminoff MJ, ed. *UpToDate*. Updated May 30, 2014. Available at: www.uptodate.com/contents/neuroleptic-malignant-syndrome. Accessed July 7, 2015

37. Meeks TW, Jeste DV. Medication-induced movement disorders. In: Tasman A, Kay J, Lieberman A, First MB, Maj M, eds. *Psychiatry*. 3rd ed. West Sussex, England: John Wiley & Sons; 2008:2142

38. Perry PJ, Wilborn CA. Serotonin syndrome vs neuroleptic malignant syndrome: a contrast of causes, diagnoses, and management. *Ann Clin Psychiatry*. 2012;24(2):155–162

39. Birmes P, Coppin D, Schmitt L, Lauque D. Serotonin syndrome: a brief review. *CMAJ*. 2003;168(11):1439–1442

40. Kant S, Liebelt E. Recognizing serotonin toxicity in the pediatric emergency department. *Pediatr Emerg Care*. 2012;28(8):817–821, quiz 822–824

41. Christensen RC. Identifying serotonin syndrome in the emergency department. *Am J Emerg Med*. 2005;23(3):406–408

42. Boyer EW, Shannon M. The serotonin syndrome. *N Engl J Med*. 2005;352(11):1112–1120

43. Isbister GK, Buckley NA, Whyte IM. Serotonin toxicity: a practical approach to diagnosis and treatment. *Med J Aust*. 2007;187(6):361–365

44. Ganz JB, Davis JL, Lund EM, Goodwyn FD, Simpson RL. Meta-analysis of PECS with individuals with ASD: investigation of targeted versus non-targeted outcomes, participant characteristics, and implementation phase. *Res Dev Disabil*. 2012;33(2):406–418

45. Sullivan M. Autism demands attention in the emergency department. *ACEP News*. April 17, 2012

46. Oster A, Bindman AB. Emergency department visits for ambulatory care sensitive conditions: insights into preventable hospitalizations. *Med Care*. 2003;41(2):198–207

47. Wilson KM, Klein JD. Adolescents who use the emergency department as their usual source of care. *Arch Pediatr Adolesc Med*. 2000;154(4):361–365

48. Klein JD, Woods AH, Wilson KM, Prospero M, Greene J, Ringwalt C. Homeless and runaway youths' access to health care. *J Adolesc Health*. 2000;27(5):331–339

49. Marcell AV, Klein JD, Fischer I, Allan MJ, Kokotailo PK. Male adolescent use of health care services: where are the boys? *J Adolesc Health*. 2002;30(1):35–43

50. Haughey MT, Calderon Y, Torres S, Nazario S, Bijur P. Identification of depression in an inner-city population using a simple screen. *Acad Emerg Med*. 2005;12(12):1221–1226

51. Horowitz LM, Bridge JA, Teach SJ, et al. Ask Suicide-Screening Questions (ASQ): a brief instrument for the pediatric emergency department. *Arch Pediatr Adolesc Med*. 2012;166(12):1170–1176

52. Newton AS, Gokiert R, Mabood N, et al. Instruments to detect alcohol and other drug misuse in the emergency department: a systematic review. *Pediatrics*. 2011;128(1). Available at: www.pediatrics.org/cgi/content/full/128/1/e180

53. Winston FK, Kassam-Adams N, Garcia-España F, Ittenbach R, Cnaan A. Screening for risk of persistent posttraumatic stress in injured children and their parents. *JAMA*. 2003;290(5):643–649

54. Horowitz L, Ballard E, Teach SJ, et al. Feasibility of screening patients with nonpsychiatric complaints for suicide risk in a pediatric emergency department: a good time to talk? *Pediatr Emerg Care*. 2010;26(11):787–792

55. King CA, O'Mara RM, Hayward CN, Cunningham RM. Adolescent suicide risk screening in the emergency department. *Acad Emerg Med*. 2009;16(11):1234–1241

56. O'Mara RM, Hill RM, Cunningham RM, King CA. Adolescent and parent attitudes toward screening for suicide risk and mental health problems in the pediatric emergency department. *Pediatr Emerg Care*. 2012;28(7):626–632

57. Pailler ME, Cronholm PF, Barg FK, Wintersteen MB, Diamond GS, Fein JA. Patients' and caregivers' beliefs about depression screening and referral in the emergency department. *Pediatr Emerg Care*. 2009;25(11):721–727

58. Williams JR, Ho ML, Grupp-Phelan J. The acceptability of mental health screening in a pediatric emergency department. *Pediatr Emerg Care*. 2011;27(7):611–615

59. Kit Delgado M, Ginde AA, Pallin DJ, Camargo CA Jr. Multicenter study of preferences for health education in the emergency department population. *Acad Emerg Med*. 2010;17(6):652–658

60. Pailler ME, Fein JA. Computerized behavioral health screening in the emergency department. *Pediatr Ann*. 2009;38(3):156–160

61. Ranney ML, Choo EK, Wang Y, Baum A, Clark MA, Mello MJ. Emergency department patients' preferences for technology-based behavioral interventions. *Ann Emerg Med*. 2012;60(2):218–27.e48

CLINICAL REPORT Guidance for the Clinician in Rendering Pediatric Care

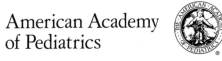

American Academy
of Pediatrics

DEDICATED TO THE HEALTH OF ALL CHILDREN™

Promoting Optimal Development: Screening for Behavioral and Emotional Problems

Carol Weitzman, MD, FAAP, Lynn Wegner, MD, FAAP, the SECTION ON DEVELOPMENTAL AND BEHAVIORAL PEDIATRICS, COMMITTEE ON PSYCHOSOCIAL ASPECTS OF CHILD AND FAMILY HEALTH, COUNCIL ON EARLY CHILDHOOD, AND SOCIETY FOR DEVELOPMENTAL AND BEHAVIORAL PEDIATRICS

abstract

By current estimates, at any given time, approximately 11% to 20% of children in the United States have a behavioral or emotional disorder, as defined in the *Diagnostic and Statistical Manual of Mental Disorders, Fifth Edition*. Between 37% and 39% of children will have a behavioral or emotional disorder diagnosed by 16 years of age, regardless of geographic location in the United States. Behavioral and emotional problems and concerns in children and adolescents are not being reliably identified or treated in the US health system. This clinical report focuses on the need to increase behavioral screening and offers potential changes in practice and the health system, as well as the research needed to accomplish this. This report also (1) reviews the prevalence of behavioral and emotional disorders, (2) describes factors affecting the emergence of behavioral and emotional problems, (3) articulates the current state of detection of these problems in pediatric primary care, (4) describes barriers to screening and means to overcome those barriers, and (5) discusses potential changes at a practice and systems level that are needed to facilitate successful behavioral and emotional screening. Highlighted and discussed are the many factors at the level of the pediatric practice, health system, and society contributing to these behavioral and emotional problems.

www.pediatrics.org/cgi/doi/10.1542/peds.2014-3716

DOI: 10.1542/peds.2014-3716

PEDIATRICS (ISSN Numbers: Print, 0031-4005; Online, 1098-4275).

SCOPE OF THE PROBLEM AND NEED FOR THIS REPORT

Behavioral and emotional problems during childhood are common, often undetected, and frequently not treated despite being responsible for significant morbidity and mortality. By current estimates, approximately 11% to 20% of children in the United States have a behavioral or emotional disorder at any given time.[1,2] Estimated prevalence rates are similar in young 2- to 5-year-old children. Developmental and behavioral health disorders are now the top 5 chronic pediatric conditions causing functional impairment.[3,4] Even greater numbers of children have behavioral or emotional problems causing impairment or distress that do not meet criteria of the *Diagnostic and Statistical Manual of Mental Disorders, Fifth Edition* for a disorder. The purpose of this report is to provide pediatricians with a rationale for and guidance to implement screening for behavioral and emotional problems in primary care settings. However, in evaluating and promoting optimal child development and well-being, the domains of development and behavior must be considered together within the context of the family. These domains are not separate constructs but rather parts of a whole. Therefore, this report emphasizes that behavioral screening must always be 1 component of a comprehensive developmental and behavioral screening program that extends through childhood and adolescence.

EPIDEMIOLOGY OF BEHAVIORAL AND EMOTIONAL DISORDERS

It is estimated that 25% to 40% of children with 1 disorder will have at least 1 additional mental health or behavioral diagnosis at a given time.[1,5,6] The most common co-occurring conditions are attention-deficit/hyperactivity disorder (ADHD) and oppositional defiant disorder, but co-occurrence of anxiety and depression is also common.

Between 37% and 39% of children will have a behavioral or emotional disorder diagnosed by 16 years of age, with the most common diagnoses being impulse control/disruptive behavior problems, anxiety, and mood disorders.[1,7,8] Between 23% and 61% of children with a diagnosis at 1 time will have a diagnosis in the future, although it is not always the same diagnosis.[1]

Approximately 50% of adults with behavioral health problems report that their disorders emerged in early adolescence.[9] Anxiety disorders and ADHD are the earliest disorders to emerge, often in the preschool and early school-age years, with substance abuse being the latest to emerge. An approximately 2- to 4-year period between symptom appearance and disorder has been demonstrated, suggesting that there may be opportunities for secondary prevention or early intervention.[6]

FACTORS AFFECTING THE EMERGENCE OF BEHAVIORAL AND EMOTIONAL PROBLEMS

In 2010, more than 1 in 5 children were reported to be living in poverty.[6,10] Economic disadvantage is among the most potent risks for behavioral and emotional problems due to increased exposure to environmental, familial, and psychosocial risks.[11–13] In families in which parents are in military service, parental deployment and return has been determined to be a risk factor for behavioral and emotional problems in children.[14] Data from the 2003 National Survey of Children's Health demonstrated a strong linear relationship between increasing number of psychosocial risks and many poor health outcomes, including social-emotional health.[15] The Adverse Childhood Experience Study surveyed 17 000 adults about early traumatic and stressful experiences. Two-thirds of respondents experienced at least 1 type of childhood psychosocial risk, and 20% experienced more than 3. Adverse early experiences were related to increased rates of health problems in adulthood including obesity and cardiovascular disease as well as substance abuse, mental health problems, and poor health-related quality of life. As the Adverse Childhood Experience Study score increased, so did the number of risk factors for the leading causes of death.[16,17] Shonkoff uses the phrase "toxic stress" to describe high cumulative psychosocial risk in the absence of supportive caregiving[18,19]; this type of unremitting stress ultimately compromises children's ability to regulate their stress response system effectively and can lead to adverse long-term structural and functional changes in the brain and elsewhere in the body. The 2012 American Academy of Pediatrics (AAP) Policy Statement "Early Childhood Adversity, Toxic Stress, and the Role of the Pediatrician: Translating Developmental Science Into Lifelong Health" advocated viewing the causes and consequences of toxic stress from the same perspective as other biologically based health impairments.[19]

POLICIES IN PLACE

In 2004, the AAP established the Task Force on Mental Health, which "articulated mental health competencies for primary care; developed guidance for addressing systemic and financial barriers to providing mental health care in primary care settings; and provided tools and strategies to assist pediatricians in applying chronic care principles to children with mental health problems."[20] The Task Force also provided guidance (through identifying tools and describing strategies) to providers on adapting current practice to include mental health care. A recent publication articulated an initial blueprint for behavioral and emotional screening in pediatric practice.[21] The current statement supports the Task Force guidance by providing the evidence supporting screening for emotional and behavioral concerns.

CURRENT STATE OF DETECTION OF BEHAVIORAL AND EMOTIONAL PROBLEMS IN PEDIATRIC SETTINGS

Behavioral and emotional problems and concerns in children and adolescents are not being reliably identified or treated in the US health system.[6,22–25] Current estimates suggest that fewer than 1 in 8 children with identified mental health problems receive treatment. Even when a child or adolescent is well known in a pediatric practice, only

50% of those with clinically significant behavioral and emotional problems are detected.[23] Other investigators have found similarly high failure of detection rates ranging from 14% to 40%.[22,24] Surveyed pediatricians, however, overwhelmingly endorse that they should be responsible for identifying children with ADHD, eating disorders, depression, substance abuse, and behavior problems.[26]

Clinicians' ability to identify developmental and behavioral problems in primary care, on the basis of clinical judgment alone in the absence of a standardized measure, has been shown to have low sensitivity, ranging from 14% to 54% and a specificity ranging from 69% to 100%.[27] Providers are less likely to identify problems in minority or non–English-speaking children and adolescents.[25]

In a study of clinicians in more than 200 practices, pediatric providers reported using a standardized measure to assess mental health problems in 20.2% of all visits, with 50.2% of providers reporting never using any formal measure.[28] Fewer than 7% of providers reported using a standardized measure during 50% or more of visits.[28]

BARRIERS TO SCREENING

Pediatricians report a lack of confidence in their training and ability to successfully manage children's behavioral and emotional problems[29] with only 13% of pediatricians reporting confidence.[30] Common barriers to adopting new screening practices in pediatrics include lack of time,[30] long waits for children to be seen by mental health providers, and lack of available mental health providers to refer children.[31,32] Liability issues have been identified as a barrier to screening and managing children with behavioral and emotional problems. Pediatricians have also raised concerns about the increasing

number of mandates outlined in practice guidelines with ever-shrinking time for health maintenance visits as a result of reimbursement pressures.[33]

AVAILABLE TOOLS TO SCREEN FOR BEHAVIOR AND EMOTIONAL PROBLEMS

Behavioral and emotional screening instruments have many of the same advantages and limitations as developmental screening instruments. They involve a time commitment for parents or guardians to complete and for staff and clinicians to score, interpret, and report the results.[32]

Screening instruments can be used to predict risk of a disorder but do not make the diagnosis. There are global (broadband) scales that may screen for several conditions, and there are domain-specific (single-condition) tools are most useful for screening for a specific problem, such as substance use or adolescent depression and suicidality.[32]

Pediatricians should be aware of the sociodemographic characteristics of populations enrolled in validation studies as they make decisions regarding any screening instruments used. Pediatricians need to consider the literacy and health literacy levels of parents, guardians, children, and adolescents completing screens, whether the instrument should be administered in English or another language, and whether the person completing the screen will need additional help.

Pediatricians should be familiar with the psychometric properties of an instrument and under what conditions reported sensitivities and specificities were obtained.[32] Like developmental screening tools, behavioral and emotional screening tools should have a sensitivity and specificity of ≥0.70.[34]

Once the patient is old enough to answer reliably, self-report versions can provide information about

feelings not noticed by outside observers, such as those associated with anxiety or depression. Most self-report versions are normed on patients 8 years and older.

The research on behavioral and emotional screening in younger children is more limited than in school-age children, but increasingly, reliable, brief measures suitable for use in primary care exist, and new ones are being developed,[35,36] making it possible to screen children and adolescents from aged 6 months through 18 years of age.

Behavior and emotional screens available in the public domain can be found in Appendix 1.

OVERCOMING BARRIERS TO SCREENING

The policy statement "The Future of Pediatrics: Mental Health Competencies for Pediatric Primary Care" outlined the skills pediatricians need in the area of mental health.[37] The AAP Task Force on Mental Health has developed materials to help pediatricians assess their current practice and readiness to change and to code accurately for mental health screening and services.[38,39] The AAP also developed a Web site providing resources and materials free of charge (http://www2.aap.org/commpeds/dochs/mentalhealth/KeyResources.html)[40] as well as "Addressing Mental Health Concerns in Primary Care: A Clinician's Toolkit,"[41] which is available for a fee.

Professional organizations, including the AAP, Society for Developmental and Behavioral Pediatrics, American Academy of Child and Adolescent Psychiatry, and National Alliance on Mental Illness, provide ongoing continuing medical education and resources.

LESSONS LEARNED FROM DEVELOPMENTAL SCREENING

Many barriers to behavioral and emotional screening are similar to those identified when developmental screening was proposed as a regular part of pediatric care. In 2006, the AAP policy statement "Identifying Infants and Young Children With Developmental Disorders in the Medical Home: An Algorithm for Screening and Surveillance"[42] was published. Since the publication of the statement, 44.8% of pediatricians reported using standardized developmental screening tools more often, and 72.2% reported using standardized autism screening tools more often.[43] National demonstration projects including the Assuring Better Child Development Screening Academy[44] and the AAP's Developmental Surveillance and Screening Policy Implementation Project[45] achieved high levels of screening in primary care. These projects provided valuable lessons about implementing a screening program (Table 1) and behavioral and emotional screening may follow similar patterns. Similar large-scale initiatives may need to be developed to determine the best practices for implementing a behavioral and emotional screening program.

GUIDANCE FOR PEDIATRICIANS

The following steps and Table 2 are designed to give pediatricians a clear road map to implement behavioral and emotional screening in practice. Although distinct from screening, pediatricians should familiarize themselves with evidence-based

programs that have been shown to promote children's social-emotional development through positive parenting,[46–51] possibly preventing the emergence of problems.

1. Readying the Practice. As was seen in developmental screening, front-end work is needed to train and prepare an office to adopt screening practices. It may be helpful to enlist the assistance of local mental health professionals or developmental-behavioral pediatricians in selecting and implementing screening procedures.

2. Identifying Resources. Before initiating a behavioral and emotional screening program, pediatricians need to determine what they will do when a child or parent has a positive screening result. Pediatricians should familiarize themselves with local resources and identify referral sources. In the absence of this, pediatricians are likely to feel frustrated and overwhelmed when they identify children and adolescents in need of services but are unable to find appropriate, high-quality treatment of them. Pediatricians will need to work with the community to advocate for more treatment and intervention services.

Increasing numbers of practices have colocated a mental health provider (eg, psychologist, licensed clinical social worker, licensed therapist) within the practice. These providers are integrated into the

practice and can provide timely assistance for behavioral emergencies as well as support the primary care provider in implementing and interpreting the office screening program.

Another model of a successful collaboration program between primary providers and child psychiatrists, the Massachusetts Child Psychiatry Access Project, promotes access to psychiatric consultation for primary care providers through a network of children's mental health collaboration teams. The overall aim is to improve access to treatment of children with mental health concerns (http://www.mcpap.com/about.asp). This type of program currently is being implemented in more than 30 states.

3. Establishing Office Routines for Screening. As with developmental screening, children should be screened at regular intervals for behavioral and emotional problems with standardized, well-validated measures beginning in infancy and continuing through adolescence. Screening beginning in the first year of life can identify disturbances in attachment, regulation, and the parent-child relationship, although the optimal approaches to screening infants and very young children are less clear-cut than screening children at older ages. Ongoing care involves maintaining a good history regarding factors that can influence the early parent-child relationships, such as discipline practice, parenting stress, psychosocial risks, and positive parenting.

Currently, developmental and behavioral/emotional screenings are viewed as separate constructs, and most well-validated measures screen for them independently. Developmental screening is commonly perceived as identifying disordered expressive and receptive language, fine and gross motor skills, self-help skills, and

TABLE 1 Lessons Learned From Implementing a Screening Program

What Promoted Screening Implementation	What Challenges Remained
• Creating an office-wide implementation system • Dividing responsibility among staff	• Consistent referral of children with failed screens • Distributing screens to children at screening ages but not to others
• Actively monitoring implementation and continuing to make changes • Choosing screens perceived to least disrupt clinic flow • Aligning screening measures with those used in community based programs	• Maintaining consistent screening practice during busy times • Coping with screening gaps due to staff turnover
	• Not screening when surveillance raised concerns • Tracking referrals through a distinct implementation system from screening • Nonadherence to the 30-mo screen because of expected nonreimbursement

TABLE 2 Steps to Implement Behavioral and Emotional Screening in Practice

1. Readying the practice
   - Describe and evaluate current efforts already in place
   - Identify a practice champion
   - Train all staff
   - Consider incremental screening and actively monitor implementation
   - Develop a screening roadmap from providing the screen through the referral process
   - Add behavior and emotional problems to the problem list and update this at each visit
   - Problem solve challenges that arise across the entire practice
   - Determine how to best publicize new screening practices to families
   - Consider additional costs for procuring screening tools, etc
   - Prepare for psychiatric emergencies that may present in the office
2. Identifying resources
   - Identify referral resources that include the following:
     - Areas of expertise
     - Hours of operation
     - Payment methods
     - Ability to treat non–English speakers
   - Develop a plan for bidirectional communication
   - Learn about emergency mental health services
   - Partner with adult providers and community resources to help parents with identified psychosocial risk
3. Establishing office routines for screening and surveillance
   - Implement screening in the first year of life and at regular intervals throughout childhood and adolescence
   - Incorporate screening for family psychosocial risks and strengths
   - Determine appropriate screening intervals for the practice (combined with or distinct from developmental screening intervals) based on things such as clinic flow, allotted time to discuss screening results, etc
   - Partner with parents to formulate a plan when there is a failed screen
   - Identify strengths of the child and communicate these to the family
   - Screen when the child, family, or provider has concerns
   - Establish a registry of children with positive screens and family psychosocial risk
   - Monitor children with significant risk factors with heightened surveillance and more frequent screening
4. Tracking referrals
   - Develop a mechanism to track progress of children referred for assessment or treatment (eg, successful referral, evaluation or initiation of treatment)
   - Collect information about families' experience with referral resources
5. Seeking payment
   - Familiarize the practice with appropriate CPT codes for screening, care plan oversight, face-to-face and non–face-to-face services and reimbursement by different insurance companies
   - Track billing and reimbursement for screening efforts
6. Fostering collaboration
   - Explore colocated or other innovative models of care and partnerships with mental health professionals

cognitive milestones, whereas behavioral and emotional screening identifies problems in areas including social-emotional regulation, mood and affect, attention, and interpersonal skills. There is a significant yet incomplete overlap between developmental and behavior problems. Studies have revealed that children with cognitive, language, and social impairments and developmental disabilities, in general, are far more likely to manifest behavioral and emotional problems.[12]

Beginning in early adolescence, screening for substance use should be implemented.[21,52] Substance use and dependence have consistently been found to be 1 of the most prevalent behavioral health diagnoses in adolescents. Identifying and treating a behavioral or emotional problem without detecting and treating co-occurring substance use will likely lead to ineffectual treatment. The US Preventive Services Task Force recommends screening all adolescents (12–18 years of age) for

depression, when systems are in place, to ensure accurate diagnosis, treatment, and follow-up.[53] Pediatricians should use targeted screening for other problems, such as suicidality or anxiety, if there is concern raised by the provider, patient, or parent or the child is at high risk.

Children's behavioral and emotional problems are frequently associated with family psychosocial risk. Family psychosocial screening can provide important information about potential protection or lack thereof for a child who may or may not yet show signs of behavioral or emotional problems. Early detection and treatment of family psychosocial risk may potentially avert the emergence of problems in the child. Only a limited number of well-validated screens suitable for use in primary care for broad screening of family psychosocial risk and family support and functioning are available, although a few show promise.[54–56] There are screening measures for specific psychosocial stressors, such as maternal depression, and these have been shown to be feasible in pediatric settings.[57,58] Family screening for psychosocial risk within pediatric settings, however, raises a number of dilemmas, including concerns about liability and payment and who is responsible for an adult's well-being after a problem is detected.[59]

4. Tracking Referrals. If the child was referred for services after screening, it is important for pediatricians to inquire as to whether referrals were completed and services were obtained or understand what barriers parents have experienced and how these can be overcome. Furthermore, it is important for pediatricians, with parental permission, to obtain information from the referral and to learn whether services obtained were effective and whether symptoms in the child have been reduced or eliminated.

This follow-up may require a separate office system than screening procedures.

5. Seeking Payment. One of the biggest "systems" hurdles facing pediatricians is the difficulty obtaining payment for screening patients for behavioral and emotional problems and for screening families for psychosocial risk and functioning. The adoption of the proposed screening and surveillance practices, may lengthen visit time to discuss results without additional payment to support that time and create significant non–face-to-face work.[60] This includes referring patients and families to appropriate resources, tracking referrals, communicating with other professionals (which may require reviewing lengthy reports and school plans), and following up with children and families. Overcoming this critical barrier is fundamental to transforming pediatric practice to a medical home model. With the advent of reimbursable billing codes for screening, including *Current Procedural Terminology* (CPT) codes 96110 and 99420, some practices are beginning to see some financial payment for the addition of screening programs. Additionally, a new CPT code for brief behavioral assessment, 96127, has been included in *CPT 2015* to allow the separate reporting of this service.

6. Fostering Collaboration. Innovative collaborations have been well described and include colocation and integrated and consultative models, such as the Massachusetts Child Psychiatry Access Project, the North Carolina Chapter AAP/NC Pediatric Society (ICARE), and the Washington Partnership Access Line.[61–64] Innovative means of consultation and collaboration will continue to evolve with emerging technology.[65] These relationships help build the capacity of pediatricians to manage various

behavioral and emotional problems in the office. This is particularly true for the management of subthreshold problems not meeting the severity level warranted to refer for treatment.

FUTURE DIRECTIONS

As medical practice continues to shift into more electronic formats, standardized screening instruments will need to be formatted for electronic health record systems, to facilitate a wide implementation of screening. Automating guidelines and scoring of screening measures, providing decision support that is integrated into electronic health records, and providing patients with opportunities for greater participation in their health care via portals into their electronic medical record have already shown promise.[66,67] Paper-and-pencil screening methods will need to be transformed into Web-based versions, smartphone apps, and waiting room tablets to successfully harness available technology.[65,68] These changes will be critical areas needing further evaluation to determine best practices.[69] Additional system challenges that will need to be addressed are included in Appendix 2.

SUMMARY

Evaluating and promoting optimal child development and well-being includes assessing developmental and behavioral domains in the context of the family. Behavioral and emotional problems are common, persistent, and cause significant functional impairment for many children and adolescents. A 2- to 4-year window may exist between initial presentation of symptoms and the development of a disorder, suggesting an opportunity to intervene before problems become more serious in children.[6] In recent years, many pediatricians have taken advantage of more widely disseminated public

domain screening tools and have used emerging computer technology to facilitate behavioral/emotional screening. There have been many examples of colocated practices, and national organizations, such as the AAP, have strongly advocated for payment for these integrated practice models. The lessons learned through developmental screening implementation have been used to make behavioral and emotional screening a more routine component of pediatric health supervision. The investments described in this report, financial and otherwise, are critical to ensure a future of thriving and strong infants, children, and adolescents who will mature into healthy adults.

LEAD AUTHORS

Carol Weitzman, MD
Lynn Mowbray Wegner, MD

CONTRIBUTING AUTHORS

Laura Joan McGuinn, MD
Alan L. Mendelsohn, MD
Patricia Gail Williams, MD
Terry Stancin, PhD

SECTION ON DEVELOPMENTAL AND BEHAVIORAL PEDIATRICS EXECUTIVE COMMITTEE, 2013–2014

Nathan J. Blum, MD, Chairperson
Michelle M. Macias, MD, Immediate Past Chairperson
Nerissa S. Bauer, MD, MPH
Carolyn Bridgemohan, MD
Edward Goldson, MD
Laura J. McGuinn, MD
Carol Weitzman, MD

LIAISONS

Pamela High, MD — *Society for Developmental and Behavioral Pediatrics*
Susan Levy, MD — *Council on Children with Disabilities*

CONSULTANT

Lynn Mowbray Wegner, MD

STAFF

Linda B. Paul, MPH

COMMITTEE ON PSYCHOSOCIAL ASPECTS OF CHILD AND FAMILY HEALTH, 2013–2014

Benjamin S. Siegel, MD, Chairperson
Michael W. Yogman, MD, Chairperson-Elect
Thresia B. Gambon, MD
Arthur Lavin, MD
LTC Keith M. Lemmon, MD

REFERENCES

1. Costello EJ, Mustillo S, Erkanli A, Keeler G, Angold A. Prevalence and development of psychiatric disorders in childhood and adolescence. *Arch Gen Psychiatry.* 2003;60(8):837–844

2. *Report of the Surgeon General's Conference on Children's Mental Health: A National Action Agenda.* Washington, DC: US Department of Health and Human Services, US Department of Education, US Department of Justice; 2000

3. Slomski A. Chronic mental health issues in children now loom larger than physical problems. *JAMA.* 2012;308(3):223–225

4. Halfon N, Houtrow A, Larson K, Newacheck PW. The changing landscape of disability in childhood. *Future Child.* 2012;22(1):13–42

5. Merikangas KR, He JP, Burstein M, et al. Lifetime prevalence of mental disorders in U.S. adolescents: results from the National Comorbidity Survey Replication —Adolescent Supplement (NCS-A). *J Am Acad Child Adolesc Psychiatry.* 2010; 49(10):980–989

6. O'Connell ME, Boat TF, Warner KE; National Research Council (US) and Institute of Medicine (US) Committee on Prevention of Mental Disorders and Substance Abuse Among Children Youth and Young Adults: Research Advances and Promising Interventions. *Preventing Mental, Emotional, and Behavioral Disorders Among Young People: Progress and Possibilities.* Washington, DC: National Academies Press; 2009. Available at: http://www.ncbi.nlm.nih.gov/books/NBK32775. Accessed November 26, 2014

7. Jaffee SR, Harrington H, Cohen P, Moffitt TE. Cumulative prevalence of psychiatric disorder in youths. *J Am Acad Child Adolesc Psychiatry.* 2005;44(5):406–407

8. Kim-Cohen J, Caspi A, Moffitt TE, Harrington H, Milne BJ, Poulton R. Prior juvenile diagnoses in adults with mental disorder: developmental follow-back of a prospective-longitudinal cohort. *Arch Gen Psychiatry.* 2003;60(7):709–717

9. Kessler RC, Berglund P, Demler O, Jin R, Merikangas KR, Walters EE. Lifetime prevalence and age-of-onset distributions of *DSM-IV* disorders in the National Comorbidity Survey Replication [published correction appears in *Arch Gen Psychiatry.* 2005;62(7):768 (Note: Merikangas, Kathleen R added)]. *Arch Gen Psychiatry.* 2005;62(6):593–602

10. Gills J. Screening practices of family physicians and pediatricians in 2 southern states. *Infants Young Child.* 2009;22(4):321–331

11. Briggs-Gowan MJ, Carter AS, Skuban EM, Horwitz SM. Prevalence of social-emotional and behavioral problems in a community sample of 1- and 2-year-old children. *J Am Acad Child Adolesc Psychiatry.* 2001;40(7):811–819

12. Qi CH, Kaiser AP. Behavior problems in preschool children from low-income families: review of the literature. *Top Early Child Spec Educ.* 2003;23(4): 188–216

13. Evans GW, Kim P. Multiple risk exposure as a potential explanatory mechanism for the socioeconomic status-health gradient. *Ann N Y Acad Sci.* 2010;1186(1): 174–189

14. Chartrand MM, Frank DA, White LF, Shope TR. Effect of parents' wartime deployment on the behavior of young children in military families. *Arch Pediatr Adolesc Med.* 2008;162(11): 1009–1014

15. Larson K, Russ SA, Crall JJ, Halfon N. Influence of multiple social risks on children's health. *Pediatrics.* 2008;121(2): 337–344

16. Felitti VJ, Anda RF, Nordenberg D, et al. Relationship of childhood abuse and household dysfunction to many of the leading causes of death in adults. The Adverse Childhood Experiences (ACE) Study. *Am J Prev Med.* 1998;14(4): 245–258

17. Anda RF, Felitti VJ, Bremner JD, et al. The enduring effects of abuse and related adverse experiences in childhood. A convergence of evidence from neurobiology and epidemiology. *Eur Arch*

Psychiatry Clin Neurosci. 2006;256(3): 174–186

18. Shonkoff JP, Garner AS; Committee on Psychosocial Aspects of Child and Family Health; Committee on Early Childhood, Adoption, and Dependent Care; Section on Developmental and Behavioral Pediatrics. The lifelong effects of early childhood adversity and toxic stress. *Pediatrics.* 2012;129(1). Available at: www.pediatrics.org/cgi/content/full/129/1/e232

19. Garner AS, Shonkoff JP; Committee on Psychosocial Aspects of Child and Family Health; Committee on Early Childhood, Adoption, and Dependent Care; Section on Developmental and Behavioral Pediatrics. Early childhood adversity, toxic stress, and the role of the pediatrician: translating developmental science into lifelong health. *Pediatrics.* 2012;129(1). Available at: www.pediatrics.org/cgi/content/full/129/1/e224

20. Foy JM; American Academy of Pediatrics Task Force on Mental Health. Enhancing pediatric mental health care: report from the American Academy of Pediatrics Task Force on Mental Health. Introduction. *Pediatrics.* 2010;125(suppl 3):S69–S74

21. American Academy of Pediatrics. Appendix S4: the case for routine mental health screening. *Pediatrics.* 2010;125 (suppl 3):S133–S139

22. Costello EJ, Edelbrock CS. Detection of psychiatric disorders in pediatric primary care: a preliminary report. *J Am Acad Child Psychiatry.* 1985;24(6): 771–774

23. Lavigne JV, Binns HJ, Christoffel KK, et al; Pediatric Practice Research Group. Behavioral and emotional problems among preschool children in pediatric primary care: prevalence and pediatricians' recognition. *Pediatrics.* 1993;91(3):649–655

24. Dulcan MK, Costello EJ, Costello AJ, Edelbrock C, Brent D, Janiszewski S. The pediatrician as gatekeeper to mental health care for children: do parents' concerns open the gate? *J Am Acad Child Adolesc Psychiatry.* 1990;29(3):453–458

25. Brown JD, Wissow LS. Screening to identify mental health problems in pediatric primary care: considerations for practice. *Int J Psychiatry Med.* 2010; 40(1):1–19

26. Stein REK, Horwitz SM, Storfer-Isser A, Heneghan A, Olson L, Hoagwood KE. Do pediatricians think they are responsible for identification and management of child mental health problems? Results of the AAP periodic survey. *Ambul Pediatr.* 2008;8(1):11–17

27. Sheldrick RC, Merchant S, Perrin EC. Identification of developmental-behavioral problems in primary care: a systematic review. *Pediatrics.* 2011;128 (2):356–363

28. Gardner W, Kelleher KJ, Pajer KA, Campo JV. Primary care clinicians' use of standardized tools to assess child psychosocial problems. *Ambul Pediatr.* 2003;3(4):191–195

29. Cunningham PJ. Beyond parity: primary care physicians' perspectives on access to mental health care. *Health Aff (Millwood).* 2009;28(3):w490–w501

30. Olson AL, Kelleher KJ, Kemper KJ, Zuckerman BS, Hammond CS, Dietrich AJ. Primary care pediatricians' roles and perceived responsibilities in the identification and management of depression in children and adolescents. *Ambul Pediatr.* 2001;1(2):91–98

31. Horwitz SM, Kelleher KJ, Stein RE, et al. Barriers to the identification and management of psychosocial issues in children and maternal depression. *Pediatrics.* 2007;119(1):e208–e218

32. Stancin T, Palermo TM. A review of behavioral screening practices in pediatric settings: do they pass the test? *J Dev Behav Pediatr.* 1997;18(3): 183–194

33. Stein MT, Plonsky C, Zuckerman B, Carey WB. Reformatting the 9-month Health Supervision Visit to enhance developmental, behavioral and family concerns. *J Dev Behav Pediatr.* 2005;26 (1):56–60

34. Glascoe FP. In: Jacobson JW, Mulick JA, Rojahn J, eds. *Developmental and Behavioral Screening: Handbook of Intellectual and Developmental Disabilities.* New York, NY: Springer Publishing Company; 2007:353–371

35. Sheldrick RC, Henson BS, Neger EN, Merchant S, Murphy JM, Perrin EC. The baby pediatric symptom checklist: development and initial validation of a new social/emotional screening instrument for very young children. *Acad Pediatr.* 2013;13(1):72–80

36. Sheldrick RC, Henson BS, Merchant S, Neger EN, Murphy JM, Perrin EC. The Preschool Pediatric Symptom Checklist (PPSC): development and initial validation of a new social/emotional screening instrument. *Acad Pediatr.* 2012;12(5):456–467

37. Committee on Psychosocial Aspects of Child and Family Health and Task Force on Mental Health. Policy statement—The future of pediatrics: mental health competencies for pediatric primary care. *Pediatrics.* 2009;124(1):410–421

38. American Academy of Pediatrics. Appendix S5: coding for the mental health algorithm steps. *Pediatrics.* 2010; 125(suppl 3):S140–S152

39. American Academy of Pediatrics. Appendix S3: mental health practice readiness inventory. *Pediatrics.* 2010;125 (suppl 3):S129–S132

40. American Academy of Pediatrics. *Children's Mental Health in Primary Care: Key AAP Resources.* 2011. Available at: http://www2.aap.org/commpeds/dochs/mentalhealth/KeyResources.html. Accessed November 26, 2014

41. Task Force on Mental Health. *Addressing Mental Health Concerns in Primary Care: A Clinician's Toolkit.* Elk Grove Village, IL: American Academy of Pediatrics; 2010

42. Council on Children With Disabilities; Section on Developmental Behavioral Pediatrics; Bright Futures Steering Committee; Medical Home Initiatives for Children With Special Needs Project Advisory Committee. Identifying infants and young children with developmental disorders in the medical home: an algorithm for developmental surveillance and screening. *Pediatrics.* 2006;118(1):405–420

43. Arunyanart A, Fenick A, Ukritchon S, Imjaijitt W, Northrup V, Weitzman C. Developmental and Autism Screening: A Survey Across Six States. *Infants Young Child.* 2012;25(3):175–187

44. Earls M. Expanding innovation through networks: the Assuring Better Child Health and Development (ABCD) Project. *N C Med J.* 2009;70(3):253–255

45. Pilowsky DJ, Wickramaratne P, Talati A, et al. Children of depressed mothers 1 year after the initiation of maternal treatment: findings from the STAR*D—child study. *Am J Psychiatry.* 2008;165(9): 1136–1147

46. Sanders MR, Markie-Dadds C, Turner KMT. *Theoretical, scientific and clinical foundations of the Triple P-Positive Parenting Program: A population approach to the promotion of parenting competence*, vol. 1. Brisbane, Australia: Parenting and Family Support Centre, The University of Queensland; 2003

47. Eyberg S. Parent-child interaction therapy. *Child Fam Behav Ther.* 1988; 10(1):33–46

48. Webster-Stratton C. The incredible years. Available at: http://www.incredibleyears.com. Accessed November 26, 2014

49. Foster EM, Olchowski AE, Webster-Stratton CH. Is stacking intervention components cost-effective? An analysis of the Incredible Years program. *J Am Acad Child Adolesc Psychiatry.* 2007; 46(11):1414–1424

50. McNeil CB, Hembree-Kigin TL. *Parent-child interaction therapy.* New York, NY: Springer Publishing Company; 2010

51. Centers for Disease Control. *Essentials for Childhood: Steps to Create Safe, Stable, and Nurturing Relationships.* Atlanta, GA: National Center for Injury Prevention and Control Division of Violence Prevention Center for Injury Prevention

52. Levy SJ, Kokotailo PK; Committee on Substance Abuse. Substance use screening, brief intervention, and referral to treatment for pediatricians. *Pediatrics.* 2011;128(5). Available at: www.pediatrics.org/cgi/content/full/128/5/e1330

53. US Preventive Services Task Force. Screening and treatment for major depressive disorder in children and adolescents: US Preventive Services Task Force Recommendation Statement. *Pediatrics.* 2009;123(4):1223–1228

54. Garg A, Butz AM, Dworkin PH, Lewis RA, Thompson RE, Serwint JR. Improving the management of family psychosocial problems at low-income children's well-child care visits: the WE CARE Project. *Pediatrics.* 2007;120(3):547–558

55. Dubowitz H, Feigelman S, Lane W, Kim J. Pediatric primary care to help prevent child maltreatment: The Safe Environment for Every Kid (SEEK) Model. *Pediatrics.* 2009;123(3):858–864

56. Perrin E. The Survey of Wellbeing of Young Children. 2012. Available at: http://www.theswyc.org. Accessed November 26, 2014

57. AAP Taskforce on Mental Health. *Mental Health Screening and Assessment Tools for Primary Care. Addressing Mental Health Concerns in Primary Care: A Clinician's Toolkit.* Elk Grove Village, IL: American Academy of Pediatrics; 2012:1–20

58. Earls MF; The Committee on Psychosocial Aspects of Child and Family Health. Incorporating Recognition and Management of Perinatal and Postpartum Depression Into Pediatric Practice. *Pediatrics.* 2010;126(5): 1032–1039

59. Chaudron LH, Szilagyi PG, Campbell AT, Mounts KO, McInerny TK. Legal and ethical considerations: risks and benefits of postpartum depression screening at well-child visits. *Pediatrics.* 2007;119(1):123–128

60. Meadows T, Valleley R, Haack MK, Thorson R, Evans J. Physician "costs" in providing behavioral health in primary care. *Clin Pediatr (Phila).* 2011;50(5): 447–455

61. Honigfeld L, Nickel M. *Integrating Behavioral Health and Primary Care: Making It Work in Four Practices in Connecticut.* Farmington, CT: Child Health and Development Institute; 2010

62. Sarvet B, Gold J, Bostic JQ, et al. Improving access to mental health care for children: the Massachusetts Child Psychiatry Access Project. *Pediatrics.* 2010;126(6):1191–1200

63. Weitzman CC, Edmonds D, Davagnino J, Briggs-Gowan M. The association between parent worry and young children's social-emotional functioning. *J Dev Behav Pediatr.* 2011;32(9):660–667

64. Fenick AM, Dorsey KB. *Brief Motivational Interviewing Training for Obesity Management in Pediatric Residency: BMI:4.* Poster presentation, Pediatric Academic Societies Annual Meeting; 2011; Boston, MA

65. Kelleher KJ, Stevens J. Evolution of child mental health services in primary care. *Acad Pediatr.* 2009;9(1):7–14

66. Anand V, Carroll AE, Downs SM. Automated primary care screening in pediatric waiting rooms. *Pediatrics.* 2012;129(5). Available at: www.pediatrics.org/cgi/content/full/129/5/e1275

67. Wald JS, Middleton B, Bloom A, et al. A patient-controlled journal for an electronic medical record: issues and challenges. *Stud Health Technol Inform.* 2004;107(pt 2):1166–1170

68. Sturner R. The Child Health and Development Interactive System (CHADIS). Paper presented at the Seventh Annual National Institutes of Health Small Business Innovation Research/Small Business Technology Transfer Research Conference; 2005

69. Horwitz SM, Hoagwood KE, Garner A, et al. No technological innovation is a panacea: a case series in quality improvement for primary care mental health services. *Clin Pediatr (Phila).* 2008;47(7):685–692

APPENDIX 1 Behavioral and Emotional Screening Measures for Use in Primary Care in the Public Domain[a]

Category	Screening Tool	Age Group	No. of items	Available Forms	Reported Psychometrics/Other	Link
				General Behavioral Screens		
Young children (0–5)	Baby Pediatric Symptom Checklist	2–17 mo	12	Parent completed	Retest reliability and internal reliability >0.7	https://sites.google.com/site/swycscreen
	Preschool Pediatric Symptom Checklist	18–60 mo	18	Parent completed		https://sites.google.com/site/swycscreen
	Strengths and Difficulties Questionnaire	3–17 y	25 items	Parent/teacher 3(4)-y-old; parent/teacher 4–10-y-old; parent/teacher follow-up forms available	Variable across cultural groups; sensitivity: 63%–94%, specificity: 88%–96%; available in >70 languages	http://www.sdqinfo.org
School-age and adolescent children	Strengths and Difficulties Questionnaire	3–17 y	25 items	Parent/teacher 4–10-y-old; parent/teacher 11–17-y-old; youth self report 11–17-y-old; parent/teacher/self follow-up forms available	Variable across cultural groups; sensitivity: 63%–94%, specificity: 88%–96%; available in >70 languages	http://www.sdqinfo.org
	Pediatric Symptom Checklist—17	4–16 y	17 items	Parent completed; youth self-report >10 y; pictorial version available	Variable psychometrics for detection of psychiatric problems; available in multiple languages	http://www.massgeneral.org/psychiatry/services/psc_home.aspx
	Pediatric Symptom Checklist—35	4–16 y	35 items	Parent completed; youth self-report >10 y; pictorial version available	Sensitivity: 80%–95%, specificity: 68%–100%; available in multiple languages	http://www.massgeneral.org/psychiatry/services/psc_home.aspx
				Psychosocial Screens		
	WE-CARE (Well-Child Care Visit, Evaluation, Community Resources, Advocacy, Referral, Education)	Parent	10 items	Parent completed		http://pediatrics.aappublications.org/content/120/3/547.full#sec-1
	Family Psychosocial Screen	Parent	~50 items	Parent completed	Variable psychometrics for detection of specific psychosocial problems; cut points for various domains recommended	http://depts.washington.edu/dbpeds/Screening%20Tools/FamPsychoSocQaire.pdf
	Survey of Wellbeing in Young Children	Parent	9 items	Parent completed	Preliminary findings show promise	https://sites.google.com/site/swycscreen/parts-of-the-swyc/family-questions
	Adverse Childhood Experience Score	Parent	10 items	Parent completed	Increasing score associated with many adverse physical and mental health outcomes	http://acestoohigh.com/got-your-ace-score
				Screens for Specific Disorders		
Parental or adolescent depression	Edinburgh Maternal Depression	Parent (mother)	10 items	Parent self-report	Sensitivity 86%; specificity 78%	http://www.fresno.ucsf.edu/pediatrics/downloads/edinburghscale.pdf
	2 Question Screen (Modification of the Patient Health Questionnaire—2	Parent, adolescents	2 items	Parent or adolescent self-report	Sensitivity: 83%–87%; specificity: 78%–92%	http://www.uphp.com/Two_Question_Screen.pdf; http://www.cqaimh.org/pdf/tool_phq2.pdf
	Patient Health Questionnaire (PHQ)—9	Parent	9 items	Parent or Adolescent self-report	Sensitivity: 88% for major depression; specificity: 88% for major depression	http://www.integration.samhsa.gov/images/res/PHQ%20-%200Questions.pdf

APPENDIX 1 Continued

Category	Screening Tool	Age Group	No. of items	Available Forms	Reported Psychometrics/Other	Link
				General Behavioral Screens		
	Center for Epidemiologic Studies Depression Scale	Parent; adolescents >14 y (modified version for children as young as 6 available)	20 items	Parent completed; youth self-report	Coefficient α >.9; sensitivity 91%; specificity 81%. Psychometrics for children <14 indicate measure may not discriminate well between depressed and nondepressed youth.	http://cesd-r.com
	Mood and Feelings Questionnaire	Has been used about children as young as 7	Short version; 9 items; long version: 34 items	Parent completed; youth self-report	Parent report version has shown a sensitivity of 75%–86% and specificity of 73%–87%	http://devepi.mc.duke.edu/mfq.html
Substance abuse	CRAFFT (Car, Relax, Alone, Forget, Friends, Trouble)	11–21 y old	Three screener questions, then 6 items	Interview of youth; youth self-report version available	Sensitivity 76%–93%, specificity 76% to 94%; available in multiple languages	http://www.ceasar-boston.org/CRAFFT
	CAGE-AID	Adolescents	4 items	Youth self-report	One or more positive answers is associated with a sensitivity of 79% and specificity of 77%, ≥2 answers 70% and 85%	http://www.integration.samhsa.gov/images/res/CAGEAID.pdf
Anxiety	Screen for Child Anxiety Related Disorders (SCARED)	≥8 y	41 items	Parent completed; youth self-report	Coefficient α: .9	http://www.psychiatry.pitt.edu/research/tools-research/assessment-instruments
	Spence Children's Anxiety Scale (SCAS)	2.5–6.5 y and 8–12 y	45 items	Parent completed 2.5–6.5 y; youth self-report 8–12 y	High internal consistency and adequate test–retest reliability in adolescents	http://www2.psy.uq.edu.au/~sues/scas
ADHD	Vanderbilt ADHD Diagnostic Rating Scales	4–18 y	55-items parent scale; 43-items teacher scale	Parent, teacher completed; follow-up forms available	Sensitivity 80%, specificity 75%, retest reliability >0.80	http://www.nichq.org/ toolkits_publications/complete_adhd/ 03VanAssesScaleParent%20Infor.pdf; http://www.brightfutures.org/ mentalhealth/pdf/professionals/ bridges/adhd.pdf http://www.adhd.net
	Strengths and Weaknesses of ADHD Symptoms (SWAN)	6–18 y	30 items (18-item available)	Parent, teacher completed		http://www.adhd.net
	SNAP-IV	6–18 y	90 items (18-item version available)	Parent, teacher completed	Coefficient α >.90; available in multiple languages	

CAGE-AID, CAGE Questions (Cut Down, Annoyed, Guilty and Eye Opener) adapted to include drug use; Swanson, Nolan and Pelham Questionnaire, Version IV (SNAP-IV).

a This list is not meant to be exhaustive but representative of a range of screening instruments suitable for primary care that are in the public domain. Psychometrics may vary based on the findings of different studies and there is considerable variability in the strength of psychometric reliability between measures.

APPENDIX 2 System Challenges

Resources	• Identify national programs to assist parents and pediatricians in identifying mental health resources such as Help Me Grow,[69] which has established a centralized call center
	• Advocate for a greater workforce of mental health providers and developmental-behavioral pediatricians
	• Advocate for additional community mental health services and ensure they are of high quality
Screening	• Develop additional well-validated screens to identify psychosocial risk
	• Develop and validate screens appropriate for use in low-literacy and non–English-speaking populations
Payment	• Advocate for payment for
	behavioral, emotional, and substance abuse screening
	non–face-to-face time including care plan oversight, complex chronic care coordination and prolonged services
	• Evaluate enhanced payment systems for medical-home practices and monitor financial viability of hiring care coordinators
	• Consider payment incentives for medical homes that include potentially enhanced reimbursement for behavioral and emotional screening, family psychosocial, or substance use screening and all follow-up care, case management, care plan oversight, and prolonged services in their capitation calculations.
	• Evaluate cost savings associated with the detection and treatment of behavioral and emotional problems
Collaboration	• Establish payment for collaborative care models that include telephone communications between providers, etc.
	• Develop efficient methods to ensure that results of community-based screening are reported to the medical home
Other	• Develop quality improvement initiatives related to behavioral and emotional screening as a part of maintenance of certification
	• Develop electronic health records that incorporate screening but maintain patient privacy regarding behavioral and emotional problems and family psychosocial stressors

Weitzman, Wegner, the Section on Developmental and Behavioral Pediatrics, Committee on Pyschosocial Aspects of Child and Family Health, Council on Early Childhood, and Society for Developmental and Behavioral Pediatrics. Promoting Optimal Development: Screening for Behavioral and Emotional Problems. Pediatrics. 2015;135(2):384–395

An error occurred in the American Academy of Pediatrics clinical report, titled "Promoting Optimal Development: Screening for Behavioral and Emotional Problems" published in the February 2015 issue of *Pediatrics* (2015;135[2]:384–395). Reference 45 should be "King TM, Tandon SD, Macias MM, et al. Implementing developmental screening and referrals: lessons learned from a national project. *Pediatrics*. 2010;125 (2):350–360". We regret the error.

doi:10.1542/peds.2015-0904

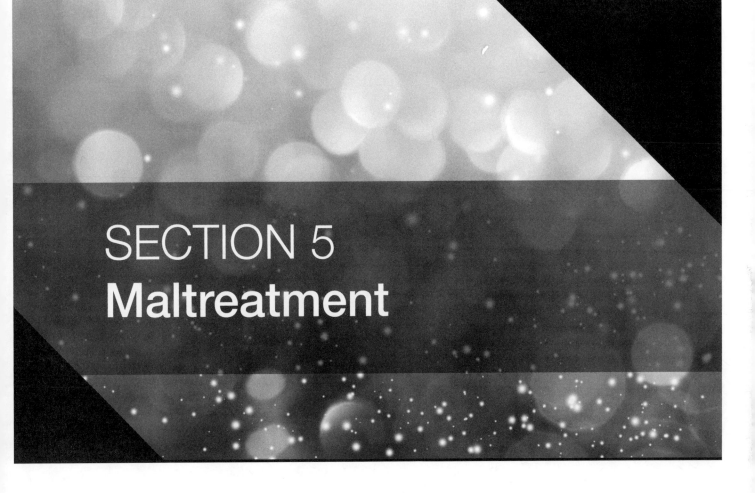

SECTION 5
Maltreatment

CLINICAL REPORT   Guidance for the Clinician in Rendering Pediatric Care

American Academy
of Pediatrics

DEDICATED TO THE HEALTH OF ALL CHILDREN™

Clinical Considerations Related to the Behavioral Manifestations of Child Maltreatment

Robert D. Sege, MD, PhD, FAAP,[a,b] Lisa Amaya-Jackson, MD, MPH, FAACAP,[c] AMERICAN ACADEMY OF PEDIATRICS Committee on Child Abuse and Neglect, Council on Foster Care, Adoption, and Kinship Care; AMERICAN ACADEMY OF CHILD AND ADOLESCENT PSYCHIATRY Committee on Child Maltreatment and Violence; NATIONAL CENTER FOR CHILD TRAUMATIC STRESS

abstract

Children who have suffered early abuse or neglect may later present with significant health and behavior problems that may persist long after the abusive or neglectful environment has been remediated. Neurobiological research suggests that early maltreatment may result in an altered psychological and physiologic response to stressful stimuli, a response that deleteriously affects the child's subsequent development. Pediatricians can assist caregivers by helping them recognize the abused or neglected child's emotional and behavioral responses associated with child maltreatment and guide them in the use of positive parenting strategies, referring the children and families to evidence-based therapeutic treatment and mobilizing available community resources.

[a]Health Resources in Action, Boston, Massachusetts; [b]Center for the Study of Social Policy, Washington District of Columbia; and [c]Department of Psychiatry & Behavioral Sciences, UCLA-Duke National Center for Child Traumatic Stress, Center for Child & Family Health, Duke University School of Medicine, Durham, North Carolina

This brief listing of the 12 Core Concepts (with abbreviated accompanying commentaries) is derived for illustrative purposes only and is used with permission from the National Child Traumatic Stress Network, Core Curriculum on Childhood Trauma Task Force. The 12 Core Concepts: Concepts for Understanding Traumatic Stress Responses in Children and Families. Los Angeles, CA, and Durham, NC: UCLA-Duke University National Center for Child Traumatic Stress; 2012. Please use the official (complete) 12 Core Concepts and their full commentaries in training and other publications, available at www.nctsn.org/resources/audiences/parents-caregivers/what-iscts/12-core-concepts. A PDF version is available from the NCTSN Learning Center for Child and Adolescent Trauma at http://learn.nctsn.org).

Drs Sege and Amaya-Jackson were each responsible for all aspects of writing and editing the document and reviewing and responding to questions and comments from committee members, reviewers, and the Board of Directors.

INTRODUCTION

Abuse or neglect during early childhood (ages birth–6 years) can endanger a child's normal development and increase the risk for long-term physical and mental health problems. Recent population surveys of adults[1] and adolescents[2] report that more than a quarter of US children have experienced abuse or neglect. Comparison of this estimate with published incidence data drawn from child welfare systems[3] suggests that most child maltreatment is undetected or unreported. Health care providers have a legal responsibility to report suspected abuse or neglect to state authorities. In addition, attention to the diagnosis of current or past maltreatment may lead to treatment decisions that will improve childhood and longer-term outcomes for children and their families.

Pediatricians and other pediatric health care providers have 2 important roles to play in helping children who have experienced maltreatment or neglect heal and achieve their developmental potential. First, pediatricians have the opportunity to ameliorate the adverse

To cite: Sege RD, Amaya-Jackson L, AAP AMERICAN ACADEMY OF PEDIATRICS Committee on Child Abuse and Neglect, Council on Foster Care, Adoption, and Kinship Care; AMERICAN ACADEMY OF CHILD AND ADOLESCENT PSYCHIATRY Committee on Child Maltreatment and Violence; NATIONAL CENTER FOR CHILD TRAUMATIC STRESS. Clinical Considerations Related to the Behavioral Manifestations of Child Maltreatment. Pediatrics. 2017;139(4):e20170100 consequences in children who are known to have experienced traumatic events, including abuse and neglect. Second, when evaluating children with problematic behavior (or behavioral disorders), they may be able to provide more accurate and effective assessment and treatment by considering the possibility of past trauma as an etiological agent. A variety of terms are used to describe the child's experience of maltreatment and its consequences; Table 1 describes many of the commonly used terms.

This report updates the 2008 clinical report from the American Academy of Pediatrics (AAP), the American Academy of Child and Adolescent Psychiatry, and the National Center for Child Traumatic Stress.[6] In the years since the original report, there have been additions to the substantial body of evidence that document the relationship between adverse experiences in early childhood and medical and psychological complications that manifest throughout childhood and adulthood. Much of the evidence concerning toxic stress and its effects is summarized in a 2012 AAP policy statement and technical report that describes the effects of early childhood stress[5,7] and in summary information available from the National Child Traumatic Stress Network.[8] This discussion of the pediatrician's approach to children who have been abused or neglected may also be best considered in the broader context of child mental health, as discussed in the forthcoming AAP policy statement and technical report "Addressing Early Childhood Emotional and Behavioral Problems."[9,10]

This report further guides the pediatrician in recognizing and managing the behavioral and mental health symptoms exhibited by maltreated children and in seeking appropriate therapy to help affected children recover in ways that may

TABLE 1 Commonly Used Terms in Trauma-Informed Care

ACEs	Adverse childhood experiences that include emotional, physical, or sexual abuse; emotional or physical neglect; domestic violence; parental substance use; parental mental illness; parental separation or divorce; or incarceration of a household member.[1]
Trauma	Psychological trauma occurs when a child experiences an intense event that threatens or causes harm to his or her emotional and physical well-being.[4]
Child traumatic stress	The intense fear and stress response occurring when children are exposed to traumatic events that overwhelm their ability to cope with what they have experienced. The 12 Core Concepts defined by the National Child Traumatic Stress Network in 2007 are key tenets for professionals to understand the impact of traumatic level adverse experiences on children (see Table 2) and provide a rationale for trauma-informed assessment and intervention.
Toxic stress	Term introduced by Garner and Shonkoff and the AAP.[5] Defined as excessive or prolonged activation of the physiologic stress response systems in the absence of the buffering protection afforded by stable, responsive relationships.
PTSD	Set of psychiatric symptoms meeting *Diagnostic and Statistical Manual of Mental Disorders, Fifth Edition*, criteria for PTSD after a person has experienced, witnessed, or learned of a close family member experiencing an event involving actual or threatened death, serious injury, or sexual violation (see text).

mitigate the consequences of child maltreatment. The report begins with brief summaries of the consequences of maltreatment, continues with a discussion of a clinical approach oriented to the pediatrician taking a particular focus on behavioral presentations, and concludes with a discussion of currently available treatment approaches.

Effects of Maltreatment: Childhood Behavior and Mental Health

Research and practice have made it clear that being a victim of maltreatment has serious negative implications for a child's mental health. Although some children recover from adversity, traumatic experiences can result in significant disruption of a child's development. Symptoms of child traumatic stress and comorbid disruptions in the parent-child relationship can present to the pediatrician in a variety of ways.[11-13]

The most trauma-specific psychiatric diagnosis associated with child maltreatment is posttraumatic stress disorder (PTSD).[14] The diagnostic criteria for PTSD in children are

described in the fifth edition of *Diagnostic and Statistical Manual of Mental Disorders, Fifth Edition* and may be summarized as follows: (1) a tendency to persistently reexperience the traumatic event through intrusive thoughts, feelings, dreams, and "flashback" recollections; (2) avoidance of stimuli associated with the event (ie, avoiding people, places, or other cues that remind the child of the traumatic event); (3) negative alterations in cognitions and mood (ie, negative beliefs and expectations about oneself or world; persistent emotions of fear, horror, anger, guilt, or shame; and detachment or estrangement); and (4) alterations in arousal and reactivity (ie, hypervigilance, exaggerated startle, and irritability or anger outbursts and reckless behavior as well as decreased attention, poor concentration, and sleep disturbance).[15]

Comorbidities with PTSD often include internalizing problems, such as depression and anxiety, and externalizing problems, including disruptive behavioral disorders (oppositional defiant and conduct disorders) as well as substance abuse and suicidal behavior.[16–21] Although maltreated children may fit the diagnostic criteria for attention-deficit/hyperactivity disorder (ADHD), a traumatic event may be the primary cause of the behavioral manifestations (including symptoms similar to ADHD) and lead to the diagnostic impression of ADHD.[22] Child abuse is a risk factor for ADHD, particularly when maltreatment occurs early in life and with recurrence.[23]

The clinical presentations of a child with a maltreatment history may include signs of intense emotional and physiologic distress, disturbed sleep, difficulty paying attention and concentrating, anger and irritability, withdrawal, repeated and intrusive thoughts, and extreme distress, particularly when confronted by experiences reminding them of the trauma.

Common examples of problematic behaviors that may be exhibited by children who have been abused, neglected, or otherwise exposed to violence include the following:

- An apparently minor stimulus may echo the previous abuse and produce a dramatic (and inappropriate) emotional reaction. Such reactions may be elicited by "trauma reminders" such as a sight, smell, sound, or other sensory input or by an action, place, or date reminiscent of the trauma. The brain becomes engaged in an exaggerated form of pattern recognition: similar patterns of stimuli call forth a similar neuroendocrine (and behavioral) response.[24,25] In some ways, this response may echo the fight-or-flight response of the initial abuse or of the trauma associated with removal from the abusive home environment.

- Maltreated children are far more often identified as "problem children" than are their peers and show higher rates of diagnoses of attention problems and violent and oppositional behaviors.[26,27] A child's hypervigilance and inability to regulate emotional states after maltreatment can result in challenging behaviors when interacting with others, often including peers.

- Behavioral responses can be exacerbated when caregivers and teachers respond to these behaviors with their own escalation; for example, warnings can be become louder and brusquer and discipline may be more strict and punitive. When the child's exaggerated emotional response elicits an escalated response from an individual, the child may mistakenly assume that his or her initial reaction was warranted. Such responses inadvertently confirm the child's mistaken impression that the world is a high-threat environment. This is, in effect, positive reinforcement for the preceding behavior—behavior that has negative consequences for the child and those in his or her environment.

It is important to recognize that children may exhibit problematic behavior long after their abuse or neglect has ended. Signs and symptoms may be delayed, may linger, and if untreated, can evolve into more problematic presentations as children age into adolescence and adulthood. In addition, children with disabilities may have different behavioral presentations, particularly among those children with intellectual disabilities.[28,29]

The exposure to trauma and other adverse childhood experiences (ACEs) that triggered these behavioral reinforcements may directly affect brain development, as described in a previous AAP technical report.[7] Of note, continued exposure to abuse or neglect can be associated with changes in the child's brain structure and physiology.[30] Such changes may be associated with impairment in the child's interactions with caregivers, whose response may further accelerate maladaptive behavioral responses.

Beyond the stress response, the effect on neurobiological factors via learning and modeling maladaptive behaviors is relevant. Children who see their primary caregivers model aggressive, violent behaviors (eg, physical abuse or domestic violence) and/or disregard others' needs (eg, neglect) often mimic these behaviors and come to believe that these are effective strategies for managing negative emotional states or for getting their own needs met.[31] In the absence of more positive modeling, these behaviors are likely to persist.

The effects of child maltreatment extend to other aspects of child health. Maltreated children are more likely to experience physical injuries, conditions that result from neglect, and failure to attend to chronic health concerns. These effects result in increased health care expenditures; a recent economic model of the effects of abuse and neglect estimated that children who have been abused or neglected account for 9% of total Medicaid expenditures for children.[32]

ACEs (Table 1) tend to cooccur, such that an individual exposed to 1 ACE is more likely to be exposed to ≥2.[33] Putnam et al[34] noted that 7 of the originally described ACEs were significantly associated with complex adult psychopathology (meeting 2–4 comorbid *Diagnostic and Statistical Manual of Mental Disorders, Fourth Edition* disorders). Sexual abuse proved the most "potent" childhood adversity in terms of synergistic multiplicative effects, especially for women. Parental psychopathology was synergistic with sexual abuse for both sexes and with physical abuse for men. Poverty, although not included in the original ACE study, was added to the analyses and proved the most potent adversity in men and was critically synergistic with several childhood adversities in predicting adult psychopathology.[34] In addition, some young children and their families may experience stress related to the effects of racism.[35] Multiple adversities in childhood are often more than additive, and some adversities have higher potency in combination with others. The cumulative effects of ACEs will need attention in not only clinical application but directives at the policy level.[36]

Understanding Behavioral Problems in Young Children Who Have Experienced Maltreatment

The child's sense of the parents' responsiveness to his or her needs is a building block of secure attachment[37] and a critical mediator of developmental success, especially under conditions of traumatic stress.[38] An attentive caregiver helps the child to build trust and learn the "give-and-take" nature of social communication. Early emotional development centers on the communication between mothers and their infants organized around face, voice, gesture, gaze, and a mutual and synergistic emotional and physiologic regulation.[39] This interactive communication also teaches the child to recognize and regulate his or her own emotions in a continuous "dance" of interaction.[40,41] With such a benefactor, the infant is secure to learn and explore. When the parent is substantially inconsistent, frightening, neglectful, or abusive, the resultant attachment can be confused and disorganized, with research indicating high predictability for later psychopathology.[37] However, even lesser degrees of impairment in the parent-child relationship can affect attachment. A caregiver who is frequently absent, preoccupied, or inconsistent interferes with the ability of the infant to feel safe. As a result, neglected infants may be more demanding, anxious, and more difficult to console[42] and evolve

into toddlers who lack enthusiasm and are easily frustrated and noncompliant.

Early brain development is sensitive to severe ongoing stress or "toxic stress." This term, coined by Garner and Shonkoff,[5] intends to relay the impact on brain anatomy and function brought about when the young child experiences chronic stress in the absence of the buffering capacity of the caregiver. In the context of child maltreatment, the lifelong effects of early childhood stress may emerge in childhood or adolescence as stress-related changes in the neuroendocrine system. For example, analysis of the Nurses' Health Study demonstrated a strong association between child physical and sexual abuse and early menarche.[43]

Effects of Maltreatment That Manifest During Adolescence

Although any of the associated impairments in childhood described previously can extend to adolescents, many of the most serious long-term effects of childhood maltreatment may become apparent as risk behaviors beginning in adolescence. In their analysis of 161 published studies, Norman and colleagues[13] concluded that "there was robust evidence of a significant association between exposure to nonsexual child maltreatment and increased likelihood of suicide attempts, sexually transmitted infections, drug use, and risky sexual behavior." Adolescents are also more likely to present with complex trauma presentations resulting from chronic victimization and/or polyvictimization that include not only PTSD and trauma-related behavioral disorders but also cognitive and emotional dysregulation with feelings of rage and shame; the impact of disrupted attachments and unstable, sometimes chaotic relationships; and impaired self-efficacy and self-perception.[44]

According to the National Survey of Adolescents,[45] neglect and emotional, physical, and sexual abuse are strong contributors to adolescent behavior disorders. Childhood neglect and emotional and sexual abuse were associated with adolescent substance abuse.[46] The investigators further noted a high rate of cooccurrence of childhood adversity in their sample: 97% of neglected respondents had at least 1 other childhood adversity, as did 96% of those who recalled physical abuse and 90% of those who recalled sexual abuse. Adolescent respondents who recalled any form of maltreatment had a mean of 4 to 5 other childhood adversities, further demonstrating the frequent cooccurrence of multiple forms of adversity.

Effects of Maltreatment Persist Into Adulthood

There is now a robust literature on the persistent effects of maltreatment on adult health; however, from the perspective of the pediatrician, the child and adolescent manifestations of trauma are most salient. Long-term follow-up of children who experienced child maltreatment demonstrated that children with ≥2 ACEs reported more somatic concerns, health problems, and poor health in general as adults.[24,47] Child maltreatment is associated with both the onset[48] and persistence[49] of adult psychiatric disorders.

Not surprisingly, children who have been abused or neglected have high lifetime health care utilization. A 2013 report from the Centers for Disease Control and Prevention showed increased cost for psychiatric care, case management, inpatient care, outpatient (clinic) care, and home health.[32] In summary, ACEs, especially child physical, sexual, and emotional abuse and neglect, lead to significantly increased risk of impairment in child development and subsequent adolescent and adult mental and physical health problems.

CLINICAL APPROACH

A child's primary care pediatrician plays an important role in identifying the psychological and biological signs and symptoms of child traumatic stress. The importance of being able to assess whether child maltreatment has occurred among children and adolescents presenting with behavioral and emotional problems cannot be overemphasized. Pediatricians who recognize the relationships of these common behavior problems to possible previous maltreatment may improve outcomes for affected children. When a previously maltreated infant or child exhibits behavior problems, especially when those problems are resistant to intervention, a confluence of emotional and maladaptive physiologic responses may be contributing to a child's presentation. The thorough evaluation of a child's behavioral symptoms includes a careful psychosocial history asking about children's exposure to early abuse, neglect, abandonment, or other traumas. In addition, histories that reveal exposure to intimate partner violence, parental substance use disorder, or parental mental health diagnoses may be relevant to understanding and treating the patient's behavioral issues. Maltreated children may benefit from a comprehensive mental health assessment, which may help determine whether further treatment would be helpful.

Although caregivers—be they birth parents, foster parents, or adoptive parents—are almost certain to face major challenges related to the child's mental and physical health needs, they may not initially realize the extent to which these problems result from the child's past experiences. Maladaptive physiologic responses to trauma and loss reminders ("triggers") are frequently misinterpreted by teachers and parents as disobedience. This misinterpretation can result in punishment and lack of understanding and guidance for the child, which further reinforces the maladaptive physiologic response.

Primary care pediatricians can counsel parents or guardians and help them better understand that the child's maladaptive response to stress may have originated as a biologically based adaptation to ACEs and other forms of trauma the child experienced and that the persisting problem behaviors are a consequence of the adversity. Caregivers can be taught that children may not feel psychologically safe, even if they are physically safe from danger from the original perpetrator. Biological, foster, and adoptive parents can learn that traumatic reminders can elicit emotional and behavioral reactions in children. When an accentuated stress response is suspected, the physician can help caregivers understand that the child's problems are more than simple defiance or willful misbehavior. Caregivers will better understand a child's behavior when they learn that a child who has suffered maltreatment may respond differently from a child who has not suffered abuse.[50] Given that a child's development, self-image, and perception of the world are affected by maltreatment, pediatric guidance to parents can include discouraging aggressive responses to aggressive behaviors (eg, corporal punishment) and explaining how noise and anger can further aggravate the child's stress reaction and lack of psychological safety. Furthermore, parents can be taught to use positive parenting strategies and to coach a child to be prepared for triggers in their environment.

In addition to primary care counseling, children with persistent or severe behavioral problems resulting from maltreatment may benefit from referral for further trauma assessment or evidence-based treatment, particularly when accompanying a history of trauma or maltreatment. Many of these behavioral symptoms can be addressed in trauma-focused psychotherapy. Whenever possible, pediatricians can help caregivers access evidence-based therapeutic treatments that can address children's emotional and behavioral problems and assist children in resuming a normal developmental trajectory. Previous reports discuss the importance of improving children's access to mental health services.[51]

Effective therapy involves reshaping the child's misperceptions, traumatic stress responses (which often include affect instability), and maladaptive coping. For example, some children may feel that they were at least partially responsible for the abuse or that their own misbehavior initiated it. Therapy may also help nonoffending caregivers examine their own behaviors, enhance parenting skills, and address worries about the child. Caregivers may have mental health symptoms that would benefit from assessment and referral for their own therapy. Adjunctive interventions often target social support and comorbidities, assist the relevant service systems to be trauma-informed, and identify and address developmental needs. Treatment of children's emotional and behavioral problems related to child maltreatment may reduce the risk of long-term consequences, including violent behavior, dangerous risk taking, and impaired interpersonal relationships,[52,53] in addition to the negative physical and mental health consequences associated with ACEs.[24]

EVIDENCE-BASED TREATMENT OF CHILDHOOD TRAUMA

Overview

Although the effects of traumatic experiences vary considerably and are often complex, trauma-specific mental health interventions have been shown to be effective. Notably, cognitive behavioral therapy (CBT) has proven effective in the treatment of childhood PTSD.[54] Recent systematic reviews reported by the Cochrane Collaborative,[55] Silverman et al,[56] Dorsey et al,[57] and a federally funded evidence synthesis on interventions for nonrelational trauma[58] each concluded that although CBT appears effective overall, there is no agreement on which particular variants of CBT are most effective.

The National Child Traumatic Stress Network[59] recommends trauma-specific treatments, including those with cognitive-behavioral approaches, for children with PTSD and related mental health symptoms (eg, anxiety, behavioral difficulties, shame) who have experienced child abuse. These therapies typically include (1) educating children and their parents about child abuse and common (psychological and physiologic) reactions of children; (2) teaching safety skills, stress management, and coping techniques and emotional-regulation skills; (3) facilitating a coherent narrative of the traumatic event(s) done in a way to desensitize the child to the fear and anxiety about what happened; (4) emotional and cognitive processing (correcting untrue or distorted ideas about how and why the trauma occurred); and (5) providing parenting strategies to assist in promoting normal development and decreasing problem behaviors.

The knowledge of trauma's underlying concepts, the emergence of evidence-based practice, and the ability to apply these practices with clinical knowledge, reasoning, and judgment skills are important. The 12 Core Concepts of Childhood Trauma (summarized in Table 2), developed by the National Child Traumatic Stress Network Core Curriculum Task Force, provide a rationale for trauma-informed assessment and intervention. The Concepts cover

a broad range of topics that assist providers as they assess, understand, and assist trauma-exposed children, families, and communities.

Individual and Parent CBT for Sexual Abuse, Physical Abuse, and Other Traumas With PTSD Symptoms

Trauma-focused cognitive behavioral therapy[60] (TFCBT), developed initially for treating child sexual abuse, is the specific evidence-based treatment of child traumatic stress symptoms (including PTSD) that has the most documented research (>10 randomized controlled trials). Mental health clinicians earn TFCBT certification as a result of participation in formal online or in-person training programs. Cohen, Deblinger, and Mannarino[61-63] demonstrated that TFCBT for sexually abused children, many of whom had other cooccurring complex presentations of traumas, was superior to supportive psychotherapy in multiple domains 3 months and 1 year after treatment.

Other CBT trials focusing on physically abused youth demonstrated significant improvements.[64,65] The TFCBT modality incorporates individual CBT and family therapy to reduce not only trauma symptoms but also the use of physical punishment and coercion.

Trauma Treatments for Young Children and Their Parents or Guardians

The approach to mental health treatment of young children is described in an AAP policy statement and technical report on this topic[9,10]; this report discusses specific treatments in the context of child abuse and neglect.

A treatment model created for children between 0 and 6 years of age living in violent households, child-parent psychotherapy focuses on the importance of nurturing a secure, growth-promoting attachment and assists the child's caregivers in being

in tune with their own reactions and in tune with their child's signals and responses to traumatic reminders. The result is a heightened sense of ability for the caregiver and positive interactions with the child on a day-to-day basis that are critical to developmental progress, particularly regarding the early foundations for emotional regulation.[31,66-68] Child-parent psychotherapy significantly improved psychiatric symptoms in both mother and child compared with other treatments.[69-71]

Parent-child interaction therapy (PCIT) works with parents and children 2 to 7 years of age to both increase positive parenting skills and decrease serious child disruptive behavior. Although there are several other parent-focused behavior management programs with strong evidence,[44] PCIT has stronger effect sizes, has the most published studies, and has shown decreased recurrence of physical abuse reports compared with parenting groups in the community (19% vs 49%).[72] One randomized controlled trial of PCIT tested individual CBT for preschoolers who had been exposed to trauma and demonstrated significant reductions in PTSD symptoms at 6 months' follow-up.[73]

Trauma Treatments for Adolescents, Including Those With Complex Presentations

A selection of treatments in child trauma are also being evaluated as part of ongoing research, many addressing polyvictimization and chronic complex trauma presentations.[44] Some share similar core components with those listed previously but may emphasize different components altogether, targeting more marked psychopathology. Although traditional CBT focuses on managing stress, fear, and changing maladaptive thoughts, these treatments focus on extreme emotional instability and self-control

TABLE 2 National Child Traumatic Stress Network Core Concepts for Childhood Traumatic Stress

1. Traumatic experiences are inherently complex.
   a. Every traumatic event is made up of different traumatic moments, each of which includes varying degrees of objective life threat, physical violation, and witnessing of injury, or death. Children's thoughts and actions (or inaction) during various moments may lead to feelings of conflict at the time and to feelings of confusion, guilt, regret, and/or anger afterward.
2. Trauma occurs within a broad context that includes children's personal characteristics, life experiences, and current circumstances.
   a. The child's own experience, personality, and environment affect his or her own appraisal of traumatic events and may act exacerbate the adverse effects of trauma.
3. Traumatic events often generate secondary adversities, life changes, and distressing reminders in children's daily lives.
   a. Children's exposure to trauma reminders can serve as additional sources of distress. Secondary adversities may significantly affect functioning in trauma survivors.
4. Children can exhibit a wide range of reactions to trauma and loss.
   a. Posttraumatic stress and grief reactions can develop over time into psychiatric disorders (eg, PTSD, separation anxiety, and depression), may disrupt major domains of child development, and reduce children's level of functioning at home, at school, and in the community.
5. Danger and safety are core concerns in the lives of traumatized children.
   a. Lack of physical and psychological safety can be magnified in a child's mind. Ensuring children's physical safety is foundational to restoring the sense of a protective shield.
6. Trauma experiences affect the family and broader caregiving systems.
   a. Caregivers' own concerns may impair their ability to support traumatized children. The ability of caregiver systems to provide support is an important contributor to children's and families' adjustment.
7. Protective and promotive factors can reduce the adverse impact of trauma.
   a. Protective factors buffer the adverse effects of trauma and its stressful aftermath, whereas promotive factors generally enhance children's positive adjustment regardless of whether risk factors are present. The presence of these factors (ie, positive attachment to a caregiver, reliable social support, environment) can enhance children's ability to resist, or to "bounce back" from adversities.
8. Trauma and posttrauma adversities can strongly influence development.
   a. Trauma and posttrauma adversities can profoundly influence children's acquisition of developmental competencies and their capacity to reach important developmental milestones. Trauma and its aftermath can lead to developmental disruptions (regressive behavior, reluctance, or inability to participate in developmentally appropriate activities), and developmental accelerations such as leaving home at an early age and engagement in precocious sexual behavior.
9. Developmental neurobiology underlies children's reactions to traumatic experiences.
   a. Children's capacities to appraise and respond to danger are linked to an evolving neurobiology of brain structures, neurophysiological pathways, and neuroendocrine systems. Traumatic experiences evoke strong biological responses that can persist and alter the normal course of neurobiological maturation. Exposure to multiple traumatic experiences carries a greater risk.
10. Culture is closely interwoven with traumatic experiences, response, and recovery.
    a. Culture can profoundly affect the ways in which children and their families respond to traumatic events, including how they express distress and disclose personal information to others.
11. Challenges to the social contract, including legal and ethical issues, affect trauma response and recovery.
    a. Traumatic experiences often constitute a violation of expectations of the child, family, community, and society. The perceived success or failure of these institutional responses may exert a profound influence on the course of children's posttrauma adjustment and on their evolving beliefs regarding family, work, and civic life.
12. Working with trauma-exposed children can evoke distress in providers that makes it more difficult for them to provide good care.
    a. Health care providers often encounter personal and professional challenges as they confront details of children's traumatic experiences and life adversities. Proper self-care is an important part of providing quality care.

dysregulation, problems in interpersonal relationships, current functioning, and social problem solving.[74]

Evidence-Based Treatments and Trauma-Informed Practices for Children in Foster Care

Attachment and Bio-behavioral Catchup (ABC intervention[75,76]) is a home-based program for toddlers. Two randomized controlled trials found that among foster care and neglect groups, the children in the ABC intervention developed secure and organized attachments.[77] Another study showed significantly lower cortisol levels and fewer behavior problems.[78]

Two additional practices are worth noting in the context of behavioral sequelae to child maltreatment. In a randomized clinical trial, Farmer et al found evidence that case workers and foster families provided structured therapeutic environments to delinquent/emotionally troubled youth showing reduced problem behaviors, likelihood of committing felonies, delinquency, and days incarcerated while increasing placement permanency.[79] In addition, the National Child Traumatic Stress

Network has created a Resource Parenting Curriculum, cofacilitated by a mental health master trainer and foster parent, to groups of foster/adoptive/kinship caregivers, to educate how trauma affects children's behavior, feelings, and attitudes and to enhance caregiver skills and techniques.[58]

Pharmacotherapy

Systematic reviews do not support the use of pharmacotherapy as a first-line treatment of pediatric PTSD. However, medications may be considered to assist children temporarily in regulating symptoms of physiologic hyperarousal, such as nightmares, sleep difficulties, and high anxiety. Although medication often can ameliorate the stress response in youth, psychopharmacologic intervention should be considered an adjunct to, rather than a substitute for, psychotherapy. Because comorbidity is quite common with PTSD, symptoms of ADHD, anxiety, and depression may be present. In particular, distinguishing between true ADHD, symptoms of PTSD and a response to a chaotic posttrauma environment may require a referral for a mental health evaluation. Emphasis on the appropriate use of trauma-focused, evidence-based treatment and coordination across the system of care when a child's case interfaces with multiple agencies may help address the overuse of medication or other less effective types of therapy.

Cultural Considerations

Physicians caring for abused and neglected children may be able to access specialized, culturally aligned treatments. For example, Bigfoot and Schmidt report the integration of trauma-focused care with traditional American Indian practices.[80]

CONCLUSIONS

In pediatric office practice, physicians and nurse practitioners are often asked to treat common behavioral problems. Children with a history of abuse, neglect, or abandonment may present to the pediatrician with symptoms including anger, aggressive behaviors, sexually reactive behaviors, depression, or difficulties sustaining attention. In many cases, the children are no longer exposed to the direct threat but present with residual behaviors that can be linked to neurophysiologic responses to their previous maltreatment. Even when the child is living in a protective

home, caregivers still may find typical parenting behavioral strategies unsuccessful. In many cases, the child's exaggerated reactions to stressful stimuli can cause the caregivers to act in ways that reinforce the child's misbehavior.

When attentive parenting appears ineffective, it is important to reflect on how early maltreatment (physical or sexual abuse, neglect, or exposure to violence and fear) can deprive the child of the tools needed to adapt to a larger social environment. In addition to denying the developing child necessary social interactions, early maltreatment can alter the normal child's neural physiology, significantly changing the expected responses to stress and affecting the child's ability to learn from experience.

The pediatrician can assist directly and in cooperation with other professionals. Pediatricians should continue to advocate for timely evaluation of children entering the foster care system, as recommended by the AAP.[81,82] Given the risks posed by early neglect and abuse, these examinations should include mental health, developmental, and cognitive screening, in addition to the usual medical assessment.[83] Unfortunately, many foster children do not receive these comprehensive evaluations.[84] Ongoing education for caregivers of previously maltreated children, especially for foster parents, can be better guided by the results of a comprehensive evaluation.[85]

Using their therapeutic relationship with the child and family, pediatricians can work to educate caregivers and help them to understand that their child's behavioral responses may differ from those of other children in the same situation. Such differences may reflect a triggered physiologic response rather than willful misbehavior or an egregious failure on the part of caregivers.[86] If such timely educational interventions

can change caregivers' perceptions, they can relieve stress and begin to stabilize the family or foster placement. Many patients with a significant history of trauma will need to be followed by mental health professionals, and the pediatrician plays an important role in referral and comanagement. By providing a medical home, the pediatrician can work longitudinally with caregivers and continue to treat symptoms that are obstructing therapy. Pediatricians can facilitate access to community resources, work closely with the child's school to address behavioral challenges to learning, and help coordinate care among specialists in other disciplines.[86]

Clinical Considerations for the Pediatrician

1. Inquiries regarding past traumatic experiences, including child abuse and neglect, may be included in the social and family histories of patients. Awareness and understanding of a child's trauma history, including child abuse and neglect, and the frequent multiplicity of trauma exposures can make a dramatic difference in the evaluation of children with behavior problems because these problems commonly occur as a result of current or previous abuse, neglect, and/or other traumatic life experiences

2. Treatment of severe or persistent behavioral consequences of child maltreatment is indicated and effective; many mental health clinicians have the training and skills needed to use these evidence-based treatment approaches.

3. Pediatricians and other pediatric health care providers are a useful resource to parents and teachers of maltreated children and may be able to assist them to better understand the behavioral consequences of past maltreatment.

4. Similar considerations apply to advising foster families and child welfare agencies in understanding the behavioral consequences of past maltreatment and the assessment and treatment of resultant mental health disorders. Pediatricians can help advise social service agencies on the common behavioral problems exhibited by children who have been maltreated and advocate for prompt referral to effective therapies for these children.

RESOURCES

Dorsey S, McLaughlin KA, Kerns SE, et al. Evidence base update for psychosocial treatments children and adolescents exposed to traumatic events [published online ahead of print October 19, 2016]. *J Clin Child Adolesc Psychol.* doi: 10.1080/15374416.2016.1220309

Amaya-Jackson L, Briggs-King E, Thompson R. Psychopathology of child maltreatment. In: Chadwick D, Alexander R, Giardino AP, Esermio-Jenssen, eds. *Chadwick's Child Maltreatment.* Vol 2. St Louis, MO: STM Learning; 2014:251–267

Cohen JA, Kelleher KJ, Mannarino AP. Identifying, treating, and referring traumatized children: the role of pediatric providers. *Arch Pediatr Adolesc Med.* 2008;162(5):447–452

Shonkoff JP, Garner AS; American Academy of Pediatrics, Committee on Psychosocial Aspects of Child and Family Health, Committee on Early Childhood Adoption, and Dependent Care, Section on Developmental and Behavioral Pediatrics. Technical report: the lifelong effects of early childhood adversity and toxic stress. *Pediatrics.* 2012;129(1). Available at: www.pediatrics.org/cgi/content/full/129/1/e232

AUTHORS

Robert D. Sege, MD, PhD, FAAP
Lisa Amaya-Jackson, MD, MPH, FAACAP

AAP COMMITTEE ON CHILD ABUSE AND NEGLECT, 2014–2016

Emalee G. Flaherty, MD, FAAP, Chairperson
Sheila M. Idzerda, MD, FAAP
Lori A. Legano, MD, FAAP
John M. Leventhal, MD, FAAP
James L. Lukefahr, MD, FAAP
Robert D. Sege, MD, PhD, FAAP

LIAISONS

Harriet MacMillan, MD, MSc, FRCPC – *American Academy of Child and Adolescent Psychiatry*
Catherine M. Nolan, MSW, ACSW – *Administration for Children, Youth and Families, Office on Child Abuse and Neglect*
Linda Anne Valle, PhD – *Centers for Disease Control and Prevention*

STAFF

Tammy Piazza Hurley, BA

AAP COUNCIL ON FOSTER CARE, ADOPTION, AND KINSHIP CARE EXECUTIVE COMMITTEE, 2014–2016

Moira A. Szilagyi, MD PhD, FAAP, Chairperson
Heather C. Forkey, MD, FAAP
David A. Harmon, MD, FAAP
Paula K. Jaudes, MD, FAAP
Veronnie Faye Jones, MD, PhD, MSPH, FAAP
Paul J Lee, MD, FAAP
Lisa M. Nalven, MD, MA, FAAP
Linda Davidson Sagor, MD MPH, FAAP
Elaine E. Schulte, MD, FAAP
Sarah H. Springer, MD, FAAP

LIAISONS

George Fouras, MD – *American Academy of Child and Adolescent Psychiatry*
Jeremy Harvey – *Foster Care Alumni of America*
Melissa Hill, MD – *Section on Medical Students, Residents, and Training Fellows*

STAFF

Mary Crane, PhD, LSW

ABBREVIATIONS

AAP: American Academy of Pediatrics
ABC intervention: attachment and bio-behavioral catchup
ACE: adverse childhood experiences
ADHD: attention-deficit/hyperactivity disorder
CBT: cognitive-behavioral therapy
PCIT: parent-child interaction therapy
PTSD: posttraumatic stress disorder
TFCBT: trauma-focused cognitive behavioral therapy

AACAP COMMITTEE ON CHILD MALTREATMENT AND VIOLENCE

Judith Cohen, MD, Co-Chair
Jeanette Scheid, MD, Co-Chair
Lisa Amaya-Jackson, MD, MPH
David Corwin, MD
Eve Spratt, MD
Harriet MacMillan, MD, Liaison American Academy of Pediatrics
Brooks Keeshin, MD
Lisa Hutchison, MD
Michael De Bellis, M.D
Nina Butler, MD
Rashmi Gupta, MD
Dayna Leplatte-Ogini, MD
Sara Pawlowski, MD
Anna Kerlek, MD

STAFF

Tony Green

NATIONAL CENTER FOR CHILD TRAUMATIC STRESS (SUBSTANCE ABUSE AND MENTAL HEALTH SERVICES ADMINISTRATION FUNDED)

Lisa Amaya-Jackson, MD, MPH
Robert Pynoos, MD, MPH
John Fairbank, PhD
Ellen Gerrity, PhD
Jenifer Maze, PhD
Mary Mount

approved by the Board of Directors. The American Academy of Pediatrics has neither solicited nor accepted any commercial involvement in the development of the content of this publication.

Clinical reports from the American Academy of Pediatrics benefit from expertise and resources of liaisons and internal (AAP) and external reviewers. However, clinical reports from the American Academy of Pediatrics may not reflect the views of the liaisons or the organizations or government agencies that they represent.

DOI: 10.1542/peds.2017-0100

Address correspondence to Robert D. Sege, MD, PhD, FAAP. E-mail: bsege@hria.org

PEDIATRICS (ISSN Numbers: Print, 0031-4005; Online, 1098-4275).

FINANCIAL DISCLOSURE: The authors have indicated they have no financial relationships relevant to this article to disclose.

FUNDING: No external funding.

POTENTIAL CONFLICT OF INTEREST: The authors have indicated they have no potential conflicts of interest to disclose.

REFERENCES

1. Felitti VJ, Anda RF, Nordenberg D, et al. Relationship of childhood abuse and household dysfunction to many of the leading causes of death in adults. The Adverse Childhood Experiences (ACE) Study. *Am J Prev Med.* 1998;14(4):245–258

2. Finkelhor D, Ormrod R, Turner H, Hamby SL. The victimization of children and youth: a comprehensive, national survey. *Child Maltreat.* 2005;10(1):5–25

3. Administration for Children, Youth, and Families, Children's Bureau. Child Maltreatment 2013. Available at: www.acf.hhs.gov/programs/cb/resource/child-maltreatment-2013. Accessed June 13, 2016

4. National Child Traumatic Stress Network. What Is Child Traumatic Stress? Available at: www.nctsnet.org/sites/default/files/assets/pdfs/what_is_child_traumatic_stress_0.pdf. Accessed January 21, 2017

5. Garner AS, Shonkoff JP; Committee on Psychosocial Aspects of Child and Family Health; Committee on Early Childhood, Adoption, and Dependent Care; Section on Developmental and Behavioral Pediatrics. Early childhood adversity, toxic stress, and the role of the pediatrician: translating developmental science into lifelong health. *Pediatrics.* 2012;129(1). Available at: www.pediatrics.org/cgi/content/full/129/1/e224

6. Stirling J Jr, Amaya-Jackson L, Amaya-Jackson L; American Academy of Pediatrics; Committee on Child Abuse and Neglect and Section on Adoption and Foster Care; American Academy of Child and Adolescent Psychiatry; National Center for Child Traumatic Stress. Understanding the behavioral and emotional consequences of child abuse. *Pediatrics.* 2008;122(3):667–673

7. Shonkoff JP, Garner AS; Committee on Psychosocial Aspects of Child and Family Health; Committee on Early Childhood, Adoption, and Dependent Care; Section on Developmental and Behavioral Pediatrics. The lifelong effects of early childhood adversity and toxic stress. *Pediatrics.* 2012;129(1). Available at: www.pediatrics.org/cgi/content/full/129/1/e232

8. Pynoos RS, Fairbank JA, Steinberg AM, et al. The National Child Traumatic Stress Network: collaborating to improve the standard of care. *Prof Psychol Res Pr.* 2008;39(4):389–395

9. American Academy of Pediatrics, Council on Early Childhood, Committee on Psychosocial Aspects of Child and Family Health, Section on Developmental and Behavioral Pediatrics. Addressing early childhood emotional and behavioral problems. *Pediatrics.* 2016;138(6):e20163023

10. Gleason MM, Goldson E, Yogman MW, American Academy of Pediatrics, Committee on Early Childhood, Committee on Psychosocial Aspects of Child and Family Health, Section on Developmental and Behavioral Pediatrics. Addressing early childhood emotional and behavioral problems. *Pediatrics.* 2016;138(6):e201630257

11. Holbrook TL, Hoyt DB, Coimbra R, Potenza B, Sise M, Anderson JP. Long-term posttraumatic stress disorder persists after major trauma in adolescents: new data on risk factors and functional outcome. *J Trauma.* 2005;58(4):764–769, discussion 769–771

12. Lansford JE, Dodge KA, Pettit GS, Bates JE, Crozier J, Kaplow J. A 12-year prospective study of the long-term effects of early child physical maltreatment on psychological, behavioral, and academic problems in adolescence. *Arch Pediatr Adolesc Med.* 2002;156(8):824–830

13. Norman RE, Byambaa M, De R, Butchart A, Scott J, Vos T. The long-term health consequences of child physical abuse, emotional abuse, and neglect: a systematic review and meta-analysis. *PLoS Med.* 2012;9(11):e1001349

14. Kearney CA, Wechsler A, Kaur H, Lemos-Miller A. Posttraumatic stress disorder in maltreated youth: a review of contemporary research and thought. *Clin Child Fam Psychol Rev.* 2010;13(1):46–76

15. American Psychiatric Association, eds. *Diagnostic and Statistical Manual of Mental Disorders.* 5th ed. Washington, DC: American Psychiatric Association Press; 2013

16. Manly JT, Kim JE, Rogosch FA, Cicchetti D. Dimensions of child maltreatment and children's adjustment: contributions of developmental timing and subtype. *Dev Psychopathol.* 2001;13(4):759–782

17. Turner HA, Finkelhor D, Ormrod R. The effect of lifetime victimization on the mental health of children and adolescents. *Soc Sci Med.* 2006;62(1):13–27

18. Lau AS, Weisz JR. Reported maltreatment among clinic-referred children: implications for presenting problems, treatment

attrition, and long-term outcomes. *J Am Acad Child Adolesc Psychiatry.* 2003;42(11):1327–1334

19. Fergusson DM, Boden JM, Horwood LJ. Exposure to childhood sexual and physical abuse and adjustment in early adulthood. *Child Abuse Negl.* 2008;32(6):607–619

20. Thompson R, Litrownik AJ, Weisbart C, Kotch JB, English DJ, Everson MD. Adolescent outcomes associated with early maltreatment and exposure to violence: the role of early suicidal ideation. *Intl J Child Adolesc Health.* 2010;3:55–66

21. Bensley LS, Spieker SJ, Van Eenwyk J, Schoder J. Self-reported abuse history and adolescent problem behaviors. II. Alcohol and drug use. *J Adolesc Health.* 1999;24(3):173–180

22. Weinstein D, Staffelbach D, Biaggio M. Attention-deficit hyperactivity disorder and posttraumatic stress disorder: differential diagnosis in childhood sexual abuse. *Clin Psychol Rev.* 2000;20(3):359–378

23. Thompson R, Tabone JK. The impact of early alleged maltreatment on behavioral trajectories. *Child Abuse Negl.* 2010;34(12):907–916

24. Bremner JD, Vythilingam M, Vermetten E, et al. Cortisol response to a cognitive stress challenge in posttraumatic stress disorder (PTSD) related to childhood abuse. *Psychoneuroendocrinology.* 2003;28(6):733–750

25. Elzinga BM, Schmahl CG, Vermetten E, van Dyck R, Bremner JD. Higher cortisol levels following exposure to traumatic reminders in abuse-related PTSD. *Neuropsychopharmacology.* 2003;28(9):1656–1665

26. Greeson JK, Briggs EC, Layne CM, et al. Traumatic childhood experiences in the 21st century: broadening and building on the ACE studies with data from the National Child Traumatic Stress Network. *J Interpers Violence.* 2014;29(3):536–556

27. Wodarski JS, Kurtz PD, Gaudin JM Jr, Howing PT. Maltreatment and the school-age child: major academic, socioemotional, and adaptive outcomes: *Soc Work.* 1990;35(6):506–513

28. Hibbard RA, Desch LW; American Academy of Pediatrics Committee on Child Abuse and Neglect; American Academy of Pediatrics Council on Children With Disabilities. Maltreatment of children with disabilities. *Pediatrics.* 2007;119(5):1018–1025

29. Ko SJ, Pynoos RS, Griffin D, Vanderbuilt D; NCTSN Trauma and IDD Expert Panel. *Road to Recovery: Supporting Children With Intellectual and Developmental Disabilities Who Have Experienced Trauma.* Los Angeles, CA and Durham, NC: National Center for Child Traumatic Stress; 2015

30. Twardosz S, Lutzker JR. Child maltreatment and the developing brain: a review of neuroscience perspectives. *Aggress Violent Behav.* 2010;15(1):59–68

31. Kolko DJ, Swenson CC. *Assessing and Treating Physically Abused Children and Their Families: A Cognitive-Behavioral Approach.* Thousand Oaks, CA: Sage Publications; 2002

32. Florence C, Brown DS, Fang X, Thompson HF. Health care costs associated with child maltreatment: impact on medicaid. *Pediatrics.* 2013;132(2):312–318

33. Dong M, Anda RF, Felitti VJ, et al. The interrelatedness of multiple forms of childhood abuse, neglect, and household dysfunction. *Child Abuse Negl.* 2004;28(7):771–784

34. Putnam KT, Harris WW, Putnam FW. Synergistic childhood adversities and complex adult psychopathology. *J Trauma Stress.* 2013;26(4):435–442

35. Priest N, Paradies Y, Trenerry B, Truong M, Karlsen S, Kelly Y. A systematic review of studies examining the relationship between reported racism and health and wellbeing for children and young people. *Soc Sci Med.* 2013;95:115–127

36. Putnam F, Harris W, Putnam K, Lieberman A, Amaya-Jackson L. Opportunities to Change the Outcomes of Traumatized Children: The Child Adversity Narratives. May 15, 2015. Available at: www.CANarratives.org. Accessed June 13, 2016

37. Bowlby J. *Attachment and Loss.* 2nd ed. New York, NY: Basic Books; 1982

38. Lieberman AF, Amaya-Jackson L. Reciprocal influences of attachment and trauma: using a dual lens in the assessment and treatment of infants, toddlers, and preschoolers. In: Berlin LJ, Ziv Y, Amaya-Jackson L, Greenberg MT, eds. *Enhancing Early Attachments: Theory, Research, Intervention and Policy.* New York, NY: Guilford Press; 2005:100–124

39. Putnam F. Developmental neurobiology of disrupted attachment: lessons from animal models and child abuse research. In: Berlin LJ, Ziv Y, Amaya-Jackson L, Greenberg MT, eds. *Enhancing Early Attachments: Theory, Research, Intervention & Policy.* New York, NY: Guilford Press; 2005:100–124

40. Greenspan SI. Comprehensive clinical approaches to infants and their families: psychodynamic and developmental perspectives. In: Meisels SJ, Shonkoff JP, eds. *Handbook of Early Childhood Intervention.* New York, NY: Cambridge University Press; 1990:150–172

41. Cicchetti D, Cohen DJ, eds. Contribution of attachment theory to developmental psychopathology., Developmental Psychopathology. Vol. 1: *Theory and Methods.* New York, NY: John Wiley & Sons; 1995:581–617

42. Egeland B, Sroufe LA, Erickson M. The developmental consequence of different patterns of maltreatment. *Child Abuse Negl.* 1983;7(4):459–469

43. Boynton-Jarrett R, Wright RJ, Putnam FW, et al. Childhood abuse and age at menarche. *J Adolesc Health.* 2013;52(2):241–247

44. Amaya-Jackson L, Derosa RR. Treatment considerations for clinicians in applying evidence-based practice to complex presentations in child trauma. *J Trauma Stress.* 2007;20(4):379–390

45. McLaughlin KA, Greif Green J, Gruber MJ, Sampson NA, Zaslavsky AM, Kessler RC. Childhood adversities and first onset of psychiatric disorders in a national sample of US adolescents. *Arch Gen Psychiatry.* 2012;69(11):1151–1160

46. Suarez LM, Belcher HM, Briggs EC, Titus JC. Supporting the need for an integrated system of care for youth with co-occurring traumatic stress and substance abuse

problems. *Am J Community Psychol.* 2012;49(3–4):430–440

47. Flaherty EG, Thompson R, Dubowitz H, et al. Adverse childhood experiences and child health in early adolescence. *JAMA Pediatr.* 2013;167(7):622–629

48. Green JG, McLaughlin KA, Berglund PA, et al. Childhood adversities and adult psychiatric disorders in the national comorbidity survey replication I: associations with first onset of DSM-IV disorders. *Arch Gen Psychiatry.* 2010;67(2):113–123

49. McLaughlin KA, Green JG, Gruber MJ, Sampson NA, Zaslavsky AM, Kessler RC. Childhood adversities and adult psychiatric disorders in the national comorbidity survey replication II: associations with persistence of DSM-IV disorders. *Arch Gen Psychiatry.* 2010;67(2):124–132

50. James B. *Handbook for the Treatment of Attachment Trauma Problems in Children.* New York, NY: The Free Press; 1994

51. Committee on Psychosocial Aspects of Child and Family Health and Task Force on Mental Health. Policy statement—the future of pediatrics: mental health competencies for pediatric primary care. *Pediatrics.* 2009;124(1):410–421

52. Styron T, Janoff-Bulman R. Childhood attachment and abuse: long-term effects on adult attachment, depression, and conflict resolution. *Child Abuse Negl.* 1997;21(10):1015–1023

53. Alexander P. The differential effects of abuse characteristics and attachment in the prediction of long-term effects of sexual abuse. *J Interpers Violence.* 1993;8(3):346–362

54. Cummings M, Berkowitz SJ, Scribano PV. Treatment of childhood sexual abuse: an updated review. *Curr Psychiatry Rep.* 2012;14(6):599–607

55. Gillies D, Taylor F, Gray C, O'Brien L, D'Abrew N. Psychological therapies for the treatment of post-traumatic stress disorder in children and adolescents. *Cochrane Database Syst Rev.* 2012;12(12):CD006726

56. Silverman WK, Ortiz CD, Viswesvaran C, et al. Evidence-based psychosocial treatments for children and adolescents exposed to traumatic events. *J Clin Child Adolesc Psychol.* 2008;37(1):156–183

57. Dorsey S, McLaughlin KA, Kerns SE, et al. Evidence base update for psychosocial treatments children and adolescents exposed to traumatic events. *J Clin Child Adolesc Psychol.* 2016;1–28

58. Forman-Hoffman VL, Zolotor AJ, McKeeman JL, et al. Comparative effectiveness of interventions for children exposed to nonrelational traumatic events. *Pediatrics.* 2013;131(3):526–539

59. National Child Traumatic Stress Network. Empirically supported treatments and promising practices. Los Angeles, CA and Durham, NC: National Center for Child Traumatic Stress; November 25, 2015. Available at: www.nctsnet.org/resources/topics/treatments-that-work/promising-practices Accessed June 13, 2016

60. Cohen J, Mannarino A, Deblinger E. *Treating Trauma and Traumatic Grief in Children and Adolescents.* New York, NY: Guilford Press; 2006

61. Cohen JA, Deblinger E, Mannarino AP, Steer RA. A multisite randomized controlled clinical trial for multiply traumatized children with sexual abuse-related PTSD symptoms. *J Am Acad Child Adolesc Psychiatry.* 2004;43(4):393–402

62. Cohen JA, Mannarino AP, Knudsen K. Treating sexually abused children: 1 year follow-up of a randomized controlled trial. *Child Abuse Negl.* 2005;29(2):135–145

63. Cohen JA, Mannarino AP, Kliethermes M, Murray LA. Trauma-focused CBT for youth with complex trauma. *Child Abuse Negl.* 2012;36(6):528–541

64. Kolko DJ. Individual cognitive behavioral treatment and family therapy for physically abused children and their offending parents: a comparison of clinical outcomes. *Child Maltreat.* 1996;1(4):322–342

65. Runyon MK, Deblinger E, Steer RA. Group cognitive behavioral treatment for parents and children at-risk for physical abuse: an initial study. *Child Fam Behav Ther.* 2010;32:196–218

66. Chaffin M, Hanson R, Saunders BE, et al. Report of the APSAC task force on attachment therapy, reactive attachment disorder, and attachment problems. *Child Maltreat.* 2006;11(1):76–89

67. Lieberman AF. Child-parent psychotherapy: a relationship-based approach to the treatment of mental health disorders in infancy and early childhood. In: Sameroff AJ, McDonough SC, Rosenblum KL, eds. *Treating Parent-Infant Relationship Problems.* New York, NY: Guilford Press; 2004:97–122

68. Hembree-Kigin TL, Bodiford McNeil C. *Parent-Child Interaction Therapy.* New York, NY: Plenum Press; 1995

69. Lieberman AF, Ghosh Ippen C, VAN Horn P. Child-parent psychotherapy: 6-month follow-up of a randomized controlled trial. *J Am Acad Child Adolesc Psychiatry.* 2006;45(8):913–918

70. Ghosh Ippen C, Harris WW, Van Horn P, Lieberman AF. Traumatic and stressful events in early childhood: can treatment help those at highest risk? *Child Abuse Negl.* 2011;35(7):504–513

71. Cicchetti D, Rogosch FA, Toth SL. Fostering secure attachment in infants in maltreating families through preventive interventions. *Dev Psychopathol.* 2006;18(3):623–649

72. Chaffin M, Funderburk B, Bard D, Valle LA, Gurwitch R. A combined motivation and parent-child interaction therapy package reduces child welfare recidivism in a randomized dismantling field trial. *J Consult Clin Psychol.* 2011;79(1):84–95

73. Scheeringa MS, Weems CF, Cohen JA, Amaya-Jackson L, Guthrie D. Trauma-focused cognitive-behavioral therapy for posttraumatic stress disorder in three-through six year-old children: a randomized clinical trial. *J Child Psychol Psychiatry.* 2011;52(8):853–860

74. Ford JD, Courtois CA, Steele K, Hart O, Nijenhuis ER. Treatment of complex posttraumatic self-dysregulation. *J Trauma Stress.* 2005;18(5):437–447

75. Cicchetti D, Rogosch FA, Toth SL. The efficacy of toddler-parent psychotherapy for fostering cognitive development in offspring of depressed mothers. *J Abnorm Child Psychol.* 2000;28(2):135–148

76. Dozier M, Lindhiem O, Ackerman J. Attachment and biobehavioral catch-up. In: Berlin L, Ziv Y, Amaya-Jackson L, Greenberg MT, eds. *Enhancing Early Attachments*. New York, NY: Guilford Press; 2005:178–194

77. Dozier M, Lindhiem O, Lewis E, Bick J, Bernard K, Peloso E. Effects of a foster parent training program on young children's attachment behaviors: preliminary evidence from a randomized clinical trial. *Child Adolesc Social Work J*. 2009;26(4):321–332

78. Dozier M, Fisher PA. Neuroscience enhanced child maltreatment interventions to improve outcomes. *Soc Res Child Dev Policy Rep*. 2014;28(1):25–27

79. Farmer EM, Burns BJ, Wagner HR, Murray M, Southerland DG. Enhancing "usual practice" treatment foster care: findings from a randomized trial on improving youths' outcomes. *Psychiatr Serv*. 2010;61(6):555–561

80. BigFoot DS, Schmidt SR. Honoring children, mending the circle: cultural adaptation of trauma-focused cognitive-behavioral therapy for American Indian and Alaska native children. *J Clin Psychol*. 2010;66(8):847–856

81. Council on Foster Care, Adoption, and Kinship Care; Committee on Adolescence, and Council on Early Childhood. Health care issues for children and adolescents in foster care and kinship care. *Pediatrics*. 2015;136(4). Available at: www.pediatrics.org/cgi/content/full/136/4/e1131

82. Szilagyi MA, Rosen DS, Rubin D, Zlotnik S; Council on Foster Care, Adoption, and Kinship Care; Committee on Adolescence, and Council on Early Childhood. Technical report: health care issues for of children and adolescents in foster care and kinship care. *Pediatrics*. 2015;136(4). Available at: www.pediatrics.org/cgi/content/full/136/4/e1142

83. American Academy of Pediatrics, Committee on Early Childhood, Adoption, and Dependent Care. American Academy of Pediatrics. Committee on Early Childhood and Adoption and Dependent Care. Developmental issues for young children in foster care. *Pediatrics*. 2000;106(5):1145–1150

84. Leslie LK, Hurlburt MS, Landsverk J, Rolls JA, Wood PA, Kelleher KJ. Comprehensive assessments for children entering foster care: a national perspective. *Pediatrics*. 2003;112(1 Pt 1):134–142

85. Greeson JK, Briggs EC, Kisiel CL, et al. Complex trauma and mental health in children and adolescents placed in foster care: findings from the National Child Traumatic Stress Network. *Child Welfare*. 2011;90(6):91–108

86. Layne CM, Strand V, Popescu M, et al. Using the core curriculum on childhood trauma to strengthen clinical knowledge in evidence-based practitioners. *J Clin Child Adolesc Psychol*. 2014;43(2):286–300

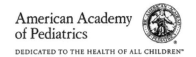

Guidance for the Clinician in
Rendering Pediatric Care

CLINICAL REPORT

Psychological Maltreatment

abstract

Psychological or emotional maltreatment of children may be the most challenging and prevalent form of child abuse and neglect. Caregiver behaviors include acts of omission (ignoring need for social interactions) or commission (spurning, terrorizing); may be verbal or nonverbal, active or passive, and with or without intent to harm; and negatively affect the child's cognitive, social, emotional, and/or physical development. Psychological maltreatment has been linked with disorders of attachment, developmental and educational problems, socialization problems, disruptive behavior, and later psychopathology. Although no evidence-based interventions that can prevent psychological maltreatment have been identified to date, it is possible that interventions shown to be effective in reducing overall types of child maltreatment, such as the Nurse Family Partnership, may have a role to play. Furthermore, prevention before occurrence will require both the use of universal interventions aimed at promoting the type of parenting that is now recognized to be necessary for optimal child development, alongside the use of targeted interventions directed at improving parental sensitivity to a child's cues during infancy and later parent-child interactions. Intervention should, first and foremost, focus on a thorough assessment and ensuring the child's safety. Potentially effective treatments include cognitive behavioral parenting programs and other psychotherapeutic interventions. The high prevalence of psychological abuse in advanced Western societies, along with the serious consequences, point to the importance of effective management. Pediatricians should be alert to the occurrence of psychological maltreatment and identify ways to support families who have risk indicators for, or evidence of, this problem. *Pediatrics* 2012;130:372–378

Roberta Hibbard, MD, Jane Barlow, DPhil, Harriet MacMillan, MD, and the Committee on Child Abuse and Neglect and AMERICAN ACADEMY OF CHILD AND ADOLESCENT PSYCHIATRY, Child Maltreatment and Violence Committee

KEY WORDS
psychological maltreatment, child abuse, emotional maltreatment, neglect, verbal abuse, development

ABBREVIATIONS
AAP—American Academy of Pediatrics
NFP—nurse family partnership

This document is copyrighted and is property of the American Academy of Pediatrics and its Board of Directors. All authors have filed conflict of interest statements with the American Academy of Pediatrics. Any conflicts have been resolved through a process approved by the Board of Directors. The American Academy of Pediatrics has neither solicited nor accepted any commercial involvement in the development of the content of this publication.

The guidance in this report does not indicate an exclusive course of treatment or serve as a standard of medical care. Variations, taking into account individual circumstances, may be appropriate.

www.pediatrics.org/cgi/doi/10.1542/peds.2012-1552

doi:10.1542/peds.2012-1552

All clinical reports from the American Academy of Pediatrics automatically expire 5 years after publication unless reaffirmed, revised, or retired at or before that time.

PEDIATRICS (ISSN Numbers: Print, 0031-4005; Online, 1098-4275).

INTRODUCTION

Psychological or emotional maltreatment of children and adolescents may be the most challenging and prevalent form of child abuse and neglect, but until recently, it has received relatively little attention. The American Academy of Pediatrics (AAP) reviewed the topic in a technical report in 2002.[1] This clinical report updates the pediatrician on current knowledge and approaches to psychological maltreatment, with guidance on its identification and effective methods of prevention and treatments/intervention.

DEFINITION

There is no universally agreed definition of psychological maltreatment or emotional maltreatment, terms that are often used interchangeably. Psychological maltreatment encompasses both the cognitive and affective components of maltreatment.[2] One of the difficulties in clearly defining what such maltreatment comprises involves the absence of a strong societal consensus on the distinction between psychological maltreatment and suboptimal parenting.[3] Exposure to psychological maltreatment is considered when acts of omission or commission inflict harm on the child's well-being, which may then be manifested as emotional distress or maladaptive behavior in the child. Psychological maltreatment is difficult to identify, in part because such maltreatment involves "a relationship between the parent and the child rather than an event or a series of repeated events occurring within the parent-child relationship."[4] Isolated incidents of behaviors identified in Table 1 do not necessarily constitute psychological abuse. Psychological maltreatment refers to a repeated pattern of parental behavior that is likely to be interpreted by a child that he or she is unloved, unwanted, or serves only instrumental purposes and/or that severely undermines the child's development and socialization.[4] Recent conceptualization[5] of psychological maltreatment focuses on the caregiver's behaviors as opposed to the disturbed behaviors in the child. Such behaviors of the caregiver include acts of omission (ignoring the need for social interaction) or commission (spurning, terrorizing); may be verbal or nonverbal, active or passive, and with or without intent to harm; and negatively affect the child's cognitive, social, emotional, and/or physical development. Table 1 summarizes the different types of psychologically abusive caregivers' behaviors across 6 main categories.[2,5]

Although the psychological components of any form of child maltreatment are key to understanding its effects, psychological maltreatment is often not recognized when other forms of maltreatment coexist.[3] When psychological maltreatment occurs alone, it can be even harder to identify, and opportunities for intervention may be missed. This form of child maltreatment is possibly the most underreported to authorities.[3,6]

DISTRIBUTION OF PSYCHOLOGICAL MALTREATMENT

A recent review of the burden and consequences of psychological abuse concluded that, although there were few studies reporting its prevalence, a number of large population-based, self-report studies in the United Kingdom and United States found that approximately 8% to 9% of women and 4% of men reported exposure to severe psychological abuse during childhood.[7] This review found even higher rates reported in Eastern Europe. A number of US surveys found that psychological and emotional maltreatment were the most frequently self-reported forms of victimization.[8]

DETERMINANTS OF PSYCHOLOGICAL MALTREATMENT

Although it is recognized that psychological maltreatment occurs in a wide range of families, it is more often associated with multiple family stresses[9] and, in particular, with factors such as family conflict, adult mental health problems, and parental substance abuse[10] that may be co-occurring.[11] For example, some parental mental health problems are associated with unpredictable and frightening behaviors, and others (particularly depression) are linked with parental withdrawal and neglect.[12,13] Similarly, in terms of family conflict, attacks on a parent almost always frighten a child, even if the child is not the direct target. Threats or actual violence as part of a pattern of aggression against one parent will sometimes exploit the other parent's or child's fears.[14,15] Children exposed to violence in the home are at disproportionate risk of injury,

TABLE 1 Types of Psychologically Abusive Behaviors by Caregivers

Spurning	• Belittling, denigrating, or other rejecting • Ridiculing for showing normal emotions • Singling out or humiliating in public
Terrorizing	• Placing in unpredictable/chaotic circumstances • Placing in recognizably dangerous situations • Having rigid/unrealistic expectations accompanied by threats if not met • Threatening/perpetrating violence against child or child's loved ones/objects
Isolating	• Confining within environment • Restricting social interactions in community
Exploiting/Corrupting	• Modeling, permitting, or encouraging antisocial or developmentally inappropriate behavior • Restricting/undermining psychological autonomy • Restricting/interfering with cognitive development
Denying emotional responsiveness	• Being detached or uninvolved; interacting only when necessary • Providing little or no warmth, nurturing, praise during any developmental period in childhood
Mental health/medical/educational neglect	• Limiting a child's access to necessary health care because of reasons other than inadequate resources • Refusing to provide for serious emotional/behavioral, physical health, or educational needs

Adapted from Hart et al[2] and Brassard et al.[5]

eating disorders, and self-harm,[16] even when they are not themselves victims of physical violence. The AAP statement "Intimate Partner Violence: The Role of the Pediatrician" deals with how such issues should be addressed.[17] Although there is a paucity of literature specifically addressing the issue of parental substance abuse and psychological maltreatment,[18] substance abuse on the part of one or both parents is associated with high rates of child maltreatment.[19,20]

ASSOCIATED IMPAIRMENT

Precisely because it interferes with a child's developmental trajectory, psychological maltreatment has been linked with disorders of attachment, developmental and educational problems, socialization problems, and disruptive behavior.[21,22] Research involving institutionalized Romanian orphans demonstrated the effects of severe emotional and sensory deprivation on later IQ, executive function and memory, psychological processing, attachment, and psychiatric disorders.[23,24] The effects of psychological maltreatment during the first 3 years of life can be particularly profound, because rapid and extensive growth of the brain and biological systems takes place during this period, and this growth is significantly influenced by the young child's environment and, in particular, the early parenting that he or she receives.[25] Psychological maltreatment also negatively affects the organization of the child's attachment to important adults in his or her life.[26,27] Longitudinal studies have shown that impairment in security of attachment is associated with a range of later problems,[27] because early parenting plays a significant role in influencing children's beliefs about themselves (ie, in terms of the extent to which they are lovable) and about themselves in relation to other people

(ie, when they have needs, people will respond appropriately to them). The research suggests that these internalized beliefs can affect children's later cognitive schemas and, thereby, their psychological adjustment.[28]

Psychological maltreatment in early childhood is also associated with insecure attachment in adulthood.[29] A recent overview of the evidence found that as the child grows older, such attachment problems interfere with a number of aspects of later functioning, including peer relations, intimacy, caregiving and caretaking, sexual functioning, conflict resolution, and relational aggression.[29] The findings from longitudinal[30] and retrospective[28] studies also suggest a strong association with psychiatric morbidity. For example, one longitudinal study found that psychological unavailability and neglect in early childhood were associated with increased social problems, delinquency, aggression, and attempted suicide in adolescents and also that most psychologically abused children received at least 1 diagnosis of mental illness, with three-quarters having comorbid conditions for 2 or more disorders. Factors that may influence the effects of the abuse include early caregiving experiences; frequency, intensity, and duration of the abuse; factors intrinsic to the child, such as behavioral and coping strategies, self-esteem, and disposition; and the availability of supportive relationships.[31] For example, although the evidence does not relate specifically to psychological maltreatment, 1 study found that boys who experienced abuse that started before 12 years of age had more serious problems (eg, arrests and severity of delinquency) compared with boys who were abused after 12 years of age.[32] Without intervention, the cycle of abuse is often repeated in the next generation.[29]

Psychological maltreatment carries a significant burden for society, as can

be seen in its effects on the health and social care systems,[33] such as the costs of educational failure, crime, and health services as a result of poor mental health.

ASSESSMENT

Psychological maltreatment poses a real challenge to pediatricians dedicated to ensuring the health and well-being of children. Pediatricians need to be alert to the possibility of psychological maltreatment and consider such exposure in any assessment of psychological and behavioral conditions in childhood. Just as history about a psychological or behavioral problem should be obtained from multiple informants whenever possible, this is also the case when considering whether a child is being exposed to psychological maltreatment. Much emphasis has been placed on appropriate skills for interviewing children about sexual abuse, but it is also important to develop approaches for asking children about their relationships with caregivers, experiences of discipline (some psychological maltreatment occurs in this context), and feelings of self-worth, safety, and being loved. Once it is possible to interview a child from a developmental standpoint and the pediatrician is comfortable doing so, an individual interview with the child becomes important for assessment of any concerns of major psychological or behavioral problems. Even very young children, once they are speaking in sentences, can often provide this information. It is important to interview children alone, away from their caregivers, because they may be experiencing maltreatment from the very caregivers who accompanied them to an appointment. The AAP resources, Bright Futures[34] and Addressing Mental Health Concerns in Primary Care, A Clinician's Toolkit[35] provide guidance that may be helpful in approaching these issues. The pediatrician needs to be aware of risk indicators for psychological maltreatment, such as parental psychiatric illness, including depression and substance abuse, among others. It is also important to be aware of the psychological maltreatment that can accompany exposure to intimate partner violence, although this is considered a separate type of maltreatment and is the focus of a previous AAP report as outlined above.[17] For children of all ages, major caregivers need to be interviewed (this should be performed individually to ensure the parent's safety when asking about such issues as intimate partner violence), and information should be gathered from teachers or child care personnel. Even brief telephone contact with school or child care personnel can be helpful in assessing a child's exposure to psychological maltreatment. Because this can be time consuming, ideally, the task of obtaining this information can be shared with another member of the pediatrician's office staff. Consultation with a pediatrician who has expertise in assessing child maltreatment or a mental health professional may assist the pediatrician in completing an assessment and plan.

Although there are no specific physical indicators for psychological maltreatment, it is essential to assess a child's growth and development, because these can be impaired in association with exposure to psychological maltreatment. The extent of impairment can vary; severe forms of psychological deprivation can be associated with psychosocial short stature, a condition of short stature or growth failure formerly known as psychosocial dwarfism.[36] Observing a child and parent(s) together can provide valuable information about the quality of their relationship and ability of a parent to respond to a child, although appropriate behavior by a parent in the context of a brief office visit does not rule out the possibility that a child is experiencing psychological maltreatment. Conversely, a single interaction that is of concern between a parent and child is generally not diagnostic of psychological maltreatment. Close clinical follow-up may be needed to clarify any issues of concern.

As outlined in the earlier technical report on this topic,[1] reporting of psychological maltreatment can be difficult. In some jurisdictions, clear indication of impairment in growth and/or development may be necessary for a child protective services agency to accept a report; detailed documentation is essential in such situations. It is important that the pediatrician record specific statements from the child, the family, and other sources and that the pediatrician is systematic in assessing the child's behavioral, psychological, and physical status in relation to the baseline assessment. For example, the pediatrician who has been providing general pediatric care to a child whose parents become involved in an extremely contentious custody/access dispute can alert the parents to the potential for the child to experience psychological trauma and can be aware of early indicators of impairment in the child. If identification for the parents of a child being exposed to potential psychological maltreatment does not lead to improvement in parenting behavior, the pediatrician can then make referrals to such services as mediation, mental health services, or child protective services. Careful follow-up is very important, because parents who are psychologically abusive may not be reliable in providing information about their child's functioning or their own response to intervention.

PREVENTION

The potential for major impairment associated with psychological maltreatment during the early years of life underscores the importance of identifying approach to intervention in infancy and toddlerhood. Prevention before occurrence involves both the use of universal interventions aimed at promoting the type of parenting that is now recognized to be necessary for optimal child development, alongside the use of targeted interventions directed at improving parental sensitivity to infant cues. This would include, for example, the recommendation that all routine contact between professionals and parents be used as an opportunity to promote sensitive and attuned parenting using a range of approaches (including media-based strategies, such as leaflets, books, and videos, among others) and to observe and identify parent-child interactions that require further intervention using targeted approaches. Although it is unknown whether these strategies actually prevent psychological maltreatment, there is preliminary evidence to suggest that the use of population strategies of this nature show promise in the prevention of child maltreatment generally.[37]

Targeted programs aimed at preventing early indicators of psychological abuse often focus on infants and younger children.[38] Much less is known about approaches to preventing psychological maltreatment in the older age groups. Specifically, maternal insensitivity to infant cues,[39] which is associated with insecure attachment, is a significant predictor of socioemotional maladaptation.[27] A meta-analysis of attachment-based interventions that ranged from home-visiting programs to parent-infant psychotherapy, found significant improvements in maternal sensitivity (d = 0.33) and infant attachment insecurity (d = 0.22).[40]

Greater effectiveness was associated with programs that included several sessions and had a clear behavioral focus. Maternal insensitivity is an important element of psychologically harmful parent-child relationships; brief focused interventions, such as those involving video feedback and attachment discussion, might improve insensitive parenting, but there is no direct evidence at this time that these interventions prevent psychological maltreatment. Furthermore, interventions to date have focused on maternal-child interactions; it is important to address paternal-child interactions as well as other significant caregiving relationships.

One targeted program that has been shown effective in preventing child maltreatment generally is the Nurse Family Partnership (NFP), an intensive home-visitation program provided by nurses to low-income first-time mothers beginning prenatally and during infancy.[41] Because the goals of the NFP include assisting women to promote healthy prenatal behaviors and parents' competent care of their children, it is possible that the NFP could prevent psychological maltreatment as part of the overall reduction in maltreatment, but its effectiveness in preventing this specific type of maltreatment has not been assessed.

TREATMENT

Despite ongoing debate about the role of formal child protection processes for dealing with psychological maltreatment,[42] there is agreement about the need to intervene early to minimize poor outcomes. It is important to consider what is known about approaches to prevent recurrence of psychological maltreatment and treat associated impairment, once it has been identified. There is a paucity of studies evaluating the effectiveness of approaches specifically designed for

parents or caregivers who psychologically abuse their children. One randomized trial compared 2 group-based cognitive-behavioral therapy parenting programs (standard and enhanced models of the Triple-P Program) aimed at psychologically abusive parents.[43] The standard program focused on child-management strategies, and the enhanced model included components to alter parental anger and misattributions. Both groups made gains, there was no actual control group, and many parents had self-referred, reducing the generalizability of the results. Parents who are psychologically abusive may not be able to recognize their own behavior and self-refer.[44] Results of another trial suggest that a preschool child-parent psychotherapy program may be beneficial in improving specific aspects of the mother-child relationship, but further research is necessary.[45] A number of innovative methods of working with parents with mental health[46] and substance misuse problems have recently been developed and evaluated.[47]

There is major need for research to develop and test effective treatments for children who have experienced psychological maltreatment, either alone or in combination with other forms of maltreatment.

GUIDANCE FOR THE PEDIATRICIAN

Psychological maltreatment is just as harmful as other types of maltreatment. Although little is known about approaches to its prevention or treatment, it is important for pediatricians to be alert to its occurrence and consider ways to support families who have risk indicators for this problem. Pediatricians should develop approaches for asking children about their relationships with caregivers, experiences of discipline and feelings of self-worth, safety, and being loved.

Bright Futures[34] and the Addressing Mental Health Concerns in Primary Care toolkit[35] are resources that can assist the pediatrician in the evaluation; however, they are not specific to psychological maltreatment.

The pediatrician should encourage parents who are experiencing mental health problems, intimate partner violence, or substance misuse to consider the effects of such conditions on their parenting and assist them in accessing appropriate resources, such as referrals to mental health professionals and substance misuse treatment programs. With respect to identification of psychological maltreatment, Rees[48] suggests that pediatricians need to be "as confident in assessing inadequate emotional care as physical and sexual abuse." This might include an assessment of parent-child interactions through the use of interviews or consultation with other clinicians, such as mental health providers, to assess the child's feelings and understanding about the situation. As with other types of child maltreatment, children showing signs of behavioral and psychological problems should be assessed to identify specific conditions, such as depression or posttraumatic stress disorder, for which there are evidence-based treatments, such as cognitive-behavioral therapy. Several trauma-specific interviews have been developed to determine whether children and adolescents presenting with mental health problems have been exposed to maltreatment.[49] To date, such instruments have been used mainly in research settings, but studies are increasingly examining their clinical applicability.

Although the evidence is limited with regard to interventions for psychological maltreatment, it is important for pediatricians to refer families for additional assessment and treatment if psychological abuse or neglect is suspected, in addition to referring to child protective services in accordance with individual state laws, and follow-up appointments should be made so that the progress of the situation can be monitored.

Another equally important aspect of responding to psychological maltreatment is professional communication; collaboration among pediatric, psychiatric, and child protective services professionals is essential in formulating a management plan for a child at risk for or experiencing psychological maltreatment. Specific goals need to be put in place, and in cases where exposure to psychological maltreatment persists, the pediatrician should advocate for the needs of the child to remain paramount. Although efforts should focus on ways to assist the family with the child remaining in the home, it is important for the pediatrician to be alert to situations in which a child's needs are better met outside the home, either on a temporary or permanent basis. Consideration of out-of-home care interventions should not be restricted to cases of physical or sexual abuse; children exposed to psychological maltreatment may also require a level of protection that necessitates removal from the parental home.

Pediatricians are uniquely positioned to educate those working in child welfare, child health care, and the judicial system about the complex needs of children exposed to psychological maltreatment. Because determination of and response to psychological maltreatment by child protective services can vary considerably across regions, pediatricians can assist child protective services workers in understanding the effects of exposure to maltreatment on the child as well as possible resources for intervention. Because less is known about psychological maltreatment and it has been recognized relatively recently compared with other subtypes of abuse and neglect, there is even less standardization of approaches to investigation and intervention by child protective services agencies. The pediatrician is well situated to advocate on behalf of the child and can take on an important liaison role with professionals in the child welfare system.

LEAD AUTHORS
Roberta Hibbard, MD
Jane Barlow, DPhil
Harriet MacMillan, MD

COMMITTEE ON CHILD ABUSE AND NEGLECT, 2011–2012
Cindy W. Christian, MD
James E. Crawford-Jakubiak, MD
Emalee G. Flaherty, MD
John M. Leventhal, MD
James L. Lukefahr, MD
Robert D. Sege MD, PhD

FORMER COMMITTEE MEMBER
Roberta Hibbard, MD

LIAISONS
Harriet MacMillan, MD – *American Academy of Child and Adolescent Psychiatry*
Catherine M. Nolan, MSW, ACSW – *Administration for Children, Youth, and Families*
Janet Saul, PhD – *Centers for Disease Control and Prevention*

STAFF
Tammy Piazza Hurley

ACKNOWLEDGMENT
The authors gratefully acknowledge the assistance of the Family Violence Prevention Unit, Public Health Agency of Canada, in the development of this paper.

REFERENCES

1. Kairys SW, Johnson CF; Committee on Child Abuse and Neglect. Technical report: the psychological maltreatment of children. *Pediatrics*. 2002;109(4). Available at: www.pediatrics.org/cgi/content/full/109/4/e68

2. Hart SN, Brassard MR, Binggeli NJ, Davidson HA. Psychological maltreatment. In: Myers JEB, Berliner LA, Briere JN, Hendrix CT, Reid TA, Jenny CA, eds. *The APSAC Handbook on Child Maltreatment*. Thousand Oaks, CA: Sage Publications; 2002:79–104

3. Trickett PK, Mennen FE, Kim K, Sang J. Emotional abuse in a sample of multiply maltreated, urban young adolescents: issues of definition and identification. *Child Abuse Negl*. 2009;33(1):27–35

4. Glaser D. Emotional abuse and neglect (psychological maltreatment): a conceptual framework. *Child Abuse Negl*. 2002;26(6-7):697–714

5. Brassard MR, Donovan KL. Defining psychological maltreatment. In: Feerick MM, Knutson JF, Trickett PK, Flanzer SM, eds. *Child Abuse and Neglect: Definitions, Classifications, and a Framework for Research*. Baltimore, MD: Paul H Brookes Publishing Co Inc; 2006:3–27

6. Barnett O, Miller-Perrin CL, Perrin RD. Child psychological maltreatment. In: Barnett O, Miller-Perrin C-L, Perrin RD, eds. *Family Violence Across the Lifespan: An Introduction*. 2nd ed. Thousand Oaks, CA: Sage Publications; 2005:151–178.

7. Gilbert R, Widom CS, Browne K, Fergusson D, Webb E, Janson S. Burden and consequences of child maltreatment in high-income countries. *Lancet*. 2009;373(9657):68–81

8. Reyome ND. Childhood emotional maltreatment and later intimate relationships: themes from the empirical literature. *J Aggress Maltreat Trauma*. 2010;19:224–242

9. Doyle C. Emotional abuse of children: issues for intervention. *Child Abuse Rev*. 2002;6:330–342.

10. Department of Health, Home Office, Department for Education and Employment. *Working Together to Safeguard Children: A Guide to Inter-agency Working to Safeguard and Promote the Welfare of Children*. London, England: The Stationery Office; 2006.

11. Stromwall LK, Larson NC, Nieri T, et al. Parents with co-occurring mental health and substance abuse conditions involved in Child Protection Services: clinical profile and treatment needs. *Child Welfare*. 2008; 87(3):95–113

12. Loh CC, Vostanis P. Perceived mother-infant relationship difficulties in postnatal depression. *Infant Child Dev.* 2004; 13:159–171

13. Foster CJ, Garber J, Durlak JA. Current and past maternal depression, maternal interaction behaviors, and children's externalizing and internalizing symptoms. *J Abnorm Child Psychol.* 2008;36(4):527–537

14. Creighton S, Russell N. *Voices from Childhood: A Survey of Childhood Experiences and Attitudes to Childrearing among Adults in the United Kingdom.* London, England: National Society for Prevention of Cruelty to Children; 1995

15. Bifulco A, Moran P. *Wednesday's Child: Research into Women's Experience of Neglect and Abuse in Childhood.* London, England: Routledge; 1998

16. World Health Organization. *World Report on Violence and Health.* Geneva, Switzerland: World Health Organization; 2002. Available at: www.who.int/violence_injury_prevention/violence/world_report. Accessed December 17, 2011

17. Thackeray JD, Hibbard R, Dowd MD; Committee on Child Abuse and Neglect; Committee on Injury, Violence, and Poison Prevention. Intimate partner violence: the role of the pediatrician. *Pediatrics.* 2010;125(5):1094–1100

18. Straussner SLA, Fewell CH. Preface. *J Soc Work Pract Addict.* 2006;6:xxi–xxviii

19. Ammerman RT, Kolko DJ, Kirisci L, Blackson TC, Dawes MA. Child abuse potential in parents with histories of substance use disorder. *Child Abuse Negl.* 1999;23(12):1225–1238

20. Chaffin M, Kelleher K, Hollenberg J. Onset of physical abuse and neglect: psychiatric substance abuse, and social risk factors from prospective community data. *Child Abuse Negl.* 1996;20(3):191–203.

21. Iwaniec D. An overview of emotional maltreatment and failure-to-thrive. *Child Abuse Rev.* 1997;6:370–388

22. Erickson M, Egeland B, Pianta R. The effects of maltreatment on the development of young children. In: Cicchetti D, Carlson V, eds. *Child Maltreatment: Theory and Research on the Causes and Consequences of Child Abuse and Neglect.* New York, NY: Cambridge University Press; 1989:647–684

23. Zeanah CH, Egger HL, Smyke AT, et al. Institutional rearing and psychiatric disorders in Romanian preschool children. *Am J Psychiatry.* 2009;166(7):777–785

24. Zeanah CH, Nelson CA, Fox NA, et al. Designing research to study the effects of institutionalization on brain and behavioral development: the Bucharest Early Intervention Project. *Dev Psychopathol.* 2003; 15(4):885–907

25. Schore AN. *Affect Regulation and the Origin of the Self: The Neurobiology of Emotional Development.* Hillsdale, NJ: Lawrence Erlbaum Associates; 1994

26. Jacobvitz D, Hazen N, Riggs S. Disorganized mental processes in mother, frightening/frightened caregiving and disorganized behavior in infancy. Paper presented at The Meeting of the Society of Research in Child Development. Washington, DC: Society of Research in Child Development; 1997

27. Sroufe LA. Attachment and development: a prospective, longitudinal study from birth to adulthood. *Attach Hum Dev.* 2005;7(4): 349–367

28. Wright MO, Crawford E, Del Castillo D. Childhood emotional maltreatment and later psychological distress among college students: the mediating role of maladaptive schemas. *Child Abuse Negl.* 2009;33(1):59–68

29. Riggs S, Kaminski P. Childhood emotional abuse, adult attachment, and depression as predictors of relational adjustment and psychological aggression. *J Aggress Maltreat Trauma.* 2010;19(4):75–104

30. Egeland B. Taking stock: childhood emotional maltreatment and developmental psychopathology. *Child Abuse Negl.* 2009;33(1):22–26

31. Iwaniec D, Larkin E, Higgins S. Research review: risks and resilience in cases of emotional abuse. *Child Fam Soc Work.* 2006;11:73–82

32. Smith CA, Thornberry TP. The relationship between childhood maltreatment and adolescent involvement in delinquency. *Criminology.* 1995;33(4):451–481

33. Glaser D, Prior V, Lynch M. *Emotional Abuse and Emotional Neglect: Antecedents, Operational Definitions and Consequences.* York, United Kingdom: BASPCAN; 2001:iii–iv.

34. Hagan JF, Shaw JS, Duncan P, eds. *Bright Futures: Guidelines for Health Supervision of Infants, Children, and Adolescents.* 3rd ed. Elk Grove Village, IL: American Academy of Pediatrics; 2008:77–107

35. American Academy of Pediatrics, Task Force on Mental Health. *Addressing Mental Health Concerns in Primary Care: A Clinician's Toolkit* [CD-ROM]. Elk Grove Village, IL: American Academy of Pediatrics; 2010

36. Muñoz-Hoyos A, Molina-Carballo A, Augustin-Morales M, et al. Psychosocial dwarfism: psychopathological aspects and putative neuroendocrine markers. *Psychiatry Res.* 2011;188(1):96–101

37. Prinz RJ, Sanders MR, Shapiro CJ, Whitaker DJ, Lutzker JR. Population-based prevention of child maltreatment: the U.S. Triple P system population trial. *Prev Sci.* 2009;10 (1):1–12

38. MacMillan HL, Wathen CN, Barlow J, Fergusson DM, Leventhal JM, Taussig HN. Interventions to prevent child maltreatment and associated impairment. *Lancet.* 2009;373(9659):250–266

39. Barlow J, Schrader-MacMillan A. *Safeguarding Children from Emotional Maltreatment: What Works?* London, England: Jessica Kingsley; 2010

40. Bakermans-Kranenburg MJ, van IJzendoorn MH, Juffer F. Less is more: meta-analyses of sensitivity and attachment interventions in early childhood. *Psychol Bull.* 2003;129(2): 195–215

41. Olds DL, Sadler L, Kitzman H. Programs for parents of infants and toddlers: recent evidence from randomized trials. *J Child Psychol Psychiatry.* 2007;48(3-4): 355–391

42. Glaser D, Prior, V. Is the term child protection applicable to emotional abuse? *Child Abuse Rev.* 1998;6:315–329

43. Sanders MR, Pidgeon AM, Gravestock F, et al. Does parental attributional retraining and anger management enhance the effects of the Triple P-Positive Parenting Program with parents at risk of child maltreatment? *Behav Ther.* 2004;35(3):513–535

44. Boulton S, Hindle D. Emotional abuse: the work of a multidisciplinary consultation group in a child psychiatric service. *Clin Child Psychol Psychiatry.* 2000;5(3):439–452

45. Toth SL, Maughan A, Manly JT, Spagnola M, Cicchetti D. The relative efficacy of two interventions in altering maltreated preschool children's representational models: implications for attachment theory. *Dev Psychopathol.* 2002;14(4):877–908

46. Slade A, Sadler LS, De Dios-Kenn C, Webb D, Currier-Ezepchick J, Mayes LC. Minding the baby a reflective parenting program. *Psychoanal Study Child.* 2005;60:74–100

47. Dawe S, Harnett P. Reducing potential for child abuse among methadone-maintained parents: results from a randomized controlled trial. *J Subst Abuse Treat.* 2007;32(4):381–390

48. Rees CA. Understanding emotional abuse. *Arch Dis Child.* 2010;95(1):59–67

49. Gilbert R, Kemp A, Thoburn J, et al. Recognising and responding to child maltreatment. *Lancet.* 2009;373(9658):167–180

SECTION 6
Mental Health Emergencies

American Academy
of Pediatrics
DEDICATED TO THE HEALTH OF ALL CHILDREN™

POLICY STATEMENT

Pediatric Mental Health Emergencies in the Emergency Medical Services System

Organizational Principles to Guide and Define the Child Care Health System and/or Improve the Health of All Children

AMERICAN ACADEMY OF PEDIATRICS
Committee on Pediatric Emergency Medicine
AMERICAN COLLEGE OF EMERGENCY PHYSICIANS
Pediatric Emergency Medicine Committee

Endorsed by the American Academy of Child and Adolescent Psychiatry and the American Academy of Family Physicians.

ABSTRACT

Emergency departments are vital in the management of pediatric patients with mental health emergencies. Pediatric mental health emergencies are an increasing part of emergency medical practice because emergency departments have become the safety net for a fragmented mental health infrastructure that is experiencing critical shortages in services in all sectors. Emergency departments must safely, humanely, and in a culturally and developmentally appropriate manner manage pediatric patients with undiagnosed and known mental illnesses, including those with mental retardation, autistic spectrum disorders, and attention-deficit/hyperactivity disorder and those experiencing a behavioral crisis. Emergency departments also manage patients with suicidal ideation, depression, escalating aggression, substance abuse, posttraumatic stress disorder, and maltreatment and those exposed to violence and unexpected deaths. Emergency departments must address not only the physical but also the mental health needs of patients during and after mass-casualty incidents and disasters. The American Academy of Pediatrics and the American College of Emergency Physicians support advocacy for increased mental health resources, including improved pediatric mental health tools for the emergency department, increased mental health insurance coverage, and adequate reimbursement at all levels; acknowledgment of the importance of the child's medical home; and promotion of education and research for mental health emergencies.

STATEMENT

PEDIATRIC mental health emergencies constitute a large and growing segment of pediatric emergency medical care. Emergency departments (EDs) play a critical role in the evaluation and management of child and adolescent patients with mental health emergencies. Community mental health resources have diminished and, in some regions, even disappeared through inpatient bed shortages, private and public health insurance changes, reorganization of state mental health programs, and shortages of pediatric-trained mental health specialists. These changes have resulted in critical shortages of inpatient and outpatient mental health services for children.[1] The ED has increasingly become the safety net for a fragmented mental health infrastructure in which the needs of children and adolescents, among the most vulnerable populations, have been insufficiently addressed.

ED staff must safely, humanely, and in a culturally sensitive manner manage patients with exacerbations of known diagnosed mental illnesses as well as those

www.pediatrics.org/cgi/doi/10.1542/peds.2006-1925

doi:10.1542/peds.2006-1925

All policy statements from the American Academy of Pediatrics automatically expire 5 years after publication unless reaffirmed, revised, or retired at or before that time.

Key Words
emergency department, mental health emergencies, school and community mental health services, medical home

Abbreviation
ED—emergency department

with mental retardation, autistic spectrum disorders, and attention-deficit/hyperactivity disorder or those who are having a behavioral crisis. They also must identify and manage patients with previously undiagnosed and/or undetected conditions such as suicidal ideation, depression, escalating aggression, substance abuse, and posttraumatic stress disorder.[2] ED personnel evaluate and treat trauma patients, physically and sexually maltreated children, and children exposed to community and domestic violence and also must deal with unexpected deaths of children in the ED. Violence-related situations may involve pediatric victims and/or pediatric-aged perpetrators of violence. In many states, adolescents can seek and receive care for mental health issues and drug/alcohol use without parental involvement, and confidentiality must be maintained unless the child is at risk of harming himself/herself or others. The ED staff must also recognize the primary support role of the family and caregivers in all phases of pediatric mental illness.

EDs play a critical role in mass-casualty occurrences and disasters, and staff must address the unique mental health needs of children during and after these events. A strong and growing body of evidence indicates that emotional and physical trauma to children can cause neurochemical and structural brain changes resulting in posttraumatic stress disorder and can affect some children into their adult lives.[1–12] Emotional trauma may be ameliorated by timely, culturally appropriate, pediatric-specific stress intervention that may be implemented in the initial hours after the trauma.[13,14]

The epidemiologic and outcome data on pediatric mental health emergencies are insufficient, but there is evidence that pediatric mental health concerns are commonly unaddressed.[15,16] Pediatric mental health emergencies are frequently not recognized as such, presenting initially as trauma or somatic complaints, and are, therefore, underrepresented in the existing data.[17–20] The challenges to an already overburdened ED "safety net" are to provide safe, humane, and culturally and developmentally sensitive triage, diagnosis, stabilization, initial management, and treatment and referral for a broad spectrum of mental health emergencies, working within a mental health infrastructure in crisis.

Pediatric mental health emergencies are best managed by a skilled, multidisciplinary team approach, including specialized screening tools, pediatric-trained mental health consultants, the availability of pediatric psychiatric facilities when hospitalization is necessary, and an outpatient infrastructure that supports pediatric mental health care, including communication back to the primary care physician and timely and appropriate ED referrals to mental health professionals.[21]

The American Academy of Pediatrics and American College of Emergency Physicians support the following actions:

1. Advocacy for adequate pediatric mental health resources in both inpatient and outpatient settings, including the availability of prompt psychiatric consultation for ED psychiatric patients and school and community mental health services, including adequate mental health screening.

2. Development of mechanisms for the ED to deal with unique pediatric mental health issues including violence in the community, physical trauma, domestic violence, child maltreatment, mass-casualty incidents and disasters, suicides and suicide attempts, and the death of a child in the ED.

3. Appropriate payment for both inpatient and outpatient pediatric mental health services.

4. Acknowledgment of the importance of the child's medical home* to his or her continued well-being, including prevention, screening, and treatment of mental health issues.[22]

5. Advocacy for comprehensive pediatric mental health insurance coverage to include provision of mental health services for the uninsured and expansion of coverage to include mental health services for those who are insured.

6. Advocacy for additional research funding dedicated to pediatric emergency mental health issues.

7. Promotion of education and research for mental health emergencies and specifically to

- expand the data on epidemiology, best practices, treatment outcomes, and cost/benefit issues for pediatric mental health emergencies in the ED;

- evaluate the adequacy of patient access to pediatric mental health services;

- evaluate children with behavioral crisis to understand gaps in primary care and community resources;

- develop mental health support networks that minimize reliance on acute crisis management;

- develop and validate accurate pediatric mental health screening tools for use in various settings and best practices for follow-up programs for pediatric mental health patients; and

- enhance the pediatric mental health curriculum for emergency medicine and pediatric residency training programs and pediatric emergency medicine fellowships.

---

* A medical home is defined as primary care that is accessible, continuous, comprehensive, family centered, coordinated, compassionate, and culturally effective.

REFERENCES

1. American Academy of Pediatrics, Committee on Child Health Financing. Scope of health care benefits from birth through age 21. *Pediatrics.* 2006;117:979–982

2. American Academy of Pediatrics, Committee on Injury and Poison Prevention. Firearm-related injuries affecting the pediatric population. *Pediatrics.* 2000;105:888–895

3. Terr LC. Childhood traumas: an outline and review. *Am J Psychiatry.* 1991;148:10–20

4. Brick ND. The neurological basis for the theory of recovered memory [research paper]. 2003. Available at: http://members. aol.com/smartnews/Neurological_Memory.htm. Accessed August 7, 2005

5. Meichenbaum D. *A Clinical Handbook/Practical Therapist Manual for Assessing and Treating Adults With Post-Traumatic Stress Disorder (PTSD).* Waterloo, Ontario, Canada: Institute Press; 1994

6. Foy DW. Introduction and description of the disorder. In: Foy DW, ed. *Treating PTSD: Cognitive-Behavioral Strategies.* New York, NY: Guilford; 1992:1–12

7. Knopp FH, Benson AR. *A Primer on the Complexities of Traumatic Memory Childhood Sexual Abuse: A Psychobiological Approach.* Brandon, VT: Safer Society Press; 1996

8. van der Kolk BA. The body keeps the score: memory and the evolving psychobiology of post traumatic stress. *Harv Rev Psychiatry.* 1994;1:253–265

9. Mukerjee M. Hidden scars. *Sci Am.* 1995;273(4):14–15

10. Winston FK, Kassam-Adams N, Vivarelli-O'Neill C, et al. Acute stress disorder symptoms in children and their parents after pediatric traffic injury. *Pediatrics.* 2002;109(6). Available at: www.pediatrics.org/cgi/content/full/109/6/e90

11. Children's Hospital of Philadelphia. Post-traumatic stress disorder may follow traffic crashes according to doctors at the Children's Hospital of Philadelphia [press release]. Available at: www.eurekalert.org/pub_releases/1999-12/CHoP-Psdm-061299. php. Accessed August 7, 2005

12. American Academy of Pediatrics. Insurance coverage of mental health and substance abuse services for children and adolescents: a consensus statement. *Pediatrics.* 2000;106: 860–862

13. Davidhizar R, Shearer R. Helping children cope with public disasters. *Am J Nurs.* 2002;102(3):26–33

14. Kalyjian A. Sri Lanka: post tsunami mental health outreach project—lessons learned. February 24, 2005. Available at: www.psichi.org/pubs/articles/article_494.asp. Accessed November 25, 2005

15. Popovic JR. 1999 National Hospital Discharge Survey: annual summary with detailed diagnosis and procedure data. *Vital Health Stat 13.* 2001;(151):i–v, 1–206

16. Olson L, Melese-d'Hospital I, Cook L, et al. Mental health problems of children presenting to emergency departments. Paper presented at: Third National Congress on Childhood Emergencies; Dallas, TX; April 15–17, 2002

17. US Consumer Product Safety Commission, Division of Hazard and Injury Data Systems. *Hospital-Based Pediatric Emergency Resource Survey*. Bethesda, MD: US Consumer Product Safety Commission; 1997

18. Seidel JS, Hornbein M, Yoshiyama K, Kuznets D, Finklestein JZ, St Geme JW Jr. Emergency medical services and the pediatric patient: are the needs being met? *Pediatrics*. 1984;73: 769–772

19. Seidel JS. Emergency medical services and the adolescent patient. *J Adolesc Health*. 1991;12:95–100

20. Sapien RE, Fullerton L, Olson LM, Broxterman KJ, Sklar DP. Disturbing trends: the epidemiology of pediatric emergency medical services use. *Acad Emerg Med*. 1999;6:232–238

21. American Academy of Pediatrics, Committee on Substance Abuse. Indications for management and referral of patients involved in substance abuse. *Pediatrics*. 2000;106: 143–148

22. American Academy of Pediatrics, Medical Home Initiatives for Children With Special Needs Project Advisory Committee. The medical home. *Pediatrics*. 2002;110:184–186

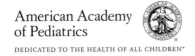

American Academy of Pediatrics
DEDICATED TO THE HEALTH OF ALL CHILDREN™

Organizational Principles to Guide and Define the Child
Health Care System and/or Improve the Health of all Children

Technical Report—Pediatric and Adolescent Mental Health Emergencies in the Emergency Medical Services System

abstract

Emergency department (ED) health care professionals often care for patients with previously diagnosed psychiatric illnesses who are ill, injured, or having a behavioral crisis. In addition, ED personnel encounter children with psychiatric illnesses who may not present to the ED with overt mental health symptoms. Staff education and training regarding identification and management of pediatric mental health illness can help EDs overcome the perceived limitations of the setting that influence timely and comprehensive evaluation. In addition, ED physicians can inform and advocate for policy changes at local, state, and national levels that are needed to ensure comprehensive care of children with mental health illnesses. This report addresses the roles that the ED and ED health care professionals play in emergency mental health care of children and adolescents in the United States, which includes the stabilization and management of patients in mental health crisis, the discovery of mental illnesses and suicidal ideation in ED patients, and approaches to advocating for improved recognition and treatment of mental illnesses in children. The report also addresses special issues related to mental illness in the ED, such as minority populations, children with special health care needs, and children's mental health during and after disasters and trauma. *Pediatrics* 2011; 127:e1356–e1366

Margaret A. Dolan, MD, Joel A. Fein, MD, MPH, and THE COMMITTEE ON PEDIATRIC EMERGENCY MEDICINE

KEY WORDS
emergency department, emergency medical services, mental health care, psychiatric illness, trauma, posttraumatic stress disorder

ABBREVIATIONS
ED—emergency department
PTSD—posttraumatic stress disorder
AAP—American Academy of Pediatrics
ACEP—American College of Emergency Physicians
EMS—emergency medical services

The guidance in this report does not indicate an exclusive course of treatment or serve as a standard of medical care. Variations, taking into account individual circumstances, may be appropriate.

BACKGROUND

Emergency department (ED) health care professionals often care for patients with previously diagnosed psychiatric illnesses who are ill, injured, or having a behavioral crisis. ED health care professionals also need to identify and manage patients with previously undiagnosed and/or undetected conditions such as suicidal ideation, depression, anxiety, psychosis, substance use and abuse, and posttraumatic stress disorder (PTSD). This report will address the roles that the ED and ED health care professionals play in emergency mental health care of children and adolescents in the United States. This technical report supports the 2006 joint statement from the American Academy of Pediatrics (AAP) and American College of Emergency Physicians (ACEP) titled "Pediatric Mental Health Emergencies in the Emergency Medical Services System."[1,2] Previous policy statements, clinical reports, and technical reports by the AAP that have addressed specific pediatric emergency mental health issues and formulated guidelines for model programs include, but are not limited to, "Adolescent Assault Victim

www.pediatrics.org/cgi/doi/10.1542/peds.2011-0522

doi:10.1542/peds.2011-0522

All technical report from the American Academy of Pediatrics automatically expire 5 years after publication unless reaffirmed, revised, or retired at or before that time.

PEDIATRICS (ISSN Numbers: Print, 0031-4005; Online, 1098-4275).

Needs: A Review of Issues and a Model Protocol" (1996),[3] "Access to Pediatric Emergency Medical Care" (2000),[4] "Child Life Services" (2006),[5] "Care of the Adolescent Sexual Assault Victim" (2008),[6] "Achieving Quality Health Services for Adolescents" (2008),[7] "Suicide and Suicide Attempts in Adolescents" (2007),[8] "Underinsurance of Adolescents" (2008),[9] "Death of a Child in the Emergency Department" (joint statement from the AAP and ACEP in 2002[10] and a supporting technical report by the same title (2005),[11] "Patient- and Family-Centered Care and the Role of the Emergency Physician Providing Care to a Child in the Emergency Department" (2006),[12] and "Family-Centered Care and the Pediatrician's Role" (2003).[13]

PSYCHIATRIC ILLNESS AND THE ED

The current and increasing concerns regarding pediatric mental health emergencies occur within the context of the overall crisis in pediatric ED care. First, there has been an increase in the prevalence of ED visits for psychiatric illness.[14–18] This situation is complicated by a shortage of inpatient and outpatient services available for patients who need mental health care and an unfunded mandate to care for these patients in an ED setting. The 1999 Surgeon General's report on mental health[19] indicated that 21% of US children 9 to 17 years of age have a diagnosable mental or addictive disorder. The National Institute of Mental Health has reported that 10% of children in the United States currently suffer from mental illness, and more than 13 million children require mental health or substance abuse services.[20,21] The World Health Organization has estimated that by the year 2020, neuropsychiatric disorders will become 1 of the 5 most common causes of morbidity, mortality, and disability for children.[22] A study at the University of Pittsburgh found that from

1979 to 1996, the rate of psychosocial problems identified in primary care visits of 4- to 15-year-olds increased from 7% to 18%.[23] Suicide in the United States currently ranks as the fourth leading cause of death for 10- to 14-year-olds and the third leading cause of death for 15- to 19-year-olds, accounting for 11.3% of all deaths in the latter age group in 2006. More than half of adolescents 13 to 19 years of age have suicidal thoughts, nearly 250 000 adolescents attempt suicide each year, and up to 10% of children attempt suicide sometime during their lives.[24–26] Of great concern is the fact that, despite its increasing prevalence, the risk of suicidal behavior in many children and adolescents is often undetected. One study found that 83% of adolescent patients who had attempted suicide were not recognized as suicidal by their primary care physicians.[27] Rotheram-Borus et al[28] reported that fewer than 50% of adolescents seen for suicidal behavior in the ED were ever referred for treatment, and, even when they were referred, compliance with treatment was low. Another study revealed that only one-fifth of these children receive necessary treatment.[21]

Patients who need mental health care can be disturbing to the routine and flow of the ED and require more resources than many medical or trauma patients. In a 2006 study, Santiago et al[29] reported that 210 patients with a median age of 14 years and requiring psychiatric evaluation spent a median of 5.7 hours in the ED. Hospital police monitored 51.9% of these patients, and 45 patients exhibited dangerous behaviors. Among children who frequently used mental health services in the ED, approximately 50% of them were seen again within 2 months of their initial visit, which suggests that patterns of recidivism are high for psychiatric patients. Repeat patients are

more likely to threaten to harm others; to have a diagnosis of adjustment, conduct, or oppositional disorder; and to be under the care of a child welfare agency. Repeat users were also significantly more likely than one-time patients to be less compliant with outpatient follow-up, be admitted to the hospital, and require more social support. These youth also have increased risk of involvement with juvenile justice; a large proportion of them have related behavioral, emotional, and cognitive disabilities and have greater difficulty remaining in residential treatment. The total proportion of children admitted to general inpatient services from the ED for mental health problems is also increasing. In Washington State, psychiatric disorders were the leading cause of adolescent hospitalization and accounted for one-third of hospital days for 5- to 19-year-olds over a 10-year period from 1994 to 2003.[30]

According to a 2004 AAP policy statement, ED overcrowding threatens access to emergency services for those who need them the most and further complicates the ability of EDs to serve the needs of patients who need mental health care and their families.[31] A 2008 report from the Centers for Disease Control and Prevention noted that ED visits increased 32% from 1996 to 2006, whereas the number of EDs decreased by 5%. Approximately one-third of EDs reported having to divert incoming patients to another ED in the previous year.[32] Boarding of patients with mental illness in the ED has many deleterious effects on the health care of those patients and others.[33] The ED is often a high-stimulation environment that is not conducive to calming agitated patients. In addition, privacy is not as easy to arrange, which leads to distraction and disruption of care for these patients and their families as well as the other ED patients.

The pediatrics section of the 2007 Institute of Medicine report on emergency services described the burgeoning problem of pediatric mental health problems in the saturated emergency medical services (EMS) system.[34] The report cited studies that have demonstrated inadequate or nonexistent screening and evaluation for children with mental health complaints, inadequate training and comfort levels for ED physicians and nurses in caring for pediatric patients with mental health complaints, suboptimal ED environment for mental health patients in crisis, and extended ED wait times for patients who need mental health care and require admission because of lack of psychiatric inpatient resources. According to the Institute of Medicine report, not only is ED use increasing, but younger patients are being seen, and depression, bipolar disorder, and anxiety are now being identified in children of elementary school age. EDs are increasingly used as the safety net for diagnosing and managing psychiatric illness in these children. The pediatric ED at Yale noted an increase of 59% in psychiatric illness-related visits between 1995 and 1999; the most common complaints were behavioral changes, ingestions, suicide attempts, and violence.[35] The Cincinnati Children's Hospital ED reported an annual increase in visits by psychiatric patients from 800 in 1995 to more than 2000 in 2004.[36] In their 1999 study of pediatric EMS usage, Sapien et al[37] found that 15% of pediatric EMS responses were for suicide, assault, or alcohol and drug intoxication, which emphasizes the need for first responders to have an informed approach to these problems. The actual number of psychiatric emergencies may be underestimated, because many children and adolescents who present with trauma may have made a suicide attempt, and vague somatic complaints may actually represent depression, PTSD, suicidal ideation, or abuse.

BARRIERS TO MENTAL HEALTH SERVICES IN THE EMS SYSTEM

Hoyle and White[38] outlined the barriers to adequate pediatric mental health services in the EMS system. These barriers can be categorized as (1) a lack of information relating to pediatric psychiatric illness, (2) limitations of the ED setting that influence timely and comprehensive evaluation, (3) need for education and training of ED staff regarding identification and management of pediatric psychiatric illness, and (4) a lack of access to and effectiveness of inpatient and outpatient mental health services.

Lack of Information Relating to Pediatric Psychiatric Illness

In a 2002 report, Horwitz et al noted, "Federal agencies' planning documents devote considerable attention to the need to understand the identification and treatment of children's behavioral and emotional issues within primary medical settings. Nevertheless, a paucity of evidence exists to demonstrate that such attention has resulted in aggressive programs of research in this area."[39] They found that adults received 15 times more research attention than did children and adolescents. Some epidemiologic data regarding psychiatric problems are available from national database sources including the National Hospital Discharge Survey, the National Hospital Ambulatory Medical Care Survey, and the National Electronic Injury Surveillance System. However, because children's psychiatric issues were largely unrecognized during the development of these databases, information regarding children and adolescents is obtained most often by extrapolation or inference. The National Hospital Discharge Survey and National Hospital Ambulatory Medical Care Survey use broad age groupings (younger than 15 and 15 through 44 years) that obfuscate the data pertinent to children and do not always subcategorize psychiatric illness or ED visits. Olson et al[40] used National Electronic Injury Surveillance System data from 10 hospitals over a 3-month period in 2000 to categorize presentations to the ED and found that psychiatric or violence-related complaints represented a relatively high proportion of pediatric ED visits.

Limitations of the ED Setting That Influence Timely and Comprehensive Evaluation

ED health care professionals recognize the difficulties in providing care to all children with psychiatric emergencies and note a lack of psychiatric specialists and inpatient and outpatient facilities and an increase in referrals from schools, primary care physicians, and mental health therapists who cannot admit patients directly from their offices.[34] These limitations, coupled with a mandate to care for all patients who present to the ED, create a difficult obligation for ED practitioners to fulfill. The Emergency Medical Treatment and Active Labor Act (EMTALA), enacted in 1985 with the purpose of protecting the rights of indigent patients seeking emergency care, requires Medicare-participating hospitals to provide a medical screening examination for all patients who present for care to the ED, regardless of the patient's ability to pay.[41] Subsequent revisions have clarified the responsibility of hospitals, EDs, and their physicians to act on this medical screening examination if the patient is determined to have an acute medical or psychiatric condition, such as suicidal ideation, by providing all ancillary services routinely available to the ED, such as a physician consultation, inpatient care, and mental health services, in a nondiscriminatory and consistent manner. This revision guarantees that hospital EDs are essentially the only place in our current health care system in which all patients with acute psychiatric illness can be guaranteed thorough evaluation.[42-44] A comprehensive emergency psychiatric examination may take several hours, and often there is no private or quiet area within the ED to facilitate effective consultations. In addition, the ED is not the optimal setting for assessing and managing patient and family anxiety, because they are crowded, noisy, and full of distressing sights and sounds that may even exacerbate some patients' symptoms or behavior. Given the declining numbers of available consultants, the formal psychiatric evaluation often begins hours after initial medical stabilization. Regulatory agencies have recognized the importance of standardized approaches toward high-risk psychiatric patients in the ED. Since January 1, 2007, the Joint Commission has required accredited organizations to conduct suicide risk assessment for any patient with a primary diagnosis or primary complaint of an emotional or behavioral disorder.[42]

Need for Education and Training of ED Staff Regarding Identification and Management of Pediatric Psychiatric Illness

Education about the causes, signs and symptoms, and optimal management of pediatric mental illness is essential for pediatric, family practice, and emergency medicine practitioners, including residents and pediatric emergency medicine fellows as well as those who practice in community hospitals. This education includes the use of appropriate mental health screening tools, appropriate discharge instructions, and mental health follow-up for depressed patients and patients who have considered or attempted suicide. However, residency

program education may be insufficient in many of these areas.[45,46]

Lack of Access to Inpatient and Outpatient Mental Health Services

Nationally, the number of adult and pediatric beds in state mental health facilities plummeted 32% between 1992 and 1998 and has since dropped significantly below 60 000, and fewer than half are allocated for acute care.[47] Media reports have highlighted the fact that these inpatient cost reductions have not been offset by outpatient expenditures, and as a consequence, the ED has more frequently become a location for nonurgent mental health complaints.[48-50] They cite the combination of fewer inpatient psychiatric beds and insufficient outpatient services, which leaves EDs to hold pediatric psychiatric patients or admit them to a medical unit with little hope of being reimbursed for that admission. This process can be resource-intensive, because these patients sometimes must be restrained and/or constantly monitored.

POTENTIAL SOLUTIONS TO THE CRISIS IN MENTAL HEALTH CARE

Solutions to the mental health care crisis are not easily found within other, nonmedical systems, which are equally unprepared to handle children with acute psychiatric illness. A nationwide survey of juvenile detention centers, the results of which were presented at a Senate hearing in July 2004, revealed that 15 000 children with psychiatric disorders were improperly incarcerated the previous year because no mental health services were available.[48] Many community health centers that traditionally provide mental health care have lost their state funding and often turn away patients or place them on long waiting lists. Schools, therefore, frequently function as the de facto mental health system for children and adolescents; 70% to 80% of schoolchildren who

need mental health services receive that care in the school setting.[51-53] School counselors are primarily funded by state and local funds, but school districts also use funds from federal programs such as the Safe and Drug-Free Schools grants that are authorized by the Elementary and Secondary Education Act, otherwise known as the No Child Left Behind Act (Pub L No. 107-110 [2002]). However, it is important to remember that this program, like other legislative mandates, depends on the vagaries of federal funding and budget cuts. Primary care physician offices are another point of contact for children and youth at which there is high potential for identifying and managing mental illness, but even when children are seen in the general medical setting, identification and management of mental illness are still challenging.[54-57] To address these issues, the AAP Task Force on Mental Health has developed algorithms to help pediatricians identify, manage, and develop safety plans for children and adolescents and offers strategies for diverting patients from the ED and referring more directly to mental health resources when available.[51] However, primary care physicians cannot do this alone. For this approach to be successful there needs to be an increase in the flow of pediatric trainees into child psychiatry training programs and a concomitant increase in payments for child psychiatric services to these program graduates. Telepsychiatry, first piloted in Britain, also offers a potential solution to the lack of mental health care providers in rural and remote areas.[58,59]

Stabilization and Management of Patients in Psychiatric Crisis

Patients who arrive with a psychiatric emergency require a rapid, thoughtful response by the ED team to assess the degree of stress and safety of the patient, provide medical stabilization, and use specific interventions to alleviate symptoms and increase safety for the patient and ED staff and other patients. During these evaluations, ED health care professionals maintain a delicate balance between maintaining patient confidentiality and engaging the external support systems that already exist for these patients. In many states, adolescents can seek and receive care for mental health issues and drug/alcohol use without parental involvement, and EDs must maintain confidentiality except if the child is at risk of harming himself or herself or others. However, the ED must also recognize the primary support role of the family and caregivers, as well as the child's primary care providers, in all phases of pediatric mental illness. In this light, ED health care professionals must encourage, but not coerce, the adolescent to allow family involvement whenever possible.

Of paramount importance is for EDs to have the capacity to provide such care within an overall system of mental health care. The most important element is establishing an effective relationship with a specialized mental health team. Team composition and availability may vary but should be predefined. When consultations are requested, the degree of urgency and the expected response time should be communicated clearly. Additional dialogue should take place after consultation to ensure that there is agreement with a treatment plan and to facilitate expeditious and appropriate disposition. Acute drug ingestions present a specific challenge in this regard and require ED health care professionals to blend the usual resuscitation protocols with psychosocial management by medical staff, social workers, psychiatrists, and security personnel. Preexisting relationships with psychiatric inpatient facilities promote efficient disposition. It is also helpful to have

familiarity with child protection laws and to establish relationships with local law enforcement and child welfare and social service agencies. School nurses, often the liaisons among family, health care professionals, and school personnel, can also be included, with appropriate consent, to help inform as well as facilitate management plans after the ED visit.[60] Adequate and appropriate physical space should be available for children and families in crisis; a private room with monitoring equipment that is out of the patient's reach is considered optimal. Patients should be within the sight of ED staff; screening for suicide risk or potential self-harm should occur, and one-to-one supervision should be provided as needed. If a patient requires medical admission or must wait in the ED for transfer to another facility, guidelines should be available for staff and faculty members in handling inpatient psychiatric patients and their family members.

On occasion, children and adolescents with psychiatric illness will require physical or chemical restraint to protect them or others from harm. The AAP and ACEP offer guidelines or policies related to patient restraint and reaffirm the need for frequent safety checks, vital-sign monitoring, evaluation of limb neurovascular status, and assistance with nutritional and bathroom needs.[61,62] It is more common for EDs to use anxiolysis and mild sedation to avoid the need for physical restraint. The decision to use physical restraints should be made by an attending physician but may be initiated by nursing staff in extenuating circumstances. Even with proper restraint, mental or cardiopulmonary status may deteriorate unexpectedly; therefore, patients in restraints should be monitored continuously with time-limited orders. The Joint Commission carefully monitors the institutional

policies around implementation and documentation of patient restraint and emphasizes that it must be used as a last resort and that the treatment is for the patient's benefit.[63,64]

The Role of the ED in Discovering Mental Illness in Children

As mentioned above, in 2007, the Joint Commission recommended a suicide risk assessment for any patient with a primary diagnosis or primary complaint of an emotional or behavioral disorder.[42] Some suicide-assessment instruments, such as the Suicidal Behavior Interview and the Suicide Intent Scale, are not options for EDs, because they are designed to be administered by trained mental health specialists or require complicated computations by clinicians.[65,66] Although there is no standard or optimal instrument that screens for suicidality, high sensitivity and rapid administration are 2 highly valued characteristics. One tool with such characteristics is the Suicidal Ideation Questionnaire (SIQ), a 30-item instrument originally designed for 10th- through 12th-grade students.[67] A 15-item instrument (SIQ-JR) is also available for students in grades 7 through 9 and has been standardized for older students as well.[68] These tools may take longer than desired in an ED setting but have strong psychometric validity and reliability. Shorter tools that are more appropriate for the ED setting have also been developed. Horowitz et al[69] demonstrated good content validity of the Risk of Suicide Questionnaire (RSQ), a brief screening tool for screening for suicidal ideation in the ED that assesses major facets for suicide risk, present and past suicidal ideation, previous self-destructive behavior, and current stressors. Folse et al[70] piloted a 2-question version of this screening tool in the pediatric emergency setting, and almost 30% of the adolescents screened positive for suicidal ideation within the previous week. The authors recommended that clinicians ask the questions: "Are you here because you tried to hurt yourself," and "In the past week have you thought about killing yourself" as an initial assessment for adolescents coming to the ED for medical care, regardless of the presenting symptoms.

Patients may exhibit "externalizing" symptoms that initially have been identified by a caregiver, teacher, health care professional, or even criminal justice personnel. However, many children with psychiatric illness do not present to the ED with overt psychiatric symptoms. It is also clear that many patients with psychiatric disorders exhibit somatic symptoms, such as headache and abdominal pain; some chronic medical illnesses, such as asthma and diabetes, can be exacerbated by stress and anxiety.[71,72] Scott et al[73] found a 30% rate of moderate or severe depression in 13- to 19-year-olds in the pediatric ED. Similarly, Rutman et al[74] found that 37% of the adolescents in a pediatric ED research study were above the threshold for depression on the Center for Epidemiologic Studies Depression Scale.

The US Preventive Services Task Force recommends screening of adolescents 12 to 18 years of age for major depressive disorder when systems are in place to ensure accurate diagnosis, psychotherapy, and follow-up.[75] Because the ED may be the only point of contact for children with undiagnosed psychiatric illness, it is imperative to have adequate resources in this setting to link patients who "screen positive" with inpatient or outpatient services. In addition, it is necessary to have efficient, culturally sensitive, and developmentally appropriate screening tools that promote the accurate detection of suicidal ideation, depression, and other psychiatric illnesses. Some investigators have adapted full-length, adult scales for use with younger populations, but they require 20 to 40 minutes to administer.[76] Some EDs have developed their own mental health screening tools to help in the evaluation of child and adolescent patients. Adolescents at the Children's Hospital of Philadelphia use computers to complete the self-administered Behavioral Health Screen for Emergency Departments, which provides their physicians and nurses with information about their risk for depression, suicidal ideation, PTSD symptoms, and substance abuse.[77,78]

Similar developments have occurred in the real-time assessment of traumatic stress in pediatric ED patients. Just like adults, children's previous adverse experiences can influence their response to acute illness and their ED visit. When children experience sustained stress attributable to traumatic experiences, neurohormones, such as cortisol, are increased. These elevated neurohormones can lead to permanent changes in their developing brain structures, such as the amygdala and hypothalamus.[79] Unrecognized and untreated, acute stress symptoms can cause lifelong behavioral and mental health problems attributable to changes in neurodevelopment and function.[80–86] Children with a history of a traumatic experience, be it from unintentional injury, violence, or sexual or physical abuse, can be expected to have more acute stress symptoms in the immediate aftermath of a specific event.[87] Shemesh et al[88] identified PTSD in 29% of the patients in a small convenience sample of pediatric patients who presented to a pediatric ED. All patients but 6 identified at least 1 previous salient traumatic event; most of the events were not immediately related to the reason for the ED presentation. Knowledge of trauma symptoms significantly altered the ED clinical management in 16% of the cases.[88] Winston and colleagues[89] have developed brief screening tools for acutely injured children and their families and have achieved some success in providing these families with practical print and Web-based management tools. Although these data suggest that early identification and management of psychological trauma and its consequences are feasible in the pediatric ED, further efforts are required to incorporate these techniques into the routine systems and processes in the ED.[90] Parents and caregivers also need education from appropriate personnel on what to expect, how to parent a traumatized child, how to know when additional help is needed, and where to find it. Information such as this can be found at sites for the National Child Traumatic Stress Network (www.nctsnet. org) and the Center for Pediatric Traumatic Stress at the Children's Hospital of Philadelphia (www.healthcaretoolbox. org).

SPECIAL ISSUES RELATED TO MENTAL ILLNESS IN THE ED

Minority Populations

Children from minority populations have less access to mental health services and are less likely to receive needed care.[91] Likely because of the complexity and cultural interpretation of psychiatric illness, the lack of proper translation when needed, even by trained interpreters, may contribute to difficulty in receiving information and following through with mental health referrals.[92] According to Rand's 2001 *Mental Health Care for Youth*,[93] 31% of white children who needed mental health services received them, compared with 22% of black and 14% of Hispanic children. In addition, the same study found that people from minority populations in treatment often receive a poorer quality of mental health care and are underrepresented in mental health research. After adjusting for other demographic factors and parent characteristics, Hispanic children with mental health problems had greater odds of having no care or unmet need compared with white children. This finding is particularly concerning given the increased suicidal ideation, depression, anxiety symptoms, and school dropout rates among Hispanic compared with white adolescents. Cultural factors, particularly around the stigma of mental illness, were noted to be important for Hispanic people. Financial factors also play a role in these disparities; although they differ according to state, these differences are more likely the result of varied state policies and health care market characteristics rather than differences in racial or ethnic makeup.[94]

Children With Special Health Care Needs

It is well known that children with special health care needs frequently have coexisting psychiatric morbidity.[95–97] For example, children with asthma and allergies are especially prone to having anxiety disorders.[98] Obesity is also associated with problems such as depression, especially in Hispanic and black children.[99] The Emergency Information Form (EIF), developed jointly by the AAP and ACEP (www.aap.org/advocacy/blankform.pdf), allows providers to include psychiatric and behavioral diagnoses for children with special health care needs and also includes information about their health care professionals, medications, and significant medical history.

Children's Mental Health During and After Disasters and Trauma

The ED is the initial source of physical care for child victims of disasters (natural or man-made) or trauma (unintentional or intentional). Many studies have demonstrated the development

of depression and PTSD in child survivors of trauma and disaster.[100–104] Unrecognized and untreated, acute and posttraumatic stress symptoms can cause lifelong behavioral and mental health problems as a result of changes in brain neurodevelopment and function. These alterations in function create a lifetime risk of subsequent poor school performance, depression, suicidal ideation or attempts, aggression, and risk-taking behaviors. Current research is ongoing to identify these at-risk children as early as possible and to develop validated interventions to cope with the stress and avoid later psychiatric morbidity. An AAP-funded Agency for Healthcare Research and Quality resource, "Pediatric Terrorism and Disaster Preparedness: A Resource for Pediatricians," includes information on children's mental health in disasters (www.ahrq.gov/research/pedprep/resource.htm).

RESEARCH AND ADVOCACY AGENDA FOR MENTAL HEALTH EMERGENCIES IN THE ED

The President's New Freedom Commission on Mental Health was convened in 2002 to study the mental health service delivery system and make recommendations to enable adults and children with emotional disturbance "live, work, and learn and participate fully in their communities." The 2003 report of the commission addressed awareness, disparities, early screening, the use of technology, and the need for research in this area. Specifically, research that focuses on the identification and management of pediatric mental health emergencies is critical for establishing best practices for screening of undiagnosed psychiatric illness, formal psychiatric evaluation in the ED setting, and engagement into community care. The development of a mental health interest group in the Pediatric Emergency Care Applied Research Network provides an ideal vehi-

cle through which to conduct much-needed large-scale studies that elucidate and evaluate identification, identification, engagement, and treatment methodologies for the emergency setting.[105] Support of funding for local and regional fatality-review teams can also promote surveillance and understanding of factors related to suicide in children and adolescents.[106] Pediatricians can also petition legislators and policy makers to increase reimbursement for mental health services for children and adolescents at all levels, including funding for Medicaid, school-based and community-center services, inpatient services, and mental health providers who provide Medicaid services. This petitioning includes encouraging private insurers to promote need-based coverage rather than fixed limits for mental health and to increase reimbursements to hospitals and consultants who provide pediatric mental health services. A recent joint statement from the American Academy of Pediatrics and the American Academy of Child and Adolescent Psychiatry outlined recommendations to insurers that could decrease the impediments to providing mental health care in the primary care setting.[107] In October 2008, Congress passed the Paul Wellstone and Pete Domenici Mental Health Parity and Addiction Equity Act of 2008 (Pub L No. 110-343).[108] The new law, which went into effect January 1, 2010, requires equity between mental health and substance abuse benefits and medical and surgical benefits in employer-sponsored group health insurance plans for companies with more than 50 employees. The law also requires equity in all financial requirements, including deductibles, copayments, coinsurance, out-of-pocket expenses, and all treatment limitations, including frequency of treatment, number of visits, days of coverage, or other similar limits. The federal legislation will not override state laws that require additional coverage and subjects the definition of mental health conditions to state law.

SUMMARY

Pediatric psychiatric emergencies constitute a large and growing segment of pediatric emergency medical care, and EDs play a critical role in the evaluation and management of these child and adolescent patients. The ED has increasingly become the safety net for a fragmented mental health infrastructure in which the needs of children and adolescents, among the most vulnerable populations, have been insufficiently addressed. Inpatient bed shortages, private and public insurance changes, and shortages of pediatric-trained mental health specialists create particular challenges in this effort. Ideally, these challenges can be addressed through a reinvigorated outpatient infrastructure that supports pediatric mental health care, advance planning for crises on a local level using community resources, and the establishment of a stronger mental health support and education network for primary care physicians. Using a skilled, culturally sensitive, multidisciplinary approach, EDs can safely and effectively manage child and adolescent patients. In addition, EDs can play a significant role in identifying and referring patients with previously undiagnosed and undetected conditions such as suicidal ideation, depression, substance abuse, and PTSD.

The 3-pronged approach of education, research, and advocacy are crucial for improving the accurate and timely ED management of childhood psychiatric illness. Education of medical students, residents, fellows, faculty members, and nurses can focus on not only rapid diagnosis and medical management but also the internal social supports and available external resources for their local service area. Researchers need to develop easy and rapid pediatric screening tools and test strategies that enlist the family and primary care physicians as partners in the effort to provide basic psychiatric care and appropriately access the mental health system. Finally, because this issue permeates almost all aspects of pediatric medicine, it is clear that pediatricians need to advocate for fairness and parity with respect to the provision and reimbursement for mental health care for children.

LEAD AUTHORS

Margaret A. Dolan, MD
Joel A. Fein, MD, MPH

COMMITTEE ON PEDIATRIC EMERGENCY MEDICINE, 2010–2011

Kathy N. Shaw, MD, MSCE, Chairperson
Alice D. Ackerman, MD, MBA
Thomas H. Chun, MD, MPH
Gregory P. Conners, MD, MPH, MBA
Nanette C. Dudley, MD
Joel A. Fein, MD, MPH
Susan M. Fuchs, MD
Brian R. Moore, MD
Steven M. Selbst, MD
Joseph L. Wright, MD, MPH

LIAISONS

Kim Bullock, MD – *American Academy of Family Physicians*
Toni K. Gross, MD, MPH – *National Association of EMS Physicians*
Tamar Magarik Haro – *AAP Department of Federal Government Affairs*
Jaclyn Haymon, MPA, RN – *EMSC National Resource Center*
David Heppel, MD – *Maternal and Child Health Bureau*

Mark A. Hostetler, MD, MPH – *American College of Emergency Physicians*
Cynthia Wright Johnson, MSN, RN – *National Association of State EMS Officials*
Lou E. Romig, MD – *National Association of Emergency Medical Technicians*
Sally K Snow, RN, BSN, CPEN – *Emergency Nurses Association*
David W. Tuggle, MD – *American College of Surgeons*
Tina Turgel, BSN, RN-C – *Maternal and Child Health Bureau*
Tasmeen Weik, DrPH, NREMT-P – *Maternal and Child Health Bureau*
Joseph L. Wright, MD, MPH – *EMSC National Resource Center*

FORMER COMMITTEE MEMBERS

Steven E. Krug, MD, Immediate Past Chairperson
Thomas Bojko, MD, MS
Margaret A. Dolan, MD
Laura S. Fitzmaurice, MD
Karen S. Frush, MD
Patricia J. O'Malley, MD
Robert E. Sapien, MD
Joan E. Shook, MD
Paul E. Sirbaugh, DO
Milton Tenenbein, MD
Loren G. Yamamoto, MD, MPH, MBA

FORMER LIAISONS

Jane Ball, RN, DrPH – *EMSC National Resource Center*
Jill M. Baren, MD – *American College of Emergency Physicians*
Kathleen Brown, MD – *American College of Emergency Physicians*
Andrew Garrett, MD, MPH – *National Association of EMS Physicians*
Dan Kavanaugh, MSW – *Maternal and Child Health Bureau/EMSC Program*
Tommy Loyacono – *National Association of Emergency Medical Technicians*
Sharon E. Mace, MD – *American College of Emergency Physicians*
Cindy Pellegrini – *AAP Department of Federal Government Affairs*
Susan Eads Role, JD, MSLS – *EMSC National Resource Center*
Ghazala Sharieff, MD – *American College of Emergency Physicians*

STAFF

Sue Tellez

REFERENCES

1. American College of Emergency Physicians. Pediatric mental health emergencies in the emergency medical services system. *Ann Emerg Med.* 2006;48(4):484–486

2. American Academy of Pediatrics, Committee on Pediatric Emergency Medicine; American College of Emergency Physicians, Pediatric Emergency Medicine Committee. Pediatric mental health emergencies in the emergency medical services system. *Pediatrics.* 2006;118(4):1764–1767

3. American Academy of Pediatrics, Task Force on Adolescent Assault Victim Needs. Adolescent assault victim needs: a review

of issues and a model protocol. *Pediatrics.* 1996;98(5):991–1001

4. American Academy of Pediatrics, Committee on Pediatric Emergency Medicine. Access to pediatric emergency medical care. *Pediatrics.* 2000;105(3 pt 1):647–649

5. American Academy of Pediatrics, Child Life Council and Committee on Hospital Care. Child life services. *Pediatrics.* 2006;118(4): 1757–1763

6. Kaufman M; American Academy of Pediatrics, Committee on Adolescence. Care of the adolescent sexual assault victim. *Pediatrics.* 2008;122(2):462–470

7. American Academy of Pediatrics, Committee on Adolescence. Achieving quality health services for adolescents. *Pediatrics.* 2008;121(6):1263–1270

8. Shain BN; American Academy of Pediatrics, Committee on Adolescence. Suicide and suicide attempts in adolescents. *Pediatrics.* 2007;120(3):669–676

9. American Academy of Pediatrics, Committee on Adolescence, Committee on Child Health Financing. Underinsurance of adolescents: recommendations for improved coverage of preventive, reproductive, and behavioral health care services. *Pediatrics.* 2009;123(1):191–196

10. American Academy of Pediatrics, Committee on Pediatric Emergency Medicine; Pediatric Emergency Medicine Committee, American College of Emergency Physicians. Death of a child in the emergency department: joint statement by the American Academy of Pediatrics and the American College of Emergency Physicians. *Pediatrics.* 2002;110(4):839–840

11. Knapp J, Mulligan-Smith D; American Academy of Pediatrics, Committee on Pediatric Emergency Medicine. Death of a child in the emergency department. *Pediatrics.* 2005;115(5):1432–1437

12. American Academy of Pediatrics, Committee on Pediatric Emergency Medicine; American College of Emergency Physicians, Pediatric Emergency Medicine Committee. Patient- and family-centered care and the role of the emergency physician providing care to a child in the emergency department. *Pediatrics.* 2006;118(5): 2242–2244

13. American Academy of Pediatrics, Committee on Hospital Care. Family-centered care and the pediatrician's role. *Pediatrics.* 2003;112(3 pt 1):691–696

14. Sills MR, Bland SD. Summary statistics for pediatric psychiatric visits to US emergency departments, 1993–1999. *Pediat-*

rics. 2002;110(4). Available at: www. pediatrics.org/cgi/content/full/110/4/e40

15. Goldstein AB, Silverman MA, Phillips S, Lichenstein R. Mental health visits in a pediatric emergency department and their relationship to the school calendar. *Pediatr Emerg Care.* 2005;21(10):653–657

16. Larkin GL, Claassen CA, Emond JA, Pelletier AJ, Camargo CA. Trends in U.S. emergency department visits for mental health conditions, 1992 to 2001. *Psychiatr Serv.* 2005; 56(6):671–677

17. Grupp-Phelan J, Harman JS, Kelleher KJ. Trends in mental health and chronic condition visits by children presenting for care at U.S. emergency departments. *Public Health Rep.* 2007;122(1):55–61

18. Mahajan P, Alpern ER, Grupp-Phelan J, et al; Pediatric Emergency Care Applied Research Network (PECARN). Epidemiology of psychiatric-related visits to emergency departments in a multicenter collaborative research pediatric network. *Pediatr Emerg Care.* 2009;25(11):715–720

19. Substance Abuse and Mental Health Services Administration, National Institute of Mental Health, Department of Health and Human Services. *Mental Health: A Report of the Surgeon General—Executive Summary.* Rockville, MD: US Department of Health and Human Services; 1999

20. US Department of Health and Human Services. *Report of the Surgeon General's Conference on Children's Mental Health: A National Action Agenda.* Washington, DC: US Department of Health and Human Services; 1999

21. National Institute of Mental Health. *Brief Notes on the Mental Health of Children and Adolescents.* Bethesda, MD: National Institute of Mental Health; 1999

22. Murray CJL, Lopez AD. *The Global Burden of Disease: A Comprehensive Assessment of Mortality and Disability From Diseases, Injuries, and Risk Factors in 1990 and Projected to 2020.* Cambridge, MA: Harvard School of Public Health, on behalf of the World Health Organization and the World Bank, Distributed by Harvard University Press; 1996

23. Gardner W, Kelleher KJ, Wasserman R, et al. Primary care treatment of pediatric psychosocial problems: a study from Pediatric Research in Office Settings and Ambulatory Sentinel Practice Network. *Pediatrics.* 2000;106(4). Available at: www.pediatrics.org/cgi/content/full/106/4/e44

24. Meehan P, Lamb J, Saltzman L, O'Carroll P. Attempted suicide among young adults: progress toward a meaningful estimate of

prevalence. *Am J Psychiatry.* 1992;149(1): 41–44

25. Pfeffer CR, Lipkins R, Plutchik R, Mizruchi M. Normal children at risk for suicidal behavior: a two-year follow up. *J Am Acad Child Adolesc Psychiatry.* 1988;27(1): 34–41

26. American Academy of Child and Adolescent Psychiatry. Summary of the practice parameters for the assessment and treatment of children and adolescents with suicidal behavior. *J Am Acad Child Adolesc Psychiatry.* 2001;40(4):495–499

27. Clark D. Suicidal behavior in childhood and adolescence: recent studies and clinical implications. *Psychiatr Ann.* 1993;23(5): 271–283

28. Rotheram-Borus M, Piacentini J, Van Rossem R, et al. Enhancing treatment adherence with a specialized emergency room program for adolescent suicide attempters. *J Am Acad Child Adolesc Psychiatry.* 1996;35(5):654–663

29. Santiago L, Tunik M, Foltin G, Mojica M. Children requiring psychiatric consultation in the pediatric emergency department: epidemiology, resource utilization, and complications. *Pediatr Emerg Care.* 2006;22(2):85–89

30. Washington State Emergency Medical Services for Children. *Hospital Emergency Departments and Children/Adolescents With Mental Health Concerns in Washington State. Final Report.* Seattle, WA: Department of Health and Human Services, Health Resources and Services Administration Emergency Medical Services for Children; 2001

31. American Academy of Pediatrics, Committee on Pediatric Emergency Medicine. Overcrowding crisis in our nation's emergency departments: is our safety net unraveling? *Pediatrics.* 2004;114(3):878–888

32. Shappert S, Rechtsteiner E. Ambulatory medical care utilization estimates for 2006. *Natl Health Stat Report.* 2008;(8): 1–29

33. Mansbach JM, Wharff E, Austin SB, Ginnis K, Woods ER. Which psychiatric patients board on the medical service? *Pediatrics.* 2003;111(6 pt 1). Available at: www. pediatrics.org/cgi/content/full/111/6/e693

34. Institute of Medicine. *Emergency Care for Children: Growing Pains.* Washington, DC: National Academies Press; 2007

35. Santucci K, Sather J, Douglas M. Psychiatry-related visits to the pediatric emergency department: a growing epidemic? [abstract]. *Pediatr Res.* 2000;47(4 suppl 2):117A

36. Cincinnati Children's Hospital Medical. *Health News Release.* November 26, 2001. Available at: www.cincinnatichildrens. org/about/news/release/2001/11-college-hill.htm. Accessed March 30, 2011

37. Sapien R, Fullerton L, Olson L, Broxterman K, Sklar D. Disturbing trends: the epidemiology of pediatric emergency medical services use. *Acad Emerg Med.* 1999;6(3): 232–238

38. Hoyle JD Jr, White LJ; Emergency Medical Services for Children; Health Resources Services Administration, Maternal and Child Health Bureau, National Association of EMS Physicians. Treatment of pediatric and adolescent mental health emergencies in the United States: current practices, models, barriers and potential solutions. *Prehosp Emerg Care.* 2003;7(1): 66–73

39. Horwitz SM, Kelleher K, Boyce T, et al. Barriers to health care research for children and youth with psychosocial problems. *JAMA.* 2002;288(12):1508–1512

40. Olson L, Melese-d'Hospital I, Cook L, et al. Mental health problems of children presenting to emergency departments. Presented at: Third National Congress on Childhood Emergencies; April 15–17, 2002; Dallas, TX

41. Linzer JF. EMTALA: a clearer road in the future? *Clin Pediatr Emerg Med* 2003;4(4): 249–255

42. The Joint Commission. *Patient Safety Goals: Behavioral Health Care.* Available at: www.jointcommission.org/behavioral_ health_care_2011_national_patient_safety_ goals/. Accessed March 30, 2011

43. Krug SE. Access and use of emergency services: inappropriate use versus unmet need. *Clin Pediatr Emerg Med.* 1999;1(1): 35–44

44. Richardson L, Hwang U. Access to care: a review of the emergency medicine literature. *Acad Emerg Med.* 2001;8(11): 1030–1036

45. Garbrick L, Levitt M, Barrett M, Graham L. Agreement between emergency physicians regarding admission decisions. *Acad Emerg Med.* 1996;3(11):1027–1030

46. Santucci KA, Sather J, Baker MD. Emergency medicine training programs' educational requirements in the management of psychiatric emergencies: current perspective. *Pediatr Emerg Care.* 2003;19(3): 154–156

47. Weiss E. Mental health care emergency looms, N. Va officials warn. *Washington Post.* 2004:B01. Available at: www. washingtonpost.com/wp-dyn/articles/

A55515-2004Nov16.html. Accessed March 25, 2011

48. Dembner A. Acutely mentally ill children face delay of care, study finds. *Boston Globe.* 2003

49. Jenkins CL. Shortages hinder aid to disabled: regions' agencies cite lack of staffing, funds. *Washington Post.* 2004: PW03

50. Pear R. Many youths reported held awaiting mental help. *New York Times.* 2004:A18. Available at: www.nytimes.com/2004/07/ 08/politics/08mental.html?pagewanted= all. Accessed March 25, 2011

51. Brener ND, Martindale J, Weist MD. Mental health and social services: results from the School Health Policies and Programs Study 2000. *J Sch Health.* 2001;71(7): 305–312

52. National Assembly on School Based Care. *Creating Access to Care for Children and Youth: SBHC Census 1998–1999.*

53. Rones M, Hoagwood K. School-based mental health services: a research review. *Clin Child Fam Psychol Rev.* 2000;3(4):223–241

54. Borowsky IW, Mozayeny S, Ireland M. Brief psychosocial screening at health supervision and acute care visits. *Pediatrics.* 2003;112(1 pt 1):129–133

55. Costello EJ, Shugart MA. Above and below the threshold: severity of psychiatric symptoms and functional impairment in a pediatric sample. *Pediatrics.* 1992;90(3): 359–368

56. Lavigne JV, Binns HJ, Christoffel KK, et al. Behavioral and emotional problems among preschool children in pediatric primary care: prevalence and pediatricians' recognition. *Pediatrics.* 1993;91(3): 649–655

57. Wells K, Stewart A, Hays R, et al. The functioning and well-being of depressed patients. results from the Medical Outcomes Study. *JAMA.* 1989;262(7):914–919

58. Monnier J, Knapp RG, Frueh BC. Recent advances in telepsychiatry: an updated review. *Psychiatr Serv.* 2003;54(12): 1604–1609

59. Norman S. The use of telemedicine in psychiatry. *J Psychiatr Ment Health Nurs.* 2006;13(6):771–777

60. American Academy of Pediatrics, Council on School Health. Role of the school nurse in providing school health services. *Pediatrics.* 2008;121(5):1052–1056

61. American Academy of Pediatrics, Committee on Pediatric Emergency Medicine. The use of physical restraint interventions for children and adolescents in the acute care setting. *Pediatrics.* 1997;99(3):497–498

62. American College of Emergency Physicians. Use of patient restraint. *Ann Emerg Med.* 1996;28(3):384

63. Joint Commission on Accreditation of Healthcare Organizations. Standards for restraint and seclusion. *Jt Comm Perspect.* 1996;16(1):RS1–RS8

64. Fein J, Daugherty R. Restraint techniques and issues. In: King C, Henretig FM *The Textbook of Pediatric Emergency Procedures.* 2nd ed. Baltimore, MD: Lippincott, Williams & Wilkins; 2005:15–22

65. Beck A, Schuyler D, Herman I. Development of suicidal intent scales. In: Beck A, Resnik H, Lettieri D *The Prediction of Suicide.* Bowie, MD: Charles Press; 1974:45–56

66. White G Jr, Murdock R, Richardson G, Ellis G, Schmidt L. Development of a tool to assess suicide risk factors in urban adolescents. *Adolescence.* 1990;25(99):655–666

67. Reynolds W. *Suicidal Ideations Questionnaire: Professional Manual.* Odessa, FL: Psychological Assessment Resources; 1988

68. Siemen J, Warrington C, Mangano E. Comparison of the Millon Adolescent Personality Inventory and the Suicide Ideation Questionnaire–Junior with an adolescent inpatient sample. *Psychol Rep.* 1994;75(2): 947–950

69. Horowitz LM, Wang PS, Koocher GP, et al. Detecting suicide risk in a pediatric emergency department: development of a brief screening tool. *Pediatrics.* 2001;107(5): 1133–1137

70. Folse V, Eich K, Hall A, Ruppmann J. Detecting suicide risk in adolescents and adults in an emergency department: a pilot study. *J Psychosoc Nurs Ment Health Serv.* 2006; 44(3):22–29

71. Matthews KA, Salomon K, Brady SS, Allen MT. Cardiovascular reactivity to stress predicts future blood pressure in adolescence. *Psychosom Med.* 2003;65(3): 410–415

72. Middlebrooks JS, Audage NC. *The Effects of Childhood Stress on Health Across the Lifespan.* Atlanta, GA: Centers for Disease Control and Prevention, National Center for Injury Prevention and Control; 2008

73. Scott E, Luxmore B, Alexander H, Fenn R, Christopher N. Screening for adolescent depression in a pediatric emergency department. *Acad Emerg Med.* 2006;13(5): 537–542

74. Rutman M, Shenassa E, Becker B. Brief screening for adolescent depressive symptoms in the emergency department. *Acad Emerg Med.* 2008;15(1):17–22

75. US Preventive Services Task Force. Screening and treatment for major de-

pressive disorder in children and adolescents: US Preventive Services Task Force recommendation statement [published correction appears in *Pediatrics*. 2009; 123(6):1611]. *Pediatrics*. 2009;123(4): 1223–1228

76. Reynolds W. Development of a semistructured clinical interview for suicidal behaviors in adolescents. *Psychol Assess*. 1990; 2(4):382–390

77. Fein JA, Pailler M, Diamond G, Wintersteen M, Tien A, Hayes K, Barg F. Self-administered, Computerized Assessment of Adolescent Mental Illness in the Pediatric ED. *Archives of Pediatric and Adolescent Medicine*. 2010;164(12):1112–1117

78. Pailler M, Fein JA. Computerized behavioral health screening in the emergency department. *Pediatr Ann*. 2009;38(3): 156–160

79. National Scientific Council on the Developing Child. Excessive stress disrupts the architecture of the developing brain. Available at: www.developingchild.net/reports. shtml. Accessed May 25, 2009

80. Brick ND. The neurological basis for the theory of recovered memory. Available at: http://ritualabuse.us/research/memory-fms/the-neurological-basis-for-the-theory-of-recovered-memory/. Accessed March 25, 2011

81. Carrion VG, Weems CF, Reiss AL. Stress predicts brain changes in children: a pilot longitudinal study on youth stress, post-traumatic stress disorder, and the hippocampus. *Pediatrics*. 2007;119(3): 509–516

82. Foy D. Introduction and description of the disorder. In: Foy DW, ed *Treating PTSD: Cognitive-Behavioral Strategies*. New York, NY: Guilford; 1992:1–12

83. Meichenbaum D. *A Clinical Handbook/Practical Therapist Manual for Assessing and Treating Adults With Post-Traumatic Stress Disorder (PTSD)*. Waterloo, Ontario, Canada: Institute Press; 1994

84. Terr L. Childhood traumas: an outline and review. *Am J Psychiatry*. 1991;148(1): 10–20

85. van der Kolk B. The body keeps the score: memory and the evolving psychobiology of post traumatic stress. *Harv Rev Psychiatry*. 1994;1(5):253–265

86. Winston FK, Kassam-Adams N, Vivarelli-O'Neill C, et al. Acute stress disorder symptoms in children and their parents after pediatric traffic injury. *Pediatrics*. 2002;

109(6). Available at: www.pediatrics.org/cgi/content/full/109/6/e90

87. Kassam-Adams N, Fein J. Posttraumatic stress disorder and injury. *Clin Pediatr Emerg Med*. 2003;4(4):148–155

88. Shemesh E, Keshavarz R, Leichtling NK, et al. Pediatric emergency department assessment of psychological trauma and posttraumatic stress. *Psychiatr Serv*. 2003;54(9):1277–1281

89. Winston FK, Kassam-Adams N, Garcia-Espana F, Ittenbach R, Cnaan A. Screening for risk of persistent posttraumatic stress in injured children and their parents. *JAMA*. 2003;290(5):643–649

90. Zatzick D, Roy-Byrne P. Developing high-quality interventions for posttraumatic stress disorder in the acute care medical setting. *Semin Clin Neuropsychiatry*. 2003; 8(3):158–167

91. Kataoka S, Zhang L, Wells K. Unmet needs for mental health care among US children: variation by ethnicity and insurance status. *Am J Psychiatry*. 2002;159(9): 1548–1555

92. Marcos L. Effects of interpreters on the evaluation of psychopathology in non-English-speaking patients. *Am J Psychiatry*. 1979;136(2):171–174

93. Sturm, Roland, Ringel JS, Stein BD, Kapur K. *Mental Health Care for Youth: Who Gets It? How Much Does It Cost? Who Pays? Where Does the Money Go?*. Santa Monica, CA: RAND Corporation, 2001. Available at: www.rand.org/pubs/research_briefs/RB4541. Accessed March 31, 2011

94. Sturm R, Ringel JS, Andreyeva T. Geographic disparities in children's mental health care. *Pediatrics*. 2003;112(4). Available at: www.pediatrics.org/cgi/content/full/112/4/e308

95. Canty-Mitchell J, Austin JK, Jaffee K, Qi RA, Swigonski N. Behavioral and mental health problems in low-income children with special health care needs. *Arch Psychiatr Nurs*. 2004;18(3):79–87

96. Ganz ML, Tendulkar SA. Mental health care services for children with special health care needs and their family members: prevalence and correlates of unmet needs [published correction appears in *Pediatrics*. 2006;118(4):1806–1807]. *Pediatrics*. 2006;117(6):2138–2148

97. Stuber M, Shemesh E, Saxe G. Posttraumatic stress responses in children with life-threatening illnesses. *Child Adolesc Psychiatr Clin N Am*. 2003;12(2):195–209

98. Chavira D, Garland A, Daley S, Hough R. The

impact of medical comorbidity on mental health and functional health outcomes among children with anxiety disorders. *J Dev Behav Pediatr*. 2008;29(5):394–402

99. BeLue R, Francis LA, Colaco B. Mental health problems and overweight in a nationally representative sample of adolescents: effects of race and ethnicity. *Pediatrics*. 2009;123(2):697–702

100. Brown EJ, Goodman RF. Childhood traumatic grief: an exploration of the construct in children bereaved on September 11. *J Clin Child Adolesc Psychol*. 2005;34(2): 248–259

101. Goenjian AK, Molina L, Steinberg AM, et al. Posttraumatic stress and depressive reactions among Nicaraguan adolescents after Hurricane Mitch. *Am J Psychiatry*. 2001; 158(5):788–794

102. Goenjian AK, Walling D, Steinberg AM, Karayan I, Najarian LM, Pynoos R. A prospective study of posttraumatic stress and depressive reactions among treated and untreated adolescents 5 years after a catastrophic disaster. *Am J Psychiatry*. 2005; 162(12):2302–2308

103. Pfefferbaum B, North C, Doughty D, et al. Trauma, grief and depression in Nairobi children after the 1998 bombing of the American embassy. *Death Stud*. 2006; 30(6):561–577

104. Zatzick D, Grossman D, Russo J, et al. Predicting posttraumatic stress symptoms longitudinally in a representative sample of hospitalized injured adolescents. *J Am Acad Child Adolesc Psychiatry*. 2006; 45(10):1188–1195

105. Dayan P, Chamberlain J, Dean JM, Maio RF, Kuppermann N. The pediatric emergency care applied research network: progress and update. *Clin Pediatr Emerg Med* 2006: 7:128–135

106. Azrael D, Hemenway D, Miller M, Barber C, Schackner R. Youth suicide: insights from 5 years of Arizona child fatality review team data. *Suicide Life-threat Behav*. 2004; 34(1):36–43

107. American Academy of Child and Adolescent Psychiatry, Task Force on Mental Health. Improving mental health services in primary care: reducing administrative and financial barriers to access and collaboration [published correction appears in *Pediatrics*. 2009;123(6):1611]. *Pediatrics*. 2009;123(4):1248–1251

108. Paul Wellstone and Pete Dominici Mental Health Parity and Addiction Equity Act, Pub L No. 110-3432008

CLINICAL REPORT   Guidance for the Clinician in Rendering Pediatric Care

American Academy
of Pediatrics

DEDICATED TO THE HEALTH OF ALL CHILDREN™

Suicide and Suicide Attempts in Adolescents

Benjamin Shain, MD, PhD, COMMITTEE ON ADOLESCENCE

Suicide is the second leading cause of death for adolescents 15 to 19 years old. This report updates the previous statement of the American Academy of Pediatrics and is intended to assist pediatricians, in collaboration with other child and adolescent health care professionals, in the identification and management of the adolescent at risk for suicide. Suicide risk can only be reduced, not eliminated, and risk factors provide no more than guidance. Nonetheless, care for suicidal adolescents may be improved with the pediatrician's knowledge, skill, and comfort with the topic, as well as ready access to appropriate community resources and mental health professionals.

abstract

Clinical reports from the American Academy of Pediatrics benefit from expertise and resources of liaisons and internal (AAP) and external reviewers. However, clinical reports from the American Academy of Pediatrics may not reflect the views of the liaisons or the organizations or government agencies that they represent.

The guidance in this report does not indicate an exclusive course of treatment or serve as a standard of medical care. Variations, taking into account individual circumstances, may be appropriate.

All clinical reports from the American Academy of Pediatrics automatically expire 5 years after publication unless reaffirmed, revised, or retired at or before that time.

DOI: 10.1542/peds.2016-1420

PEDIATRICS (ISSN Numbers: Print, 0031-4005; Online, 1098-4275).

FINANCIAL DISCLOSURE: The author has indicated he does not have a financial relationship relevant to this article to disclose.

FUNDING: No external funding.

POTENTIAL CONFLICT OF INTEREST: The author has indicated he has no potential conflicts of interest to disclose.

To cite: Shain B and AAP COMMITTEE ON ADOLESCENCE. Suicide and Suicide Attempts in Adolescents. *Pediatrics.* 2016;138(1):e20161420

INTRODUCTION

The number of adolescent deaths that result from suicide in the United States had been increasing dramatically during recent decades until 1990, when it began to decrease modestly. From 1950 to 1990, the suicide rate for adolescents 15 to 19 years old increased by 300%,[1] but from 1990 to 2013, the rate in this age group decreased by 28%.[2] In 2013, there were 1748 suicides among people 15 to 19 years old.[2] The true number of deaths from suicide actually may be higher, because some of these deaths may have been recorded as "accidental."[3] Adolescent boys 15 to 19 years old had a completed suicide rate that was 3 times greater than that of their female counterparts,[2] whereas the rate of suicide attempts was twice as high among girls than among boys, correlating to girls tending to choose less lethal methods.[4] The ratio of attempted suicides to completed suicides among adolescents is estimated to be 50:1 to 100:1.[5]

Suicide affects young people from all races and socioeconomic groups, although some groups have higher rates than others. American Indian/Alaska Native males have the highest suicide rate, and black females have the lowest rate of suicide. Sexual minority youth (ie, lesbian, gay, bisexual, transgender, or questioning) have more than twice the rate of suicidal ideation.[6] The 2013 Youth Risk Behavior Survey of students in grades 9 through 12 in the United States indicated that during the 12 months before the survey, 39.1% of girls and 20.8% of boys felt sad or hopeless almost every day for at least 2 weeks in a row, 16.9% of girls and 10.3% of boys had planned a suicide attempt, 10.6% of girls and 5.4% of boys had attempted suicide, and 3.6% of girls and 1.8% of boys had made a suicide attempt that required medical attention.[7]

The leading methods of suicide for the 15- to 19-year age group in 2013 were suffocation (43%), discharge of firearms (42%), poisoning (6%), and falling (3%).[2] Particular attention should be given to access to firearms, because reducing firearm access may prevent suicides. Firearms in the home, regardless of whether they are kept unloaded or stored locked, are associated with a higher risk of completed adolescent suicide.[8,9] However, in another study examining firearm security, each of the practices of securing the firearm (keeping it locked and unloaded) and securing the ammunition (keeping it locked and stored away from the firearm) were associated with reduced risk of youth shootings that resulted in unintentional or self-inflicted injury or death.[10]

Youth seem to be at much greater risk from media exposure than adults and may imitate suicidal behavior seen on television.[11] Media coverage of an adolescent's suicide may lead to cluster suicides, with the magnitude of additional deaths proportional to the amount, duration, and prominence of the media coverage.[11] A prospective study found increased suicidality with exposure to the suicide of a schoolmate.[12] Newspaper reports about suicide were associated with an increase in adolescent suicide clustering, with greater clustering associated with article front-page placement, mention of suicide or the method of suicide in the article title, and detailed description in the article text about the individual

or the suicide act.[13] More research is needed to determine the psychological mechanisms behind suicide clustering.[14,15] The National Institute of Mental Health suggests best practices for media and online reporting of deaths by suicide.[16]

ADOLESCENTS AT INCREASED RISK

Although no specific tests are capable of identifying a suicidal person, specific risk factors exist.[11,17] The health care professional should use care in interpreting risk factors, however, because risk factors are common, whereas suicide is infrequent. Of importance, the lack of most risk factors does not make an adolescent safe from suicide. Fixed risk factors include: family history of suicide or suicide attempts; history of adoption[18,19]; male gender; parental mental health problems; lesbian, gay, bisexual, or questioning sexual orientation; transgender identification; a history of physical or sexual abuse; and a previous suicide attempt. Personal mental health problems that predispose to suicide include sleep disturbances,[20] depression, bipolar disorder, substance intoxication and substance use disorders, psychosis, posttraumatic stress disorder, panic attacks, a history of aggression, impulsivity, severe anger, and pathologic Internet use (see *Internet Use* section). In particular, interview studies showed a marked higher rate of suicidal behavior with the presence of psychotic symptoms.[21] A prospective study found a 70-fold increase of acute suicidal behavior in adolescents with psychopathology that included psychosis.[22] By definition, nonsuicidal self-injury (NSSI) does not include intent to die, and risk of death is deliberately low. Nonetheless, NSSI is a risk factor for suicide attempts[23,24] and suicidal ideation.[25] More than 90% of adolescent suicide victims met criteria for a psychiatric disorder

before their death. Immediate risk factors include agitation, intoxication, and a recent stressful life event. More information is available from the American Academy of Child and Adolescent Psychiatry[26] and Gould et al.[11]

Social and environmental risk factors include bullying, impaired parent–child relationship, living outside of the home (homeless or in a corrections facility or group home), difficulties in school, neither working nor attending school, social isolation, and presence of stressful life events, such as legal or romantic difficulties or an argument with a parent. An unsupported social environment for lesbian, gay, bisexual, and transgender adolescents, for example, increases risk of suicide attempts.[27] Protective factors include religious involvement and connection between the adolescent and parents, school, and peers.[26]

Bullying

Bullying has been defined as having 3 elements: aggressive or deliberately harmful behavior (1) between peers that is (2) repeated and over time and (3) involves an imbalance of power, for example, related to physical strength or popularity, making it difficult for the victim to defend himself or herself.[28] Behavior falls into 4 categories: direct-physical (eg, assault, theft), direct-verbal (eg, threats, insults, name-calling), indirect-relational (eg, social exclusion, spreading rumors), and cyberbullying.[29] The 2013 Youth Risk Behavior Survey of students in grades 9 through 12 in the United States indicated that during the 12 months before the survey, 23.7% of girls and 15.6% of boys were bullied on school property, 21.0% of girls and 8.5% of boys were electronically bullied, and 8.7% of girls and 5.4% of boys did not go to school 1 day in the past 30 because they felt unsafe at or to or from school.[7] Studies have focused on 3 groups: those who were victims, those who were bullies, and those who were both victims and bullies (bully/victims).[30]

Reviewing 31 studies, Klomek et al[29] found a clear relationship between both bullying victimization and perpetration and suicidal ideation and behavior in children and adolescents. Females were at risk regardless of frequency, whereas males were at higher risk only with frequent bullying. A review by Arseneault et al[31] cited evidence that bullying victimization is associated with severe baseline psychopathology, as well as individual characteristics and family factors, and that the psychopathology is made significantly worse by the victimization. Being the victim of school bullying or cyberbullying is associated with substantial distress, resulting in lower school performance and school attachment.[32] Suicidal ideation and behavior were greater in those bullied with controlling for age, gender, race/ethnicity, and depressive symptomology.[33] Suicidal ideation and behavior were increased in victims and bullies and were highest in bully/victims.[34] Similar increases in suicide attempts were found comparing face-to-face bullying with cyberbullying, both for victims and bullies.[35]

Bullying predicts future mental health problems. Bullying behavior at 8 years of age was associated with later suicide attempts and completed suicides,[36] although among boys, frequent perpetration and victimization was not associated with attempts and completions after controlling for conduct and depressive symptoms. Among girls, frequent victimization was associated with later suicide attempts and completions even after controlling for conduct and depressive symptoms. High school students with the highest psychiatric impairment 4 years later were those who had been identified as at-risk for

suicide *and* experiencing frequent bullying behavior. Copeland et al[30] found that children and adolescents involved in bullying behavior had the worst outcomes when they were both bullies and victims, leading to depression, anxiety, and suicidality (suicidality only among males) as adults. Assessment for adolescents with psychopathology, other signs of emotional distress, or unusual chronic complaints should include screening for participation in bullying as victims or bullies.

Internet Use

Pathologic Internet use correlates with suicidal ideation and NSSI.[37] Self-reported daily use of video games and Internet exceeding 5 hours was strongly associated with higher levels of depression and suicidality (ideation and attempts) in adolescents.[38] A more specific problem is that adolescents with suicidal ideation may be at particular risk for searching the Internet for information about suicide-related topics.[39] Suicide-related searches were found to be associated with completed suicides among young adults.[40] Prosuicide Web sites and online suicide pacts facilitate suicidal behavior, with adolescents and young adults at particular risk.[37]

A number of factors diminish the exposure of prosuicide Web sites. Web site results from the search term, "suicide," are predominantly of institutional origin, with content largely related to research and prevention. Although there are a substantial number of sites from private senders (these sites are often antimedical, antitreatment, and pro-suicide,[41] including sites that advocate suicide or describe methods in detail[42]), suicide research and prevention sites tend to come up in searches more commonly. Clicking on links within each site keeps the reader in the site, strengthening the site's position. Methods sites and overtly prosuicide sites are

more isolated, decentralized, and unfocused; these are less prevalent among the first 100 search results, perhaps related to a recent and deliberate strategy by the internet search engines (eg, search engine optimization).[41]

Learning of another's suicide online may be another risk factor for youth.[43] Exposure to such information is through online news sites (44%), social networking sites (25%), online discussion forums (15%), and video Web sites (15%). Social networking sites have particular importance, because these may afford information on suicidal behavior of social contacts that would not otherwise be available. Fortunately, exposure to information from social networking sites does not appear related to changes in suicidal ideation, with increased exposure mitigated by greater social support. Participation in online forums, however, was associated with increases in suicidal ideation, possibly related to anonymous discussions about mental health problems. For example, suicide attempts by susceptible individuals appear to have been encouraged by such conversations.[44,45]

INTERVIEWING THE ADOLESCENT

Primary care pediatricians should be comfortable screening patients for suicide, mood disorders, and substance abuse and dependence. Ask about emotional difficulties and use of drugs and alcohol, identify lack of developmental progress, and estimate level of distress, impairment of functioning, and level of danger to self and others. Depression screening instruments shown to be valid in adolescents include the Patient Health Questionnaire (PHQ)-9 and PHQ-2.[46] If needed, a referral should be made for appropriate mental health evaluation and treatment. In areas where the resources necessary to make a timely mental health referral are lacking, pediatricians are encouraged to obtain extra training and become competent in providing a more in-depth assessment.

Suicidal ideation may be assessed by directly asking or screening via self-report. Self-administered scales can be useful for screening, because adolescents may disclose information about suicidality on self-report that they deny in person. Scales, however, tend to be oversensitive and underspecific and lack predictive value. Adolescents who endorse suicidality on a scale should be assessed clinically. Screening tools useable in a primary care setting have not been shown to have more than limited ability to detect suicide risk in adolescents,[47] consistent with the findings of an earlier review.[48] Instruments studied in adolescent groups with high prevalence of suicidal ideation and behavior showed sensitivity of 52% to 87% and specificity of 60% to 85%; the results are only generalizable to high-risk populations.[49,50] Suicide screening, at least in the school setting, does not appear to cause thoughts of suicide or other psychiatric symptoms in students.[51,52]

One approach to initiate a confidential inquiry into suicidal thoughts or concerns is to ask a general question, such as, "Have you ever thought about killing yourself or wished you were dead?" The question is best placed in the middle or toward the end of a list of questions about depressive symptoms. Regardless of the answer, the next question should be, "Have you ever done anything on purpose to hurt or kill yourself?" If the response to either question is positive, the pediatrician should obtain more detail (eg, nature of past and present thoughts and behaviors, time frame, intent, who knows and how they found out). Inquiry should include suicide plans ("If you were to kill yourself, how would you do it?"), whether there are firearms in the

home, and the response of the family. No data indicate that inquiry about suicide precipitates the behavior, even in high-risk students.[51]

The adolescent should be interviewed separately from the parent, because the patient may be more likely to withhold important information in the parent's presence. Information should also be sought from parents and others as appropriate. Although confidentiality is important in adolescent health care, for adolescents at risk to themselves or others, safety takes precedence over confidentiality; the adolescent should have this explained by the pediatrician so that he or she understands that at the onset. Pediatricians need to inform appropriate people, such as parent(s) and other providers, when they believe an adolescent is at risk for suicide and to share with the adolescent that there is a need to break confidentiality because of the risk of harm to the adolescent. As much as is possible, the sequence of events that preceded the threat should be determined, current problems and conflicts should be identified, and the degree of suicidal intent should be assessed. In addition, pediatricians should assess individual coping resources, accessible support systems, and attitudes of the adolescent and family toward intervention and follow-up.[53] Questions should also be asked to elicit known risk factors. Note that it is acceptable and, in some cases, more appropriate for the patient to be referred to a mental health specialist to access the degree of suicide intent and relevant factors such as coping mechanisms and support systems.

Care in interviewing needs to be taken, because abrupt, intrusive questions could result in a reduction of rapport and a lower likelihood of the adolescent sharing mental health concerns. This is especially true during a brief encounter for an

unrelated concern. Initial questions should be open-ended and relatively nonthreatening. Examples include "Aside from [already stated non–mental health concern], how have you been doing?" "I know that a lot of people your age have a lot going on. What kinds of things have been on your mind or stressing you lately?" "How have things been going with [school, friends, parents, sports]?" When possible, more detailed questions should then follow, particularly during routine care visits or when a mental health concern is stated or suspected.

Suicidal thoughts or comments should never be dismissed as unimportant. Statements such as, "You've come really close to killing yourself," may, if true, acknowledge the deep despair of the youth and communicate to the adolescent that the interviewer understands how serious he or she has felt about dying. Such disclosures should be met with reassurance that the patient's pleas for assistance have been heard and that help will be sought.

Serious mood disorders, such as major depressive disorder or bipolar disorder, may present in adolescents in several ways.[54] Some adolescents may come to the office with complaints similar to those of depressed adults, having symptoms, such as sad or down feelings most of the time, crying spells, guilty or worthless feelings, markedly diminished interest or pleasure in most activities, significant weight loss or weight gain or increase or decrease in appetite, insomnia or hypersomnia, fatigue or loss of energy, diminished ability to think or concentrate, and thoughts of death or suicide. The pediatrician should also look for adolescent behaviors that are characteristic of symptoms (Table 1).[54] Some adolescents may present with irritability rather than depressed mood as the main manifestation. Other adolescents present for an acute care visit with somatic symptoms, such as abdominal pain, chest pain, headache, lethargy, weight loss, dizziness and syncope, or other nonspecific symptoms[55] Others present with behavioral problems, such as truancy, deterioration in academic performance, running away from home, defiance of authorities, self-destructive behavior, vandalism, substance use disorder, sexual acting out, and delinquency.[56] Typically, symptoms of depression, mania, or a mixed state (depression and mania coexisting or rapidly alternating) can be elicited with careful questioning but may not be immediately obvious. The American Academy of Pediatrics (AAP) provides more information about adolescent bipolar disorder and the role of the pediatrician in screening, diagnosis, and management.[57]

At well-adolescent visits, adolescents who show any evidence of psychosocial or adaptive difficulties should be assessed regularly for mental health concerns and also asked about suicidal ideation, physical and sexual abuse, bullying, substance use, and sexual orientation. Depression screening is now recommended for all adolescents between the ages of 11 and 21 years of age in the third edition of *Bright Futures*.[58] The AAP developed a resource, "Addressing Mental Health Concerns in Primary Care: A Clinician's Toolkit," which is available for a fee.[59] The AAP also developed a Web site that provides resources and materials free of charge.[60] Identification and screening at acute care visits, when possible, is desirable, because mental health problems may manifest more strongly at these times.

MANAGEMENT OF THE SUICIDAL ADOLESCENT

Management depends on the degree of acute risk. Unfortunately, no one can accurately predict suicide, so

TABLE 1 Depressive Symptoms and Examples in Adolescents[54]

Signs and Symptoms of Major Depressive Disorder	Signs of Depression Frequently Seen in Youth
Depressed mood most of the day	Irritable or cranky mood; preoccupation with song lyrics that suggest life is meaningless
Decreased interest/enjoyment in once-favorite activities	Loss of interest in sports, video games, and activities with friends
Significant wt loss/gain	Failure to gain wt as normally expected; anorexia or bulimia; frequent complaints of physical illness (eg, headache, stomach ache)
Insomnia or hypersomnia	Excessive late-night TV; refusal to wake for school in the morning
Psychomotor agitation/retardation	Talk of running away from home or efforts to do so
Fatigue or loss of energy	Persistent boredom
Low self-esteem; feelings of guilt	Oppositional and/or negative behavior
Decreased ability to concentrate; indecisive	Poor performance in school; frequent absences
Recurrent thoughts of death or suicidal ideation or behavior	Recurrent suicidal ideation or behavior (threats of suicide, writing about death; giving away favorite toys or belongings)

even experts can only determine who is at higher risk. Intent is a key issue in the determination of risk. Examples of adolescents at high risk include: those with a plan or recent suicide attempt with a high probability of lethality; stated current intent to kill themselves; recent suicidal ideation or behavior accompanied by current agitation or severe hopelessness; and impulsivity and profoundly dysphoric mood associated with bipolar disorder, major depression, psychosis, or a substance use disorder. An absence of factors that indicate high risk, especially in the presence of a desire to receive help and a supportive family, suggests a lower risk but not necessarily a low risk. Low risk is difficult to determine. For example, an adolescent who has taken 8 ibuprofen tablets may have thought that it was a lethal dose and may do something more lethal the next time. Alternatively, the adolescent may have known that 8 ibuprofen tablets is not lethal and took the pills as a rehearsal for a lethal attempt. In the presence of a recent suicide attempt, the lack of current suicidal ideation may also be misleading if none of the factors that led to the attempt have changed or the reasons for the attempt are not understood. The benefit of the doubt is generally

on safety in the management of the suicidal adolescent.

The term "suicide gesture" should not be used, because it implies a low risk of suicide that may not be warranted. "Suicide attempt" is a more appropriate term for any deliberately self-harmful behavior or action that could reasonably be expected to produce self-harm and is accompanied by some degree of intent or desire for death as well as thinking by the patient at the time of the behavior that the behavior had even a small possibility of resulting in death. In a less-than-forthcoming patient, intent may be inferred by the lethality of the behavior, such as ingesting a large number of pills, or by an affirmative answer to a question such as, "At the time of your action, would you have thought it okay if you had died?"

Adolescents who initially may seem at low risk, joke about suicide, or seek treatment of repeated somatic complaints may be asking for help the only way they can. Their concerns should be assessed thoroughly. Adolescents who are judged to be at low risk of suicide should still receive close follow-up, referral for a timely mental health evaluation, or both if they should have any significant degree of dysfunction or distress from emotional or behavioral symptoms.

For adolescents who seem to be at moderate or high risk of suicide or have attempted suicide, arrangements for immediate mental health professional evaluation should be made during the office visit. Options for immediate evaluation include hospitalization, transfer to an emergency department, or a same-day appointment with a mental health professional.

Intervention should be tailored to the adolescent's needs. Adolescents with a responsive and supportive family, little likelihood of acting on suicidal impulses (eg, thought of dying with no intent or plan for suicide), and someone who can take action if there is mood or behavior deterioration may require only outpatient treatment.[17] In contrast, adolescents who have made previous attempts, exhibit a high degree of intent to commit suicide, show evidence of serious depression or other psychiatric illness, engage in substance use or have an active substance use disorder, have low impulse control, or have families who are unwilling to commit to counseling are at high risk and may require psychiatric hospitalization.

Although no controlled studies have been conducted to prove that admitting adolescents at high risk to a psychiatric unit saves lives,[17] likely the safest course of action is hospitalization, thereby placing the adolescent in a safe and protected environment. An inpatient stay will allow time for a complete medical and psychiatric evaluation with initiation of therapy in a controlled setting as well as arrangement of appropriate mental health follow-up care.

Pediatricians can enhance continuity of care and adherence to treatment recommendations by maintaining contact with suicidal adolescents even after referrals are made. Collaborative care is encouraged, because it has been shown to result in greater reduction of depressive symptoms in a primary care setting.[61] Recommendations should include that all firearms are removed from the home, because adolescents may still find access to locked guns stored in their home, and that medications, both prescription and over-the-counter, are locked up. Vigorous treatment of the underlying psychiatric disorder is important in decreasing short-term and long-term risk of suicide. Although asking the adolescent to agree to a contract against suicide has not been proven effective in preventing suicidal behavior,[17] the technique may still be helpful in assessing risk in that refusal to agree either not to harm oneself or to tell a specified person about intent to harm oneself is ominous. In addition, safety planning may help guide a patient and his or her family in what steps to take in moments of distress to ensure patient safety.

Working with a suicidal adolescent can be very difficult for those who are providing treatment. Suicide risk can only be reduced, not eliminated, and risk factors provide no more than guidance. Much of the information regarding risk factors is subjective and must be elicited from the adolescent, who may have his or her own agenda. Just as importantly, pediatricians need to be aware of their personal reactions to prevent interference in evaluation and treatment and overreaction or underreaction.

ANTIDEPRESSANT MEDICATIONS AND SUICIDE

The Food and Drug Administration (FDA) directive of October 2004 and heavy media coverage changed perceptions of antidepressant medications, and not favorably. The FDA directed pharmaceutical companies to label all antidepressant medications distributed in the United States with a "black-box warning" to alert health care providers to an increased risk of suicidality (suicidal thinking and behavior) in children and adolescents being treated with these agents. The FDA did not prohibit the use of these medications in youth but called on clinicians to balance increased risk of suicidality with clinical need and to monitor closely "for clinical worsening, suicidality, or unusual changes in behavior."[62] The warning particularly stressed the need for close monitoring during the first few months of treatment and after dose changes.

The warning by the FDA was prompted by a finding that in 24 clinical trials that involved more than 4400 child and adolescent patients and 9 different antidepressant medications, spontaneously reported suicidal ideation or behavior was present in 4% of subjects who were receiving medication and in just half that (2%) of subjects who were receiving a placebo. No completed suicides occurred during any of the studies. In the same studies, however, only a slight reduction of suicidality was found when subjects were asked directly at each visit about suicidal ideation and behavior, which was considered a contradictory finding. The method of asking directly does not rely on spontaneous reports and is considered to be more reliable than the spontaneous events report method used by the FDA to support the black-box warning.[63] In addition, a reanalysis of the data including 7 additional studies and using a more conservative model showed only a trivial 0.7% increase in the risk of suicidal ideation or behavior in those receiving antidepressant medications.[64]

Subsequent studies have addressed the validity of the black-box warning and suggest that, for appropriate youth, the risk of not prescribing antidepressant medication is significantly higher than the risk of prescribing. Gibbons et al[65] conducted a reanalysis of all sponsor-conducted randomized controlled trials of fluoxetine and venlafaxine, which included 12 adult, 4 geriatric, and 4 youth studies of fluoxetine and 21 adult trials of venlafaxine. Adult and geriatric patients treated with both medications showed decreased suicidal thoughts and behaviors, an effect mediated by the decreases of depressive symptoms with treatment. No significant treatment effect on suicidal thoughts and behaviors was found with youth treated with fluoxetine, although depressive symptoms in fluoxetine-treated patients decreased more quickly than symptoms in patients receiving placebo. There was no overall greater rate of suicidal thoughts and behaviors in the treatment groups versus the placebo groups. The finding of increased suicidal ideation and behavior in the treatment groups that formed the basis of the FDA black-box warning on antidepressant use in children and adolescents was not found in this reanalysis of the fluoxetine studies. More importantly, these reanalyses demonstrated the efficacy of fluoxetine in the treatment of depression in youth. Patients in all age and drug groups had significantly greater improvement relative to patients in placebo groups, with youth having the largest differential rate of remission over 6 weeks—46.6% of patients receiving fluoxetine versus 16.5% of those receiving placebo.[66]

Suicidal ideation and behavior are common, and suicides are vastly less common, which makes it difficult to relate a change in one to a change in the other.[63] Examining all available observational studies, Dudley et al[67] found that recent exposure to selective serotonin reuptake inhibitor medications was rare (1.6%) for young people who died by suicide, supporting the conclusion that most of the suicide victims did not have the potential benefit of antidepressants at the time of their deaths. The study suggests that whether antidepressants increase suicidal

thoughts or behaviors in adolescents, few actual suicides are related to current use of the medications.

Several studies showed a negative correlation between antidepressant prescribing and completed adolescent suicide. The 28% decrease in completed suicides in the 10- to 19-year-old age group from 1990 to 2000 may have been at least partly a result of the increase in youth antidepressant prescribing over the same time period. Analyzing US data by examining prescribing and suicide in each of 588 2-digit zip code zones showed a significant ($P < .001$) 0.23-per-100 000 annual decrease in adolescent suicide with every 1% increase in antidepressant prescribing.[68] A second study analyzed county-level data during the period from1996 to1998 and found that higher selective serotonin reuptake inhibitor prescription rates significantly correlated with lower suicide rates among children and adolescents 5 to 14 years of age.[69] Using a decision analysis model, Cougnard et al[70] calculated that antidepressant treatment of children and adolescents would prevent 31.9% of suicides of depressed subjects, similar to findings in the adult (32.2%) and geriatric (32.3%) age groups.

The FDA advisory panel was aware that the black-box warning could have the unintended effect of limiting access to necessary and effective treatment[63] and reported that prescriptions of antidepressants for children and adolescents decreased by 19% in the third quarter of 2004 and 16% in the fourth quarter compared with the year before.[71] Claims data for Tennessee Medicaid showed a 33% reduction of new users of antidepressants 21 months after the black-box warning.[72] US national managed care data showed reduced diagnosing of pediatric depression and a 58% reduction of antidepressant prescribing compared with what was predicted by the preadvisory trend.[73] Decreased

antidepressant prescribing was also seen with chart review.[74] Most of the reductions in diagnosing and prescribing were related to substantial reductions by primary care providers, with these reductions persisting through 2007.[75] Studies differed as to whether there was[76] or was not[73,74] a compensatory increase of psychotherapy treatment during the same time period.

Concern was expressed that the reduction of antidepressant prescribing may be related to the increase in US youth suicides from 2003 to 2004 after a decade of steady declines.[77] Gibbons et al[78] found that antidepressant prescribing for youth decreased by 22% in both the United States and the Netherlands the year after the black-box warnings in both countries and a reduction in prescribing was observed across all ages. From 2003 to 2004, the youth suicide rate in the United States increased by 14%; from 2003 to 2005, the youth suicide rate in the Netherlands increased by 49%. Across age groups, data showed a significant inverse correlation between prescribing and change in suicide rate. The authors suggested that the warnings could have had the unintended effect of increasing the rate of youth suicide.[78] Examining health insurance claims data for 1.1 million adolescents, 1.4 million young adults, and 5 million adults, the rate of psychotropic medication poisonings, a validate proxy for suicide attempts, was found to have increased significantly in adolescents (21.7%) and young adults (33.7%), but not in adults (5.2%), in the second year after the FDA black-box warning, corresponding with decreases in antidepressant prescribing (adolescents, –31.0%; young adults, –24.3%; adults, –14.5%).[79]

Regardless of whether the use of antidepressant medications changes the risk of suicide, depression is an important suicide risk factor, and careful monitoring of adolescents' mental health and behavioral status is critically important, particularly when initiating or changing treatment. Furthermore, despite the aforementioned new information, the FDA has not removed or changed the black-box warning; the warning should be discussed with parents or guardians and appropriately documented. The American Psychiatric Association and the American Academy of Child and Adolescent Psychiatry recommended a monitoring approach[63] that enlists the parents or guardians in the responsibility for monitoring and individualizing the frequency and nature of monitoring to the needs of the patient and the family. This approach potentially increases the effectiveness of monitoring and provides greater flexibility, thus reducing a barrier to prescribing. Warning signs for family members to contact the prescribing physician are listed in Table 2.[63]

SUMMARY

1. Adolescent suicide is an important public health problem.

2. Knowledge of risk factors, particularly mood disorders, psychosis, and bullying victimization and perpetration, may assist in the identification of adolescents who are at higher risk.

3. It is important to know and use appropriate techniques for interviewing potentially suicidal adolescents.

4. Mood disorders predisposing adolescents to suicide have a variety of presentations.

5. Management options depend on the degree of suicide risk.

6. Treatment with antidepressant medication is important when indicated.

TABLE 2 Treatment With Antidepressant Medication: Warning Signs for Family Members To Contact the Physician

New or more frequent thoughts of wanting to die
Self-destructive behavior
Signs of increased anxiety/panic, agitation, aggressiveness, impulsivity, insomnia, or irritability
New or more involuntary restlessness (akathesia), such as pacing or fidgeting
Extreme degree of elation or energy
Fast, driven speech
New onset of unrealistic plans or goals

ADVICE FOR PEDIATRICIANS

1. Ask questions about mood disorders, use of drugs and alcohol, suicidal thoughts, bullying, sexual orientation, and other risk factors associated with suicide in routine history taking throughout adolescence. Know the risk factors (eg, signs and symptoms of depression) associated with adolescent suicide and screen routinely for depression. Consider using a depression screening instrument, such as the PHQ-9 or PHQ-2, at health maintenance visits from 11 to 21 years of age and as needed at acute care visits.[46]

2. Educate yourself and your patients about the benefits and risks of antidepressant medications. Patients with depression should be carefully monitored, with appropriately frequent appointments and education of the family regarding warning signs for when to call you, especially after the initiation of antidepressant medication treatment and with dose changes. Recent studies suggest that, for appropriate youth, the benefits of antidepressant medications outweigh the risks.

3. Recognize the medical and psychiatric needs of the suicidal adolescent and work closely with families and health care professionals involved in the management and follow-up of youth who are at risk or have attempted suicide. Develop working relationships with emergency departments and colleagues in child and adolescent psychiatry, clinical psychology, and other mental health professions to optimally evaluate and manage the care of adolescents who are at risk for suicide. Because mental and physical health services are often provided through different systems of care, extra effort is necessary to ensure good communication, continuity, and follow-up through the medical home.

4. Because resources for adolescents and physicians vary by community, become familiar with local, state, and national resources that are concerned with treatment of psychopathology and suicide prevention in youth, including local hospitals with psychiatric units, mental health agencies, family and children's services, crisis hotlines, and crisis intervention centers. Compile the names and contact information of local mental health resources and providers and make that information available to patients/families when needed.

5. Because there is great variation among general pediatricians in training and comfort with assessing and treating patients with mental health problems, as well as in access to appropriate mental health resources, consider additional training and ongoing education in diagnosing and managing adolescent mood disorders, especially if practicing in an underserved area.

Pediatricians with fewer resources still have an important role in screening, comanaging with mental health professionals, and referring patients when necessary (as recommended in *Bright Futures, Fourth Edition*).

6. During routine evaluations and where consistent with state law, ask whether firearms are kept in the home and discuss with parents the increased risk of adolescent suicide with the presence of firearms. Specifically for adolescents at risk for suicide, advise parents to remove guns and ammunition from the house and secure supplies of prescription and over-the-counter medications.

LEAD AUTHOR

Benjamin Shain, MD, PhD

COMMITTEE ON ADOLESCENCE, 2014-2015

Paula K. Braverman, MD, Chairperson
William P. Adelman, MD
Elizabeth M. Alderman, MD, FSHAM
Cora C. Breuner, MD, MPH
David A. Levine, MD
Arik V. Marcell, MD, MPH
Rebecca F. O'Brien, MD

LIAISONS

Laurie L. Hornberger, MD, MPH – *Section on Adolescent Health*
Margo Lane, MD, FRCPC – *Canadian Pediatric Society*
Julie Strickland, MD – *American College of Obstetricians and Gynecologists*
Benjamin Shain, MD, PhD – *American Academy of Child and Adolescent Psychiatry*

STAFF

Karen Smith
James Baumberger, MPP

ABBREVIATIONS

AAP: American Academy of Pediatrics
FDA: Food and Drug Administration
NSSI: nonsuicidal self-injury
PHQ: Patient Health Questionnaire

REFERENCES

1. O'Carroll PW, Potter LB, Mercy JA. Programs for the prevention of suicide among adolescents and young adults. *MMWR Recomm Rep.* 1994;43(RR-6):1–7

2. Centers for Disease Control and Prevention. CDC Wonder [database]: mortality query. Available at: http://wonder.cdc.gov. Accessed April 24, 2015

3. American Psychiatric Association, Committee on Adolescence. *Adolescent Suicide.* Washington, DC: American Psychiatric Press; 1996

4. Grunbaum JA, Kann L, Kinchen S, et al; Centers for Disease Control and Prevention. Youth risk behavior surveillance--United States, 2003. [published corrections appear in *MMWR Morb Mortal Wkly Rep.* 2004;53(24):536 and *MMWR Morb Mortal Wkly Rep.* 2005;54(24):608] *MMWR Surveill Summ.* 2004;53(2):1–96

5. Husain SA. Current perspective on the role of psychological factors in adolescent suicide. *Psychiatr Ann.* 1990;20(3):122–127

6. Committee On Adolescence. Office-based care for lesbian, gay, bisexual, transgender, and questioning youth. *Pediatrics.* 2013;132(1):198–203

7. Kann L, Kinchen S, Shanklin SL, et al; Centers for Disease Control and Prevention (CDC). Youth risk behavior surveillance--United States, 2013. *MMWR Suppl.* 2014;63(4):1–168

8. Brent DA, Perper JA, Allman CJ, Moritz GM, Wartella ME, Zelenak JP. The presence and accessibility of firearms in the homes of adolescent suicides. A case-control study. *JAMA.* 1991;266(21):2989–2995

9. American Academy of Pediatrics, Committee on Injury and Poison Prevention. Firearm injuries affecting the pediatric population. *Pediatrics.* 1992;89(4 pt 2):788–790

10. Grossman DC, Mueller BA, Riedy C, et al. Gun storage practices and risk of youth suicide and unintentional firearm injuries. *JAMA.* 2005;293(6):707–714

11. Gould MS, Greenberg T, Velting DM, Shaffer D. Youth suicide risk and preventive interventions: a review of the past 10 years. *J Am Acad Child Adolesc Psychiatry.* 2003;42(4):386–405

12. Swanson SA, Colman I. Association between exposure to suicide and suicidality outcomes in youth. *CMAJ.* 2013;185(10):870–877

13. Gould MS, Kleinman MH, Lake AM, Forman J, Midle JB. Newspaper coverage of suicide and initiation of suicide clusters in teenagers in the USA, 1988-96: a retrospective, population-based, case-control study. *Lancet Psychiatry.* 2014;1(1):34–43

14. Haw C, Hawton K, Niedzwiedz C, Platt S. Suicide clusters: a review of risk factors and mechanisms. *Suicide Life Threat Behav.* 2013;43(1):97–108

15. Ali MM, Dwyer DS, Rizzo JA. The social contagion effect of suicidal behavior in adolescents: does it really exist? *J Ment Health Policy Econ.* 2011;14(1):3–12

16. National Institute of Mental Health. Recommendations for reporting on suicide. Available at: www.nimh.nih.gov/health/topics/suicide-prevention/recommendations-for-reporting-on-suicide.shtml. Accessed July 27, 2015

17. American Academy of Child and Adolescent Psychiatry. Practice parameter for the assessment and treatment of children and adolescents with suicidal behavior. *J Am Acad Child Adolesc Psychiatry.* 2001;40(7 Suppl):24S–51S

18. Slap G, Goodman E, Huang B. Adoption as a risk factor for attempted suicide during adolescence. *Pediatrics.* 2001;108(2). Available at: http://pediatrics.aappublications.org/content/108/2/e30

19. Keyes MA, Malone SM, Sharma A, Iacono WG, McGue M. Risk of suicide attempt in adopted and nonadopted offspring. *Pediatrics.* 2013;132(4):639–646

20. Goldstein TR, Bridge JA, Brent DA. Sleep disturbance preceding completed suicide in adolescents. *J Consult Clin Psychol.* 2008;76(1):84–91

21. Kelleher I, Lynch F, Harley M, et al. Psychotic symptoms in adolescence index risk for suicidal behavior: findings from 2 population-based

case-control clinical interview studies. *Arch Gen Psychiatry.* 2012;69(12):1277–1283

22. Kelleher I, Corcoran P, Keeley H, et al. Psychotic symptoms and population risk for suicide attempt: a prospective cohort study. *JAMA Psychiatry.* 2013;70(9):940–948

23. Asarnow JR, Porta G, Spirito A, et al. Suicide attempts and nonsuicidal self-injury in the treatment of resistant depression in adolescents: findings from the TORDIA study. *J Am Acad Child Adolesc Psychiatry.* 2011;50(8):772–781

24. Wilkinson PO. Nonsuicidal self-injury: a clear marker for suicide risk. *J Am Acad Child Adolesc Psychiatry.* 2011;50(8):741–743

25. Cox LJ, Stanley BH, Melhem NM, et al. Familial and individual correlates of nonsuicidal self-injury in the offspring of mood-disordered parents. *J Clin Psychiatry.* 2012;73(6):813–820

26. American Academy of Child and Adolescent Psychiatry Web site. Available at: www.aacap.org. Accessed July 27, 2015

27. Hatzenbuehler ML. The social environment and suicide attempts in lesbian, gay, and bisexual youth. *Pediatrics.* 2011;127(5):896–903

28. Olweus D. Bullying at school: basic facts and effects of a school based intervention program. *J Child Psychol Psychiatry.* 1994;35(7):1171–1190

29. Brunstein Klomek A, Sourander A, Gould M. The association of suicide and bullying in childhood to young adulthood: a review of cross-sectional and longitudinal research findings. *Can J Psychiatry.* 2010;55(5):282–288

30. Copeland WE, Wolke D, Angold A, Costello EJ. Adult psychiatric outcomes of bullying and being bullied by peers in childhood and adolescence. *JAMA Psychiatry.* 2013;70(4):419–426

31. Arseneault L, Bowes L, Shakoor S. Bullying victimization in youths and mental health problems: 'much ado about nothing'? *Psychol Med.* 2010;40(5):717–729

32. Schneider SK, O'Donnell L, Stueve A, Coulter RW. Cyberbullying, school bullying, and psychological distress: a regional census of high school students. *Am J Public Health.* 2012;102(1):171–177

33. Kaminski JW, Fang X. Victimization by peers and adolescent suicide in three US samples. *J Pediatr.* 2009;155(5):683–688

34. Winsper C, Lereya T, Zanarini M, Wolke D. Involvement in bullying and suicide-related behavior at 11 years: a prospective birth cohort study. *J Am Acad Child Adolesc Psychiatry.* 2012;51(3):271–282.e3

35. Hinduja S, Patchin JW. Bullying, cyberbullying, and suicide. *Arch Suicide Res.* 2010;14(3):206–221

36. Klomek AB, Sourander A, Niemelä S, et al. Childhood bullying behaviors as a risk for suicide attempts and completed suicides: a population-based birth cohort study. *J Am Acad Child Adolesc Psychiatry.* 2009;48(3):254–261

37. Durkee T, Hadlaczky G, Westerlund M, Carli V. Internet pathways in suicidality: a review of the evidence. *Int J Environ Res Public Health.* 2011;8(10):3938–3952

38. Messias E, Castro J, Saini A, Usman M, Peeples D. Sadness, suicide, and their association with video game and internet overuse among teens: results from the youth risk behavior survey 2007 and 2009. *Suicide Life Threat Behav.* 2011;41(3):307–315

39. Katsumata Y, Matsumoto T, Kitani M, Takeshima T. Electronic media use and suicidal ideation in Japanese adolescents. *Psychiatry Clin Neurosci.* 2008;62(6):744–746

40. Hagihara A, Miyazaki S, Abe T. Internet suicide searches and the incidence of suicide in young people in Japan. *Eur Arch Psychiatry Clin Neurosci.* 2012;262(1):39–46

41. Westerlund M, Hadlaczky G, Wasserman D. The representation of suicide on the Internet: implications for clinicians. *J Med Internet Res.* 2012;14(5):e122

42. Kemp CG, Collings SC. Hyperlinked suicide: assessing the prominence and accessibility of suicide websites. *Crisis.* 2011;32(3):143–151

43. Dunlop SM, More E, Romer D. Where do youth learn about suicides on the Internet, and what influence does this have on suicidal ideation? *J Child Psychol Psychiatry.* 2011;52(10):1073–1080

44. Becker K, Schmidt MH. Internet chat rooms and suicide. *J Am Acad Child Adolesc Psychiatry.* 2004;43(3):246–247

45. Becker K, Mayer M, Nagenborg M, El-Faddagh M, Schmidt MH. Parasuicide online: Can suicide websites trigger suicidal behaviour in predisposed adolescents? *Nord J Psychiatry.* 2004;58(2):111–114

46. Allgaier AK, Pietsch K, Frühe B, Sigl-Glöckner J, Schulte-Körne G. Screening for depression in adolescents: validity of the patient health questionnaire in pediatric care. *Depress Anxiety.* 2012;29(10):906–913

47. O'Connor E, Gaynes BN, Burda BU, Soh C, Whitlock EP. Screening for and treatment of suicide risk relevant to primary care: a systematic review for the U.S. Preventive Services Task Force. *Ann Intern Med.* 2013;158(10):741–754

48. Peña JB, Caine ED. Screening as an approach for adolescent suicide prevention. *Suicide Life Threat Behav.* 2006;36(6):614–637

49. Thompson EA, Eggert LL. Using the suicide risk screen to identify suicidal adolescents among potential high school dropouts. *J Am Acad Child Adolesc Psychiatry.* 1999;38(12):1506–1514

50. Holi MM, Pelkonen M, Karlsson L, et al. Detecting suicidality among adolescent outpatients: evaluation of trained clinicians' suicidality assessment against a structured diagnostic assessment made by trained raters. *BMC Psychiatry.* 2008;8:97

51. Gould MS, Marrocco FA, Kleinman M, et al. Evaluating iatrogenic risk of youth suicide screening programs: a randomized controlled trial. *JAMA.* 2005;293(13):1635–1643

52. Robinson J, Pan Yuen H, Martin C, et al. Does screening high school students for psychological distress, deliberate self-harm, or suicidal ideation cause distress--and is it acceptable? An Australian-based study. *Crisis.* 2011;32(5):254–263

53. King RA; American Academy of Child and Adolescent Psychiatry. Practice parameters for the psychiatric assessment of children and adolescents. *J Am Acad Child Adolesc Psychiatry.* 1997;36(10 Suppl):4S–20S

54. American Psychiatric Association. *Diagnostic and Statistical Manual of Mental Disorders (DS-5).* 5th ed. Washington, DC: American Psychiatric Association; 2013

55. Wolraich ML, Felice ME, Drotar D, eds. *The Classification of Child and Adolescent Mental Diagnoses in Primary Care: Diagnostic and Statistical Manual for Primary Care (DSM-PC), Child and Adolescent Version.* Elk Grove Village, IL: American Academy of Pediatrics; 1996

56. Birmaher B, Brent D, Bernet W, et al; AACAP Work Group on Quality Issues. Practice parameter for the assessment and treatment of children and adolescents with depressive disorders. *J Am Acad Child Adolesc Psychiatry.* 2007;46(11):1503–1526

57. Shain BN; COMMITTEE ON ADOLESCENCE. Collaborative role of the pediatrician in the diagnosis and management of bipolar disorder in adolescents. *Pediatrics.* 2012;130(6). Available at: http://pediatrics.aappublications.org/content/130/6/e1725

58. American Acadamy of Pediatrics. *Bright Futures: Guidelines for Health Supervision of Infants, Children, and Adolescents.* 4th ed. 2016, In press.

59. American Academy of Pediatrics, Task Force on Mental Health. *Addressing Mental Health Concerns in Primary Care: A Clinician's Toolkit.* Elk Grove Village, IL: American Academy of Pediatrics; 2010

60. American Academy of Pediatrics. Mental health initiatives. Available at: https://www.aap.org/en-us/advocacy-and-policy/aap-health-initiatives/Mental-Health/Pages/Primary-Care-Tools.aspx. Accessed July 27, 2015

61. Richardson LP, Ludman E, McCauley E, et al. Collaborative care for adolescents with depression in primary care: a randomized clinical trial. *JAMA.* 2014;312(8):809–816

62. US Food and Drug Administration. FDA public health advisory: suicidality in children and adolescents being treated with antidepressant medications. Available at: www.fda.gov/Safety/MedWatch/SafetyInformation/SafetyAlertsforHumanMedicalProducts/ucm155488.htm. Accessed July 27, 2015

63. American Psychiatric Association and American Academy of Child and Adolescent Psychiatry. The use of medication in treating childhood and adolescent depression: information for physicians. Available at: www.parentsmedguide.org/physiciansmedguide.pdf. Accessed July 27, 2015

64. Bridge JA, Iyengar S, Salary CB, et al. Clinical response and risk for reported suicidal ideation and suicide attempts in pediatric antidepressant treatment: a meta-analysis of randomized controlled trials. *JAMA.* 2007;297(15):1683–1696

65. Gibbons RD, Brown CH, Hur K, Davis J, Mann JJ. Suicidal thoughts and behavior with antidepressant treatment: reanalysis of the randomized placebo-controlled studies of fluoxetine and venlafaxine. *Arch Gen Psychiatry.* 2012;69(6):580–587

66. Gibbons RD, Hur K, Brown CH, Davis JM, Mann JJ. Benefits from antidepressants: synthesis of 6-week patient-level outcomes from double-blind placebo-controlled randomized trials of fluoxetine and venlafaxine. *Arch Gen Psychiatry.* 2012;69(6):572–579

67. Dudley M, Goldney R, Hadzi-Pavlovic D. Are adolescents dying by suicide taking SSRI antidepressants? A review of observational studies. *Australas Psychiatry.* 2010;18(3):242–245

68. Olfson M, Shaffer D, Marcus SC, Greenberg T. Relationship between antidepressant medication treatment and suicide in adolescents. *Arch Gen Psychiatry.* 2003;60(10):978–982

69. Gibbons RD, Hur K, Bhaumik DK, Mann JJ. The relationship between antidepressant prescription rates and rate of early adolescent suicide. *Am J Psychiatry.* 2006;163(11):1898–1904

70. Cougnard A, Verdoux H, Grolleau A, Moride Y, Begaud B, Tournier M. Impact of antidepressants on the risk of suicide in patients with depression in real-life conditions: a decision analysis model. *Psychol Med.* 2009;39(8):1307–1315

71. Kilgore C. Dropoff seen in prescribing of antidepressants. Clinical Psychiatry News. 2005;33(3):1–6

72. Kurian BT, Ray WA, Arbogast PG, Fuchs DC, Dudley JA, Cooper WO. Effect of regulatory warnings on antidepressant prescribing for children and adolescents. *Arch Pediatr Adolesc Med.* 2007;161(7):690–696

73. Libby AM, Brent DA, Morrato EH, Orton HD, Allen R, Valuck RJ. Decline in treatment of pediatric depression after FDA advisory on risk of suicidality with SSRIs. *Am J Psychiatry.* 2007;164(6):884–891

74. Singh T, Prakash A, Rais T, Kumari N. Decreased use of antidepressants in youth after US Food and Drug Administration black box warning. *Psychiatry (Edgmont).* 2009;6(10):30–34

75. Libby AM, Orton HD, Valuck RJ. Persisting decline in depression treatment after FDA warnings. *Arch Gen Psychiatry.* 2009;66(6):633–639

76. Valluri S, Zito JM, Safer DJ, Zuckerman IH, Mullins CD, Korelitz JJ. Impact of the 2004 Food and Drug Administration pediatric suicidality warning on antidepressant and psychotherapy treatment for new-onset depression. *Med Care.* 2010;48(11):947–954

77. Rosack J. Impact of FDA warning questioned in suicide rise. *Psychiatric News.* 2007;42(5):1–4

78. Gibbons RD, Brown CH, Hur K, et al. Early evidence on the effects of regulators' suicidality warnings on SSRI prescriptions and suicide in children and adolescents. *Am J Psychiatry.* 2007;164(9):1356–1363

79. Lu CY, Zhang F, Lakoma MD, et al. Changes in antidepressant use by young people and suicidal behavior after FDA warnings and media coverage: quasi-experimental study. *BMJ.* 2014;348:g3596

SECTION 7
Special Pediatric Populations and Support

POLICY STATEMENT Organizational Principles to Guide and Define the Child Health Care System and/or Improve the Health of all Children

American Academy
of Pediatrics

DEDICATED TO THE HEALTH OF ALL CHILDREN™

Ensuring Comprehensive Care and Support for Transgender and Gender-Diverse Children and Adolescents

Jason Rafferty, MD, MPH, EdM, FAAP, COMMITTEE ON PSYCHOSOCIAL ASPECTS OF CHILD AND FAMILY HEALTH, COMMITTEE ON ADOLESCENCE, SECTION ON LESBIAN, GAY, BISEXUAL, AND TRANSGENDER HEALTH AND WELLNESS

abstract

As a traditionally underserved population that faces numerous health disparities, youth who identify as transgender and gender diverse (TGD) and their families are increasingly presenting to pediatric providers for education, care, and referrals. The need for more formal training, standardized treatment, and research on safety and medical outcomes often leaves providers feeling ill equipped to support and care for patients that identify as TGD and families. In this policy statement, we review relevant concepts and challenges and provide suggestions for pediatric providers that are focused on promoting the health and positive development of youth that identify as TGD while eliminating discrimination and stigma.

INTRODUCTION

In its dedication to the health of all children, the American Academy of Pediatrics (AAP) strives to improve health care access and eliminate disparities for children and teenagers who identify as lesbian, gay, bisexual, transgender, or questioning (LGBTQ) of their sexual or gender identity.[1,2] Despite some advances in public awareness and legal protections, youth who identify as LGBTQ continue to face disparities that stem from multiple sources, including inequitable laws and policies, societal discrimination, and a lack of access to quality health care, including mental health care. Such challenges are often more intense for youth who do not conform to social expectations and norms regarding gender. Pediatric providers are increasingly encountering such youth and their families, who seek medical advice and interventions, yet they may lack the formal training to care for youth that identify as transgender and gender diverse (TGD) and their families.[3]

This policy statement is focused specifically on children and youth that identify as TGD rather than the larger LGBTQ population, providing brief, relevant background on the basis of current available research

Department of Pediatrics, Hasbro Children's Hospital, Providence, Rhode Island; Thundermist Health Centers, Providence, Rhode Island; and Department of Child Psychiatry, Emma Pendleton Bradley Hospital, East Providence, Rhode Island

Dr Rafferty conceptualized the statement, drafted the initial manuscript, reviewed and revised the manuscript, approved the final manuscript as submitted, and agrees to be accountable for all aspects of the work.

Policy statements from the American Academy of Pediatrics benefit from expertise and resources of liaisons and internal (AAP) and external reviewers. However, policy statements from the American Academy of Pediatrics may not reflect the views of the liaisons or the organizations or government agencies that they represent.

The guidance in this statement does not indicate an exclusive course of treatment or serve as a standard of medical care. Variations, taking into account individual circumstances, may be appropriate.

All policy statements from the American Academy of Pediatrics automatically expire 5 years after publication unless reaffirmed, revised, or retired at or before that time.

To cite: Rafferty J, AAP COMMITTEE ON PSYCHOSOCIAL ASPECTS OF CHILD AND FAMILY HEALTH, AAP COMMITTEE ON ADOLESCENCE, AAP SECTION ON LESBIAN, GAY, BISEXUAL, AND TRANSGENDER HEALTH AND WELLNESS. Ensuring Comprehensive Care and Support for Transgender and Gender-Diverse Children and Adolescents. *Pediatrics.* 2018;142(4): e20182162

TABLE 1 Relevant Terms and Definitions Related to Gender Care

Term	Definition
Sex	An assignment that is made at birth, usually male or female, typically on the basis of external genital anatomy but sometimes on the basis of internal gonads, chromosomes, or hormone levels
Gender identity	A person's deep internal sense of being female, male, a combination of both, somewhere in between, or neither, resulting from a multifaceted interaction of biological traits, environmental factors, self-understanding, and cultural expectations
Gender expression	The external way a person expresses their gender, such as with clothing, hair, mannerisms, activities, or social roles
Gender perception	The way others interpret a person's gender expression
Gender diverse	A term that is used to describe people with gender behaviors, appearances, or identities that are incongruent with those culturally assigned to their birth sex; gender-diverse individuals may refer to themselves with many different terms, such as transgender, nonbinary, genderqueer,[7] gender fluid, gender creative, gender independent, or noncisgender. "Gender diverse" is used to acknowledge and include the vast diversity of gender identities that exists. It replaces the former term, "gender nonconforming," which has a negative and exclusionary connotation.
Transgender	A subset of gender-diverse youth whose gender identity does not match their assigned sex and generally remains persistent, consistent, and insistent over time; the term "transgender" also encompasses many other labels individuals may use to refer to themselves.
Cisgender	A term that is used to describe a person who identifies and expresses a gender that is consistent with the culturally defined norms of the sex they were assigned at birth
Agender	A term that is used to describe a person who does not identify as having a particular gender
Affirmed gender	When a person's true gender identity, or concern about their gender identity, is communicated to and validated from others as authentic
MTF; affirmed female; trans female	Terms that are used to describe individuals who were assigned male sex at birth but who have a gender identity and/or expression that is asserted to be more feminine
FTM; affirmed male; trans male	Terms that are used to describe individuals who were assigned female sex at birth but who have a gender identity and/or expression that is asserted to be more masculine
Gender dysphoria	A clinical symptom that is characterized by a sense of alienation to some or all of the physical characteristics or social roles of one's assigned gender; also, gender dysphoria is the psychiatric diagnosis in the *DSM-5*, which has focus on the distress that stems from the incongruence between one's expressed or experienced (affirmed) gender and the gender assigned at birth.
Gender identity disorder	A psychiatric diagnosis defined previously in the *DSM-IV* (changed to "gender dysphoria" in the *DSM-5*); the primary criteria include a strong, persistent cross-sex identification and significant distress and social impairment. This diagnosis is no longer appropriate for use and may lead to stigma, but the term may be found in older research.
Sexual orientation	A person's sexual identity in relation to the gender(s) to which they are attracted; sexual orientation and gender identity develop separately.

This list is not intended to be all inclusive. The pronouns "they" and "their" are used intentionally to be inclusive rather than the binary pronouns "he" and "she" and "his" and "her." Adapted from Bonifacio HJ, Rosenthal SM. Gender variance and dysphoria in children and adolescents. *Pediatr Clin North Am.* 2015;62(4):1001–1016. Adapted from Vance SR Jr, Ehrensaft D, Rosenthal SM. Psychological and medical care of gender nonconforming youth. *Pediatrics.* 2014;134(6):1184–1192. DSM-5, *Diagnostic and Statistical Manual of Mental Disorders, Fifth Edition*; DSM-IV, *Diagnostic and Statistical Manual of Mental Disorders, Fourth Edition*; FTM, female to male; MTF, male to female.

and expert opinion from clinical and research leaders, which will serve as the basis for recommendations. It is not a comprehensive review of clinical approaches and nuances to pediatric care for children and youth that identify as TGD. Professional understanding of youth that identify as TGD is a rapidly evolving clinical field in which research on appropriate clinical management is limited by insufficient funding.[3,4]

DEFINITIONS

To clarify recommendations and discussions in this policy statement, some definitions are provided. However, brief descriptions of human behavior or identities may not capture nuance in this evolving field.

"Sex," or "natal gender," is a label, generally "male" or "female," that is typically assigned at birth on the basis of genetic and anatomic characteristics, such as genital anatomy, chromosomes, and sex hormone levels. Meanwhile, "gender identity" is one's internal sense of who one is, which results from a multifaceted interaction of biological traits, developmental influences, and environmental conditions. It may be male, female, somewhere in between, a combination of both, or neither (ie, not conforming to a binary conceptualization of gender). Self-recognition of gender identity develops over time, much the same way as a child's physical body does. For some people, gender identity can be fluid, shifting in different contexts. "Gender expression"

refers to the wide array of ways people display their gender through clothing, hair styles, mannerisms, or social roles. Exploring different ways of expressing gender is common for children and may challenge social expectations. The way others interpret this expression is referred to as "gender perception" (Table 1).[5,6]

These labels may or may not be congruent. The term "cisgender" is used if someone identifies and expresses a gender that is consistent with the culturally defined norms of the sex that was assigned at birth. "Gender diverse" is an umbrella term to describe an ever-evolving array of labels that people may apply when their gender identity, expression, or even perception does not conform to the norms and stereotypes others expect of their assigned sex. "Transgender" is usually reserved for a subset of such youth whose gender identity does not match their assigned sex and generally remains persistent, consistent, and insistent over time. These terms are not diagnoses; rather, they are personal and often dynamic ways of describing one's own gender experience.

Gender identity is not synonymous with "sexual orientation," which refers to a person's identity in relation to the gender(s) to which they are sexually and romantically attracted. Gender identity and sexual orientation are distinct but interrelated constructs.[8] Therefore, being transgender does not imply a sexual orientation, and people who identify as transgender still identify as straight, gay, bisexual, etc, on the basis of their attractions. (For more information, *The Gender Book*, found at www.thegenderbook.com, is a resource with illustrations that are used to highlight these core terms and concepts.)

EPIDEMIOLOGY

In population-based surveys, questions related to gender identity are rarely asked, which makes it difficult to assess the size and characteristics of the population that is TGD. In the 2014 Behavioral Risk Factor Surveillance System of the Centers for Disease Control and Prevention, only 19 states elected to include optional questions on gender identity. Extrapolation from these data suggests that the US prevalence of adults who identify as transgender or "gender nonconforming" is 0.6% (1.4 million), ranging from 0.3% in North Dakota to 0.8% in Hawaii.[9] On the basis of these data, it has been estimated that 0.7% of youth ages 13 to 17 years (~150 000) identify as transgender.[10] This number is much higher than previous estimates, which were

extrapolated from individual states or specialty clinics, and is likely an underestimate given the stigma regarding those who openly identify as transgender and the difficulty in defining "transgender" in a way that is inclusive of all gender-diverse identities.[11]

There have been no large-scale prevalence studies among children and adolescents, and there is no evidence that adult statistics reflect young children or adolescents. In the 2014 Behavioral Risk Factor Surveillance System, those 18 to 24 years of age were more likely than older age groups to identify as transgender (0.7%).[9] Children report being aware of gender incongruence at young ages. Children who later identify as TGD report first having recognized their gender as "different" at an average age of 8.5 years; however, they did not disclose such feelings until an average of 10 years later.[12]

MENTAL HEALTH IMPLICATIONS

Adolescents and adults who identify as transgender have high rates of depression, anxiety, eating disorders, self-harm, and suicide.[13–20] Evidence suggests that an identity of TGD has an increased prevalence among individuals with autism spectrum disorder, but this association is not yet well understood.[21,22] In 1 retrospective cohort study, 56% of youth who identified as transgender reported previous suicidal ideation, and 31% reported a previous suicide attempt, compared with 20% and 11% among matched youth who identified as cisgender, respectively.[13] Some youth who identify as TGD also experience gender dysphoria, which is a specific diagnosis given to those who experience impairment in peer and/or family relationships, school performance, or other aspects of their life as a consequence of the

incongruence between their assigned sex and their gender identity.[23]

There is no evidence that risk for mental illness is inherently attributable to one's identity of TGD. Rather, it is believed to be multifactorial, stemming from an internal conflict between one's appearance and identity, limited availability of mental health services, low access to health care providers with expertise in caring for youth who identify as TGD, discrimination, stigma, and social rejection.[24] This was affirmed by the American Psychological Association in 2008[25] (with practice guidelines released in 2015[8]) and the American Psychiatric Association, which made the following statement in 2012:

Being transgender or gender variant implies no impairment in judgment, stability, reliability, or general social or vocational capabilities; however, these individuals often experience discrimination due to a lack of civil rights protections for their gender identity or expression.... [Such] discrimination and lack of equal civil rights is damaging to the mental health of transgender and gender variant individuals.[26]

Youth who identify as TGD often confront stigma and discrimination, which contribute to feelings of rejection and isolation that can adversely affect physical and emotional well-being. For example, many youth believe that they must hide their gender identity and expression to avoid bullying, harassment, or victimization. Youth who identify as TGD experience disproportionately high rates of homelessness, physical violence (at home and in the community), substance abuse, and high-risk sexual behaviors.[5,6,12,27–31] Among the 3 million HIV testing events that were reported in 2015, the highest percentages of new infections were among women who identified as transgender[32] and were also at particular risk for not knowing their HIV status.[30]

GENDER-AFFIRMATIVE CARE

In a gender-affirmative care model (GACM), pediatric providers offer developmentally appropriate care that is oriented toward understanding and appreciating the youth's gender experience. A strong, nonjudgmental partnership with youth and their families can facilitate exploration of complicated emotions and gender-diverse expressions while allowing questions and concerns to be raised in a supportive environment.[5] In a GACM, the following messages are conveyed:

- transgender identities and diverse gender expressions do not constitute a mental disorder;

- variations in gender identity and expression are normal aspects of human diversity, and binary definitions of gender do not always reflect emerging gender identities;

- gender identity evolves as an interplay of biology, development, socialization, and culture; and

- if a mental health issue exists, it most often stems from stigma and negative experiences rather than being intrinsic to the child.[27,33]

The GACM is best facilitated through the integration of medical, mental health, and social services, including specific resources and supports for parents and families.[24] Providers work together to destigmatize gender variance, promote the child's self-worth, facilitate access to care, educate families, and advocate for safer community spaces where children are free to develop and explore their gender.[5] A specialized gender-affirmative therapist, when available, may be an asset in helping children and their families build skills for dealing with gender-based stigma, address symptoms of anxiety or depression, and reinforce the child's overall resiliency.[34,35] There is a limited but growing body

of evidence that suggests that using an integrated affirmative model results in young people having fewer mental health concerns whether they ultimately identify as transgender.[24,36,37]

In contrast, "conversion" or "reparative" treatment models are used to prevent children and adolescents from identifying as transgender or to dissuade them from exhibiting gender-diverse expressions. The Substance Abuse and Mental Health Services Administration has concluded that any therapeutic intervention with the goal of changing a youth's gender expression or identity is inappropriate.[33] Reparative approaches have been proven to be not only unsuccessful[38] but also deleterious and are considered outside the mainstream of traditional medical practice.[29,39–42] The AAP described reparative approaches as "unfair and deceptive."[43] At the time of this writing,* conversion therapy was banned by executive regulation in New York and by legislative statutes in 9 other states as well as the District of Columbia.[44]

Pediatric providers have an essential role in assessing gender concerns and providing evidence-based information to assist youth and families in medical decision-making. Not doing so can prolong or exacerbate gender dysphoria and contribute to abuse and stigmatization.[35] If a pediatric provider does not feel prepared to address gender concerns when they occur, then referral to a pediatric or mental health provider with more expertise is appropriate. There is little research on communication and efficacy with transfers in care for youth who identify as TGD,

particularly from pediatric to adult providers.

DEVELOPMENTAL CONSIDERATIONS

Acknowledging that the capacity for emerging abstract thinking in childhood is important to conceptualize and reflect on identity, gender-affirmation guidelines are being focused on individually tailored interventions on the basis of the physical and cognitive development of youth who identify as TGD.[45] Accordingly, research substantiates that children who are prepubertal and assert an identity of TGD know their gender as clearly and as consistently as their developmentally equivalent peers who identify as cisgender and benefit from the same level of social acceptance.[46] This developmental approach to gender affirmation is in contrast to the outdated approach in which a child's gender-diverse assertions are held as "possibly true" until an arbitrary age (often after pubertal onset) when they can be considered valid, an approach that authors of the literature have termed "watchful waiting." This outdated approach does not serve the child because critical support is withheld. Watchful waiting is based on binary notions of gender in which gender diversity and fluidity is pathologized; in watchful waiting, it is also assumed that notions of gender identity become fixed at a certain age. The approach is also influenced by a group of early studies with validity concerns, methodologic flaws, and limited follow-up on children who identified as TGD and, by adolescence, did not seek further treatment ("desisters").[45,47] More robust and current research suggests that, rather than focusing on who a child will become, valuing them for who they are, even at a young age, fosters secure attachment and resilience, not only for the child but also for the whole family.[5,45,48,49]

---

* For more information regarding state-specific laws, please contact the AAP Division of State Government Affairs at stgov@aap.org.

MEDICAL MANAGEMENT

Pediatric primary care providers are in a unique position to routinely inquire about gender development in children and adolescents as part of recommended well-child visits[50] and to be a reliable source of validation, support, and reassurance. They are often the first provider to be aware that a child may not identify as cisgender or that there may be distress related to a gender-diverse identity. The best way to approach gender with patients is to inquire directly and nonjudgmentally about their experience and feelings before applying any labels.[27,51]

Many medical interventions can be offered to youth who identify as TGD and their families. The decision of whether and when to initiate gender-affirmative treatment is personal and involves careful consideration of risks, benefits, and other factors unique to each patient and family. Many protocols suggest that clinical assessment of youth who identify as TGD is ideally conducted on an ongoing basis in the setting of a collaborative, multidisciplinary approach, which, in addition to the patient and family, may include the pediatric provider, a mental health provider (preferably with expertise in caring for youth who identify as TGD), social and legal supports, and a pediatric endocrinologist or adolescent-medicine gender specialist, if available.[6,28] There is no prescribed path, sequence, or end point. Providers can make every effort to be aware of the influence of their own biases. The medical options also vary depending on pubertal and developmental progression.

Clinical Setting

In the past year, 1 in 4 adults who identified as transgender avoided a necessary doctor's visit because of fear of being mistreated.[31] All clinical office staff have a role in affirming a patient's gender identity. Making flyers available or displaying posters related to LGBTQ health issues, including information for children who identify as TGD and families, reveals inclusivity and awareness. Generally, patients who identify as TGD feel most comfortable when they have access to a gender-neutral restroom. Diversity training that encompasses sensitivity when caring for youth who identify as TGD and their families can be helpful in educating clinical and administrative staff. A patient-asserted name and pronouns are used by staff and are ideally reflected in the electronic medical record without creating duplicate charts.[52,53] The US Centers for Medicare and Medicaid Services and the National Coordinator for Health Information Technology require all electronic health record systems certified under the Meaningful Use incentive program to have the capacity to confidentially collect information on gender identity.[54,55] Explaining and maintaining confidentiality procedures promotes openness and trust, particularly with youth who identify as LGBTQ.[1] Maintaining a safe clinical space can provide at least 1 consistent, protective refuge for patients and families, allowing authentic gender expression and exploration that builds resiliency.

Pubertal Suppression

Gonadotrophin-releasing hormones have been used to delay puberty since the 1980s for central precocious puberty.[56] These reversible treatments can also be used in adolescents who experience gender dysphoria to prevent development of secondary sex characteristics and provide time up until 16 years of age for the individual and the family to explore gender identity, access psychosocial supports, develop coping skills, and further define appropriate treatment goals. If pubertal suppression treatment is suspended, then endogenous puberty will resume.[20,57,58]

Often, pubertal suppression creates an opportunity to reduce distress that may occur with the development of secondary sexual characteristics and allow for gender-affirming care, including mental health support for the adolescent and the family. It reduces the need for later surgery because physical changes that are otherwise irreversible (protrusion of the Adam's apple, male pattern baldness, voice change, breast growth, etc) are prevented. The available data reveal that pubertal suppression in children who identify as TGD generally leads to improved psychological functioning in adolescence and young adulthood.[20,57–59]

Pubertal suppression is not without risks. Delaying puberty beyond one's peers can also be stressful and can lead to lower self-esteem and increased risk taking.[60] Some experts believe that genital underdevelopment may limit some potential reconstructive options.[61] Research on long-term risks, particularly in terms of bone metabolism[62] and fertility,[63] is currently limited and provides varied results.[57,64,65] Families often look to pediatric providers for help in considering whether pubertal suppression is indicated in the context of their child's overall well-being as gender diverse.

Gender Affirmation

As youth who identify as TGD reflect on and evaluate their gender identity, various interventions may be considered to better align their gender expression with their underlying identity. This process of reflection, acceptance, and, for some, intervention is known as "gender affirmation." It was formerly referred to as "transitioning," but many view the process as an affirmation and acceptance of who they have always been rather than a transition

TABLE 2 The Process of Gender Affirmation May Include ≥1 of the Following Components

Component	Definition	General Age Range[a]	Reversibility[a]
Social affirmation	Adopting gender-affirming hairstyles, clothing, name, gender pronouns, and restrooms and other facilities	Any	Reversible
Puberty blockers	Gonadotropin-releasing hormone analogues, such as leuprolide and histrelin	During puberty (Tanner stage 2–5)[b]	Reversible[c]
Cross-sex hormone therapy	Testosterone (for those who were assigned female at birth and are masculinizing); estrogen plus androgen inhibitor (for those who were assigned male at birth and are feminizing)	Early adolescence onward	Partially reversible (skin texture, muscle mass, and fat deposition); irreversible once developed (testosterone: Adam's apple protrusion, voice changes, and male pattern baldness; estrogen: breast development); unknown reversibility (effect on fertility)
Gender-affirming surgeries	"Top" surgery (to create a male-typical chest shape or enhance breasts); "bottom" surgery (surgery on genitals or reproductive organs); facial feminization and other procedures	Typically adults (adolescents on case-by-case basis[d])	Not reversible
Legal affirmation	Changing gender and name recorded on birth certificate, school records, and other documents	Any	Reversible

[a] Note that the provided age range and reversibility is based on the little data that are currently available.

[b] There is limited benefit to starting gonadotropin-releasing hormone after Tanner stage 5 for pubertal suppression. However, when cross-sex hormones are initiated with a gradually increasing schedule, the initial levels are often not high enough to suppress endogenous sex hormone secretion. Therefore, gonadotropin-releasing hormone may be continued in accordance with the Endocrine Society Guidelines.[68]

[c] The effect of sustained puberty suppression on fertility is unknown. Pubertal suppression can be, and often is indicated to be, followed by cross-sex hormone treatment. However, when cross-sex hormones are initiated without endogenous hormones, then fertility may be decreased.[68]

[d] Eligibility criteria for gender-affirmative surgical interventions among adolescents are not clearly defined between established protocols and practice. When applicable, eligibility is usually determined on a case-by-case basis with the adolescent and the family along with input from medical, mental health, and surgical providers.[68–71]

from 1 gender identity to another. Accordingly, some people who have gone through the process prefer to call themselves "affirmed females, males, etc" (or just "females, males, etc"), rather than using the prefix "trans-." Gender affirmation is also used to acknowledge that some individuals who identify as TGD may feel affirmed in their gender without pursuing medical or surgical interventions.[7,66]

Supportive involvement of parents and family is associated with better mental and physical health outcomes.[67] Gender affirmation among adolescents with gender dysphoria often reduces the emphasis on gender in their lives, allowing them to attend to other developmental tasks, such as academic success, relationship building, and future-oriented planning.[64] Most protocols for gender-affirming interventions incorporate World Professional Association of Transgender

Health[35] and Endocrine Society[68] recommendations and include ≥1 of the following elements (Table 2):

1. Social Affirmation: This is a reversible intervention in which children and adolescents express partially or completely in their asserted gender identity by adapting hairstyle, clothing, pronouns, name, etc. Children who identify as transgender and socially affirm and are supported in their asserted gender show no increase in depression and only minimal (clinically insignificant) increases in anxiety compared with age-matched averages.[48] Social affirmation can be complicated given the wide range of social interactions children have (eg, extended families, peers, school, community, etc). There is little guidance on the best approach (eg, all at once, gradual, creating new social networks, or affirming within existing networks, etc). Pediatric providers

can best support families by anticipating and discussing such complexity proactively, either in their own practice or through enlisting a qualified mental health provider.

2. Legal Affirmation: Elements of a social affirmation, such as a name and gender marker, become official on legal documents, such as birth certificates, passports, identification cards, school documents, etc. The processes for making these changes depend on state laws and may require specific documentation from pediatric providers.

3. Medical Affirmation: This is the process of using cross-sex hormones to allow adolescents who have initiated puberty to develop secondary sex characteristics of the opposite biological sex. Some changes are partially reversible if hormones are stopped, but others become

irreversible once they are fully developed (Table 2).

4. Surgical Affirmation: Surgical approaches may be used to feminize or masculinize features, such as hair distribution, chest, or genitalia, and may include removal of internal organs, such as ovaries or the uterus (affecting fertility). These changes are irreversible. Although current protocols typically reserve surgical interventions for adults,[35,68] they are occasionally pursued during adolescence on a case-by-case basis, considering the necessity and benefit to the adolescent's overall health and often including multidisciplinary input from medical, mental health, and surgical providers as well as from the adolescent and family.[69–71]

For some youth who identify as TGD whose natal gender is female, menstruation, breakthrough bleeding, and dysmenorrhea can lead to significant distress before or during gender affirmation. The American College of Obstetrics and Gynecology suggests that, although limited data are available to outline management, menstruation can be managed without exogenous estrogens by using a progesterone-only pill, a medroxyprogesterone acetate shot, or a progesterone-containing intrauterine or implantable device.[72] If estrogen can be tolerated, oral contraceptives that contain both progesterone and estrogen are more effective at suppressing menses.[73] The Endocrine Society guidelines also suggest that gonadotrophin-releasing hormones can be used for menstrual suppression before the anticipated initiation of testosterone or in combination with testosterone for breakthrough bleeding (enables phenotypic masculinization at a lower dose than if testosterone is used alone).[68] Masculinizing hormones in natal female patients may lead to a cessation of menses, but unplanned pregnancies have been reported, which emphasizes the need for ongoing contraceptive counseling with youth who identify as TGD.[72]

HEALTH DISPARITIES

In addition to societal challenges, youth who identify as TGD face several barriers within the health care system, especially regarding access to care. In 2015, a focus group of youth who identified as transgender in Seattle, Washington, revealed 4 problematic areas related to health care:

1. safety issues, including the lack of safe clinical environments and fear of discrimination by providers;

2. poor access to physical health services, including testing for sexually transmitted infections;

3. inadequate resources to address mental health concerns; and

4. lack of continuity with providers.[74]

This study reveals the obstacles many youth who identify as TGD face in accessing essential services, including the limited supply of appropriately trained medical and psychological providers, fertility options, and insurance coverage denials for gender-related treatments.[74]

Insurance denials for services related to the care of patients who identify as TGD are a significant barrier. Although the Office for Civil Rights of the US Department of Health and Human Services explicitly stated in 2012 that the nondiscrimination provision in the Patient Protection and Affordable Care Act includes people who identify as gender diverse,[75,76] insurance claims for gender affirmation, particularly among youth who identify as TGD, are frequently denied.[54,77] In 1 study, it was found that approximately 25% of individuals who identified as transgender were denied insurance coverage because of being transgender.[31] The burden of covering medical expenses that are not covered by insurance can be financially devastating, and even when expenses are covered, families describe high levels of stress in navigating and submitting claims appropriately.[78] In 2012, a large gender center in Boston, Massachusetts, reported that most young patients who identified as transgender and were deemed appropriate candidates for recommended gender care were unable to obtain it because of such denials, which were based on the premise that gender dysphoria was a mental disorder, not a physical one, and that treatment was not medically or surgically necessary.[24] This practice not only contributes to stigma, prolonged gender dysphoria, and poor mental health outcomes,[77] but it may also lead patients to seek nonmedically supervised treatments that are potentially dangerous.[24] Furthermore, insurance denials can reinforce a socioeconomic divide between those who can finance the high costs of uncovered care and those who cannot.[24,77]

The transgender youth group in Seattle likely reflected the larger TGD population when they described how obstacles adversely affect self-esteem and contribute to the perception that they are undervalued by society and the health care system.[74,77] Professional medical associations, including the AAP, are increasingly calling for equity in health care provisions regardless of gender identity or expression.[1,8,23,72] There is a critical need for investments in research on the prevalence, disparities, biological underpinnings, and standards of care relating to gender-diverse populations. Pediatric providers who work with state government and insurance officials can play an essential role in advocating for stronger nondiscrimination policies and improved coverage.

There is a lack of quality research on the experience of youth of color who identify as transgender. One theory suggests that the intersection of racism, transphobia, and sexism may result in the extreme marginalization that is experienced among many women of color who identify as transgender,[79] including rejection from their family and dropping out of school at younger ages (often in the setting of rigid religious beliefs regarding gender),[80] increased levels of violence and body objectification,[81] 3 times the risk of poverty compared with the general population,[31] and the highest prevalence of HIV compared with other risk groups (estimated as high as 56.3% in 1 meta-analysis).[30] One model suggests that pervasive stigma and oppression can be associated with psychological distress (anxiety, depression, and suicide) and adoption of risk behaviors by such youth to obtain a sense of validation toward their complex identities.[79]

FAMILY ACCEPTANCE

Research increasingly suggests that familial acceptance or rejection ultimately has little influence on the gender identity of youth; however, it may profoundly affect young people's ability to openly discuss or disclose concerns about their identity. Suppressing such concerns can affect mental health.[82] Families often find it hard to understand and accept their child's gender-diverse traits because of personal beliefs, social pressure, and stigma.[49,83] Legitimate fears may exist for their child's welfare, safety, and acceptance that pediatric providers need to appreciate and address. Families can be encouraged to communicate their concerns and questions. Unacknowledged concerns can contribute to shame and hesitation in regard to offering support and understanding,[84]

which is essential for the child's self-esteem, social involvement, and overall health as TGD.[48,85–87] Some caution has been expressed that unquestioning acceptance per se may not best serve questioning youth or their families. Instead, psychological evidence suggests that the most benefit comes when family members and youth are supported and encouraged to engage in reflective perspective taking and validate their own and the other's thoughts and feelings despite divergent views.[49,82]

In this regard, suicide attempt rates among 433 adolescents in Ontario who identified as "trans" were 4% among those with strongly supportive parents and as high as 60% among those whose parents were not supportive.[85] Adolescents who identify as transgender and endorse at least 1 supportive person in their life report significantly less distress than those who only experience rejection. In communities with high levels of support, it was found that nonsupportive families tended to increase their support over time, leading to dramatic improvement in mental health outcomes among their children who identified as transgender.[88]

Pediatric providers can create a safe environment for parents and families to better understand and listen to the needs of their children while receiving reassurance and education.[83] It is often appropriate to assist the child in understanding the parents' concerns as well. Despite expectations by some youth with transgender identity for immediate acceptance after "coming out," family members often proceed through a process of becoming more comfortable and understanding of the youth's gender identity, thoughts, and feelings. One model suggests that the process resembles grieving, wherein the family separates from their expectations for their child to embrace a new reality. This process may proceed through stages of shock,

denial, anger, feelings of betrayal, fear, self-discovery, and pride.[89] The amount of time spent in any of these stages and the overall pace varies widely. Many family members also struggle as they are pushed to reflect on their own gender experience and assumptions throughout this process. In some situations, youth who identify as TGD may be at risk for internalizing the difficult emotions that family members may be experiencing. In these cases, individual and group therapy for the family members may be helpful.[49,78]

Family dynamics can be complex, involving disagreement among legal guardians or between guardians and their children, which may affect the ability to obtain consent for any medical management or interventions. Even in states where minors may access care without parental consent for mental health services, contraception, and sexually transmitted infections, parental or guardian consent is required for hormonal and surgical care of patients who identify as TGD.[72,90] Some families may take issue with providers who address gender concerns or offer gender-affirming care. In rare cases, a family may deny access to care that raises concerns about the youth's welfare and safety; in those cases, additional legal or ethical support may be useful to consider. In such rare situations, pediatric providers may want to familiarize themselves with relevant local consent laws and maintain their primary responsibility for the welfare of the child.

SAFE SCHOOLS AND COMMUNITIES

Youth who identify as TGD are becoming more visible because gender-diverse expression is increasingly admissible in the media, on social media, and in schools and communities. Regardless of whether a youth with a gender-diverse identity ultimately identifies as transgender, challenges exist in nearly every social context, from lack of understanding to outright rejection, isolation, discrimination, and victimization. In the US Transgender Survey of nearly 28 000 respondents, it was found that among those who were out as or perceived to be TGD between kindergarten and eighth grade, 54% were verbally harassed, 24% were physically assaulted, and 13% were sexually assaulted; 17% left school because of maltreatment.[31] Education and advocacy from the medical community on the importance of safe schools for youth who identify as TGD can have a significant effect.

At the time of this writing,* only 18 states and the District of Columbia had laws that prohibited discrimination based on gender expression when it comes to employment, housing, public accommodations, and insurance benefits. Over 200 US cities have such legislation. In addition to basic protections, many youth who identify as TGD also have to navigate legal obstacles when it comes to legally changing their name and/or gender marker.[54] In addition to advocating and working with policy makers to promote equal protections for youth who identify as TGD, pediatric providers can play an important role by developing a familiarity with local laws and organizations that provide social work and legal assistance to youth who identify as TGD and their families.

School environments play a significant role in the social and emotional development of children. Every child has a right to feel safe

* For more information regarding state-specific laws, please contact the AAP Division of State Government Affairs at stgov@ aap.org.

and respected at school, but for youth who identify as TGD, this can be challenging. Nearly every aspect of school life may present safety concerns and require negotiations regarding their gender expression, including name/pronoun use, use of bathrooms and locker rooms, sports teams, dances and activities, overnight activities, and even peer groups. Conflicts in any of these areas can quickly escalate beyond the school's control to larger debates among the community and even on a national stage.

The formerly known Gay, Lesbian, and Straight Education Network (GLSEN), an advocacy organization for youth who identify as LGBTQ, conducts an annual national survey to measure LGBTQ well-being in US schools. In 2015, students who identified as LGBTQ reported high rates of being discouraged from participation in extracurricular activities. One in 5 students who identified as LGBTQ reported being hindered from forming or participating in a club to support lesbian, gay, bisexual, or transgender students (eg, a gay straight alliance, now often referred to as a genders and sexualities alliance) despite such clubs at schools being associated with decreased reports of negative remarks about sexual orientation or gender expression, increased feelings of safety and connectedness at school, and lower levels of victimization. In addition, >20% of students who identified as LGBTQ reported being blocked from writing about LGBTQ issues in school yearbooks or school newspapers or being prevented or discouraged by coaches and school staff from participating in sports because of their sexual orientation or gender expression.[91]

One strategy to prevent conflict is to proactively support policies and protections that promote inclusion and safety of all students. However, such policies are far from

consistent across districts. In 2015, GLSEN found that 43% of children who identified as LGBTQ reported feeling unsafe at school because of their gender expression, but only 6% reported that their school had official policies to support youth who identified as TGD, and only 11% reported that their school's antibullying policies had specific protections for gender expression.[91] Consequently, more than half of the students who identified as transgender in the study were prevented from using the bathroom, names, or pronouns that aligned with their asserted gender at school. A lack of explicit policies that protected youth who identified as TGD was associated with increased reported victimization, with more than half of students who identified as LGBTQ reporting verbal harassment because of their gender expression. Educators and school administrators play an essential role in advocating for and enforcing such policies. GLSEN found that when students recognized actions to reduce gender-based harassment, both students who identified as transgender and cisgender reported a greater connection to staff and feelings of safety.[91] In another study, schools were open to education regarding gender diversity and were willing to implement policies when they were supported by external agencies, such as medical professionals.[92]

Academic content plays an important role in building a safe school environment as well. The 2015 GLSEN survey revealed that when positive representations of people who identified as LGBTQ were included in the curriculum, students who identified as LGBTQ reported less hostile school environments, less victimization and greater feelings of safety, fewer school absences because of feeling unsafe, greater feelings of connectedness to their school community, and an increased interest in high school graduation and postsecondary education.[91] At the time of this writing,* 8 states had laws that explicitly forbade teachers from even discussing LGBTQ issues.[54]

MEDICAL EDUCATION

One of the most important ways to promote high-quality health care for youth who identify as TGD and their families is increasing the knowledge base and clinical experience of pediatric providers in providing culturally competent care to such populations, as recommended by the recently released guidelines by the Association of American Medical Colleges.[93] This begins with the medical school curriculum in areas such as human development, sexual health, endocrinology, pediatrics, and psychiatry. In a 2009–2010 survey of US medical schools, it was found that the median number of hours dedicated to LGBTQ health was 5, with one-third of US medical schools reporting no LGBTQ curriculum during the clinical years.[94]

During residency training, there is potential for gender diversity to be emphasized in core rotations, especially in pediatrics, psychiatry, family medicine, and obstetrics and gynecology. Awareness could be promoted through the inclusion of topics relevant to caring for children who identify as TGD in the list of core competencies published by the American Board of Pediatrics, certifying examinations, and relevant study materials. Continuing education and maintenance of certification activities can include topics relevant to TGD populations as well.

* For more information regarding state-specific laws, please contact the AAP Division of State Government Affairs at stgov@ aap.org.

RECOMMENDATIONS

The AAP works toward all children and adolescents, regardless of gender identity or expression, receiving care to promote optimal physical, mental, and social well-being. Any discrimination based on gender identity or expression, real or perceived, is damaging to the socioemotional health of children, families, and society. In particular, the AAP recommends the following:

1. that youth who identify as TGD have access to comprehensive, gender-affirming, and developmentally appropriate health care that is provided in a safe and inclusive clinical space;

2. that family-based therapy and support be available to recognize and respond to the emotional and mental health needs of parents, caregivers, and siblings of youth who identify as TGD;

3. that electronic health records, billing systems, patient-centered notification systems, and clinical research be designed to respect the asserted gender identity of each patient while maintaining confidentiality and avoiding duplicate charts;

4. that insurance plans offer coverage for health care that is specific to the needs of youth who identify as TGD, including coverage for medical, psychological, and, when indicated, surgical gender-affirming interventions;

5. that provider education, including medical school, residency, and continuing education, integrate core competencies on the emotional and physical health needs and best practices for the care of youth who identify as TGD and their families;

6. that pediatricians have a role in advocating for, educating, and developing liaison relationships with school districts and other community organizations to promote acceptance and inclusion of all children without fear of harassment, exclusion, or bullying because of gender expression;

7. that pediatricians have a role in advocating for policies and laws that protect youth who identify as TGD from discrimination and violence;

8. that the health care workforce protects diversity by offering equal employment opportunities and workplace protections, regardless of gender identity or expression; and

9. that the medical field and federal government prioritize research that is dedicated to improving the quality of evidence-based care for youth who identify as TGD.

LEAD AUTHOR

Jason Richard Rafferty, MD, MPH, EdM, FAAP

CONTRIBUTOR

Robert Garofalo, MD, FAAP

COMMITTEE ON PSYCHOSOCIAL ASPECTS OF CHILD AND FAMILY HEALTH, 2017–2018

Michael Yogman, MD, FAAP, Chairperson
Rebecca Baum, MD, FAAP
Thresia B. Gambon, MD, FAAP
Arthur Lavin, MD, FAAP
Gerri Mattson, MD, FAAP
Lawrence Sagin Wissow, MD, MPH, FAAP

LIAISONS

Sharon Berry, PhD, LP – *Society of Pediatric Psychology*
Ed Christophersen, PhD, FAAP – *Society of Pediatric Psychology*
Norah Johnson, PhD, RN, CPNP-BC – *National Association of Pediatric Nurse Practitioners*
Amy Starin, PhD, LCSW – *National Association of Social Workers*
Abigail Schlesinger, MD – *American Academy of Child and Adolescent Psychiatry*

STAFF

Karen S. Smith
James Baumberger

ACKNOWLEDGMENTS

We thank Isaac Albanese, MPA, and Jayeson Watts, LICSW, for their thoughtful reviews and contributions.

ABBREVIATIONS

AAP: American Academy of Pediatrics
GACM: gender-affirmative care model
GLSEN: Gay, Lesbian, and Straight Education Network
LGBTQ: lesbian, gay, bisexual, transgender, or questioning
TGD: transgender and gender diverse

DOI: https://doi.org/10.1542/peds.2018-2162

Address correspondence to Jason Rafferty, MD, MPH, EdM, FAAP. E-mail: Jason_Rafferty@mail.harvard.edu

PEDIATRICS (ISSN Numbers: Print, 0031-4005; Online, 1098-4275).

REFERENCES

1. Levine DA; Committee on Adolescence. Office-based care for lesbian, gay, bisexual, transgender, and questioning youth. *Pediatrics.* 2013;132(1). Available at: www.pediatrics.org/cgi/content/full/132/1/e297

2. American Academy of Pediatrics Committee on Adolescence. Homosexuality and adolescence. *Pediatrics.* 1983;72(2):249–250

3. Institute of Medicine; Committee on Lesbian Gay Bisexual, and Transgender Health Issues and Research Gaps and Opportunities. *The Health of Lesbian, Gay, Bisexual, and Transgender People: Building a Foundation for Better Understanding.* Washington, DC: National Academies Press; 2011. Available at: https://www.ncbi.nlm.nih.gov/books/NBK64806. Accessed May 19, 2017

4. Deutsch MB, Radix A, Reisner S. What's in a guideline? Developing collaborative and sound research designs that substantiate best practice recommendations for transgender health care. *AMA J Ethics.* 2016;18(11):1098–1106

5. Bonifacio HJ, Rosenthal SM. Gender variance and dysphoria in children and adolescents. *Pediatr Clin North Am.* 2015;62(4):1001–1016

6. Vance SR Jr, Ehrensaft D, Rosenthal SM. Psychological and medical care of gender nonconforming youth. *Pediatrics.* 2014;134(6):1184–1192

7. Richards C, Bouman WP, Seal L, Barker MJ, Nieder TO, T'Sjoen G. Non-binary or genderqueer genders. *Int Rev Psychiatry.* 2016;28(1):95–102

8. American Psychological Association. Guidelines for psychological practice with transgender and gender nonconforming people. *Am Psychol.* 2015;70(9):832–864

9. Flores AR, Herman JL, Gates GJ, Brown TNT. *How Many Adults Identify as Transgender in the United States.* Los Angeles, CA: The Williams Institute; 2016

10. Herman JL, Flores AR, Brown TNT, Wilson BDM, Conron KJ. *Age of Individuals Who Identify as Transgender in the United States.* Los Angeles, CA: The Williams Institute; 2017

11. Gates GJ. *How Many People are Lesbian, Gay, Bisexual, and Transgender?* Los Angeles, CA: The Williams Institute; 2011

12. Olson J, Schrager SM, Belzer M, Simons LK, Clark LF. Baseline physiologic and psychosocial characteristics of transgender youth seeking care for gender dysphoria. *J Adolesc Health.* 2015;57(4):374–380

13. Almeida J, Johnson RM, Corliss HL, Molnar BE, Azrael D. Emotional distress

among LGBT youth: the influence of perceived discrimination based on sexual orientation. *J Youth Adolesc.* 2009;38(7):1001–1014

14. Clements-Nolle K, Marx R, Katz M. Attempted suicide among transgender persons: the influence of gender-based discrimination and victimization. *J Homosex.* 2006;51(3):53–69

15. Colizzi M, Costa R, Todarello O. Transsexual patients' psychiatric comorbidity and positive effect of cross-sex hormonal treatment on mental health: results from a longitudinal study. *Psychoneuroendocrinology.* 2014;39:65–73

16. Haas AP, Eliason M, Mays VM, et al. Suicide and suicide risk in lesbian, gay, bisexual, and transgender populations: review and recommendations. *J Homosex.* 2011;58(1):10–51

17. Maguen S, Shipherd JC. Suicide risk among transgender individuals. *Psychol Sex.* 2010;1(1):34–43

18. Connolly MD, Zervos MJ, Barone CJ II, Johnson CC, Joseph CL. The mental health of transgender youth: advances in understanding. *J Adolesc Health.* 2016;59(5):489–495

19. Grossman AH, D'Augelli AR. Transgender youth and life-threatening behaviors. *Suicide Life Threat Behav.* 2007;37(5):527–537

20. Spack NP, Edwards-Leeper L, Feldman HA, et al. Children and adolescents with gender identity disorder referred to a pediatric medical center. *Pediatrics.* 2012;129(3):418–425

21. van Schalkwyk GI, Klingensmith K, Volkmar FR. Gender identity and autism spectrum disorders. *Yale J Biol Med.* 2015;88(1):81–83

22. Jacobs LA, Rachlin K, Erickson-Schroth L, Janssen A. Gender dysphoria and co-occurring autism spectrum disorders: review, case examples, and treatment considerations. *LGBT Health.* 2014;1(4):277–282

23. American Psychiatric Association. *Diagnostic and Statistical Manual of Mental Disorders.* 5th ed. Arlington, VA: American Psychiatric Association; 2013

24. Edwards-Leeper L, Spack NP. Psychological evaluation and medical treatment of transgender youth in an interdisciplinary "Gender Management Service" (GeMS) in a major pediatric center. *J Homosex.* 2012;59(3):321–336

25. Anton BS. Proceedings of the American Psychological Association for the legislative year 2008: minutes of the annual meeting of the Council of Representatives, February 22–24, 2008, Washington, DC, and August 13 and 17, 2008, Boston, MA, and minutes of the February, June, August, and December 2008 meetings of the Board of Directors. *Am Psychol.* 2009;64(5):372–453

26. Drescher J, Haller E; American Psychiatric Association Caucus of Lesbian, Gay and Bisexual Psychiatrists. *Position Statement on Discrimination Against Transgender and Gender Variant Individuals.* Washington, DC: American Psychiatric Association; 2012

27. Hidalgo MA, Ehrensaft D, Tishelman AC, et al. The gender affirmative model: what we know and what we aim to learn. *Hum Dev.* 2013;56(5):285–290

28. Tishelman AC, Kaufman R, Edwards-Leeper L, Mandel FH, Shumer DE, Spack NP. Serving transgender youth: challenges, dilemmas and clinical examples. *Prof Psychol Res Pr.* 2015;46(1):37–45

29. Adelson SL; American Academy of Child and Adolescent Psychiatry (AACAP) Committee on Quality Issues (CQI). Practice parameter on gay, lesbian, or bisexual sexual orientation, gender nonconformity, and gender discordance in children and adolescents. *J Am Acad Child Adolesc Psychiatry.* 2012;51(9):957–974

30. Herbst JH, Jacobs ED, Finlayson TJ, McKleroy VS, Neumann MS, Crepaz N; HIV/AIDS Prevention Research Synthesis Team. Estimating HIV prevalence and risk behaviors of transgender persons in the United States: a systematic review. *AIDS Behav.* 2008;12(1):1–17

31. James SE, Herman JL, Rankin S, Keisling M, Mottet L, Anafi M. *The Report of the 2015 U.S. Transgender Survey.* Washington, DC: National Center for Transgender Equality; 2016

32. Centers for Disease Control and Prevention. *CDC-Funded HIV Testing:* *United States, Puerto Rico, and the U.S. Virgin Islands.* Atlanta, GA: Centers for Disease Control and Prevention; 2015. Available at: https://www.cdc.gov/hiv/pdf/library/reports/cdc-hiv-funded-testing-us-puerto-rico-2015.pdf. Accessed August 2, 2018

33. Substance Abuse and Mental Health Services Administration. *Ending Conversion Therapy: Supporting and Affirming LGBTQ Youth.* Rockville, MD: Substance Abuse and Mental Health Services Administration; 2015

34. Korell SC, Lorah P. An overview of affirmative psychotherapy and counseling with transgender clients. In: Bieschke KJ, Perez RM, DeBord KA, eds. *Handbook of Counseling and Psychotherapy With Lesbian, Gay, Bisexual, and Transgender Clients.* 2nd ed. Washington, DC: American Psychological Association; 2007:271–288

35. World Professional Association for Transgender Health. *Standards of Care for the Health of Transsexual, Transgender, and Gender Nonconforming People.* 7th ed. Minneapolis, MN: World Professional Association for Transgender Health; 2011. Available at: https://www.wpath.org/publications/soc. Accessed April 15, 2018

36. Menvielle E. A comprehensive program for children with gender variant behaviors and gender identity disorders. *J Homosex.* 2012;59(3):357–368

37. Hill DB, Menvielle E, Sica KM, Johnson A. An affirmative intervention for families with gender variant children: parental ratings of child mental health and gender. *J Sex Marital Ther.* 2010;36(1):6–23

38. Haldeman DC. The practice and ethics of sexual orientation conversion therapy. *J Consult Clin Psychol.* 1994;62(2):221–227

39. Byne W. Regulations restrict practice of conversion therapy. *LGBT Health.* 2016;3(2):97–99

40. Cohen-Kettenis PT, Delemarre-van de Waal HA, Gooren LJ. The treatment of adolescent transsexuals: changing insights. *J Sex Med.* 2008;5(8):1892–1897

41. Bryant K. Making gender identity disorder of childhood: historical lessons for contemporary debates. *Sex Res Soc Policy.* 2006;3(3):23–39

42. World Professional Association for Transgender Health. *WPATH De-Psychopathologisation Statement.* Minneapolis, MN: World Professional Association for Transgender Health; 2010. Available at: https://www.wpath.org/policies. Accessed April 16, 2017

43. American Academy of Pediatrics. AAP support letter conversion therapy ban [letter]. 2015. Available at: https://www.aap.org/en-us/advocacy-and-policy/federal-advocacy/Documents/AAPsupportletterconversiontherapyban.pdf. Accessed August 1, 2018

44. Movement Advancement Project. *LGBT Policy Spotlight: Conversion Therapy Bans.* Boulder, CO: Movement Advancement Project; 2017. Available at: http://www.lgbtmap.org/policy-and-issue-analysis/policy-spotlight-conversion-therapy-bans. Accessed August 6, 2017

45. Ehrensaft D, Giammattei SV, Storck K, Tishelman AC, Keo-Meier C. Prepubertal social gender transitions: what we know; what we can learn—a view from a gender affirmative lens. *Int J Transgend.* 2018;19(2):251–268

46. Olson KR, Key AC, Eaton NR. Gender cognition in transgender children. *Psychol Sci.* 2015;26(4):467–474

47. Olson KR. Prepubescent transgender children: what we do and do not know. *J Am Acad Child Adolesc Psychiatry.* 2016;55(3):155–156.e3

48. Olson KR, Durwood L, DeMeules M, McLaughlin KA. Mental health of transgender children who are supported in their identities. *Pediatrics.* 2016;137(3):e20153223

49. Malpas J. Between pink and blue: a multi-dimensional family approach to gender nonconforming children and their families. *Fam Process.* 2011;50(4):453–470

50. Hagan JF Jr, Shaw JS, Duncan PM, eds. *Bright Futures: Guidelines for Health Supervision of Infants, Children, and Adolescents.* 4th ed. Elk Grove, IL: American Academy of Pediatrics; 2016

51. Minter SP. Supporting transgender children: new legal, social, and medical approaches. *J Homosex.* 2012;59(3):422–433

52. AHIMA Work Group. Improved patient engagement for LGBT populations: addressing factors related to sexual orientation/gender identity for effective health information management. *J AHIMA.* 2017;88(3):34–39

53. Deutsch MB, Green J, Keatley J, Mayer G, Hastings J, Hall AM; World Professional Association for Transgender Health EMR Working Group. Electronic medical records and the transgender patient: recommendations from the World Professional Association for Transgender Health EMR Working Group. *J Am Med Inform Assoc.* 2013;20(4):700–703

54. Dowshen N, Meadows R, Byrnes M, Hawkins L, Eder J, Noonan K. Policy perspective: ensuring comprehensive care and support for gender nonconforming children and adolescents. *Transgend Health.* 2016;1(1):75–85

55. Cahill SR, Baker K, Deutsch MB, Keatley J, Makadon HJ. Inclusion of sexual orientation and gender identity in stage 3 meaningful use guidelines: a huge step forward for LGBT health. *LGBT Health.* 2016;3(2):100–102

56. Mansfield MJ, Beardsworth DE, Loughlin JS, et al. Long-term treatment of central precocious puberty with a long-acting analogue of luteinizing hormone-releasing hormone. Effects on somatic growth and skeletal maturation. *N Engl J Med.* 1983;309(21):1286–1290

57. Olson J, Garofalo R. The peripubertal gender-dysphoric child: puberty suppression and treatment paradigms. *Pediatr Ann.* 2014;43(6):e132–e137

58. de Vries AL, Steensma TD, Doreleijers TA, Cohen-Kettenis PT. Puberty suppression in adolescents with gender identity disorder: a prospective follow-up study. *J Sex Med.* 2011;8(8):2276–2283

59. Wallien MS, Cohen-Kettenis PT. Psychosexual outcome of gender-dysphoric children. *J Am Acad Child Adolesc Psychiatry.* 2008;47(12):1413–1423

60. Waylen A, Wolke D. Sex 'n' drugs 'n' rock 'n' roll: the meaning and social consequences of pubertal timing. *Eur J Endocrinol.* 2004;151(suppl 3):U151–U159

61. de Vries AL, Klink D, Cohen-Kettenis PT. What the primary care pediatrician needs to know about gender incongruence and gender dysphoria in children and adolescents. *Pediatr Clin North Am.* 2016;63(6):1121–1135

62. Vlot MC, Klink DT, den Heijer M, Blankenstein MA, Rotteveel J, Heijboer AC. Effect of pubertal suppression and cross-sex hormone therapy on bone turnover markers and bone mineral apparent density (BMAD) in transgender adolescents. *Bone.* 2017;95:11–19

63. Finlayson C, Johnson EK, Chen D, et al. Proceedings of the working group session on fertility preservation for individuals with gender and sex diversity. *Transgend Health.* 2016;1(1):99–107

64. Kreukels BP, Cohen-Kettenis PT. Puberty suppression in gender identity disorder: the Amsterdam experience. *Nat Rev Endocrinol.* 2011;7(8):466–472

65. Rosenthal SM. Approach to the patient: transgender youth: endocrine considerations. *J Clin Endocrinol Metab.* 2014;99(12):4379–4389

66. Fenway Health. *Glossary of Gender and Transgender Terms.* Boston, MA: Fenway Health; 2010. Available at: http://fenwayhealth.org/documents/the-fenway-institute/handouts/Handout_7-C_Glossary_of_Gender_and_Transgender_Terms__fi.pdf. Accessed August 16, 2017

67. de Vries AL, McGuire JK, Steensma TD, Wagenaar EC, Doreleijers TA, Cohen-Kettenis PT. Young adult psychological outcome after puberty suppression and gender reassignment. *Pediatrics.* 2014;134(4):696–704

68. Hembree WC, Cohen-Kettenis PT, Gooren L, et al. Endocrine treatment of gender-dysphoric/gender-incongruent persons: an endocrine society clinical practice guideline. *J Clin Endocrinol Metab.* 2017;102(11):3869–3903

69. Milrod C, Karasic DH. Age is just a number: WPATH-affiliated surgeons' experiences and attitudes toward

vaginoplasty in transgender females under 18 years of age in the United States. *J Sex Med.* 2017;14(4):624–634

70. Milrod C. How young is too young: ethical concerns in genital surgery of the transgender MTF adolescent. *J Sex Med.* 2014;11(2):338–346

71. Olson-Kennedy J, Warus J, Okonta V, Belzer M, Clark LF. Chest reconstruction and chest dysphoria in transmasculine minors and young adults: comparisons of nonsurgical and postsurgical cohorts. *JAMA Pediatr.* 2018;172(5):431–436

72. Committee on Adolescent Health Care. Committee opinion no. 685: care for transgender adolescents. *Obstet Gynecol.* 2017;129(1):e11–e16

73. Greydanus DE, Patel DR, Rimsza ME. Contraception in the adolescent: an update. *Pediatrics.* 2001;107(3):562–573

74. Gridley SJ, Crouch JM, Evans Y, et al. Youth and caregiver perspectives on barriers to gender-affirming health care for transgender youth. *J Adolesc Health.* 2016;59(3):254–261

75. Sanchez NF, Sanchez JP, Danoff A. Health care utilization, barriers to care, and hormone usage among male-to-female transgender persons in New York City. *Am J Public Health.* 2009;99(4):713–719

76. Transgender Law Center. *Affordable Care Act Fact Sheet.* Oakland, CA: Transgender Law Center; 2016. Available at: https://transgenderlawcenter.org/resources/health/aca-fact-sheet. Accessed August 8, 2016

77. Nahata L, Quinn GP, Caltabellotta NM, Tishelman AC. Mental health concerns and insurance denials among transgender adolescents. *LGBT Health.* 2017;4(3):188–193

78. Grant JM, Mottet LA, Tanis J, Harrison J, Herman JL, Keisling M. *Injustice at Every Turn: A Report of the National Transgender Discrimination Survey.* Washington, DC: National Center for Transgender Equality and National Gay and Lesbian Task Force; 2011 Available at: http://www.thetaskforce.org/static_

html/downloads/reports/reports/ntds_full.pdf. Accessed August 6, 2018

79. Sevelius JM. Gender affirmation: a framework for conceptualizing risk behavior among transgender women of color. *Sex Roles.* 2013;68(11–12):675–689

80. Koken JA, Bimbi DS, Parsons JT. Experiences of familial acceptance-rejection among transwomen of color. *J Fam Psychol.* 2009;23(6):853–860

81. Lombardi EL, Wilchins RA, Priesing D, Malouf D. Gender violence: transgender experiences with violence and discrimination. *J Homosex.* 2001;42(1):89–101

82. Wren B. 'I can accept my child is transsexual but if I ever see him in a dress I'll hit him': dilemmas in parenting a transgendered adolescent. *Clin Child Psychol Psychiatry.* 2002;7(3):377–397

83. Riley EA, Sitharthan G, Clemson L, Diamond M. The needs of gender-variant children and their parents: a parent survey. *Int J Sex Health.* 2011;23(3):181–195

84. Whitley CT. Trans-kin undoing and redoing gender: negotiating relational identity among friends and family of transgender persons. *Sociol Perspect.* 2013;56(4):597–621

85. Travers R, Bauer G, Pyne J, Bradley K, Gale L, Papadimitriou M; Trans PULSE; Children's Aid Society of Toronto; Delisle Youth Services. *Impacts of Strong Parental Support for Trans Youth: A Report Prepared for Children's Aid Society of Toronto and Delisle Youth Services.* Toronto, ON: Trans PULSE; 2012. Available at: http://transpulseproject.ca/wp-content/uploads/2012/10/Impacts-of-Strong-Parental-Support-for-Trans-Youth-vFINAL.pdf

86. Ryan C, Russell ST, Huebner D, Diaz R, Sanchez J. Family acceptance in adolescence and the health of LGBT young adults. *J Child Adolesc Psychiatr Nurs.* 2010;23(4):205–213

87. Grossman AH, D'augelli AR, Frank JA. Aspects of psychological resilience among transgender youth. *J LGBT Youth.* 2011;8(2):103–115

88. McConnell EA, Birkett M, Mustanski B. Families matter: social support and mental health trajectories among lesbian, gay, bisexual, and transgender youth. *J Adolesc Health.* 2016;59(6):674–680

89. Ellis KM, Eriksen K. Transsexual and transgenderist experiences and treatment options. *Fam J Alex Va.* 2002;10(3):289–299

90. Lamda Legal. *Transgender Rights Toolkit: A Legal Guide for Trans People and Their Advocates.* New York, NY: Lambda Legal; 2016 Available at: https://www.lambdalegal.org/publications/trans-toolkit. Accessed August 6, 2018

91. Kosciw JG, Greytak EA, Giga NM, Villenas C, Danischewski DJ. *The 2015 National School Climate Survey: The Experiences of Lesbian, Gay, Bisexual, Transgender, and Queer Youth in Our Nation's Schools.* New York, NY: GLSEN; 2016. Available at: https://www.glsen.org/article/2015-national-school-climate-survey. Accessed August 8, 2018

92. McGuire JK, Anderson CR, Toomey RB, Russell ST. School climate for transgender youth: a mixed method investigation of student experiences and school responses. *J Youth Adolesc.* 2010;39(10):1175–1188

93. Association of American Medical Colleges Advisory Committee on Sexual Orientation, Gender Identity, and Sex Development. In: Hollenback AD, Eckstrand KL, Dreger A, eds. *Implementing Curricular and Institutional Climate Changes to Improve Health Care for Individuals Who Are LGBT, Gender Nonconforming, or Born With DSD: A Resource for Medical Educators.* Washington, DC: Association of American Medical Colleges; 2014. Available at: https://members.aamc.org/eweb/upload/Executive LGBT FINAL.pdf. Accessed August 8, 2018

94. Obedin-Maliver J, Goldsmith ES, Stewart L, et al. Lesbian, gay, bisexual, and transgender-related content in undergraduate medical education. *JAMA.* 2011;306(9):971–977

CLINICAL REPORT   Guidance for the Clinician in Rendering Pediatric Care

American Academy of Pediatrics

DEDICATED TO THE HEALTH OF ALL CHILDREN™

Health and Mental Health Needs of Children in US Military Families

CDR Chadley R. Huebner, MD, MPH, FAAP, SECTION ON UNIFORMED SERVICES, COMMITTEE ON PSYCHOSOCIAL ASPECTS OF CHILD AND FAMILY HEALTH

abstract

Children in US military families share common experiences and unique challenges, including parental deployment and frequent relocation. Although some of the stressors of military life have been associated with higher rates of mental health disorders and increased health care use among family members, there are various factors and interventions that have been found to promote resilience. Military children often live on or near military installations, where they may attend Department of Defense–sponsored child care programs and schools and receive medical care through military treatment facilities. However, many families live in remote communities without access to these services. Because of this wide geographic distribution, military children are cared for in both military and civilian medical practices. This clinical report provides a background to military culture and offers practical guidance to assist civilian and military pediatricians caring for military children.

Department of Pediatrics, Naval Medical Center, San Diego, California

Dr Huebner was responsible for revising and writing this clinical report with consideration of the input of all reviewers and the board of directors and approved the final manuscript as submitted.

The views expressed herein are those of the author and do not necessarily reflect the official policy or position of the Department of the Navy, Department of Defense, or the US Government.

DOI: https://doi.org/10.1542/peds.2018-3258

Address correspondence to Chadley R. Huebner, MD, MPH, FAAP. E-mail: chadley74@yahoo.com

PEDIATRICS (ISSN Numbers: Print, 0031-4005; Online, 1098-4275).

Copyright © 2019 by the American Academy of Pediatrics

FINANCIAL DISCLOSURE: The author has indicated he has no financial relationships relevant to this article to disclose.

To cite: Huebner CR, AAP SECTION ON UNIFORMED SERVICES, AAP COMMITTEE ON PSYCHOSOCIAL ASPECTS OF CHILD AND FAMILY HEALTH. Health and Mental Health Needs of Children in US Military Families. *Pediatrics.* 2019;143(1):e20183258

INTRODUCTION

Children who are military connected have unique needs and experiences compared with peers of the same age. These experiences often include frequent moves, prolonged separations, and deployments of family members. Although these challenges may be familiar to military and civilian health care providers working at military treatment facilities, up to 50% of children who are military connected receive care in the civilian sector.[1–3] The American Academy of Pediatrics (AAP) clinical report "Health and Mental Health Needs of Children in US Military Families" was published in 2013 to assist pediatric health care providers who care for military children who have been affected by deployment.[4] In that report, the cycle of deployment was described as well as the common reactions to deployment and the effects of wartime deployment on children at different developmental stages. Age-based recommendations were provided to assist family members, and additional resources were provided to assist pediatricians.

Since the publication of the last AAP clinical report, military families continue to be significantly challenged by deployments and various stressors associated with military life. Many children in military families live in settings remote from a military community, and civilian health care providers are faced with caring for military children in their practices. This updated clinical report is intended to provide a background of the military culture, to serve as a tool to help navigate the military health care system, and to provide resources that may assist families and the broader health care community, especially during periods of transition and relocation.

DEMOGRAPHICS

The Department of Defense (DOD) remains the nation's largest government agency and employer; 1.3 million men and women serve on active duty, 818 000 in the National Guard and Reserve and more than 2 million military retirees.[5,6] Active duty personnel are members of the US Armed Forces who serve in a full-time duty status. Approximately 88% of active duty forces are stationed in the continental United States and US territories, whereas the remainder are stationed at installations throughout the world but primarily in East Asia (5%) and Europe (5.1%).[5] According to the DOD, military personnel are composed of 17.7% officers with an average age of 34.6 years and 82.3% enlisted personnel with an average age of 27.1 years.[5,7] Most enlisted personnel have a high school diploma, and 8% have a bachelor's degree or higher; the majority of officers (85%) have a bachelor's degree or higher.[5]

Approximately 58% of the 2.2 million members serving on active duty and the National Guard and Reserve have families, and 40% have at least 2 children.[1,3] There are an estimated

1.7 million children of active duty and reserve military personnel, of whom 37.8% are 0 to 5 years of age, 31.6% are 6 to 11 years of age, and 23.8% are 12 to 18 years of age.[5] When including active duty personnel, reserve personnel, and veterans, it is estimated that there are 4 million children who are military connected, with the largest group age ≤5 years.[7]

MILITARY CULTURE

The military is a well-defined institution with a distinct hierarchy and organizational structure. Service members come from ethnically and geographically diverse backgrounds and join the military for a variety of reasons, including the propensity to serve, educational benefits, and financial motivations.[8] Redmond et al[9] described the military workplace culture as a unique environment with unifying characteristics, including discipline, self-sacrifice, cohesiveness, and emphasis on core values. Military service is associated with numerous traditions and common experiences that engender a sense of camaraderie among members who have proudly served.

Military personnel are a relatively young workforce, are more likely to marry young, and have a high proportion of children that are of preschool age.[10] Military personnel are generally paid favorably in comparison with their civilian equivalents; however, additional stressors of the military lifestyle, such as relocation, results in spousal underemployment and unemployment.[11] Military life is often defined by prolonged separation and frequent moves, with many simultaneous stressors in a short time.[10]

Children growing up in military families often share common experiences with each other, such as living on base or post, attending DOD schools, frequent moves, and prolonged separations from a parent.

These experiences create a common bond and camaraderie among peers. This sense of identity may be influential in later career choices because children of veterans are more likely than their civilian peers to enlist.[12]

Conversely, military children may feel heightened pressure to conform, behave, and wear their parent's military rank.[1] Davis et al[2] reported that early research portrayed the military family as authoritarian with children who were behaviorally challenged; however, subsequent research has revealed no psychosocial differences from nonmilitary families. Padden and Agazio[13] described 4 major stressors for military children: relocation, family separation, adaptation to danger, and a unique military culture. Socioeconomic challenges include financial stressors among junior enlisted personnel[14] and rates of food insecurity similar to the national average.[15]

RELOCATION

One of the most common aspects of military life is frequent relocation. Active duty personnel receive orders to their respective duty stations for a tour of duty, which is generally 2 to 3 years in length. These orders may be designated as accompanied or unaccompanied, in which the former authorizes dependents' travel and sponsorship at the new duty station and the latter does not. Unaccompanied orders are generally 1 to 2 years in length and are often a result of the nature of the assignment or a dependent family member having medical needs that exceed the capabilities of the local military medical treatment facility.

Military families are geographically mobile, moving at a rate 2.4 times more frequent than that of their civilian counterparts.[7,10,16] Military children may experience a move every 2 to 4 years and can transition between schools up to 9 times by the age of 18 years.[1,17] Because of the frequent mobility, there is often a lack of continuity of health care[1] and limited employment opportunities for nonmilitary spouses.[10]

In a large population study of military youth, there were increased mental health encounters if a geographic move occurred in the past year.[18] This study also revealed that adolescents who were affected had increased psychiatric hospitalizations and emergency department visits. Because families often move away from extended family support, they often refer to the military community as a surrogate family that provides a support network.

Although children of reservists are typically geographically more stable than their active duty counterparts, they often live in nonmilitary communities without resources or knowledge specific to the military.[1] They may feel isolated from the community,[10] and services may not be as readily available.[2] Veteran families may also feel isolated and have challenges when transitioning to civilian communities,[10] where familiar military programs may not exist and there may no longer be access to many of the benefits that were associated with active duty service.[12]

Although moves may be stressful, Clever and Segal[10] asserted that some research has demonstrated increased resilience in military children, including decreased school problems and enhanced development of positive attitudes about moves.[19] Protective factors may include effective support systems, such as living in a military community and military programs designed to address relocation challenges, which may include family newcomer orientations, command sponsorship programs, and programs intended to assist children in connecting with peers at the prospective duty station before the move.

DEPLOYMENT

One of the characteristics of military life that is well known to the public is deployment. Research has found that more than 2 million children of military families have had a parent deployed since 2001.[1] Service members may be deployed to areas throughout the world in support of combat operations or peacekeeping missions for periods ranging from several weeks to more than a year. During this time, family members often remain at home to adapt to life without the military service member or temporarily move to areas where they may have support from extended family members.

The deployment cycle, as described by Pincus et al,[20] consists of 5 stages (predeployment, deployment, sustainment, redeployment, and postdeployment) that each present various emotional challenges to family members. Recommendations to assist family members during each of these stages have been offered by various authors[4,13,20] and serve as a valuable framework for pediatricians caring for children affected by deployment.

Impact of Deployment

Multiple studies have explored the effects of deployment on families and children who are military connected. The stressors associated with deployment, including prolonged family separation, potential injury or death of a service member, and traumatic experiences, can have a cumulative negative effect on the entire family unit. Aranda et al[21] found that 1 in 4 military children have an emotional-behavioral challenge associated with deployment. One study revealed an 11% increase in mental and behavioral health outpatient visits in children 3 to 8 years of age during parental deployment.[22] An additional study evaluating the effect of deployment on children 5 to 12 years of age showed increased child

psychosocial morbidity with parental stress and decreased morbidity with military supports.[3]

A 2014 systematic review explored literature examining the impact of parental deployment–related mental health problems on children's outcomes.[23] Of the 42 studies reviewed, the authors found that outcomes were negatively affected by caregiver stress and mental health, and there was evidence of increased child maltreatment and substance abuse. The authors found that family communication was a protective factor, and interventions should be aimed at addressing these challenges. Another 2015 systematic review revealed that a child's age and development, parental mental health and coping abilities, available resources, and resilience factors influenced coping abilities in children affected by military deployment.[24]

Mustillo et al[25] evaluated the timing and duration of deployment on children ages 10 years and younger and whether deployment was associated with any particular type of emotional-behavioral disorder. The authors identified increased anxiety in children ages 3 to 5 years if there was a recent long deployment. For older children ages 6 to 10 years, there was evidence of a long-term impact of parental deployment at the time of their birth, including more peer problems and behavioral problems. This study and others suggested differential effects on the basis of developmental age.[4,26] In a telephone survey involving children 11 to 17 years of age and their home caregivers, increased length of deployment and poor mental health of the caregiver who was not deployed was associated with more challenges for children in dealing with the deployment.[27] Another study of 6- to 12-year-old children and their civilian parent who was not deployed demonstrated increased depression and externalizing symptoms associated with parental distress and cumulative length of parental combat deployment as well as increased anxiety symptoms.[28] The aforementioned research was focused on the immediate effects of wartime deployment, and more longitudinal studies are needed to assess the long-term effects.[29]

Deployment Interventions

Given the challenges associated with deployment, numerous programs have been established to assist service members and their families. Nelson et al[7] described several family-based intervention programs that have been established to increase resilience, combat stress, and improve family functioning: Families OverComing Under Stress,[30] After Deployment: Adaptive Parenting Tools,[31] and the STRoNG Intervention for families with young children.[32] Additional programs that may assist families with younger children in preparing for the stress of the deployment cycle include Sesame Workshop's Talk, Listen, Connect initiative[33] and child-parent psychotherapy–based interventions.[34]

Health Care Use

Research has revealed various challenges associated with deployment, including a decline in academics, increased behavioral problems during deployment, increased emergency and specialist visits, and somatic symptoms.[1,35] A systematic review of 26 studies found an association between increased deployment-related stress and mental health problems in parents and young children as well as increased use of mental health resources.[36] One of these studies demonstrated an increase in outpatient and well-child visits during deployment for children of married parents, which may be attributed to the effect of deployment-related stress on the spouse who was not deployed.[37]

Conversely, the authors found decreased visits for children of single parents, which may be attributed to a decreased effect of deployment on a nonparent caregiver or lack of familiarity navigating the health care system. Another study showed an increase in specialist visits and antidepressant and/or anxiolytic medication use among children during deployment. Additionally, a shift from military treatment facilities to civilian facilities during deployment was observed, which may be indicative of a temporary family relocation while the active duty service member was deployed.[38] Finally, research has shown a 7% increase in outpatient visits for children younger than 2 years during the deployment of a parent[37] as well as an increased effect of deployment on children if it occurred during the developmental or attachment period.[39]

Abuse and/or Neglect

Deployment and relocation stressors are concerning for an increased risk of child maltreatment.[40] Cozza et al[41] demonstrated an increased risk of neglect among deployed families compared with families that were never deployed, and a systematic review found an increased risk of child maltreatment, including neglect and physical abuse.[36] Furthermore, there is an increased risk at the time of redeployment,[1] making it important to continue to provide resources once a service member who was deployed returns.

Various programs are available to assist families with abuse prevention, and there are also resources available if abuse has occurred, including the Family Advocacy Program (FAP).[42] FAP professionals interact with families in a variety of ways, including parent workshops and support programs, and conduct investigations when allegations of abuse are made. Because civilian providers may not be aware of the

FAP, they may report concerns about child maltreatment to local child protective services without also notifying the local FAP office. Wood et al[40] found that only 42% of cases of medically diagnosed maltreatment were reported to the FAP, compared with 90% reported to child protective services, meaning that many families do not receive timely and appropriate military-specific services.

The DOD has various programs to support families with young children. The New Parent Support Program is an FAP that uses licensed clinicians, nurses, and home-visiting specialists to serve families with young children. A variety of services are available through this program, including home visits, parenting classes, and linkages to community and DOD resources. More information on this valuable program may be found at http://www.militaryonesource. mil/-/the-new-parent-support-program.[43]

RESILIENCE

Despite many of the inherent challenges of military life, multiple studies indicate increased resilience among children who are military connected. Easterbrooks et al[44] noted that most research on military children is focused on deficits rather than the strengths and supports that promote resilience. The authors cite several studies that describe positive outcomes, including enhanced family bonding during deployment, resilience through shared experiences, and enhanced social connections. Aranda et al[21] found that although school-aged children had increased psychosocial morbidity during parental wartime deployment, they had lower baseline psychosocial symptoms than those of civilian peers. Resilience is key in all phases of deployment, and effective support networks may improve coping skills.[2] There is usually not a difference in psychological symptoms in military children during nondeployed seasons, although there may be a "dose effect" with repeated deployments.[21]

Research has examined factors that promote resilience. Parental mental health and parental adjustment to deployment may impact a child's resilience[11]; therefore, it is important to consider the family dynamic when caring for military children. A longitudinal study across the deployment cycle found that socialization with other military children during a deployment was a protective factor that led to better functioning.[45] An ecological model[46] that includes various systems of influence on an individual, such as family and community, has been suggested as a framework to identify the effects of military deployment and separations on children,[26,47] and effective interventions to promote resilience should be designed and tailored at each level.

CHILD CARE AND EDUCATION

Child Care System

The DOD runs the nation's largest employee-sponsored child care system, which consists of 900 child development centers, 300 school-age care program sites, 4500 family child care homes, and subsidized civilian child care.[48] Child development centers are located on most military installations throughout the world and provide child care to children from ages 6 weeks to 5 years. School-age care programs are available for children ages 5 to 12 years and are typically located at schools or youth centers. Additional child care services may be provided in other settings, including on- or off-base child care homes, providing more flexible hours and servicing a wider age range. Services at DOD-sponsored child care sites are income based, and some families may receive subsidies for civilian child care if space is unavailable through military care centers and if they meet specific income qualifications.[48]

Despite the immensity of the child care system, a 2008 study by the RAND Corporation revealed that only a small fraction of the military population was reached by these programs.[49] In this study, only 7% of military members were served by child development centers, and fewer than half of families with children younger than 6 years of age were using DOD-sponsored child care. Child development centers were found to be costlier and less flexible than other options, such as family child care homes. An increased awareness of the various child care options can assist families who are seeking child care arrangements, and additional information may be found at http://www.militaryonesource.mil/-/military-child-care-programs.[50]

Education System

Approximately 13% of children with an active duty parent attend a Department of Defense Education Activity (DODEA) school.[7] DODEA operates 166 schools for 72 000 children enrolled in kindergarten through 12th grade; is located in 7 states, 11 countries, and 2 territories; and also provides support for 1.2 million students who are military connected in public schools in the United States.[51,52] DODEA schools are accredited by the Commission on Accreditation and School Improvement and use a comprehensive curriculum and standardized assessments, including the National Assessment of Educational Progress.[52]

Although continuity of education through DODEA provides many advantages for transient military children, the vast majority of military children attend civilian schools. Astor et al[53] referenced research that revealed that the average military student attends 9 schools between kindergarten and 12th grade.[54] The authors remarked that civilian schools may be less familiar with the needs of military children. Because of increased risks of academic challenges and social problems,[55] it is recommended that military children are provided a supportive environment, which can serve as a protective factor. To facilitate the challenges civilian schools may encounter with military issues, there is a partnership grant with DODEA and public schools to assist civilian schools[11] with children who are military connected. School liaison officers serve as a valuable resource and are available near military installations worldwide (http://www.dodea.edu/Partnership/schoolLiaisonOfficers.cfm).[56]

MILITARY HEALTH SYSTEM

The Military Health System is a global health care delivery system dedicated to supporting the nation's military mission.[57] It is a single-payer umbrella system[2] that serves 9.4 million beneficiaries at an annual cost of approximately $50 billion.[57,58] The Assistant Secretary of Defense for Health Affairs oversees the Defense Health Agency, which manages regional Tricare contracts and the centralized Military Health System while integrating direct and purchased health care systems.[59] Each service branch is responsible for ensuring medical readiness of its operational forces and provides direct health care to beneficiaries at 54 inpatient hospitals and 377 ambulatory clinics throughout the world.[57]

There are multiple Tricare plans available. Eligibility is dependent on service status and enrollment in the Defense Enrollment Eligibility Reporting System. All health care plans are in compliance with the coverage requirements for the Affordable Care Act.[60] The most recent changes to Tricare occurred on January 1, 2018, with several changes to health plans, coverage limits, and regional contractors.[61] Most dependents of active duty members are enrolled in the Tricare Prime program if they live in Prime Service Areas, usually near a military treatment facility.[62] This is a managed care option in which beneficiaries receive direct care at military facilities or from network providers and generally do not pay out of pocket.[58] Tricare Select (Formerly Tricare Standard and Extra) is a fee-for-service plan with deductibles and cost sharing that is available to beneficiaries who do not meet eligibility for Prime or choose not to enroll in Prime and generally receive purchased care through network providers outside of military treatment facilities.[58,63]

There are different Tricare regions throughout the United States administered by a managed care support contractor.[64] Tricare-authorized providers can work directly with the managed care support contractor for claims processing and any management assistance. Additional information for providers can be found at www.tricare.mil/Providers.[64]

MILITARY CHILDREN WITH SPECIAL HEALTH CARE NEEDS

Approximately 220 000 active duty and reserve military personnel have a family member with special needs,[65] including 20% of children who are military connected.[66] In fiscal year 2015, 1.79 million children ages 6 months to 21 years were enrolled in the Military Health System, 17.3% of whom had noncomplex chronic needs and 5.6% of whom had complex chronic needs.[57]

Although subspecialty care may be available at military treatment facilities, children with special health care needs often receive services through civilian network providers, who may be unfamiliar with the

military system. In a survey of military family support providers, the most common challenges included navigating systems, child behavioral problems, parental stress and child care, relocation, and the therapy and/or insurance referral process.[65,67] To assist parents of children with special needs, the Office of Community Support for Military Families with Special Needs published the DOD *Special Needs Tool Kit: Birth to 18*.[68] This resource provides valuable information for families navigating early intervention programs and special education services, relocating, accessing Tricare benefits, and connecting to support services.

In addition, the Office of Special Needs provides an early intervention and special education directory to assist families with transitions during relocation to different communities, which is available through the Military OneSource Web site (www.militaryonesource.mil).[69] For military children located overseas who qualify for early intervention services, Educational and Developmental Intervention Services provides comprehensive developmental services, including early childhood special education, speech therapy, occupational therapy, physical therapy, social work, and child psychology. For children ages 3 to 21 years who qualify for special education services, DODEA schools provide special education services while collaborating with Educational and Developmental Intervention Services for medically related services in the school setting.

Exceptional Family Member Program

The Exceptional Family Member Program (EFMP) is a DOD program that provides services for families with special health care or educational needs. There are currently more than 128 000 military family members enrolled in the EFMP,[47,70] with approximately two-thirds of these being children

and youth.[65] Any active duty family member with a chronic medical condition or special education need should be enrolled in the EFMP. In a survey of EFMP family support providers across all branches, the largest proportion of disabilities cited included autism spectrum disorders and attention-deficit/hyperactivity disorder.[23,65]

For children of an active duty service member with a chronic medical condition, a DD Form 2792 documenting medical diagnoses and therapeutic needs is required from their pediatrician and should be taken by the family to their respective EFMP service coordinator to complete the enrollment process. The educational form (DD Form 2792-1) should be completed by an early intervention program or school special education program provider if the child is receiving Individuals with Disabilities Education Act Part C or Part B services, respectively. An EFMP quick reference guide is available on the Military OneSource Web site (www.militaryonesource.mil) and may be used to guide families and providers when enrolling in the EFMP. Enrollment in the EFMP is mandatory for dependents of active duty members and ensures that medical and educational needs can be met when service members are considered for various duty stations.

Overseas Screening

Overseas suitability screening (OSS) is a process that active duty service members and their family members undergo once they are identified for an overseas assignment. Because of limited medical service capabilities in overseas environments, OSS reviewers take these factors into consideration when making a determination. Families undergoing this process should bring required OSS and EFMP paperwork to their provider for completion and return these to their screening coordinator.

If a determination is made by the receiving overseas medical facility that the patient's medical needs exceed local capability and capacity or if the environment may exacerbate a medical condition, then the service member may receive unaccompanied orders to the overseas location or may be reconsidered for an alternative duty assignment in an area with the required services to preserve family cohesiveness and avoid unnecessary costs for early returns because of lack of available services.

EXTENDED CARE HEALTH OPTION

The Tricare Extended Care Health Option (ECHO) program is a supplemental benefit for active duty family members with a qualifying condition, such as autism spectrum disorders, intellectual disability, serious physical disabilities, and neuromuscular developmental conditions.[71] It is a monthly cost share based on the sponsor's rank that ranges from $25 to $250 per month, with an annual coverage limit of $36 000.[71] Services covered by ECHO may include durable medical equipment, in-home medical services, rehabilitative services, respite care, and transportation.[71] ECHO eligibility is contingent on enrollment in the EFMP.

AUTISM CARE DEMONSTRATION

Military children with autism spectrum disorders are eligible for applied behavioral analysis (ABA) therapy through the Tricare Autism Care Demonstration (ACD).[72] Eligibility for dependents of active duty members and some activated reservists is contingent on EFMP and ECHO enrollment, whereas dependents of retirees are eligible for ACD services without EFMP and ECHO enrollment. Once a diagnosis of autism is received, a referral for ABA therapy is placed to the regional

Tricare contractor, who will then authorize an initial 6 months of ABA therapy.[67] The ACD provides services totaling $195 million in yearly expenditures,[57] with cost shares and copayments dependent on the family's Tricare health plan.[72]

Military families with children with autism spectrum disorders face challenges, including delays in reestablishing therapeutic services and lack of provider continuity because of relocation.[57,73] Given the unique burdens of military families, recommendations are to identify autism spectrum disorders in children early, have a tiered menu of services available, and consider telehealth options for parent training.[74,75] In addition, early identification and improving access to early intervention may be cost-effective measures to ensure sustainability of the military autism benefit.[76]

SUGGESTIONS FOR PEDIATRICIANS CARING FOR MILITARY CHILDREN

Cultural Competency

Most US medical students will care for a patient who is military connected in their career. Prospective military physicians who receive medical training through the F. Edward Hébert School of Medicine at the Uniformed Services University of the Health Sciences or civilian medical schools through the Health Professions Scholarship Program are exposed early in their careers to military medicine through clerkships and research opportunities. Furthermore, military residency programs have served a vital role in training military physicians to serve our nation in operational settings and military treatment facilities throughout the world.

Although military physicians are familiar with military culture and the military medical system, their civilian colleagues may not have received

similar training opportunities. Gleeson and Hemmer[77] have recommended competency training in medical schools, including military history taking, providing opportunities for clinical rotations through military treatment facilities, and encouraging medical students who are military connected to share their experiences in medical schools. Graduate medical education as well as printed and online information may serve as effective routes for increased cultural competency.[74]

Research indicates that 56% of providers outside of military treatment facilities do not ask for the military status of families,[78] and recommendations have been made for community capacity building through increased cultural awareness, asking families about military status, and implementation of clinical practice measures aimed at improving coordination of care between health care systems.[79] To assist providers, the Department of Veterans Affairs has created the Veterans Affairs Community Provider Toolkit,[80] which provides additional information on military culture.

Screening

Given the increased stressors associated with the military lifestyle and the associated behavioral risks, incorporating a behavioral screening tool can assist the pediatrician in the office setting. The Pediatric Symptom Checklist was used in 1 study during parental deployment and revealed increased internalizing behaviors, externalizing behaviors, and school problems.[21] The AAP, in a recent clinical report, recommends behavioral and emotional screening as a routine component in pediatric practice, and references multiple resources available on its Web site (http://www2.aap.org/commpeds/dochs/mentalhealth/KeyResources.html).[81]

Although broad-scale behavioral screening tools are effective, a mechanism to identify military children in practice would be a helpful adjunct. Chandra and London[29] recommend routinely identifying children who are military connected in practices as well as taking a military history at intake.[23] A school identifier has been proposed to assist in school-district resourcing for military students,[11] and schools may serve as a primary resource for pediatricians to identify issues that may influence the academic, social, and behavioral health of children in military families. The Have You Ever Served in the Military? campaign by the American Academy of Nursing designed a pocket card to assist clinicians caring for veterans.[82] An expanded American Academy of Nursing initiative, I Serve 2, has been launched to identify military children in practice by asking the question, "Do you have a parent who has or is serving in the military?" and to provide a modified pocket guide to assist clinicians caring for military children.[1] Furthermore, Hisle-Gorman et al[39] have also suggested not only asking families about their military status but also directly asking about deployment schedules and parental health as well as gaining familiarization with local support systems for military families.

Advocacy

Efforts to advocate for military children can occur at many levels. Lester and Flake[47] note that military children are influenced by many factors, and understanding these systems from an ecological framework may influence outcomes. In addition to the individual- and family-based interactions discussed in this report, advocacy efforts can occur at the community and national level. There have been several large-scale legislative actions and national campaigns in support of military children and their families,

including the Military Family Act of 1985 and Joining Forces.[2] April has been designated as the Month of the Military Child, during which time awareness is brought to the forefront. The *Eunice Kennedy Shriver* National Institute of Child Health and Human Development and the HSC Foundation sponsored a conference in April 2014 to raise awareness for children with special health care needs who are military connected and provided an excellent summary of the latest challenges and research surrounding the military child.[66] (conference summary can be found at: https://www.nichd. nih.gov/news/resources/spotlight/ 120214-military-families). Aronson et al[65] have stressed that health care professionals, schools, and communities should proactively reach out to military families.

Psychosocial support resources are also available to assist families that may be affected by disasters or grief and bereavement. Two AAP clinical reports are available to assist pediatricians: "Providing Psychosocial Support to Children and Families in the Aftermath of Disasters and Crises"[83] and "Supporting the Grieving Child and Family."[84]

Navigating the Military Health System

This clinical report provides a review of the current literature and identifies some of the programs available for children with connections to the military. One of the key ways providers can assist military families is through effectively navigating the military health care system and coordinating with community agencies and local support networks. The following list provides general recommendations that may provide additional assistance to providers caring for children who are military connected.

RECOMMENDATIONS

Screening

1. Establish a clinical process to identify children who are military connected and document it in the electronic medical record.

2. Take a thorough military history, including parental deployment history, relocation, and parental mental health.

3. Integrate an evidence-based behavioral and emotional rating scale in your practice to identify children who are at risk.

Deployment

1. Gain familiarization with the deployment cycle and common reactions to deployment.

2. Provide a linkage to community-based resources for families of service members who are deployed, including mental health services and evidence-based intervention programs that promote resilience:

   a. Families OverComing Under Stress (http://focusproject. org),

   b. After Deployment: Adaptive Parenting Tools (ADAPT): http://www.cehd.umn.edu/ fsos/research/adapt/default. asp,[31]

   c. STRoNG Intervention for families with young children,[32] and

   d. Sesame Workshop's Talk, Listen, Connect initiative: http://www.sesameworkshop. org/what-we-do/our-initiatives/military-families/.[33]

Relocation

1. Help new families in the local community connect with local military resources and community agencies.

2. Prepare families for an upcoming move through online resources for spouses at Military

OneSource[85] (militaryonesource.mil/for-spouses) and for children at Military Kids Connect (militarykidsconnect.dcoe.mil/).

3. Work with local schools to implement a program identifying military children and provide resources to assist with transitions.

Special Needs

1. For children with special health care needs, complete EFMP paperwork and ask the family member to turn in the completed copy to their local EFMP office. The EFMP Quick Reference Guide, which includes the DD Form 2792 to be completed by the medical provider, may be found on the Military OneSource Web site at: http://download.militaryonesource.mil/12038/MOS/ResourceGuides/EFMP-QuickReferenceGuide.pdf.[86]

2. Provide families with contact information for the ECHO program to assist with any additional coverage that may not be afforded by the Tricare benefit.

3. Additional resources that are valuable in assisting families with children with special needs include:

   a. the EFMP special needs tool kit,[68] (http://download.militaryonesource.mil/12038/EFMP/PTK_SCORs/ParentToolkit_Apr2014.pdf), and

   b. Specialized Training of Military Parents (http://stompproject.blogspot.com).

Tricare

1. For providers interested in becoming a Tricare-approved provider, refer to the Tricare Web site for additional information at https://tricare.mil/Providers.[64]

2. For assistance with navigating Tricare, contact information for regional contractors can be found at https://tricare.mil/Providers.[64]

3. Generally, prior authorization or referrals are not required of Tricare beneficiaries for initial outpatient mental health care with providers who are Tricare authorized.[87] Pediatricians can assist families connecting with an authorized Tricare provider by referring them to www.tricare.mil/findaprovider.[88]

4. Please refer to the following for additional Tricare information:

   a. Tricare Prime (https://tricare.mil/Plans/HealthPlans/Prime),[62]

   b. Tricare Select (https://tricare.mil/Plans/HealthPlans/TS),[63] and

   c. Tricare Mental Health Care (https://tricare.mil/mentalhealth).[89]

Overseas Screening

1. Pediatricians can work with overseas screening coordinators by completing any requested forms and providing an up-to-date assessment of a patient's medical needs.

2. Overseas hospitals frequently publish possible disqualifying conditions on their Web sites, which can help families be prepared and manage expectations.

3. In the case of an overseas screening denial, pediatricians can clarify any concerns with the overseas screening office and provide any additional documentation as needed to facilitate a thorough review of the case.

Additional Resources

1. Comprehensive resources for pediatricians and families:

   a. Military OneSource (www.militaryonesource.mil) and

   b. The National Military Family Association (www.militaryfamily.org).

2. New parent support:

   a. The New Parent Support Program (http://www.militaryonesource.mil/-/the-new-parent-support-program)[43] and

   b. Zero to Three (https://www.zerotothree.org/resources/series/honoring-our-babies-and-toddlers#the-resources).

3. Education:

   a. the Military Child Education Coalition (www.militarychild.org) and

   b. DODEA (www.dodea.edu).

4. Child care: Military Child Care (www.militarychildcare.com);

5. Autism:

   a. Operation Autism (www.operationautismonline.org) and

   b. Autism Care Demonstration: https://tricare.mil/Plans/SpecialPrograms/ACD/GettingCare.[90]

6. Advocacy:

   a. AAP Section on Uniformed Services (https://www.aap.org/en-us/about-the-aap/Committees-Councils-Sections/Section-on-Uniformed-Services/Pages/default.aspx) and

   b. Clearinghouse for Military Family Readiness (www.militaryfamilies.psu.edu).

ACKNOWLEDGMENT

The author would like to thank Lisa Serow for reviewing the report from a parent's perspective.

LEAD AUTHOR

CDR Chadley R. Huebner, MD, MPH, FAAP

ABBREVIATIONS

AAP: American Academy of Pediatrics
ABA: applied behavioral analysis
ACD: Autism Care Demonstration
DOD: Department of Defense
DODEA: Department of Defense Education Activity
ECHO: Extended Care Health Option
EFMP: Exceptional Family Member Program
FAP: Family Advocacy Program
OSS: overseas suitability screening

FUNDING: No external funding.

POTENTIAL CONFLICT OF INTEREST: The author has indicated he has no potential conflicts of interest to disclose.

REFERENCES

1. Rossiter AG, Dumas MA, Wilmoth MC, Patrician PA. "I Serve 2": meeting the needs of military children in civilian practice. *Nurs Outlook.* 2016;64(5):485–490

2. Davis BE, Blaschke GS, Stafford EM. Military children, families, and communities: supporting those who serve. *Pediatrics.* 2012;129(suppl 1):S3–S10

3. Flake EM, Davis BE, Johnson PL, Middleton LS. The psychosocial effects of deployment on military children. *J Dev Behav Pediatr.* 2009;30(4):271–278

4. Siegel BS, Davis BE; Committee on Psychosocial Aspects of Child and Family Health; Section on Uniformed Services. Health and mental health needs of children in US military families. *Pediatrics.* 2013;131(6). Available at: www.pediatrics.org/cgi/content/full/131/6/e2002

5. Department of Defense. 2016 demographics. Profile of the military community. Available at: http://download.militaryonesource.mil/12038/MOS/Reports/2016-Demographics-Report.pdf. Accessed June 7, 2018

6. Department of Defense. Our story. Available at: https://www.defense.gov/About/. Accessed July 17, 2017

7. Nelson SC, Baker MJ, Weston CG. Impact of military deployment on the development and behavior of children. *Pediatr Clin North Am.* 2016;63(5):795–811

8. Woodruff T, Kelty R, Segal DR. Propensity to serve and motivation to enlist among American combat soldiers. *Armed Forces Soc.* 2016;32(3):353–366

9. Redmond SA, Wilcox SL, Campbell S, et al. A brief introduction to the military workplace culture. *Work.* 2015;50(1):9–20

10. Clever M, Segal DR. The demographics of military children and families. *Future Child.* 2013;23(2):13–39

11. Cozza SJ, Lerner RM, Haskins R. Social policy report. Military and veteran families and children: policies and programs for health maintenance and positive development. 2014. Available at: https://www.srcd.org/sites/default/files/documents/spr283_final.pdf. Accessed September 23, 2017

12. Sherman MD. Children of military veterans: an overlooked population. Available at: https://www.srcd.org/sites/default/files/documents/spr283_final.pdf. Accessed September 6, 2017

13. Padden D, Agazio J. Caring for military families across the deployment cycle. *J Emerg Nurs.* 2013;39(6):562–569

14. Hosek J, Wadsworth SM. Economic conditions of military families. *Future Child.* 2013;23(2):41–59

15. Wax SG, Stankorb SM. Prevalence of food insecurity among military households with children 5 years of age and younger. *Public Health Nutr.* 2016;19(13):2458–2466

16. Cooney R, De Angelis K, Segal MW. Moving with the military: race, class, and gender differences in the employment consequences of tied migration. *Race, Gender & Class.* 2011;18(1/2):360–384

17. National Military Family Association. Education revolution: Their right. Our fight. Available at: https://www.militaryfamily.org/info-resources/education/education-revolution/. Accessed July 19, 2017

18. Millegan J, McLay R, Engel C. The effect of geographic moves on mental healthcare utilization in children. *J Adolesc Health.* 2014;55(2):276–280

19. Weber EG, Weber DK. Geographic relocation frequency, resilience, and military adolescent behavior. *Mil Med.* 2005;170(7):638–642

20. Pincus SH, House R, Christenson J, Adler LE. The emotional cycle of deployment: a military family perspective. *US Army Med Dep J.* 2001;2(5):15–23

21. Aranda MC, Middleton LS, Flake E, Davis BE. Psychosocial screening in children with wartime-deployed parents. *Mil Med.* 2011;176(4):402–407

22. Gorman GH, Eide M, Hisle-Gorman E. Wartime military deployment and increased pediatric mental and behavioral health complaints. *Pediatrics.* 2010;126(6):1058–1066

23. Creech SK, Hadley W, Borsari B. The impact of military deployment and reintegration on children and parenting: a systematic review. *Prof Psychol Res Pr.* 2014;45(6):452–464

24. Bello-Utu CF, DeSocio JE. Military deployment and reintegration: a systematic review of child coping. *J Child Adolesc Psychiatr Nurs.* 2015;28(1):23–34

25. Mustillo S, Wadsworth SM, Lester P. Parental deployment and well-being in children: results from a new study of military families. *J Emot Behav Disord.* 2015;24(2):82–91

26. Masten AS. Competence, risk, and resilience in military families: conceptual commentary. *Clin Child Fam Psychol Rev.* 2013;16(3):278–281

27. Chandra A, Lara-Cinisomo S, Jaycox LH, et al. Children on the homefront: the experience of children from military families. *Pediatrics.* 2010;125(1):16–25

28. Lester P, Peterson K, Reeves J, et al. The long war and parental combat deployment: effects on military children and at-home spouses.
J Am Acad Child Adolesc Psychiatry. 2010;49(4):310–320

29. Chandra A, London AS. Unlocking insights about military children and families. *Future Child.* 2013;23(2):187–198

30. FOCUS Project. FOCUS: Resilience training for military families. Available at: http://focusproject.org/. Accessed August 29, 2017

31. University of Minnesota. ADAPT - after deployment: adaptive parenting tools. Available at: www.cehd.umn.edu/fsos/research/adapt/default.asp. Accessed September 3, 2017

32. Rosenblum KL, Muzik M. STRoNG intervention for military families with young children. *Psychiatr Serv.* 2014;65(3):399

33. Sesame Workshop. Talk, listen, connect: arming military families with love, laughter, and practical tools for deployment. Available at: www.sesameworkshop.org/what-we-do/our-initiatives/military-families/. Accessed September 3, 2017

34. Osofsky JD, Chartrand MM. Military children from birth to five years. *Future Child.* 2013;23(2):61–77

35. Johnson HL, Ling CG. Caring for military children in the 21st century. *J Am Assoc Nurse Pract.* 2013;25(4):195–202

36. Trautmann J, Alhusen J, Gross D. Impact of deployment on military families with young children: a systematic review. *Nurs Outlook.* 2015;63(6):656–679

37. Eide M, Gorman G, Hisle-Gorman E. Effects of parental military deployment on pediatric outpatient and well-child visit rates. *Pediatrics.* 2010;126(1):22–27

38. Larson MJ, Mohr BA, Adams RS, et al. Association of military deployment of a parent or spouse and changes in dependent use of health care services. *Med Care.* 2012;50(9):821–828

39. Hisle-Gorman E, Harrington D, Nylund CM, Tercyak KP, Anthony BJ, Gorman GH. Impact of parents' wartime military deployment and injury on young children's safety and mental health. *J Am Acad Child Adolesc Psychiatry.* 2015;54(4):294–301

40. Wood JN, Griffis HM, Taylor CM, et al. Under-ascertainment from healthcare settings of child abuse events among children of soldiers by the U.S. Army Family Advocacy Program. *Child Abuse Negl.* 2017;63:202–210

41. Cozza SJ, Whaley GL, Fisher JE, et al. Deployment status and child neglect types in the U.S. Army. *Child Maltreat.* 2018;23(1):25–33

42. Military OneSource. The Family Advocacy Program. Available at: www.militaryonesource.mil/-/the-family-advocacy-program. Accessed September 3, 2017

43. Military OneSource. The new parent support program. Available at: http://www.militaryonesource.mil/-/the-new-parent-support-program. Accessed November 18, 2018

44. Easterbrooks MA, Ginsburg K, Lerner RM. Resilience among military youth. *Future Child.* 2013;23(2):99–120

45. Meadows SO, Tanielian T, Karney B, et al. The Deployment Life Study: longitudinal analysis of military families across the deployment cycle. *Rand Health Q.* 2017;6(2):7

46. Bronfenbrenner U, Morris PA. The bioecological model of human development. In: Damon W, Lerner RM, eds. *Handbook of Child Psychology.* Vol. 1. 6th ed. Hoboken, NJ: John Wiley & Sons, Inc; 2007

47. Lester P, Flake E. How wartime military service affects children and families. *Future Child.* 2013;23(2):121–141

48. Floyd L, Phillips DA. Child care and other support programs. *Future Child.* 2013;23(2):79–97

49. Zellman GL, Gates SM, Cho M, Shaw R. Options for improving the military child care system. 2008. Available at: https://www.rand.org/content/dam/rand/pubs/occasional_papers/2008/RAND_OP217.sum.pdf. Accessed July 28, 2017

50. Military OneSource. Military child care programs. Available at: http://www.militaryonesource.mil/-/military-child-care-programs. Accessed November 18, 2018

51. Department of Defense Education Activity. Community strategic plan volume 1: school years 2013/14–2017/18. 2013. Available at: www.

dodea.edu/CSP/upload/CSP_130703.
pdf. Accessed July 28, 2017

52. Department of Defense Education
Activity. About DoDEA - DoDEA schools
worldwide. Available at: www.dodea.
edu/aboutDoDEA/today.cfm. Accessed
June 8, 2018

53. Astor RA, De Pedro KT, Gilreath TD,
Esqueda MC, Benbenishty R. The
promotional role of school and
community contexts for military
students. Clin Child Fam Psychol Rev.
2013;16(3):233–244

54. Kitmitto S, Huberman M, Blankenship
C, Hannan S, Norris D, Christenson B.
Educational options and performance
of military-connected school districts
research study – final report.
2011. Available at: www.dodea.edu/
Partnership/upload/AIR-Research-
Study-2011.pdf. Accessed September 3,
2017

55. Chandra A, Martin LT, Hawkins SA,
Richardson A. The impact of parental
deployment on child social and
emotional functioning: perspectives
of school staff. J Adolesc Health.
2010;46(3):218–223

56. US Department of Defense Education
Activity. School liaison officers.
Available at: http://www.dodea.edu/
Partnership/schoolLiaisonOfficers.cfm.
Accessed November 18, 2018

57. Defense Health Agency. Evaluation
of the TRICARE program: Fiscal year
2017 report to Congress. Available at:
https://health.mil/Reference-Center/
Reports/2017/06/08/Evaluation-of-the-
TRICARE-Program. Accessed June 25,
2017

58. Task Force on Defense Personnel.
Health, Health Care, and a High-
Performance Force. Washington, DC:
Bipartisan Policy Center; 2017

59. Military Health System. Defense Health
Agency. Available at: http://health.mil/
dha. Accessed August 17, 2017

60. Tricare. Plan finder. Available at:
https://www.tricare.mil/Home/Plans/
PlanFinder. Accessed August 17, 2017

61. Tricare. About us - changes. Available
at: https://tricare.mil/changes.
Accessed February 4, 2018

62. Tricare. TRICARE Prime. Available at:
https://tricare.mil/Plans/HealthPlans/
Prime. Accessed February 4, 2018

63. Tricare. TRICARE Select. Available at:
https://tricare.mil/Plans/HealthPlans/
TS. Accessed February 4, 2018

64. Military Health System. Information for
TRICARE providers. Available at: https://
tricare.mil/Providers. Accessed August
17, 2017

65. Aronson KR, Kyler SJ, Moeller JD,
Perkins DF. Understanding military
families who have dependents
with special health care and/or
educational needs. Disabil Health J.
2016;9(3):423–430

66. Eunice Kennedy Shriver National
Institute of Child Health and Human
Development. Military-connected
children with special health care
needs and their families. 2014.
Available at: https://www.nichd.nih.
gov/news/resources/spotlight/120214-
military-families. Accessed November
18, 2018

67. Tricare. Getting care. Available at:
https://www.tricare.mil/Plans/
SpecialPrograms/ACD/GettingCare.
Accessed July 31, 2017

68. Department of Defense. Special
needs parent tool kit: birth to 18.
2014. Available at: http://download.
militaryonesource.mil/12038/EFMP/
PTK_SCORs/ParentToolkit_Apr2014.pdf.
Accessed September 23, 2017

69. Military OneSource. Education
directory for children with special
needs. Available at: http://apps.
militaryonesource.mil/MOS/f?p=
EFMP_DIRECTORY:HOME:0. Accessed
September 3, 2017

70. Department of Defense. Annual
Report to the Congressional Defense
Committees on Support for Military
Families with Special Needs.
Washington, DC: Department of
Defense; 2015

71. Tricare. Extended care health option.
2016. Available at: https://tricare.mil/-/
media/Files/TRICARE/Publications/
FactSheets/ECHO_FS.ashx. Accessed
July 31, 2017

72. Tricare. Autism care demonstration.
2016. Available at: https://www.tricare.
mil/Plans/SpecialPrograms/ACD.
Accessed July 31, 2017

73. Davis JM, Finke EH. The experience of
military families with children with
autism spectrum disorders during

relocation and separation. J Autism
Dev Disord. 2015;45(7):2019–2034

74. Meyer E. Case report: military
subcultural competency. Mil Med.
2013;178(7):e848–e850

75. Davis JM, Finke E, Hickerson B. Service
delivery experiences and intervention
needs of military families with children
with ASD. J Autism Dev Disord.
2016;46(5):1748–1761

76. Klin A, Wetherby AM, Woods J, et al.
Toward innovative, cost-effective,
and systemic solutions to improve
outcomes and well-being of
military families affected by autism
spectrum disorder. Yale J Biol Med.
2015;88(1):73–79

77. Gleeson TD, Hemmer PA. Providing
care to military personnel and their
families: how we can all contribute.
Acad Med. 2014;89(9):1201–1203

78. Kilpatrick DG, Best CL, Smith DW, Kudler
H, Cornelison-Grant V. Serving Those
Who Have Served: Educational Needs
of Health Care Providers Working
With Military Members, Veterans,
and Their Families. Charleston, SC:
Medical University of South Carolina
Department of Psychiatry, National
Crime Victims Research and Treatment
Center; 2011

79. Kudler H, Porter RI. Building
communities of care for military
children and families. Future Child.
2013;23(2):163–185

80. Community Provider Toolkit. Welcome
to the community provider toolkit.
Available at: https://www.mentalhealth.
va.gov/communityproviders/index.asp.
Accessed August 29, 2017

81. Weitzman C, Wegner L; Section on
Developmental and Behavioral
Pediatrics; Committee on Psychosocial
Aspects of Child and Family Health;
Council on Early Childhood; Society
for Developmental and Behavioral
Pediatrics; American Academy
of Pediatrics. Promoting optimal
development: screening for behavioral
and emotional problems [published
correction appears in Pediatrics.
2015;135(2):946]. Pediatrics.
2015;135(5):384–395

82. Have You Ever Served in the Military?
Pocket card & posters. Available
at: www.haveyoueverserved.com/

pocket-card--posters.html. Accessed August 22, 2017

83. Schonfeld DJ, Demaria T; Disaster Preparedness Advisory Council; Committee on Psychosocial Aspects of Child and Family Health. Providing psychosocial support to children and families in the aftermath of disasters and crises. *Pediatrics*. 2015;136(4). Available at: www.pediatrics.org/cgi/content/full/136/4/e1120

84. Schonfeld DJ, Demaria T; Committee on Psychosocial Aspects of Child and Family Health; Disaster Preparedness Advisory Council. Supporting the

grieving child and family. *Pediatrics*. 2016;138(3):e20162147

85. Military OneSource. For spouses. Available at: www.militaryonesource.mil/for-spouses. Accessed November 18, 2018

86. Military OneSource. Quick reference guide. Available at: http://download.militaryonesource.mil/12038/MOS/ResourceGuides/EFMP-QuickReferenceGuide.pdf. Accessed November 18, 2018

87. Tricare. Mental health care and substance use disorder services.

2017. Available at: https://tricare.mil/-/media/Files/TRICARE/Publications/FactSheets/Mental_Health_FS.ashx. Accessed September 4, 2017

88. Tricare. Find a doctor. Available at: www.tricare.mil/findaprovider. Accessed November 18, 2018

89. Tricare. Mental health care. Available at: https://tricare.mil/mentalhealth. Accessed November 18, 2018

90. Tricare. Getting care. Available at: https://tricare.mil/Plans/SpecialPrograms/ACD/GettingCare. Accessed November 18, 2018

CLINICAL REPORT   Guidance for the Clinician in Rendering Pediatric Care

American Academy
of Pediatrics

DEDICATED TO THE HEALTH OF ALL CHILDREN™

Helping Children and Families Deal With Divorce and Separation

George J. Cohen, MD, FAAP, Carol C. Weitzman, MD, FAAP, COMMITTEE ON PSYCHOSOCIAL ASPECTS OF CHILD AND FAMILY HEALTH, SECTION ON DEVELOPMENTAL AND BEHAVIORAL PEDIATRICS

abstract

For the past several years in the United States, there have been more than 800 000 divorces and parent separations annually, with over 1 million children affected. Children and their parents can experience emotional trauma before, during, and after a separation or divorce. Pediatricians can be aware of their patients' behavior and parental attitudes and behaviors that may indicate family dysfunction and that can indicate need for intervention. Age-appropriate explanation and counseling for the child and advice and guidance for the parents, as well as recommendation of reading material, may help reduce the potential negative effects of divorce. Often, referral to professionals with expertise in the social, emotional, and legal aspects of the separation and its aftermath may be helpful for these families.

Clinical reports from the American Academy of Pediatrics benefit from expertise and resources of liaisons and internal (AAP) and external reviewers. However, clinical reports from the American Academy of Pediatrics may not reflect the views of the liaisons or the organizations or government agencies that they represent.

The guidance in this report does not indicate an exclusive course of treatment or serve as a standard of medical care. Variations, taking into account individual circumstances, may be appropriate.

All clinical reports from the American Academy of Pediatrics automatically expire 5 years after publication unless reaffirmed, revised, or retired at or before that time.

DOI: 10.1542/peds.2016-3020

PEDIATRICS (ISSN Numbers: Print, 0031-4005; Online, 1098-4275).

Copyright © 2016 by the American Academy of Pediatrics

FINANCIAL DISCLOSURE: The authors have indicated they do not have a financial relationship relevant to this article to disclose.

FUNDING: No external funding.

POTENTIAL CONFLICT OF INTEREST: The authors have indicated they have no potential conflicts of interest to disclose.

To cite: Cohen GJ, Weitzman CC, AAP COMMITTEE ON PSYCHOSOCIAL ASPECTS OF CHILD AND FAMILY HEALTH, AAP SECTION ON DEVELOPMENTAL AND BEHAVIORAL PEDIATRICS. Helping Children and Families Deal With Divorce and Separation. *Pediatrics.* 2016;138(6):e20163020

INTRODUCTION

Every year, more than 1 million American children experience the divorce or separation of their parents. Poverty, lower levels of parent education, and parents being children of divorce can be factors in divorce.[1] Parents of children with chronic or serious illnesses and neurodevelopmental disorders such as cancer and autism spectrum disorders are often at higher risk of divorce, although some studies have shown this is not always the case.[2] The separation itself is usually the culmination of other stressors in the family to which the child has been exposed; parental conflict and tension often precede and may lead to behavior problems in the child.[1]

Many children show behavior changes in the first year of parent separation. Although most adjustment problems resolve in 2 to 3 years after the separation,[1] the child's sense of loss may last for years, with exacerbation on holidays, birthdays, and other special events. Adjustment to a new living situation, continuing parental tensions, and alienation can cause distress in the child.[3,4]

CHILDREN'S REACTIONS

Children's manifestations of reaction to parental divorce are related to many factors, including the stage of development of the child,[5] the parents' ability to focus on the child's needs and feelings, the child's temperament, and the child's and parents' pre- and postseparation psychosocial functioning.[1,3]

Infants

Although infants cannot understand the separation, they react to changes in routine and caregivers and the break in attachment. They may be fussier, irritable, or listless and have sleep and feeding disturbances. At approximately 6 months of age, normal separation and stranger anxiety may be increased.[6–9]

Toddlers

Separation anxiety is a frequent manifestation of distress at this age, and children may be reluctant to separate from parents even in familiar settings, such as child care or a grandparent's home. Developmental regression, including loss of toileting and language skills, is not uncommon. Eating and sleep disorders are also common.[10,11]

Preschool-Aged Children

At this age, children do not understand the permanence of the separation and will repeatedly ask for the absent parent. They may be demanding and defiant and may have sleeping and eating problems as well as regression in developmental milestones. They often test and manipulate differences in limit setting by the 2 parents. By age 4 to 5 years, they may blame themselves for the separation, begin acting out, have nightmares, have more reluctance to separate, and fear that they may be abandoned.[1,3]

School-Aged Children

Self-blame and asking and fantasizing about the reunion of the parents are not uncommon. At this age, mood and behavior changes, such as withdrawal and anger, are frequent, school performance may decline, and the child may feel abandoned by the parent no longer living in the home.[1,3]

Adolescents

Although by this age, children may understand some of the reasons for the family breakup, they may still have difficulty accepting the situation and may try to take on adult roles.[1,3,8,9] They may de-idealize 1 or both parents and still believe that they can reunite the parents. Aggressive delinquent behavior, withdrawal, substance abuse, inappropriate sexual behavior, and poor school performance are frequent responses to the change in family structure.[12] Suicidal ideation is increased in junior high school–aged boys of separated mothers[13] and is more frequent in men than in women of divorced parents.[14] Girls living with divorced fathers are more likely to make suicide attempts than girls living with their divorced mothers.[15]

Parents' Reactions

Parents also suffer negative effects of separation and divorce. Mothers are likely to feel stressed and humiliated, to use alcohol, and to seek mental health services compared with divorced fathers. Mothers' problems can persist for prolonged periods after divorce. However, fathers often feel alienated, seem less accepting of their children, and may become depressed and anxious and abuse substances. Grandparents, too, may feel a decreased quality of relationship with their grandchildren, especially in relation to custody arrangements that favor their ex–son-in-law or ex–daughter-in-law.[3]

MODIFYING FACTORS

Different situations and activities can have different effects on the children of divorce and separation. However, if the parent does not understand the child's individual need, the child is likely to be frustrated and demonstrate externalizing behaviors, such as tantrums, oppositional behavior, and general acting out.[10] Moving away from a familiar milieu may be a negative factor in the child's adjustment; children who move away from their former home are likely to feel more distress. As adolescents, girls show more hostility and boys are less hostile when they moved as children with the custodial father.[16]

Paternal Involvement

Nonresidential fathers believed they were more involved with their children than was perceived by the custodial mother but also felt a more negative change over time in their relationship with the children. The custodial mother's feelings about the relationship with her children were less likely to change.[17] Prolonged legal action in the divorce leads to worse coparenting relationships and more negative feelings in the father. However, if the father is the initiator of the divorce, he is likely to feel more fulfilled in his parenting role.[18] If the child spends more time living with the father after the separation, the child-father relationship is likely to be more positive regardless of continuing parental conflict.[19] Fathers' greater involvement with their sons has been shown to be important for the sons' development. The father's behavior and reactions to the separation, however, are specific areas that often require professional involvement.[20,21]

Children who end up living in nonnuclear (ie, other than 2 married parents) families are more likely to have a higher incidence of poor health, learning difficulties, attention-deficit/hyperactivity disorder, emotional and behavioral difficulties, and emergency department visits than those in nuclear families.[22] Interventions, such as counseling of the mother, that foster positive changes in the mother-child relationship and consistent discipline practices have resulted in increased coping efficacy in children at 6 months and at 6 years after the intervention, including in divorced, separated, and single-parent families.[23]

Financial Considerations

Low-income families are more likely to separate, and if the mother is in a new relationship, there is often a decrease in supportive coparenting.[24] When there is parental separation, fathers usually have more financial resources than the mothers. This disparity tends to increase the inequality of money available for children and thus results in a significant increase in child poverty.[25] After divorce, women are more likely than men to face significant financial challenges, receive public assistance, lose health insurance, and have decreased earning potential. In the recent US Census Bureau report on marriage, 28% of children in divorced families lived below the poverty threshold, compared with 15.9% of the total population. This situation puts children of divorced parents at a higher risk of a number of adverse outcomes.[26]

History of Child Abuse

Divorce in a family with a history of child abuse is related to a greater incidence of conduct disorder, posttraumatic stress disorder, and suicide attempts in children than does either divorce or child abuse alone.[27]

Family Conflict

Legal sources suggest that mandated parenting classes, recommended by divorce courts, could improve outcomes for all members of the family.[1] Adolescents' rating of family harmony predicted their own self-image and emotional development. Ten years after the divorce, daughters of high-conflict families reported more depression. Wariness regarding relationships was higher in children from divorced homes or homes with parental conflict.[28] Alienation of the child and the targeted parent is a frequent problem that needs practical professional input to correct the negative effects on all parties.[29] The father's reactions and behavior to the separation is a specific area that needs professional involvement.[19]

The divorce patterns of service members and veterans further highlight the potential positive effects of the support for families that the military provides. While they are in the military, couples are less likely to divorce than their civilian counterparts. Once they leave the military, however, this trend reverses. Veterans are 3 times as likely to be divorced as those who have never served in the military. Research indicates that the military environment protects families from the stresses that often lead to divorce and that veterans' marriages become less stable once they leave the supportive military setting.[30,31]

Legal Considerations

The legal profession reports that there is momentum building for more focus on the child in divorce disputes.[32] Courts and legislators also are looking at divorce as a sign of problems in parenting and the need to improve education of parents about the effects on the child of parental discord.[33] Attention can be given to the child's reactions as he or she becomes an adolescent and also to the changes in parents' lives.[34] Legal research internationally is looking at past, present, and future relocation as related to children in divorced and separated families.[35] Research suggests that previous moves and changes in family structure may cause more psychological risk to children.

Although not a common aspect of pediatric practice, pediatricians may be subpoenaed by a court or asked by a parent to provide testimony in a child custody hearing. In such circumstances, pediatricians should be cognizant of the following information. A "subpoena" is a legal document that notifies a witness that he or she is needed to present evidence in court. A subpoena might require testimony (subpoena ad testificandum), the production of documents (subpoena duces tecum), or both. Because a subpoena suspends typical rules regarding medical confidentiality, it is important for the pediatrician to read carefully what disclosures are commanded (and therefore allowed) by the subpoena. A provider receiving a subpoena for a medical record that he or she did not create should notify the attorney issuing the subpoena of the appropriate custodian instead of disclosing the record. On receiving any subpoena, the wisest course is to call the attorney who issued the subpoena and discuss with that attorney what testimony or documents are required and what facts or opinions the attorney hopes to elicit.

If a pediatrician is requested by a parent (or a particular party to a custody hearing) to provide testimony, in furtherance of the best interests of children of divorced families and maintenance of good physician-family relationships it may be prudent for the pediatrician to defer those requests to child-abuse pediatric experts (where available) or consult with them before providing any testimony. It is important for the pediatrician to remember that he or she should consider himself or herself an impartial educator of the court about the topic of his or her expertise. A physician has an ethical obligation to provide accurate, unbiased testimony based on sound scientific principles.[36] Pediatricians should make every effort to avoid taking sides and testifying on behalf of either parent about the appropriateness of parenting skills. One should seek legal advice from hospital-based forensic teams to explore alternative responses to a subpoena to testify. In the long term, the child's relationship with the pediatrician is best served by maintaining good relationships with both parents if possible.

When providing testimony in court, the court may deem the pediatrician as a "fact" or "expert" witness. If the pediatrician is providing only "fact" testimony, then exploration/ questions into the physician's qualifications are unnecessary, and a "fact" witness will provide testimony only to the specific facts that the witness has seen, heard, felt, etc. If the pediatrician is to be deemed an "expert" witness, then a formal courtroom procedure of qualifying the witness as an "expert" will be conducted. This legal procedure is a series of questions that demonstrates to the court that the witness has sufficient training, research, writing, professional activities, or other qualifications to serve as an "expert." Being qualified as an expert on a particular subject matter entitles the expert to offer opinions in court.[37] One need not be the foremost authority on the subject matter nor understand every nuance of the subject to qualify.[38]

The best preparation for any kind of court testimony is to be thoroughly familiar with the medical facts of the case. Although many courts will permit a witness to refer to notes during testimony, the witness should be able to recite the basic facts of the case (patient's name, age, dates seen, high points of the history, and injuries found) from memory. The expert should be familiar with the patient's entire chart, because questions may be asked about the patient's medical conditions unrelated to the issue of custody. If the pediatrician is asked to opine about a matter with which he or she is uncomfortable (ie, rendering

TABLE 1 American Academy of Pediatrics–Recommended Qualifications for Physician Expert Witnesses

1. Licensed in the state where the expert practices medicine.
2. Board certification in the area relevant to the testimony.
3. Actively engaged in clinical practice of medicine relevant to the testimony.
4. Unless retired from clinical practice, most of a physician's professional time should not be devoted to expert witness work. If retired, a physician should only testify on cases that occurred when he or she was in active practice.

an abuse or neglect diagnosis), the pediatrician may either confer with a specialist in that field (ie, a child-abuse pediatrician) before providing that testimony or inform the court of his or her discomfort in rendering a formal opinion on that subject matter. It is important that the pediatrician be cognizant of not providing irresponsible testimony.[39] Irresponsible testimony includes testimony for which the expert is insufficiently qualified or testimony based on idiosyncratic theories that have either not been substantiated by well-conducted medical studies or have not gained wide acceptance in the medical community.[36] Recommendations from the American Academy of Pediatrics for expert witnesses are listed in Table 1.[36]

THE LEGAL FRAMEWORK

Divorce is a legal term that means the dissolution or legal conclusion of a marriage. For children of married parents, the divorce process includes legal protections for children. For unmarried parents, state laws may provide similar protections for children through a custody/ visitation action. Specifically, family courts during a divorce or custody/ visitation action are charged with determining and securing the best interests of children. This assessment includes the financial and psychosocial needs of the children and typically leads to an agreement or order specifying the amount of time children will spend with each parent and which parent (or parents) is responsible for decision-making

with regard to education, health care, family values, and related matters. Some states have marital equivalents such as civil unions or domestic partnerships. Children of parents in civil union or domestic partnership relationships ideally should have the same legal protections as children born to married parents. The nonmedical literature has reported on the variability of legal decisions in cases involving same-sex parents and their children.[40]

The touchstone for determining whether a person who raises a child has a legal status as parent to that child is biology, marriage, or adoption. Although parenthood status is usually straightforward, circumstances in which parenthood status and parental rights are unclear may involve complex issues of law. A person with a biological or legal adoptive relationship to a child is that child's legal parent. Similarly, a person whose spouse bears a child is presumed to be a parent of that child. In any case involving a relationship dissolution involving a biological, marital, or adoptive parent, a court is expected to assess the best interests of the child.

A person who raises a child but who does not have a legal relationship to that child through biology, marriage, or adoption may not have the same protections for a continued relationship with the child despite the fact that the effect on the child can be as significant.[1] The courts have increasingly found ways to protect such relationships by recognizing them as psychological, de facto, or equitable parenting relationships.

These developments vary state by state. As families that formed through the expanding capacity of human reproductive technology separate and divorce, there will continue to be legal challenges and areas without legal precedent regarding custody determinations of the child.

Another area that is important to consider that is far more common than divorce is the issue of the separation of nonmarried heterosexual partners. In 2006, approximately 38% of all births were to nonmarried women. Although nearly 50% of partners were living together at the time of the child's birth, approximately 45% were separated 5 years later. Less attention is often given to these separations as when there is a legal divorce, but the psychological effect on children is likely as significant.[41]

THE PEDIATRICIAN'S ROLE

Prevention

Pediatricians may only learn about divorce or separation from the children's behavioral changes, family moves, and changes in family financial responsibility. Inquiring about family stressors, including parental difficulties, can be a routine part of the pediatric health supervision visit, as noted in the third edition of *Bright Futures*.[42] When pediatricians counsel the family regarding issues of child development and behavior, areas of marital discord or stress are often uncovered. Being aware of these stressors and referring for marital counseling are appropriate and may preserve the marital relationship. Pediatricians are encouraged to consider their own attitudes, religious beliefs, and ethical positions concerning divorce, especially if they have experienced divorce in their own families. Being as objective as possible in counseling children and parents is important. If the separation appears to be definite,

early interventions, such as referral to a family counselor, may decrease parental hostility and assist the child and parents in coping with family disruptions to come.

In cases of marital discord, the potential role of pediatricians includes carefully considering the child's physical and emotional needs and communicating this to parents, listening to each parent's perspective, and suggesting that they consider consulting a marriage/divorce counselor to develop strategies to address the discord or to help the child through the dissolution of the marriage. A positive, neutral relationship with both parents after a divorce and being the child's advocate are appropriate goals.

Anticipatory Guidance

The pediatrician can assess the child's reactions, the parents' reactions and levels of hostility, their abilities to understand and meet the child's physical and emotional needs, their support systems, and any indication of parental mental illness or possible substance use.[43,44] Understanding the child's experience of divorce is essential if the pediatrician is to advise the family. The works of several authors can be particularly helpful.[8,35,45–48] Wallerstein[49] correctly notes that the family divorce is a process, not simply a single event. Consequently, a child's understanding of and adjustment to divorce or separation occurs in stages.

Acute parental separation, which may precede the legal divorce by months or years, is typically the time of highest vulnerability for the child. Parental distress is high. One parent may be physically absent and often temporarily lost to the child. The custodial parent may find parenting responsibilities more difficult because of his or her own distress. At a time when children's needs are increased, parents are at an emotional disadvantage and are

often less emotionally available and less able to address the needs of their children.

Decreasing school performance, behavioral difficulties, social withdrawal, and somatic complaints are common reactions of children and accompaniments of divorce that require intervention. A heightened level of sadness is typical, and depression is not uncommon in both children and parents.[8,9]

A parent conference at this stage might be scheduled. The pediatrician can meet with the parents together, ideally, or separately, if necessary, to assess the current situation and to assist in future planning for the children's needs. It is important that pediatricians establish appropriate boundaries with parents at this point, clearly informing them that their role is to understand and meet the child's needs as much as possible, and that the pediatrician is unwilling to take sides in a contentious divorce or be a conduit of information between parents. However, if a pediatrician becomes concerned that living with a particular parent presents a significant risk of current or future abuse or neglect for the child, the pediatrician should make a report to child protective services. If a pediatrician is uncertain whether the family psychosocial dynamics pose sufficient risk to warrant a report to child protective services, it may be prudent to consult a local child-abuse pediatrician. The pediatrician can offer each parent an opportunity to discuss the separation as it affects the child.

The discussion can begin by inquiring how each member of the family is doing at this time of family stress and transition. Do both parents have adequate support systems, such as extended family, clergy, or a personal physician to help meet their own physical and emotional needs? Are there supports that can help parents in their parenting roles? What is the apparent emotional reaction of the children? It may be helpful to interpret these reactions to the parents on the basis of the child's developmental level and perspective.

Pediatricians can help parents understand their children's reactions and encourage them to discuss the divorce process with their children. Parents can be helped to answer the children's questions honestly at their level of understanding. The children's routines of school, extracurricular activities, contact with family and friends, discipline, and responsibilities ideally should remain as normal and unchanged as possible. Children can be given permission for their feelings and opportunities to express them. Children must understand that they did not cause the divorce and cannot bring the parents back together. It is hoped that they can be told that each parent will continue to love and care for them, but if they cannot be provided with this reassurance, pediatricians can help the involved parent develop strategies to help the child articulate feelings of loss and identify resources to assist the child. The pediatrician can offer families pertinent written material on divorce directed at parents and children (see the reading lists at the end of this report). These resources can be informative for the pediatrician as well. Ideally, children would not be "put in the middle" between divorcing or divorced parents, such as being asked to provide information about 1 parent to the other or when 1 or both parents are seen to be demonizing the other parent. These situations can result in children feeling disloyal to a parent and feeling that they need to choose 1 parent over the other and can result in feelings of guilt, sorrow, and anger. If this is happening, pediatricians need to be comfortable having frank, nonjudgmental, and open discussions with parents and exploring ways to help the family manage these challenges.

Custody options can be discussed, and the parents' plan may be explored. It may be helpful to remind parents that professional help can aid them in a nonbiased evaluation of the situation and approaches to resolution. If there are legal issues, including custody, finding an attorney who considers the child's best interest of highest importance is essential. Legal custody and parental rights and responsibilities can vary in their physical and legal arrangements, from sole 1-parent custody, to various forms of shared arrangements, to equal or joint custody.[3] Varying statutory requirements exist to protect the interests of children.

More important for the child's mental health than the type of custody is the quality of parenting that the child receives from each parent through the divorce and postdivorce periods as well as the child's own resilience. Regardless of the type of custody arrangement, it is important that the pediatrician be informed in writing by both parents of who has legal permission for access to the child's medical record, who is responsible for informed consent, who is to pay for the child's health care, and with whom the pediatrician may discuss health information about the child in accordance with regulations of the Health Insurance Portability and Accountability Act. If the noncustodial parent has legal visiting rights and access to health information, it is important that immunization and other pertinent health records be given to both parents in case of an emergency or urgent situation. Any conflict between parents about these issues should be resolved in accordance with legal custody agreements and may require written authorization by both parents. In an emergency situation, the pediatrician can always act to protect the child. It is a good idea for parents to inform the child's school of the change in

the family structure, request that report cards be sent to both parents, and identify which parent has the authority to grant permission for the child's school-related activities. For additional guidance, pediatricians can refer to the existing American Academy of Pediatrics' clinical report "Consent by Proxy for Nonurgent Pediatric Care."[50]

Long-term Follow-up

Although many children have long-lasting emotional and adjustment problems associated with their parents' divorce, most adjust and function well over time, particularly those who have supportive relationships and are well adjusted before the separation/divorce. Professional counseling may be necessary and has shown to be effective in helping children adjust to divorce and separation.[34,37,38,51,52] It is important that pediatricians recognize that a divorce is a process and not an event; substantive periods of change during the process can demand new adjustments on the part of children and parents. Although the legal divorce is an important issue for parents, it may be insignificant to a younger child who knows little of the legal process or very significant for the older child who experiences further proof that his parents will not reconcile. Among troublesome issues for children may be the parents' dating and sexual activities. Parental discretion and truthfulness are important for the maintenance of respect for the parents. Stepfamilies introduce another adjustment challenge for children and their parents.

As children develop and mature, their emotions, behaviors, and needs with regard to the divorce are likely to change. A custody arrangement that made sense for a younger child may need adjustment for a preadolescent or adolescent. For adolescents, with their advancing maturity, awakening sexuality, and important steps toward their own adulthood, their parents' divorce is reinterpreted and may require rediscussion and readjustment. Many behavioral and emotional reactions from the separation can be reawakened at times of subsequent loss, at anniversaries, with the child's advancing maturity, and with the need to adjust to new and different family structures.[49] Ideally, the pediatrician will be able to maintain a professional relationship with both parents so as to continue to help them care for their children in a comfortable and positive manner.

SUGGESTIONS FOR ASSISTING CHILDREN AND FAMILIES

1. Be alert to warning signs of dysfunctional marriage or coparenting relationships and impending separation. Consider inquiring orally or by written questionnaire about family changes or problems at each visit.

2. Discuss family functioning in anticipatory guidance and offer advice pertinent to divorce, as appropriate. Remind parents that what they do during and after a divorce is very important in terms of their child's adjustment.

3. Always be the child's advocate, offering support and age-appropriate advice to the child and parents regarding reactions to divorce, especially guilt, anger, sadness, and perceived loss of love. The child needs to be reassured that he or she did not cause the separation and cannot solve the problem.

4. Establish clear boundaries around divorce and define what role a pediatrician can play in divorce. Try to maintain positive relationships with both parents by not taking sides with 1 parent or the other. If there is concern for an ongoing or future abusive or neglectful situation, referral to child protective services is indicated. If a pediatrician is uncertain whether his or her statutory obligation to report has been met, discussion of the case-specific situation with a child-abuse pediatrician may be prudent. Encourage open discussion about separation and divorce with and between parents, emphasizing ways to help the child adjust to the situation and identifying appropriate reading materials.

5. Refer families to mental health and child-oriented resources with expertise in divorce if necessary.

READINGS FOR PARENTS

1. Barnes RG. *You're Not My Daddy: Winning the Heart of Your Stepchild.* Grand Rapids, MI: Zondervan Publishing House; 1997

2. Benedek EP, Brown CF. *How to Help Your Child Overcome Your Divorce.* Washington, DC: American Psychiatric Press; 1995

3. Davis RF, Borns NF. *Solo Dad Survival Guide: Raising Your Kids on Your Own.* Chicago, IL: Contemporary Books; 1999

4. Engber A, Klungness L. *The Complete Single Mother: Reassuring Answers to Your Most Challenging Concerns.* Holbrook, MA: Adams Media; 2000

5. Ricci I. *Mom's House, Dad's House: A Complete Guide for Parents Who Are Separated, Divorced or Remarried.* New York, NY: Simon & Schuster; 1997

6. Stahl PM. *Parenting After Divorce: Resolving Conflicts.* Atascadera, CA: Impact Publishers; 2007

7. Stoner KE. *Divorce Without Court.* Berkeley, CA: Nolo, Inc; 2006

8. Teyber E. *Helping Children Cope With Divorce.* New York, NY: John Wiley & Sons; 2001

9. Zero to Three. *Talking to Very Young Children About Divorce.* Washington, DC: Zero to Three; 2012. Available at: http://main. zerotothree.org/site/DocServer/ ONE_PAGE_FINAL_5-14-12.pdf? docID=13461

10. Emery RE. *The Truth About Children and Divorce.* New York, NY: Viking-Penguin; 2004

11. Long N, Forehand R. *Making Divorce Easier on Your Children.* New York, NY: McGraw Hill; 2002

READINGS FOR CHILDREN

1. Blume J. *It's Not the End of the World.* Scarsdale, NY: Bradbury Press; 1972

2. Cole J. *How Do I Feel About My Parents' Divorce?* Brookfield, CT: The Millbrook Press; 1998

3. Holyoke N. *A Smart Girl's Guide to Her Parents' Divorce.* Middleton, WI: American Girl Publishing Co; 2009

4. Lindsay JW. *Do I Have A Daddy?* Buena Park, CA: Morning Glory Express; 2000

5. Rogers F. *Let's Talk About It: Divorce.* New York, NY: G.P. Putnam Sons; 1996

6. Rogers F. *Let's Talk About It: Step Families.* New York, NY: G.P. Putnam Sons; 1997

LEAD AUTHORS

George J. Cohen, MD, FAAP
Carol C. Weitzman, MD, FAAP

COMMITTEE ON PSYCHOSOCIAL ASPECTS OF CHILD AND FAMILY HEALTH, 2015–2016

Michael Yogman, MD, FAAP, Chairperson
Nerissa Bauer, MD, MPH, FAAP
Thresia B. Gambon, MD, FAAP
Arthur Lavin, MD, FAAP
Keith M. Lemmon, MD, FAAP
Gerri Mattson, MD, FAAP

Jason Richard Rafferty, MD
Lawrence Sagin Wissow, MD, MPH, FAAP

LIAISONS

Sharon Berry, PhD, LP – *Society of Pediatric Psychology*
Terry Carmichael, MSW – *National Association of Social Workers*
Ed Christophersen, PhD, FAAP – *Society of Pediatric Psychology*
Norah Johnson, PhD, RN, CPNP-BC – *National Association of Pediatric Nurse Practitioners*
Leonard Read Sulik, MD, FAAP – *American Academy of Child and Adolescent Psychiatry*

CONSULTANT

George J. Cohen, MD, FAAP

STAFF

Stephanie Domain, MS

SECTION ON DEVELOPMENTAL AND BEHAVIORAL PEDIATRICS EXECUTIVE COMMITTEE, 2015–2016

Nathan J. Blum, MD, FAAP, Chairperson
Michelle M. Macias, MD, FAAP, Immediate Past Chairperson
Nerissa S. Bauer, MD, MPH, FAAP
Carolyn Bridgemohan, MD, FAAP
Edward Goldson, MD, FAAP
Laura J. McGuinn, MD, FAAP
Peter J. Smith, MD, MA, FAAP
Carol C. Weitzman, MD, FAAP
Stephen H. Contompasis, MD, FAAP, Web site Editor
Damon R. Korb, MD, FAAP, Discussion Board Moderator
Michael I. Reiff, MD, FAAP, Newsletter Editor
Robert G. Voigt, MD, FAAP, Program Chairperson

LIAISONS

Pamela C. High, MD, MS, FAAP – *Society for Developmental and Behavioral Pediatrics*
Beth Ellen Davis, MD, MPH, FAAP – *Council on Children With Disabilities*

STAFF

Linda Paul, MPH

REFERENCES

1. Kleinsorge C, Covitz LM. Impact of divorce on children: developmental considerations. *Pediatr Rev.* 2012;33(4):147–154; quiz: 154–155

2. Urbano RC, Hodapp RM. Divorce in families of children with Down syndrome: a population-based study. *Am J Ment Retard.* 2007;112(4):261–274

3. Cohen GJ; American Academy of Pediatrics Committee on Psychosocial Aspects of Child and Family Health.

Helping children and families deal with divorce and separation. *Pediatrics.* 2002;110(5):1019–1023

4. Darnall D. The psychosocial treatment of parental alienation. *Child Adolesc Psychiatr Clin N Am.* 2011;20(3):479–494

5. Lansford JE. Parental divorce and children's adjustment. *Perspect Psychol Sci.* 2009;4(2):140–152

6. Wallerstein JS, Kelly JB. The effects of parental divorce: experiences of the preschool child. *J Am Acad Child Psychiatry.* 1975;14(4):600–616

7. Wallerstein JS, Kelly JB. The effects of parental divorce: experiences of the child in later latency. *Am J Orthopsychiatry.* 1976;46(2):256–269

8. Clarke-Stewart KA, Vandell DL, McCartney K, Owen MT, Booth C. Effects of parental separation and divorce on very young children. *J Fam Psychol.* 2000;14(2):304–326

9. Clarke-Stewart KA, Brentano C. *Divorce: Causes and Consequences.* New Haven, CT: Yale University Press; 2006

10. Mrazek D, Garrison W. *A to Z Guide to Your Child's Behavior.* New York, NY: Putnam Publishing Group; 1993

11. Canada Department of Justice, Research and Statistics Division. The effects of divorce on children: a selected literature review. Ottawa, Canada: Canada Department of Justice; 1997. Available at: www.justice.gc.ca/eng/rp-pr/fl-lf/divorce/wd98_2-dt98_2/wd98_2.pdf. Accessed June 17, 2015

12. Sentse M, Ormel J, Veenstra R, Verhulst FC, Oldehinkel AJ. Child temperament moderates the impact of parental separation on adolescent mental health: The Trails Study. *J Fam Psychol.* 2011;25(1):97–106

13. Hayatbakhsh MR, Najman JM, Jamrozik K, Mamun AA, Williams GM, Alati R. Changes in maternal marital status are associated with young adults' cannabis use: evidence from a 21-year follow-up of a birth cohort. *Int J Epidemiol.* 2006;35(3):673–679

14. Ang RP, Ooi YP. Impact of gender and parents' marital status on adolescents' suicidal ideation. *Int J Soc Psychiatry.* 2004;50(4):351–360

15. Lizardi D, Thompson RG, Keyes K, Hasin D. Parental divorce, parental depression, and gender differences in adult offspring suicide attempt. *J Nerv Ment Dis.* 2009;197(12):899–904

16. Braver SL, Ellman IM, Fabricius WV. Relocation of children after divorce and children's best interests: new evidence and legal considerations. *J Fam Psychol.* 2003;17(2):206–219

17. Pruett MK, Williams TY, Insabella G, Little TD. Family and legal indicators of child adjustment to divorce among families with young children. *J Fam Psychol.* 2003;17(2):169–180

18. Baum N. Divorce process variables and the co-parental relationship and parental role fulfillment of divorced parents. *Fam Process.* 2003;42(1):117–131

19. Fabricius WV, Luecken LJ. Postdivorce living arrangements, parent conflict, and long-term physical health correlates for children of divorce. *J Fam Psychol.* 2007;21(2):195–205

20. Hetherington EM, Stanley-Hagan M. The adjustment of children with divorced parents: a risk and resiliency perspective. *J Child Psychol Psychiatry.* 1999;40(1):129–140

21. Kruk E. Parental and social institutional responsibilities to children's needs in the divorce transition: fathers' perspectives. *J Mens Stud.* 2010;18(2):159–178

22. Blackwell DL. Family structure and children's health in the United States: findings from the National Health Interview Survey, 2001-2007. *Vital Health Stat 10.* 2010; (246):1–166

23. Vélez CE, Wolchik SA, Tein JY, Sandler I. Protecting children from the consequences of divorce: a longitudinal study of the effects of parenting on children's coping processes. *Child Dev.* 2011;82(1):244–257

24. Kamp Dush CM, Kotila LE, Schoppe-Sullivan SJ. Predictors of supportive coparenting after relationship dissolution among at-risk parents. *J Fam Psychol.* 2011;25(3):356–365

25. Lerman R. The impact of the changing US family structure on child poverty and income inequality. *Economica.* 1996;63(250 suppl):119–139

26. Elliot DB, Simmons T. *Marital Events of Americans 2009. The American Community Survey Reports.* Washington, DC: US Census Bureau; 2011

27. Afifi TO, Boman J, Fleisher W, Sareen J. The relationship between child abuse, parental divorce, and lifetime mental disorders and suicidality in a nationally representative adult sample. *Child Abuse Negl.* 2009;33(3):139–147

28. Burns A, Dunlop R. Parental marital quality and family conflict: longitudinal effects on adolescents from divorcing and non-divorcing families. *J Divorce Remarriage.* 2002;37(1–2):57–74

29. Andre K, Baker AJL. Working with alienated children and their targeted parents; suggestions for sound practices for mental health professionals. *Ann Am Psychother Assoc.* 2008;11:10–17

30. Hogan PF, Seifert RF. Marriage and the military: evidence that those who serve marry earlier and divorce earlier. *Armed Forces Soc.* 2010;36(3):420–438

31. Karney BR, Crown JA. *Families Under Stress: An Assessment of Data, Theory, and Research on Marriage and Divorce in the Military. MG-599-OSD.* Arlington, VA: Rand Corporation; 2007. http://www.rand.org/pubs/monographs/MG599.html. http://www.rand.org/pubs/monographs/MG599.html. Accessed June 17, 2015

32. Elrod LD. National and international momentum builds for more child focus in relocation disputes. *Fam Law Q.* 2010;44(3):341–374

33. Schaefer T. Saving children or blaming parents? Lessons from mandated parenting classes. *Columbia J Gend Law.* 2010;19(2):491–537

34. Lux JG. Growing pains that cannot be ignored: automatic reevaluation of custody arrangements at child's adolescence. *Fam Law Q.* 2010;44(3):445–468

35. Taylor N, Freeman M. International research on relocation: past, present and future. *Fam Law Q.* 2010;44(3):317–339

36. Committee on Medical Liability and Risk Management. Policy statement: expert witness participation in civil and criminal proceedings. *Pediatrics.* 2009;124(1):428–438

37. Legal Information Institute. Article VII. Opinions and Expert Testimony. Rule 703: Bases of an Expert. Available at: www.law.cornell.edu/rules/fre/rule_703. Accessed June 17, 2015

38. *State v Wakisaka*, 78 P3d 317, 333 (2003)

39. Chadwick DL, Krous HF. Irresponsible testimony by medical experts in cases involving the physical abuse and neglect of children. *Child Maltreat.* 1997;2(4):313–321

40. Silverstein & Ostovitz LLC. Same-sex parents' standing in Maryland custody determination. Available at: http://mddivorce.com/2013/08/28/same-sex-parents-standing-in-maryland-custody-determinations.html. Accessed July 26, 2015

41. Melnyk BM, Alpert-Gillis LJ. Coping with marital separation: smoothing the transition for parents and children. *J Pediatr Health Care.* 1997;11(4):165–174

42. Hagan J, Shaw J, Duncan P, eds. *Bright Futures: Guidelines for Health Supervision of Infants, Children, and Adolescents.* 3rd ed. Elk Grove Village, IL: American Academy of Pediatrics; 2008

43. Amato P, Doruis C. Fathers, children, and divorce. In: Lamb M, ed. *The Role of the Father in Child Development.* Hoboken, NJ: John Wiley & Sons; 2010:177–200

44. Delaney SE. Divorce mediation and children's adjustment to parental divorce. *Pediatr Nurs.* 1995;21(5):434–437

45. Pruett KD, Pruett MK. "Only God decides": young children's perceptions of divorce and the legal system. *J Am Acad Child Adolesc Psychiatry.* 1999;38(12):1544–1550

46. Emery RE, Laumann-Billings L. Practical and emotional consequences of parental divorce. *Adolesc Med.* 1998;9(2):271–282, vi

47. Wallerstein JS, Johnston JR. Children of divorce: recent findings regarding long-term effects and recent studies of joint and sole custody. *Pediatr Rev.* 1990;11(7):197–204

48. Whiteside MF, Becker BJ. Parental factors and the young child's postdivorce adjustment: a meta-analysis with implications for parenting arrangements. *J Fam Psychol.* 2000;14(1):5–26

49. Wallerstein JS. Children of divorce: the psychological tasks of the child. *Am J Orthopsychiatry.* 1983;53(2):230–243

50. McAbee GN; American Academy of Pediatrics Committee on Medical Liability and Risk Management. Consent by proxy for nonurgent pediatric care. *Pediatrics.* 2010;126(5):1022–1031

51. Allen KR. Ambiguous loss after lesbian couples with children break up: a case for same gender divorce. *Fam Relat.* 2007;56(2):175–183

52. Sammons WA, Lewis J. Helping children survive divorce. *Contemp Pediatr.* 2001;18(3):103–114

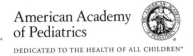

American Academy of Pediatrics
DEDICATED TO THE HEALTH OF ALL CHILDREN™

Organizational Principles to Guide and Define the Child
Health Care System and/or Improve the Health of all Children

POLICY STATEMENT

The Pediatrician's Role in Family Support and Family Support Programs

abstract

Children's social, emotional, and physical health; their developmental trajectory; and the neurocircuits that are being created and reinforced in their developing brains are all directly influenced by their relationships during early childhood. The stresses associated with contemporary American life can challenge families' abilities to promote successful developmental outcomes and emotional health for their children. Pediatricians are positioned to serve as partners with families and other community providers in supporting the well-being of children and their families. The structure and support of families involve forces that are often outside the agenda of the usual pediatric health supervision visits. Pediatricians must ensure that their medical home efforts promote a holistically healthy family environment for all children. This statement recommends opportunities for pediatricians to develop their expertise in assessing the strengths and stresses in families, in counseling families about strategies and resources, and in collaborating with others in their communities to support family relationships. *Pediatrics* 2011;128:e1680–e1684

INTRODUCTION

The health and welfare of children depend on the ability of their families, supported by systems in their communities, to foster positive emotional and physical development. Recent scientific research confirms that brain growth and neurophysiologic development during the first years of life respond directly to the environmental influences of early emotional relationships. The neurologic pathways produced then have profound effects on the behaviors of children and adolescents and affect their interactions within their families and extended society across the life course. The enormous effect the family has on this developmental process led the American Academy of Pediatrics (AAP) to make the "promotion of nurturing families for all children" a priority among AAP resolutions in 1993 and 1994 and, subsequently, to develop the AAP Task Force on the Family. The task force published a thorough and extensive report in 2003 that informs pediatricians and guides policy-makers regarding the effect that family has on children's functioning and the expectations for pediatricians to promote optimal family functioning for their patients.[1] Pediatricians play a unique role as family health advisors during the formative period of a child's development and during crucial developmental stages throughout childhood and adolescence. Pediatricians need expertise in working with families to identify strengths, stresses, and needs and to identify priorities and

COMMITTEE ON EARLY CHILDHOOD, ADOPTION, AND DEPENDENT CARE

KEY WORDS
family support, social emotional health, counseling, community resources

ABBREVIATION
AAP—American Academy of Pediatrics

www.pediatrics.org/cgi/doi/10.1542/peds.2011-2664

doi:10.1542/peds.2011-2664

All policy statements from the American Academy of Pediatrics automatically expire 5 years after publication unless reaffirmed, revised, or retired at or before that time.

PEDIATRICS (ISSN Numbers: Print, 0031-4005; Online, 1098-4275).

goals with families. They also need to develop expertise in counseling skills and knowledge regarding community-based resources to offer strategies and resources to families. The structure and support of families involve forces that are often outside the agenda of the usual pediatric health supervision visits. Pediatricians must ensure that their medical home efforts promote a holistically healthy family environment for all children.[2]

CHANGES IN FAMILIES

Stresses accompanying contemporary American life can challenge families' efforts to promote successful developmental and emotional outcomes for their children. The structure of families and patterns of family life in the United States have changed profoundly in the past quarter century. Five percent of all births in 1960 were to unmarried women; this figure increased to almost 37% by 2005.[3] Since 1960, the divorce rate has more than doubled[4]; 40% to 50% of all first-time marriages end in divorce.[5] Divorce rates seem to have leveled overall since the 1980s, but factors exist that increase the risk for some couples (eg, lower educational level or younger age at the time of marriage).[6] Although remarriage rates are high, more than one-third of remarried couples divorce again.[7] As a consequence, approximately 14% more children are now living in 1-parent households than approximately 40 years ago (25.8% in 2007 versus 11.8% in 1968).[8]

Another change in family life is that, by 2005, approximately 63% of all mothers with preschool-aged children were in the labor force, which reflects a two-fold increase since 1970.[9] Three-fourths of the mothers of school-aged children work.[10] In 2-parent households, this means a marked increase in homes in which both parents work.

Despite the majority of American mothers being in the workforce, half of female-led single-parent households lived below the poverty level in 2004.[9] A decline in the purchasing power of family income and the lack of comparable wages for women have added to the stress on families. Social disparities have also contributed to the growing percentage of children who live in poverty, and poverty is the strongest predictor of poorer health and well-being for children.[1,11] Residential mobility has separated many families from the natural support systems provided by their extended families, which may leave parents feeling socially isolated and prevents the intergenerational transmission of cultural and community-specific advice and support. Economic and social inequalities have led to increasingly impoverished neighborhoods, more working families living in or near poverty, and weakening of community ties. Longer hours away from their children, disconnection from close extended family support, and disintegration of traditional community interdependence all reduce the time, energy, and external supports available for rearing healthy children. The stress and speed of social change has weakened the support systems for many American families.[12]

RESILIENCE IN FAMILIES

Despite these enormous pressures working against families, intact and successful families do exist. Although it is evident that the risk of poorer outcomes for children is lowest among 2-parent households,[13] there is not a specific family constellation that makes poor outcomes inevitable. How a family influences children's outcomes is embedded within the interactions among its members. Table 1 lists characteristics that positively contribute to a family's success in raising children and, ultimately, to communities and society.[14]

TABLE 1 Characteristics of Successful Families[14]

Clear, open, and frequent communication
Encouragement of individual members
Expressing appreciation
Commitment to family
Religious or spiritual orientation
Social connectedness to external resources
Ability to adapt to stressors
Clear roles within the family
Time together that is of high quality and quantity

SUPPORT PROGRAMS: WHAT PEDIATRICIANS NEED TO KNOW

Social institutions have begun to offer various family support services to help parents carry out essential functions on behalf of their children. Many pediatricians have perinatal exposure to families who need community-based support for a variety of reasons, and all community pediatricians begin providing comprehensive health services for children as soon as they are discharged from the newborn nursery. Many pediatricians are already familiar with some types of family support programs. Examples of successful programs include prenatal and infant home visitor programs, comprehensive early childhood education programs (eg, Early Head Start, Head Start), early screening and referral programs, crisis care programs, parent support and/or education groups, early reading and parental literacy, and early intervention programs for children with special needs (eg, Individuals With Disabilities Education Act, Part C).[1,10,15–18] Because of significant variability regarding the effectiveness of available support programs, pediatricians should be aware of the evidence base for different types of programs and, specifically, the programs available in their communities. Home visitation programs, for example, can lead to improvements for families (eg, detecting postpartum depression, reducing the frequency of unintentional injury, improving parenting skills), but the relative effect depends on the qualities of the program; for example, programs that use professionals (ie, nurses) rather than paraprofessionals[19] and programs targeted at specific populations (eg, infants born prematurely) have more measurable effects on child outcomes.[20]

Many comprehensive, community-based family support programs have been established around the country. These programs aim to support family relationships and promote parental competencies and behaviors that contribute to parental and infant/child/adolescent health and development. The best programs offer a spectrum of services that involve informal and structured groups. Topics may include information on child development, personal growth, family relationships, parenting education, peer support groups, parent-child activities, early developmental screening, community referral and follow-up, job skills training, and/or adult education, especially language and literacy education.[21,22] Services should be available to all families regardless of economic or ethnic background. The programs operate on the premise that no family is entirely self-sufficient and that most can benefit from some external support.[23] Pediatricians should search for, become familiar with, and refer families to high-quality family support services in their communities.

Some schools are providing after-school programs for children whose parents cannot be at home when classes end; others are providing school-based or associated health services to ensure that children receive timely health care and counseling. School curricula have expanded to include topics such as conflict resolution, sex education, and community service. Some employers offer family-oriented benefits such as flexible work hours, shared jobs, and child care. Religious congregations in some commu-

nities have developed a full array of social services and supports. The Family and Medical Leave Act of 1993 is an example of government acting in support of families, as are more established programs such as the Supplemental Nutrition Program for Women, Infants, and Children (WIC) and Temporary Assistance for Needy Families (TANF).

PRINCIPLES OF FAMILY SUPPORT PROGRAMS

High-quality programs operate on the following principles[1,24,25]:

- The primary responsibility for the development and well-being of children lies within the family.

- Families are part of a community, and support should be provided in the context of community life and through collaborative links with community resources.

- The kinds of support provided should be determined by individual and community needs. Although participation should be voluntary, it should be encouraged for at-risk families such as those led by single and/or socially isolated parents and those living in poverty.

- Support offered by friends, neighbors, and community-based resources is as vital as access to professional support services. Families are resources for themselves, for other families, and for communities and programs.

- The support given should enhance the strengths found within the family unit and among family members and empower families to use those strengths. The aim of support is to strengthen the family unit and the community while preventing alienation and family dysfunction.

- Support is available for all families and provided with an awareness of and sensitivity toward the culture,

race, and native language of families and communities.

Family support programs play an important and, in some instances, essential role in promoting the positive functioning of families and ensuring the well-being of children. Their effectiveness, at least with certain populations (eg, low-income families, young single mothers, low birth weight infants, children with behavioral problems, children with special health care needs) is well documented.[17,20,26] All families need knowledge, skills, and support to raise their children and to foster normal growth, development, and learning. The AAP encourages public policies, professional practices, and personal behavior that support the caregiving role of families, advocate comprehensive approaches to child health and encourage prevention and early intervention strategies oriented toward the family.

RECOMMENDATIONS

1. Pediatricians should be aware of the increasing number of families experiencing stress and should learn to recognize situations (eg, maternal depression) that interfere with successful child rearing. The AAP *Bright Futures* guidelines recommend using open-ended questions to screen for and assess family stress during health supervision visits, with sample questions provided to probe for stressors such as parental depression, domestic violence, separation/divorce, and substance abuse. In addition, *Bright Futures* has a chapter titled "Promoting Family Support," which outlines the importance of family development to a child's overall growth and development.[27]

2. As medical homes, pediatric practices should collaborate with patients and their caregivers and provide family-centered care with an

awareness of cultural diversity. By having open and ongoing relationships with parents, pediatricians can facilitate discussions; monitor and guide developmental progress; address parental concerns; and support parental care, capacities, and needs. Focus should be on fostering those characteristics (Table 1) known to be associated with successful family functioning.

3. Pediatricians should interview families with a real awareness of the significant influence that family factors (socioeconomic status, discipline style, cultural beliefs, parental health and mental health, etc) have on children's development and behavior.[28] Continuing medical education programs on pediatric family interviewing and psychosocial issues in pediatric practice can enhance the pediatrician's skills and opportunities for counseling families. As recommended by the Task Force on the Family, the AAP advocates for pediatricians to have "adequate time, resources, billing options, and reimbursement to provide family-oriented care."[1]

4. Pediatricians can provide family support by engaging in a relationship with parents based on collaboration and shared decision-making so that parents feel and become more competent. The AAP provides pediatricians with guidance for supporting families in the prevention of violence and injury and the enhancement of parent-child communication on the basis of individual families' needs in the Connected Kids program (www.aap.org/ConnectedKids/ClinicalGuide.pdf). This collaboration with parents might also be in the form of parent councils and other partnerships that allow parents to provide input to practices and programs.

5. Pediatrician counseling of parents should include considering the needs and resources of the family and helping them benefit from the support of members of extended family and the community.

6. Pediatricians should work to identify, develop, refer to, and participate in community-based family support programs to help parents secure the knowledge, skills, support and strategies they need to raise their children. Having information easily available for families within the pediatric office that includes information and schedules of parenting classes, volunteer and community organizations incorporating family participation, and child care resources is also extremely helpful. The Maternal and Child Health Library provides an online directory to assist families and health providers to locate services within their own communities (www.mchlibrary.info/KnowledgePaths/kp_community.html).

7. Pediatricians should actively participate in sustaining the social capacity of their communities through their personal participation in local recreational, social, educational, civic, or philanthropic activities and associations. By participating in community-based family support programs, pediatricians

can provide technical advice on health and safety aspects of services, serve as a source of professional information for families, and learn from these programs how best to contribute to the healthy development of children, families, and communities.

8. Pediatricians need to work within their communities to develop plans for identifying and coordinating care for families in need of more extensive social support services. An opportunity the AAP provides that might support pediatricians in this endeavor is the Community Access to Child Health (CATCH) program. CATCH provides pediatricians funding, training, technical assistance, and networking opportunities to ensure that all children have access to needed health care services within their communities.[29]

LEAD AUTHOR

Jill J. Fussell, MD

COMMITTEE ON EARLY CHILDHOOD, ADOPTION, AND DEPENDENT CARE, 2010–2011

Pamela C. High, MD, Chairperson
Elaine Donoghue, MD
Jill J. Fussell, MD
Mary Margaret Gleason, MD
Paula K. Jaudes, MD
Veronnie F. Jones, MD
David M. Rubin, MD
Elaine E. Schulte, MD, MPH

CONTRIBUTING AUTHOR

Chet D. Johnson, MD

LIAISONS

Claire Lerner, LCSW – *Zero to Three*
Jennifer Sharma, MA – *Child Welfare League of America*

STAFF

Mary Crane, PhD, LSW

REFERENCES

1. American Academy of Pediatrics, Task Force on the Family. Family pediatrics: report of the Task Force on the Family. *Pediatrics.* 2003;111(6 pt 2):1541–1571

2. Rushton FE. *Family Support in Community Pediatrics.* Westport, CT: Praeger; 1998:53

3. Martin JA, Hamilton BE, Sutton PD, et al; Centers for Disease Control and Prevention, National Center for Health Statistics National Vital Statistics System. Births: final data for 2005. *Natl Vital Stat Rep.* 2007;56(6):1–103. Available at: www.cdc.gov/nchs/data/nvsr/nvsr56/nvsr56_06.pdf. Accessed January 22, 2010

4. US Bureau of the Census. *Statistical Abstract of the United States, 1991: The National Data Book.* 111th ed. Washington, DC: US Department of Commerce, Bureau of the Census; 1991

5. Schoen R, Standish N. The retrenchment of marriage in the US. *Popul Dev Rev*. 2001; 27(3):555–563

6. Raley RK, Bumpass L. The topography trends of the divorce plateau: level and trends in union stability in the United States after 1980. *Demogr Res*. 2003;8(8):245–260. Available at: www.demographic-research.org/Volumes/Vol8/8. Accessed January 22, 2010

7. Bramlett MD, Mosher WD. Cohabitation, marriage, divorce, and remarriage in the United States. *Vital Health Stat 23*. 2002; (22):1–93. Available at: www.cdc.gov/nchs/data/series/sr_23/sr23_022.pdf. Accessed January 22, 2010

8. US Bureau of the Census. Marital status and living arrangements. Available at: www.census.gov/population/socdemo/hh-fam/cps2007/tabC2-all.xls. Accessed January 22, 2010

9. US Department of Health and Human Services, Maternal and Child Health Bureau. *Child Health USA 2006*. Rockville, MD: US Department of Health and Human Services; 2008. Available at: http://mchb.hrsa.gov/chusa_06. Accessed January 22, 2010

10. Children's Defense Fund. *The State of America's Children 2005 Report*. Washington, DC: Children's Defense Fund; 2005. Available at: www.childrensdefense.org/child-research-data-publications/data/state-of-americas-children-2005-report.html. Accessed January 22, 2010

11. Zlotnick C. Community versus individual level indicators to identify pediatric health care needs. *J Urban Health*. 2007;84(1): 45–59

12. Ninety-seventh American Assembly. *Strengthening American Families: Reweaving the Social Tapestry*. New York, NY: American Assembly; 2000

13. McLanahan S, Sandefur G. *Growing Up With a Single Parent: What Hurts, What Helps*. Cambridge, MA: Harvard University Press; 1994

14. Krysan M, Moore KA, Zill N. *Research on Successful Families*. Washington, DC: US Department of Health and Human Services; 1990. Available at: www.aspe.hhs.gov/daltcp/Reports/ressucfa.htm. Accessed January 22, 2010

15. Barlow J, Stewart-Brown S. Behavior problems and group-based parent education programs. *J Dev Behav Pediatr*. 2000;21(5): 356–370

16. High PC; American Academy of Pediatrics, Committee on Early Childhood Adoption and Dependent Care, Council on School Health. School readiness. *Pediatrics*. 2008;121(4). Available at: www.pediatrics.org/cgi/content/full/121/4/e1008

17. Shonberg SK, Anderson SJ, Bays JA, et al. The role of home-visitation programs in improving health outcomes for children and families. *Pediatrics*. 1998;101(3 pt 1): 486–489

18. Center for the Study of Social Policy. *Strengthening Families Through Early Child Care and Education: Protective Factors Literature Review—Early Care and Education Programs and the Prevention of Child Abuse and Neglect*. Washington, DC: Doris Duke Charitable Foundation/Center for the Study of Social Policy; 2004

19. Macmillan HL, Wathen CN, Barlow J, Fergusson DM, Leventhal JM, Taussig HN. Interventions to prevent child maltreatment and associated impairment. *Lancet*. 2009; 373(9659):250–266

20. American Academy of Pediatrics, Council on Community Pediatrics. The role of preschool home-visiting programs in improving children's developmental and health outcomes. *Pediatrics*. 2009;123(2):598–603

21. Layzer JI, Goodson BD, Bernstein L, Price C. *National Evaluation of Family Support Programs Final Report Volume A: The Meta-analysis*. Cambridge, MA: Abt Associates Inc; 2001.

22. Weiss H, Halpern R. *Community-based Family Support and Education Programs: Something Old or Something New?* New York, NY: Columbia University, School of Public Health, National Center for Children in Poverty; 1991.

23. US Department of Health and Human Services, Administration for Children and Families, US Advisory Board on Child Abuse and Neglect. *Neighbors Helping Neighbors: A New National Strategy for the Protection of Children*. 4th report. Washington, DC: US Department of Health and Human Services; 1993. Available at: http://eric.ed.gov/ERICDocs/data/ericdocs2sql/content_storage_01/0000019b/80/14/72/d3.pdf. Accessed January 22, 2010

24. Langford J, Wolf KG. *Guidelines for Family Support Practice*. 2nd ed. Chicago, IL: Family Resource Coalition; 2001

25. Manalo V. Understanding practice principles and service delivery: the implementation of a community-based family support program. *Child Youth Serv Rev*. 2008;30(8): 928–941

26. Seitz V, Rosenbaum LK, Apfel NH. Effects of family support intervention: a ten-year follow-up. *Child Dev*. 1985;56(2):376–391

27. Hagan JF, Shaw JS, Duncan PM, eds. *Bright Futures: Guidelines for Health Supervision of Infants, Children, and Adolescents*. 3rd ed. Elk Grove Village, IL: American Academy of Pediatrics; 2008

28. Coleman W. Family-focused pediatrics: a primary care family systems approach to psychosocial problems. *Curr Probl Pediatr Adolesc Health Care*. 2002;32(8):260–305

29. American Academy of Pediatrics. Medical home. Available at: www.aap.org/catch/funding.htm. Accessed January 22, 2010

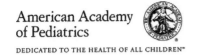

American Academy
of Pediatrics
DEDICATED TO THE HEALTH OF ALL CHILDREN™

Organizational Principles to Guide and Define the Child
Health Care System and/or Improve the Health of all Children

POLICY STATEMENT

Providing Care for Children and Adolescents Facing Homelessness and Housing Insecurity

abstract

Child health and housing security are closely intertwined, and children without homes are more likely to suffer from chronic disease, hunger, and malnutrition than are children with homes. Homeless children and youth often have significant psychosocial development issues, and their education is frequently interrupted. Given the overall effects that homelessness can have on a child's health and potential, it is important for pediatricians to recognize the factors that lead to homelessness, understand the ways that homelessness and its causes can lead to poor health outcomes, and when possible, help children and families mitigate some of the effects of homelessness. Through practice change, partnership with community resources, awareness, and advocacy, pediatricians can help optimize the health and well-being of children affected by homelessness. *Pediatrics* 2013;131:1206–1210

INTRODUCTION

An estimated 1.6 million children, or nearly 1 in 45 American children, experienced homelessness in 2010.[1] Although a national economic downturn and an increase in housing foreclosures contribute to family homelessness, additional adversity and risk factors often contribute to this complex problem. Children affected by homelessness may experience a variety of challenges to their health because of difficulty accessing health care, inadequate nutrition, education interruptions, trauma, and family dynamics. By recognizing these challenges, pediatricians can help improve the care of these children in practices and communities.

DEFINING AND MEASURING HOMELESSNESS

The US Department of Education defines a homeless individual as "(A) an individual who lacks a fixed, regular, and adequate nighttime residence . . . and (B) includes (i) children and youths who are sharing the housing of other persons due to loss of housing, economic hardship, or a similar reason; are living in motels, hotels, trailer parks, or camping grounds due to the lack of alternative accommodations; are living in emergency or transitional shelters; are abandoned in hospitals; or are awaiting foster care placement; (ii) children and youths who have a primary nighttime residence that is a public or private place not designed for or ordinarily used as

COUNCIL ON COMMUNITY PEDIATRICS

KEY WORDS
homelessness, housing insecurity, children, adolescents, pediatrician, health, poverty, toxic stress

This article was written by members of the American Academy of Pediatrics. It does not represent the views of the US government or any US government agency.

This document is copyrighted and is property of the American Academy of Pediatrics and its Board of Directors. All authors have filed conflict of interest statements with the American Academy of Pediatrics. Any conflicts have been resolved through a process approved by the Board of Directors. The American Academy of Pediatrics has neither solicited nor accepted any commercial involvement in the development of the content of this publication.

The recommendations in this statement do not indicate an exclusive course of treatment or serve as a standard of medical care. Variations, taking into account individual circumstances, may be appropriate.

All policy statements from the American Academy of Pediatrics automatically expire 5 years after publication unless reaffirmed, revised, or retired at or before that time.

www.pediatrics.org/cgi/doi/10.1542/peds.2013-0645

doi:10.1542/peds.2013-0645

PEDIATRICS (ISSN Numbers: Print, 0031-4005; Online, 1098-4275).

Copyright © 2013 by the American Academy of Pediatrics

a regular sleeping accommodation for human beings ...; (iii) children and youths who are living in cars, parks, public spaces, abandoned buildings, substandard housing, bus or train stations, or similar settings; and (iv) migratory children who qualify as homeless for the purposes of this subtitle because the children are living in circumstances described in clauses (i) through (iii)."[2]

Measuring the homeless population is difficult, and there are no definitive counts of homeless persons in the United States. The US Census Bureau does not currently attempt to estimate the total homeless population; however, the US Department of Housing and Urban Development collects data on shelter usage and makes point-in-time estimates of homelessness. The 2011 Annual Homeless Assessment Report to Congress estimates that approximately 1.5 million homeless people used an emergency shelter or transitional housing during 2010–2011, and on a single night in January 2011, 636 017 people were homeless. From 2007 to 2011, the number of children in shelters increased by 1.9% and families with children comprised 35.8% of the total sheltered population in 2011. In addition, from 2007 to 2011, the number of families that moved from stable housing arrangements to the shelter system increased by 38.5%.[3] These estimates did not include homeless persons who were unsheltered or living temporarily with other families. The incidence of homelessness in the United States in a given year is thought to be much higher.

RISK FACTORS

Although all populations experience homelessness, some populations are disproportionately affected. Major risk factors for homelessness among parents include unemployment, substance abuse, mental illness, previous military service, and a previous history of domestic violence or physical or sexual abuse.[4] An analysis of homelessness in a national cohort of US adolescents revealed that poor family relationship quality, school adjustment problems, and victimization during adolescence were each independent predictors of homelessness in adulthood.[5] Among homeless youth, a sexual orientation other than heterosexual and a history of foster care placement and school expulsion are all potential predictors of homelessness as well.[6,7] Racial and ethnic minorities are significantly overrepresented in the sheltered homeless population. In 2011, 71.9% of sheltered families were racial minorities.[3] Recognition of these risk factors is an important part of understanding and supporting homeless children and families.

Homeless children and families often experience a number of negative exposures and life events that create a cumulative risk for poor health outcomes. For example, children who live in poverty, are exposed to violence, or experience food insecurity also have poor health care service attainment, increased emergency department utilization, and overall poor health outcomes, independent of housing status.[8,9] However, these risks can be additionally compounded by homelessness. A series of studies on adverse childhood experiences has shown that multiple toxic stressors that begin in childhood can have long-term adverse effects on a child's neurobiological make-up, cognitive ability, mental health, and ability to manage stressors as an adult.[10,11] It is therefore important to understand and address these stressors both separately and in totality.

HEALTH EFFECTS OF HOMELESSNESS

Homelessness and housing insecurity negatively impact child health and development in many ways. Homeless children have shown higher rates of acute and chronic health problems than low-income children with homes. Cross-sectional surveys conducted in the 1990s reveal increased rates of multiple infectious, respiratory, gastrointestinal, and dermatologic diseases and otitis media, diarrhea, bronchitis, scabies, lice, and dental caries.[12,13] Both the prevalence and severity of asthma are markedly increased among homeless children, and homeless children suffer from higher rates of accidents and injuries than low-income children with homes.[12,14] In an evaluation completed in a school-based health center, homeless children were 2.5 times more likely to have health problems and 3 times more likely to have severe health problems than children with homes.[15] Children without a stable home are more likely to skip meals, worry about the availability of food, and consume foods with low nutritional quality and high fat content.[16,17] As a result, they suffer from high rates of malnutrition, stunting, and obesity.[8,18] Homeless children are at an increased risk of abuse, exposure to violence, and psychological trauma. Emotional distress, developmental delays, and decreased academic achievement are all more common in this population.[19–21] Speech and language deficits lead to significantly decreased literacy rates in school-aged children.[19,21] Homeless children may experience frequent moves that interrupt their education and impact school performance. In a study in elementary school students, homeless children scored lower on math and reading achievement tests than low-income students living in homes.[21] A study in homeless adolescents who received crisis services at a homeless shelter revealed just 34% of those students attained a high school diploma or general equivalency diploma (GED) by 18 years of age.[22]

Unaccompanied homeless and runaway youth differ from homeless children in families. They are more often separated from their families and more frequently exposed to violence and exploitation. Unaccompanied homeless youth are more likely to engage in high-risk sexual behaviors, have teenage pregnancies, engage in drug use, experience mood and anxiety disorders, and face violence than youth with homes.[23,24]

ACCESS TO HOUSING

Homeless families face many barriers to accessing appropriate housing. In the 2012 Hunger and Homelessness Survey conducted by the US Conference of Mayors, 64% of the surveyed cities reported that shelters turn away families with children experiencing homelessness because of lack of available beds.[25] Access to shelters is challenging in urban settings and rural communities. Although homeless families are more likely to be sheltered than individuals, age and gender restrictions in many shelters often lead to family separations. Homeless mothers are also more likely than housed mothers to have their children separated from them by the child welfare system.[26]

ACCESS TO HEALTH CARE

Children and families in unstable housing often receive fragmented health care and rely on the emergency department as a primary source of care.[27] Some of the barriers that prevent homeless children and families from accessing optimal care include the following:

- difficulty obtaining affordable, accessible, and coordinated health care services;
- frequent and unpredictable changes in living circumstances that prevent timely presentation for care, follow-up,

and communications with health care providers;

- inadequate access to storage places for medication and medical supplies; and
- potential exposure to violence or fear of violence that limits freedom.

Despite these barriers, pediatricians can support homeless children. By partnering with community resources and making changes in practice, pediatricians have the opportunity to help families establish a stable source of quality health care, improve family dynamics, and obtain housing and needed services. Addressing these barriers has been shown to have a positive effect on the health outcomes of those who have experienced homelessness.[21,22,28,29]

RECOMMENDATIONS

The following recommendations address how pediatricians can help improve the health of homeless children through practice strategies.

1. Pediatricians should help homeless children increase access to health care services by promoting and, when possible, facilitating Medicaid enrollment to eligible children and families.

2. Pediatricians should familiarize themselves with best practices for care of homeless populations and the management of chronic diseases in homeless populations.

3. Pediatricians should optimize acute care visits to best resolve patient concerns and provide comprehensive care when possible. For example, pediatricians can update immunizations if a patient is significantly behind rather than having him or her schedule a separate appointment.

4. Pediatricians should seek to identify the issues of homelessness and housing insecurity in their patient

populations. Pediatricians can use methods such as routine screening on intake and making note of frequent address changes or a history of scattered care provision.

5. Pediatricians should seek to identify underlying causes of homelessness in specific families and help facilitate connection to appropriate resources. This may include asking sensitive questions about unemployment, intimate partner violence, substance abuse, and sexual and gender identity issues. Supporting families to address these difficult issues in addition to their housing needs is critical to improving child health and development.

6. Pediatricians should partner with families to develop care plans that acknowledge barriers posed by homelessness. This can involve a variety of innovations, such as making a communications plan that takes into consideration patient access to telephone and mail services, assisting with transportation through vouchers, offering more flexible office visit scheduling, and prescribing the most affordable treatments available. Pediatricians can also learn about the availability of mobile health services in communities to facilitate care that is convenient for homeless children and families.

7. Pediatricians should become familiar with government and community-based services that assist families with unmet social and economic needs. These include such programs as Temporary Assistance for Needy Families (TANF), Special Nutrition Assistance for Nutrition (SNAP), and the Special Supplemental Nutrition Program for Women, Infants, and Children (WIC). Medical-legal partnerships and local departments of health

and human services are also helpful resources.

8. Pediatricians should support and assist in the development of shelter-based care, including partnering with mental health, dental, and other health programs when possible.

9. Pediatricians can learn about the causes and prevalence of homelessness in their communities. The State Report Card on Child Homelessness (www.homelesschildrenameric.org) issued by the National Coalition on Family Homelessness (www.familyhomelessness.org) is one of many good resources.

Pediatricians and the American Academy of Pediatrics can advocate for the needs of homeless children and families in the following ways:

1. Support local, state, and federal policies that lead to increased availability of low-income, transitional, and permanent housing.

2. Support policies and programs, such as the "Homelessness Prevention and Rapid Re-Housing Program," that aim to quickly place families in stable, permanent housing rather than a continuum of emergency and temporary housing. Permanent housing has been demonstrated to be more cost-effective and more stabilizing for families, who can be exposed to significant trauma while experiencing homelessness.

3. Support violence protection policies such as the Family Violence Prevention and Services Act and Child Abuse Prevention and Treatment Act, which provide substantial funding for shelter in addition to social services and legal aid for victims of family violence.

4. Support creative approaches to providing stable health insurance to homeless and unemployed populations, and promote strategies that enable homeless families to enroll and maintain health coverage without requiring a permanent address.

5. Support policies to eliminate any barriers for children without addresses to enroll in school.

6. Support local, state, and federal policies that provide child care vouchers for homeless families.

7. Support reformation of the foster care system to allow longer time in foster care, increased resources for maintaining families when children are aging out of foster care, and greater resources toward training/supporting foster children as they transition into independent adulthood.

Homelessness is a complex issue that presents a number of challenges for children and families. Pediatricians can support all children who are impacted, by implementing practice-level strategies and engaging in advocacy to promote their health and well-being.

LEAD AUTHOR

Melissa A. Briggs, MD, MPH

COUNCIL ON COMMUNITY PEDIATRICS, 2011–2012

Deise C. Granado-Villar, MD, MPH, Chairperson
Benjamin A. Gitterman, MD, Vice Chairperson
Jeffrey M. Brown, MD, MPH
Lance A. Chilton, MD
William H. Cotton, MD
Thresia B. Gambon, MD
Peter A. Gorski, MD, MPA
Colleen A. Kraft, MD
Alice A. Kuo, MD, PhD
Gonzalo J. Paz-Soldan, MD
Barbara Zind, MD

LIAISONS

Benjamin Hoffman, MD – Chairperson, *Indian Health Special Interest Group*
Melissa A. Briggs, MD – *Section on Medical Students, Residents, and Fellowship Trainees*
Frances J. Dunston, MD, MPH
Charles R. Feild, MD, MPH – Chairperson, *Prevention and Public Health Special Interest Group*
M. Edward Ivancic, MD – Chairperson, *Rural Health Special Interest Group*
David M. Keller, MD – Chairperson, *Community Pediatrics Education and Training Special Interest Group*

STAFF

Camille Watson, MS

REFERENCES

1. The National Center on Family Homelessness. America's youngest outcasts 2010: state report card on child homelessness. Available at: www.FamilyHomelessness.org. Accessed January 30, 2013

2. McKinney-Vento Act §725(2), 42USC 11435 (2) (2002)

3. US Department of Housing and Urban Development. The 2011 annual homeless assessment report to Congress. Washington, DC: US Department of Housing and Urban Development, Office of Community Planning and Development; 2011. Available at: https://www.onecpd.info/resources/documents/2011AHAR_FinalReport.pdf. Accessed January 30, 2013

4. US Department of Housing and Urban Development. The 2010 annual homeless assessment report to Congress. Washington, DC: US Department of Housing and Urban Development, Office of Community Planning and Development; 2010. Available at: www.hurhre.info/documents/2010 HomelessAssessmentReport.pdf. Accessed January 30, 2013

5. van den Bree MB, Shelton K, Bonner A, Moss S, Thomas H, Taylor PJ. A longitudinal population-based study of factors in adolescence predicting homelessness in young adulthood. *J Adolesc Health*. 2009;45(6): 571–578

6. US Interagency Council on Homelessness. Opening doors: federal strategic plan to

prevent and end homelessness. Washington, DC: US Interagency Council on Homelessness; 2010. Available at: www.ich.gov/PDF/Opening-Doors_2010_FSPPreventEndHomeless.pdf. Accessed January 30, 2013

7. Cook R. *A National Evaluation of Title IV-E Foster Care Independent Living Programs for Youth, Phase 2.* Rockville, MD: Westat Inc; 1991

8. Ma CT, Gee L, Kushel MB. Associations between housing instability and food insecurity with health care access in low-income children. *Ambul Pediatr.* 2008;8(1):50–57

9. Park JM, Fertig AR, Allison PD. Physical and mental health, cognitive development, and health care use by housing status of low-income young children in 20 American cities: a prospective cohort study. *Am J Public Health.* 2011;101(suppl 1):S255–S261

10. Anda RF, Felitti VJ, Bremner JD, et al. The enduring effects of abuse and related adverse experiences in childhood: a convergence of evidence from neurobiology and epidemiology. *Eur Arch Psychiatry Clin Neurosci.* 2006;256(3):174–186

11. Shonkoff JP, Garner AS; Committee on Psychosocial Aspects of Child and Family Health; Committee on Early Childhood, Adoption, and Dependent Care; Section on Developmental and Behavioral Pediatrics. The lifelong effects of early childhood adversity and toxic stress. *Pediatrics.* 2012;129(1). Available at: www.pediarics.org/cgi/content/full/129/1/e232

12. Weinreb L, Goldberg R, Bassuk E, Perloff J. Determinants of health and service use patterns in homeless and low-income housed children. *Pediatrics.* 1998;102(3 pt 1):554–562

13. Karr C, Kline S. Homeless children: what every clinician should know. *Pediatr Rev.* 2004;25(7):235–241

14. McLean DE, Bowen S, Drezner K, et al. Asthma among homeless children: undercounting and undertreating the underserved. *Arch Pediatr Adolesc Med.* 2004;158(3):244–249

15. Berti LC, Zylbert S, Rolnitzky L. Comparison of health status of children using a school-based health center for comprehensive care. *J Pediatr Health Care.* 2001;15(5):244–250

16. Wood DL, Valdez RB, Hayashi T, Shen A. Health of homeless children and housed, poor children. *Pediatrics.* 1990;86(6):858–866

17. Smith C, Richards R. Dietary intake, overweight status, and perceptions of food insecurity among homeless Minnesotan youth. *Am J Hum Biol.* 2008;20(5):550–563

18. Wiecha JL, Dwyer JT, Dunn-Strohecker M. Nutrition and health services needs among the homeless. *Public Health Rep.* 1991;106(4):364–374

19. Rubin DH, Erickson CJ, San Agustin M, Cleary SD, Allen JK, Cohen P. Cognitive and academic functioning of homeless children compared with housed children. *Pediatrics.* 1996;97(3):289–294

20. Zima BT, Wells KB, Freeman HE. Emotional and behavioral problems and severe academic delays among sheltered homeless children in Los Angeles County. *Am J Public Health.* 1994;84(2):260–264

21. Obradović J, Long JD, Cutuli JJ, et al. Academic achievement of homeless and highly mobile children in an urban school district: longitudinal evidence on risk, growth, and resilience. *Dev Psychopathol.* 2009;21(2):493–518

22. Barber CC, Fonagy P, Fultz J, Simulinas M, Yates M. Homeless near a thousand homes: outcomes of homeless youth in a crisis shelter. *Am J Orthopsychiatry.* 2005;75(3):347–355

23. Edidin JP, Ganim Z, Hunter SJ, Karnik NS. The mental and physical health of homeless youth: a literature review. *Child Psychiatry Hum Dev.* 2012;43(3):354–375

24. Thompson SJ, Bender KA, Lewis CM, Watkins R. Runaway and pregnant: risk factors associated with pregnancy in a national sample of runaway/homeless female adolescents. *J Adolesc Health.* 2008;43(2):125–132

25. US Conference of Mayors. *Hunger and Homelessness Survey: A Status Report on Hunger and Homelessness in America's Cities. A 25-City Survey.* Washington, DC: US Conference of Mayors; 2012

26. Cowal K, Shinn M, Weitzman BC, Stojanovic D, Labay L. Mother-child separations among homeless and housed families receiving public assistance in New York City. *Am J Community Psychol.* 2002;30(5):711–730

27. Morris DM, Gordon JA. The role of the emergency department in the care of homeless and disadvantaged populations. *Emerg Med Clin North Am.* 2006;24(4):839–848

28. Martinez TE, Burt MR. Impact of permanent supportive housing on the use of acute care health services by homeless adults. *Psychiatr Serv.* 2006;57(7):992–999

29. Sadowski LS, Kee RA, VanderWeele TJ, Buchanan D. Effect of a housing and case management program on emergency department visits and hospitalizations among chronically ill homeless adults: a randomized trial. *JAMA.* 2009;301(17):1771–1778

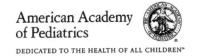

POLICY STATEMENT

Providing Care for Immigrant, Migrant, and Border Children

abstract

This policy statement, which recognizes the large changes in immigrant status since publication of the 2005 statement "Providing Care for Immigrant, Homeless, and Migrant Children," focuses on strategies to support the health of immigrant children, infants, adolescents, and young adults. Homeless children will be addressed in a forthcoming separate statement ("Providing Care for Children and Adolescents Facing Homelessness and Housing Insecurity"). While recognizing the diversity across and within immigrant, migrant, and border populations, this statement provides a basic framework for serving and advocating for all immigrant children, with a particular focus on low-income and vulnerable populations. Recommendations include actions needed within and outside the health care system, including expansion of access to high-quality medical homes with culturally and linguistically effective care as well as education and literacy programs. The statement recognizes the unique and special role that pediatricians can play in the lives of immigrant children and families. Recommendations for policies that support immigrant child health are included. *Pediatrics* 2013;131:e2028–e2034

COUNCIL ON COMMUNITY PEDIATRICS

KEY WORDS
immigrant, migrant, border, underserved communities

ABBREVIATIONS
CHIP—Children's Health Insurance Program

www.pediatrics.org/cgi/doi/10.1542/peds.2013-1099

doi:10.1542/peds.2013-1099

PEDIATRICS (ISSN Numbers: Print, 0031-4005; Online, 1098-4275).

INTRODUCTION

Many children in immigrant communities face multiple barriers to accessing comprehensive, affordable, and culturally and linguistically effective health care services. Some of these barriers include poverty, fear and stigma, high mobility, limited English proficiency, little information or misunderstandings about how the US health care system works, and lack of insurance and/or access to care. Many children of immigrant families belong to racial and ethnic minority groups that face health status disparities resulting from complex determinants that are exacerbated by children's living circumstances. Inadequate availability of basic necessities, such as housing, and lack of information regarding previous medical care are among the persistent challenges faced by these vulnerable families. For some, the fear of violence or harassment because of their immigrant status compounds their already fragile living conditions. For many within this population, care can be episodic, fragmented, and oriented to care of acute conditions.[1] Although many children in these circumstances face similar challenges, there are some differences of experiences among migrant and border immigrant subgroups (see Fig 1).

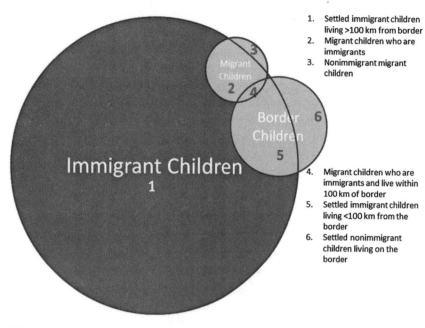

1. Settled immigrant children living >100 km from border
2. Migrant children who are immigrants
3. Nonimmigrant migrant children
4. Migrant children who are immigrants and live within 100 km of border
5. Settled immigrant children living <100 km from the border
6. Settled nonimmigrant children living on the border

FIGURE 1

Representation of the populations of immigrant, border, and migrant children: separate and overlapping groups.

DEFINITIONS

"Immigrant children" are defined as children who are foreign-born or children born in the United States who live with at least 1 parent who is foreign-born.[2]

Many immigrant children are in migrant families that move across the country seeking seasonal or temporary employment in a variety of industries. "Migrant children" may work in the industries in which their family members are employed and move frequently because of changes in their parents' employment. Migrant families are often located in areas that have many agricultural workers and/or where rapid growth is occurring.

"Border children" are those who live within 100 km of the US-Mexico border.[3] Immigrant children have a significant presence in the border states of Arizona, California, New Mexico, and Texas. Many border children are of Mexican origin, and a significant number are US citizens whose ancestors have been US citizens for generations. For the purposes of this discussion,

only children living north of the Mexican border are described, although many children south of the border share similar characteristics. Children living along the Canadian border are not discussed in this statement, because there is far less immigration across that border and discrete immigrant communities there have been rare.

DEMOGRAPHICS

Immigrant children represent the fastest growing segment of the US population. One in every 4 children in the United States, approximately 18.4 million children, live in an immigrant family. Eighty-nine percent of these children are born in the United States and are US citizens.[4] Immigrant children accounted for most of the US child population growth over the past decade. Although 64% of all children of immigrants live in 6 states (California, Texas, New York, Florida, Illinois, and New Jersey), immigrant children are dispersed throughout the country. Since 1990, the largest growth in percentage

of immigrant children has occurred in North Carolina, Nevada, Georgia, and Arkansas.[5] Families immigrate for a variety of reasons that may include seeking opportunity, fleeing war/chaos, or escaping persecution.

Pediatricians may be surprised by the high degree of diversity of the immigrant population and by the variety of immigrant communities within their midst, such as Haitians in Florida and eastern Virginia or Somali families in Seattle and Minneapolis. Hmong families are present in the Central Valley of California.[6] In response to the growth of these immigrant communities, some health care and social/community service providers have begun providing culturally appropriate care and services.

Approximately 43% of immigrant children have parents of Mexican origin, and 20% are of Central American descent. An estimated 22% of immigrant children have parents of Asian or Middle Eastern origin. Fifteen percent of children have parents with origins in Africa, Central and Eastern Europe, Western Europe, Canada, and Australia.[7] Given this rapid demographic growth, most pediatricians will provide care for immigrant children in their practices.

COMMON CHALLENGES FOR IMMIGRANT, MIGRANT, AND BORDER CHILDREN

All 3 groups of children face a variety of challenges to their health and well-being, including poverty, lack of health insurance, low educational attainment, substandard housing, and language barriers.

Poverty is a strong determinant of child well-being and is very common among immigrant children. Poverty is closely linked to negative physical, developmental, and mental health–related outcomes.[8] A family's socioeconomic status has a direct effect on its ability to access high-quality health care services and to achieve good health, social, and emotional outcomes. In 2010, 30% of children in immigrant families lived below the federal poverty level, compared with 19% of children with US-born parents.[4] This is despite the fact that immigrant children are more likely to live in 2-parent families and have parents who work and work more hours compared with parents of US-born children.[9] Immigrant children tend to live in larger families, with 19% having 4 or more siblings, compared with 14% of US-born families.[10] Housing is often substandard and/or overcrowded for these families.

Lack of health care coverage is more common among children in each of these groups than for nonimmigrant children. Children of immigrants are nearly twice as likely to be uninsured (15%) as are children of nonimmigrant families (8%).[4] Many of the immigrant children who are uninsured are eligible for Medicaid or the Children's Health Insurance Program (CHIP) but are not enrolled. Many immigrant parents fear that accessing services for their eligible children will lead them to be considered a "public charge" (a person dependent on the government for the expenses of living[11]) and worry about how that may negatively affect their immigration status and prospects. They may also fear that agencies offering assistance will share information with immigration enforcement agencies. Other families may not be aware of their children's eligibility for coverage. These same reasons may affect parents' ability and willingness to access other programs and benefits that their children may be eligible for, such as the Special Supplemental Nutrition Program for Women, Infants, and Children; Supplemental Nutrition Assistance Program; the Temporary Assistance for Needy Families program; and Supplemental Security Income.

Current federal law allows states to apply waiting periods for up to 5 years for legal permanent residents to become eligible for Medicaid coverage. Medicaid also excludes undocumented children from all but emergency health care. Although states may choose to cover children sooner, waiting periods can exacerbate the lack of health insurance coverage for immigrant children. The Affordable Care Act of 2010 (Pub L No. 111-148) also restricts the access to health insurance exchanges of children and adults who are undocumented immigrants.[12]

Language and communication barriers may impede medical care for many children in each of these 3 groups. Although many immigrant children speak English, their parents may not, creating a barrier that can prevent families from accessing health services and/or causing inadequate communication with health care providers. Without access to qualified medical interpreters in health care settings, language barriers can place English-speaking children in the difficult position of interpreting between health care providers and their family members. Use of children and other family members as untrained interpreters should be avoided. These challenges can result in major barriers to accessing health care and decreased satisfaction with services received. Providing care to families with limited English proficiency without appropriate medical interpretation services can ultimately lead to a higher incidence of medical errors when delivering care.[13]

Educational levels and health literacy are often lower among parents of immigrant, border, and migrant families than among native-born US families. Thirty-one percent of immigrant children have a mother without a high school education; the proportion of fathers without a high school education is similar.[4] It is important to note

that the level of maternal education is an important determinant of child health. Lower education levels are associated with lower health literacy. Low health literacy creates a barrier for patients in understanding medical information and is associated with poor health outcomes.

Health Status and Health Disparities

Although immigrant children may be vulnerable to many risk factors for poorer health outcomes, some groups of immigrant children enjoy a healthier infancy than expected. For example, Latino families have a relatively low incidence of low birth weight, preterm birth, and infant mortality compared with children of US-born parents.[4] This phenomenon has been called the "healthy immigrant phenomenon."[9] Immigrant mothers are more likely to breastfeed their infants than mothers born in the United States.[14] Immigrant children also seem to benefit from some additional protective factors, such as growing up in 2-parent or extended families,[9] as well as close identification with the cultural and spiritual practices of their family and community. In addition, as they grow up, immigrant children may also display relatively better adjustment and behavior in school compared with nonimmigrant peers. This phenomenon has been shown to fade with increased length of stay in the United States and is, therefore, an infrequent protective factor for health outcomes.

On the other hand, the health of immigrant children as a group is, in some respects, worse than US-born children. For example, they are less likely to be perceived by their parents to be in excellent/good health and are less likely to have a usual source of medical care and to obtain specialty care when needed.[15] They also have less access to dental care, despite the fact that they have a higher prevalence of dental caries.[16] The Affordable Care Act excluded undocumented immigrants from health care coverage made available through the Act, leaving that group of adults and children as the largest group who still will not have health insurance after the changes of 2014.[12]

Immigrant children who are foreign-born may not have been screened at birth for congenital syphilis, hemoglobinopathies, hearing deficits, and inborn errors of metabolism. In comparison with US-born children, they also have lower immunization rates, especially for vaccines that are not routinely administered in their countries of origin. Some children may lack immunization records. Foreign-born immigrant children have a higher incidence or prevalence of some infectious diseases, such as tuberculosis, hepatitis A, amebiasis, and parasitosis.[17] Immigrant children with asthma are less likely to be prescribed the recommended preventive medications.[18] Immigrant families may be uniquely vulnerable to mental health problems and experience high levels of stress, depression, grief, and traumatic events compared with nonimmigrant families.[19] Additionally, many experience the stress of family separation, in which some of the siblings or, in some cases, 1 or both of the parents do not reside in this country with them.

Development, Early Education, and School Success

Many immigrant, migrant, and border children also experience educational disparities compared with US-born children. As noted, immigrant children may enjoy a healthy start as infants but may experience developmental stagnation as toddlers compared with non-immigrant children.[20]

In general, children who grow up in bilingual homes should attain major language developmental milestones at the normally expected times. At the same time, children raised in homes with impoverished language have a greater chance of being delayed in language acquisition, whether their families are monolingual or bilingual. When language delays are suspected in children growing up in limited English proficiency households, they present complex evaluation and intervention issues. When in doubt about a suspected language delay in a bilingual child, timely referral to a knowledgeable, bilingual speech and language pathologist is ideal.

Many immigrant children have less access to quality early education programs and are less likely to be enrolled in preschool programs, such as Head Start.[4] Once enrolled in school, cultural and linguistic barriers between parents and schools can lead to decreased family interaction and involvement. As they advance in their schooling, children in immigrant families are less likely to graduate from high school than are their non-immigrant peers.[4]

Fear and Discrimination

Immigrant children and families may face discrimination and be fearful of attitudes and behaviors of the people they interact with outside their communities, including health care providers, which can reduce access to health care and lead to negative child health outcomes. Families may face anti-immigrant sentiment. Fear and discrimination can exacerbate a feeling of isolation and contribute to mental health problems, such as child and family depression, leaving these populations vulnerable.

Family Separation

Immigrant children may have 1 or more undocumented family members. An undocumented immigrant lacks the proper records and identification to live in the United States.[21] Immigration enforcement and related policies can lead to the sudden removal of an undocumented parent or other key family member without notice or preparation. Children whose parents are taken into custody and/or deported have been shown to experience mental and emotional health problems, including sleeping and eating disturbances, anxiety, depression, poor school performance, and other types of distress. Forced separations because of immigration enforcement can also result in the loss of family income and have been shown to result in family housing and food instability.[22] This can negatively affect a child's safety, health, and development.

FACTORS SPECIFIC TO MIGRANT CHILDREN

A large number of migrant children are also immigrants. For that reason, virtually all of the points made earlier about immigrant children may also apply to those who are migrants. Because of their migration patterns, migrant children are even more likely to lack medical coverage and a medical home than other immigrant children. They are also more likely to be socially, culturally, and linguistically isolated because of their mobile lifestyle.

Many migrant children face a panoply of health problems related to their living and working conditions, including workplace injuries, substandard housing, and unreliable transportation.[23] These factors can contribute to higher rates of respiratory tract and ear infections, bacterial and viral gastroenteritis, tuberculosis, nutritional deficiencies, intestinal parasites, skin infections, dental problems, lead and pesticide exposure, and undiagnosed congenital anomalies.[24] Additionally, at times, migrant adolescents travel on their own from 1 job site to another, putting them at increased risk of many health-related problems.

FACTORS SPECIFIC TO BORDER CHILDREN

Immigrant children living at the US-Mexico border share almost all of the characteristics of other immigrant children but may experience additional challenges. Children who have crossed the border to enter the United States may have experienced trauma in the form of threat of death, abuse, and exploitation that leave serious psychological scars. Once in the United States, these children may experience an enhanced fear of a family member's deportation, imprisonment, or abuse because of documentation status. Children and families who have recently crossed the border can also experience difficulty adapting to the new cultural environment of the United States and experience stress from the absence of an extended family (including a parent or head of household) that is located in another country. Border children may be even more stigmatized or mistreated by the nonimmigrant populations living nearby, as their families are falsely presumed to take advantage of scarce resources and not pay taxes.

Many border communities are poor and lacking in resources, including medical care. In general, border communities lack sufficient numbers of primary care pediatricians, and those present may lack appropriate cultural and linguistic capacity to serve minority border children. In addition, primary care providers bear an especially high proportion of Medicaid, CHIP, and self-pay patients, with few privately insured patients to whom costs may be shifted. As a consequence of these deficiencies and because of high costs of medical care in the United States, families living close

to the border may use medical care and pharmaceutical resources south of the border.

RECOMMENDATIONS

Immigrant children represent a considerable part of the economic and social future of the nation. It is in the national interest that we work to ensure that all children within the United States, including immigrant, border, and migrant children, grow up physically and developmentally healthy. The future prosperity and well-being of the United States depends on the health and vitality of all of its children, without exception. The following recommendations address how pediatricians can help support immigrant child health in practice.

1. Pediatricians and the American Academy of Pediatrics should advocate for health insurance coverage for every child and every individual living in the United States, as lack of coverage for any family member affects the health of the entire family.[25] This advocacy should focus on expanding access to quality health care within a medical home. Barriers to enrollment must be addressed, including the removal of any waiting periods for documented immigrant children to enroll into coverage. Efforts must also address barriers to enrollment for children who are potentially eligible for Medicaid and CHIP but not enrolled. Simplified enrollment for both programs and federal or state funding for those who are not currently eligible for Medicaid or CHIP is also essential.

2. The provision of comprehensive, coordinated, culturally and linguistically effective care, and continuous health services provided in a quality medical home should be integral to all efforts on behalf

of immigrant children.[26] This is especially critical for children with chronic health care needs and emotional or behavioral health problems. Private and public insurance payers should pay for qualified medical interpretation services.

3. Pediatricians caring for immigrant children should evaluate immunization adequacy and should conduct careful developmental surveillance and screening at regular intervals as recommended by the American Academy of Pediatrics.[27] Appropriate referral for early intervention services or psychoeducational evaluation should be initiated as soon as a concern is identified.

4. Pediatricians should recognize the barriers to health that are faced by immigrant children and take these barriers into account while providing care. They should inquire about beliefs and practices related to health, illness, and disability, as well as traditional healing practices and medication use while obtaining a patient's medical history. Knowledge, attitude, and skill development in culturally and linguistically effective practices and cross-cultural communication should be part of every pediatrician's professional agenda.

5. Pediatricians should be knowledgeable about the unique emotional, behavioral, mental, and physical health advantages and problems that may be faced by immigrant children, including those related to family separation. Appropriate screening to identify family, environmental, and social circumstances, as well as biological factors, should be incorporated into routine pediatric assessments, such as in Bright Futures history forms.

6. Pediatricians should have access to information regarding federal, state, and community programs that can serve as resources to at-risk children and families. Culturally relevant programs that address social and economic challenges, such as food and housing security, English literacy, and legal services, are particularly important. Medical-legal partnerships should be supported to help immigrant families with these issues.

7. Pediatricians should play a key role in helping immigrant parents assess and review the educational progress of the child and encouraging parents to become involved in and interact with teachers and the school community. If a child exhibits difficulty or academic underachievement, pediatricians are in a unique position to advocate for the child and encourage and help parents to obtain appropriate evaluation and intervention from the school system.

8. Pediatricians should routinely use available screening and diagnostic protocols for evaluating foreign-born children for infectious diseases and other medical conditions when providing care for newly arrived immigrant children.[28] Additional screenings, including lead, vision, and hearing screenings, should be considered whether required for school entry or not.

9. Pediatricians should advocate for an array of culturally effective early intervention services, including the establishment of evidence-based early literacy promotion programs, such as Reach Out and Read, in immigrant, border, and migrant communities. Because reading is such an important skill, these programs are important tools for improving the school readiness of all children, just as fostering health literacy in parents is important to the well-being of their children.

10. Pediatricians should use their positions of respect in communities to promote the value of diversity and inclusion and to advocate for children and families of all backgrounds.

Given the challenging circumstances many immigrant children face because of their family's immigration status, the following recommendations address how immigration policies can support child health and well-being.

11. The health, well-being, and safety of children should be prioritized in all immigration proceedings. Whenever possible, the separation of a child from his or her family and home environment should be prevented, and family reunions should be expedited.

12. In no circumstances should a child have to represent himself or herself in an immigration proceeding.

13. Health care facilities should be safe settings for immigrant children and families to access health care. Medical records and health care facilities should not be used in any immigration enforcement action.

LEAD AUTHORS
Lance A. Chilton, MD
Gilbert A. Handal, MD
Gonzalo J. Paz-Soldan, MD

COUNCIL ON COMMUNITY PEDIATRICS EXECUTIVE COMMITTEE, 2011–2012
Deise C. Granado-Villar, MD, MPH, Chairperson
Benjamin A. Gitterman, MD, Vice Chairperson
Jeffrey M. Brown, MD, MPH
Lance A. Chilton, MD
William H. Cotton, MD
Thresia B. Gambon, MD
Peter A. Gorski, MD, MPA
Colleen A. Kraft, MD
Alice A. Kuo, MD, PhD
Gonzalo J. Paz-Soldan, MD
Barbara Zind, MD

CONTRIBUTOR
Ricky Choi, MD, MPH – *Chairperson, Special Interest Group on Immigrant Health*

LIAISONS
Benjamin Hoffman, MD – *Chairperson, Indian Health Special Interest Group*
Melissa A. Briggs, MD – *Section on Medical Students, Residents, and Fellowship Trainees*
Frances J. Dunston, MD, MPH – *Commission to End Health Care Disparities*
Charles R. Feild, MD, MPH – *Chairperson, Prevention and Public Health Special Interest Group*
M. Edward Ivancic, MD – *Chairperson, Rural Health Special Interest Group*
David M. Keller, MD – *Chairperson, Community Pediatrics Education and Training Special Interest Group*

STAFF
Camille Watson, MS

REFERENCES

1. Okie S. Immigrants and health care—at the intersection of two broken systems. *N Engl J Med.* 2007;357(6):525–529

2. Child Trends. Immigrant children. Available at: www.childtrendsdatabank.org/?q=node/333. Accessed July 19, 2012

3. United States-Mexico Border Health Commission. What is defined as the border region? Available at: www.borderhealth.org/show_faq.php?id=16. Accessed July 19, 2012

4. Foundation for Child Development. Children in immigrant families: essential to America's future. Available at: http://fcd-us.org/node/1232. Accessed July 19, 2012

5. Fortuny K, Ajay C. *Children of Immigrants: Growing National and State Diversity. Brief 5.* Washington, DC: The Urban Institute; 2011

6. Fadiman A. *The Spirit Catches You and You Fall Down: A Hmong Child, Her American Doctors, and the Collision of Two Cultures.* New York, NY: Noonday Press; 1998

7. Fortuny K, Hernandez DJ, Ajay C. *Young Children of Immigrants: The Leading Edge of America's Future. Brief 3.* Washington, DC: The Urban Institute; 2010

8. Conroy K, Sandel M, Zuckerman B. Poverty grown up: how childhood socioeconomic status impacts adult health. *J Dev Behav Pediatr.* 2010;31(2):154–160

9. Mendoza FS. Health disparities and children in immigrant families: a research agenda. *Pediatrics.* 2009;124(suppl 3): S187–S195

10. Lansford JE, Deater-Deckard K, Bornstein MH, eds. *Immigrant Families in Contemporary Society.* New York, NY: Guilford Press; 2007

11. US Citizenship and Immigration Services. Public Charge Fact Sheet, April 2011. Available at: www.uscis.gov/portal/site/uscis/menuitem. 5af9bb95919f35e66f614176543f6d1a/? vgnextoid=775d23cbea6bf210VgnVCM 100000082ca60aRCRD&vgnextchannel=8a2f6 d26d17df110VgnVCM1000004718190aRCRD. Accessed July 19, 2012

12. National Immigration Law Center. How are immigrants included in health care reform? Washington, DC: National Immigration Law Center; April 2010. Available at: www.nilc.org/contact_us.html. Accessed July 19, 2012

13. Flores G, Laws MB, Mayo SJ, et al. Errors in medical interpretation and their potential clinical consequences in pediatric encounters. *Pediatrics.* 2003;111(1):6–14

14. Singh GK, Kogan MD, Dee DL. Nativity/ immigrant status, race/ethnicity, and socioeconomic determinants of breastfeeding initiation and duration in the United States, 2003. *Pediatrics.* 2007;119(1 suppl 1):S38–S46

15. Capps R, Fix M, Ost J, Reardon-Anderson J, Passel JS. *The Health and Well-Being of Young Children of Immigrants.* Washington, DC: The Urban Institute; 2004

16. Liu J, Probst JC, Martin AB, Wang JY, Salinas CF. Disparities in dental insurance coverage and dental care among US children: the National Survey of Children's Health. *Pediatrics.* 2007;119(suppl 1):S12–S21

17. Strine TW, Barker LE, Mokdad AH, Luman ET, Sutter RW, Chu SY. Vaccination coverage of foreign-born children 19 to 35 months of age: findings from the National Immunization Survey, 1999-2000. *Pediatrics.* 2002;110 (2 pt 1):e15

18. Tienda M, Haskin R. Immigrant children: introducing the issue. *Immigrant Children.* 2011;21(1):3–18

19. Kupersmidt JB, Martin SL. Mental health problems of children of migrant and seasonal farm workers: a pilot study. *J Am Acad Child Adolesc Psychiatry.* 1997;36(2): 1–9

20. Fuller B, Bridges M, Bein E, et al. The health and cognitive growth of Latino toddlers: at risk or immigrant paradox? *Matern Child Health J.* 2009;13(6):755–768

21. Legal Information Institute. Immigration law: an overview. Available at: www.law. cornell.edu/wex/Immigration. Accessed July 19, 2012

22. Chaudry A, Capps R, Pedroza JM, Castenada RM, Santos R, Scott MM. *Facing Our Future: Children in the Aftermath of Immigration Enforcement.* Washington, DC: The Urban Institute; 2010

23. McLaurin J, ed; American Academy of Pediatrics. *Guidelines for the Care of Migrant Farmworker's Children.* Elk Grove Village, IL: American Academy of Pediatrics; 2000

24. Migrant Clinician's Network. Children's health. Available at: www.migrantclinician. org/issues/childrens-health.html. Accessed July 19, 2012

25. Ku L, Broaddus M. *Coverage for Parents Helps Children, Too.* Washington, DC: Center on Budget and Policy Priorities; 2006

26. American Academy of Pediatrics Committee on Pediatric Workforce. Culturally effective pediatric care: education and training issues. *Pediatrics.* 1999;103(1):167–170

27. Hagan JF, Jr, Shaw JS, Duncan P, eds. *Bright Futures: Guidelines for Health Supervision of Infants, Children, and Adolescents.* 3rd ed. Elk Grove Village, IL: American Academy of Pediatrics; 2008

28. Pickering LK, Baker CJ, Kimberlin DW, Long SS, eds; American Academy of Pediatrics. *Red Book: 2012 Report of the Committee on Infectious Diseases.* 29th ed. Elk Grove Village, IL: American Academy of Pediatrics; 2012

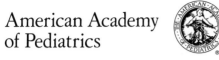

CLINICAL REPORT   Guidance for the Clinician in Rendering Pediatric Care

Providing Psychosocial Support to Children and Families in the Aftermath of Disasters and Crises

David J. Schonfeld, MD, FAAP, Thomas Demaria, PhD, the DISASTER PREPAREDNESS ADVISORY COUNCIL AND COMMITTEE ON PSYCHOSOCIAL ASPECTS OF CHILD AND FAMILY HEALTH

www.pediatrics.org/cgi/doi/10.1542/peds.2015-2861

DOI: 10.1542/peds.2015-2861

Accepted for publication Jul 30, 2015

PEDIATRICS (ISSN Numbers: Print, 0031-4005; Online, 1098-4275).

abstract

Disasters have the potential to cause short- and long-term effects on the psychological functioning, emotional adjustment, health, and developmental trajectory of children. This clinical report provides practical suggestions on how to identify common adjustment difficulties in children in the aftermath of a disaster and to promote effective coping strategies to mitigate the impact of the disaster as well as any associated bereavement and secondary stressors. This information can serve as a guide to pediatricians as they offer anticipatory guidance to families or consultation to schools, child care centers, and other child congregate care sites. Knowledge of risk factors for adjustment difficulties can serve as the basis for mental health triage. The importance of basic supportive services, psychological first aid, and professional self-care are discussed. Stress is intrinsic to many major life events that children and families face, including the experience of significant illness and its treatment. The information provided in this clinical report may, therefore, be relevant for a broad range of patient encounters, even outside the context of a disaster. Most pediatricians enter the profession because of a heartfelt desire to help children and families most in need. If adequately prepared and supported, pediatricians who are able to draw on their skills to assist children, families, and communities to recover after a disaster will find the work to be particularly rewarding.

INTRODUCTION

Disasters are "one-time or ongoing events of human or natural cause that lead groups of people to experience stressors including the threat of death, bereavement, disrupted social support systems, and insecurity of basic human needs such as food, water, housing, and access to close family members."[1] In a representative sample of more than 2000 US children 2 through 17 years of age, nearly 14% were reported to have been exposed to a disaster in their lifetime, with more than 4% of disasters occurring in the past year.[1] Disasters, thereby, affect the lives of millions of children every year, whether through natural disasters, such as earthquakes, hurricanes, tornadoes, fires, or floods; human-made disasters, such as industrial accidents, war, or terrorism; or as a result of pandemics or other naturally occurring disease outbreaks. Children are particularly vulnerable to the effects of disasters and other traumatic events because of a lack of experience, skills, and resources to be able to independently meet their developmental, social-emotional, mental, and behavioral health needs.[2,3] Disasters also have the potential to cause short- and long-term effects on the psychological functioning, emotional adjustment, health, and developmental trajectory of children, which even may have implications for their health and psychological functioning in adulthood; children, as a group, are among those most at risk for psychological trauma and behavioral difficulties after a disaster.[4]

Pediatricians and other pediatric health care providers are in an excellent position to (1) encourage families and communities to prepare for potential disasters; (2) provide support to children and families in the immediate aftermath of a disaster, as well as throughout the recovery process; (3) share advice and strategies with caregivers on how to promote and support children's adjustment, coping, and resilience; (4) provide timely triage to identify and refer children with or at considerable risk of developing adjustment difficulties to appropriate services; (5) serve as a consultant to schools, child care centers, and other child congregate care sites on preparedness, response, and recovery efforts; and (6) advocate at the local, state, and national levels for a state of preparedness and services to meet the needs of children affected by disasters.[3] Stress is intrinsic to many major life events that children and families face, including the experience

of significant illness and its treatment. The information provided in this clinical report may, therefore, be relevant for a broad range of patient encounters, even outside the context of a disaster.

Emotional distress also may interfere with the accurate reporting of symptoms and may even mimic physical conditions. Effective management of medical conditions may be compromised, thereby reducing the quality of pediatric care provided both in the aftermath of disasters and in situations involving patient/family distress. Despite the increased call for psychosocial support in the aftermath of a disaster, surveys of practicing pediatricians consistently indicate that most pediatricians perceive themselves to be unprepared to address the needs of children in such crises.[5,6] This clinical report presents information about children's common adjustment reactions to disasters, their risk factors for addressing and dealing with challenges, and practical strategies to help patients and families increase coping skills and resiliency.

CREATE A SAFE HEALTH CARE ENVIRONMENT IN THE AFTERMATH OF A DISASTER

Sites that may deliver care in the aftermath of a disaster should be designed to minimize the likelihood of contributing additional stress to children. When delivering medical care, attempts should be made to minimize the use of invasive or painful procedures or treatments and provide appropriate sedation or analgesia whenever required. Parents and family members should remain with children to the extent possible throughout the evaluation and treatment process, provided that they are able to cope with their own discomfort or distress. Parents may be guided in supporting their children, such as by using coping strategies they have found effective in

the past (eg, distraction or attention-refocusing techniques, like a calming touch or use of gentle humor). Parents should be allowed to temporarily leave the examination room if they are feeling overwhelmed, but should notify the child before leaving that they will be in an adjacent area and that the pediatrician or nurse will remain with them for a few minutes until they return.

Practical steps can be taken to minimize children's exposure to frightening images and sounds that may compound their distress or serve as triggers or reminders of a disaster. Doors/curtains in the health care setting should be closed to reduce exposure to others who are injured or in pain. Televisions in waiting, examination, and inpatient rooms can be turned off if they are broadcasting coverage of the crisis event. Staff members are encouraged to remember that children can often overhear and understand their conversations.

Parents and doctors can provide explanations about medical treatments and care in positive terms that emphasize how these interventions are intended to keep children safe and/or help them feel better. Potential risks may be presented in supportive ways, for example, "We are going to put this belt around your waist so that you remain safe and secure in the ambulance," rather than "We will put this belt on so that you don't go flying out of the ambulance if we have to stop quickly on the way to the hospital." This advice is relevant even outside the context of a disaster.[7]

COMMON ADJUSTMENT REACTIONS OF CHILDREN TO DISASTERS

The effect of a disaster on each individual child varies depending on a number of factors, including (1) the nature of the event and the amount of death, destruction, and disruption; (2) the degree of personal involvement of children and their families; (3) the duration of time before children's daily environment, and that of the overall community, returns to a safe, predictable, and comfortable routine; (4) whether the stressor is a 1-time or chronic event; (5) the level of coping ability of the children's caregivers; (6) the children's preexisting mental health, developmental level, and baseline resiliency and coping skills; and (7) the nature of the secondary stressors and losses that follow the crisis event. In communities recovering from a disaster, it is therefore often helpful for pediatricians not only to inquire about children's symptoms, but also to ask families about what children were exposed to as a result of the disaster, what they understand about what has happened to their community, any ongoing stressors that may complicate recovery, and additional questions that explore and identify these risk factors (see Table 1).

Most children who are experiencing adjustment difficulties after a disaster may demonstrate no observable symptoms. Children might try to avoid revealing concerns and complaints to not seem odd and not further burden adults in their lives who are having difficulty coping as well. Even children suffering from posttraumatic stress disorder (PTSD) may go undetected unless pediatricians screen or directly inquire about symptoms and adjustment. One of the core criteria of PTSD is an active avoidance of thinking about or talking about the triggering event and one's associated reactions to that event. Making the diagnostic process even more difficult, most of the symptoms of an acute stress disorder or PTSD may not be externally expressed at all (eg, intrusive thoughts). As a result, parents, teachers, and other caregivers tend to underestimate the level of children's distress after a disaster and overestimate their resilience, especially if relying on the observation of overt behaviors rather

TABLE 1 Common Symptoms of Adjustment Reactions in Children after a Disaster[24]

Sleep problems: difficulty falling or staying asleep, frequent night awakenings or difficulty awakening in the morning, nightmares, or other sleep disruptions.

Eating problems: loss of appetite or increased eating.

Sadness or depression: may result in a reluctance to engage in previously enjoyed activities or a withdrawal from peers and adults.

Anxiety, worries, or fears: children may be concerned about a repetition of the traumatic event (eg, become afraid during storms after surviving a tornado) or show an increase in unrelated fears (eg, become more fearful of the dark even if the disaster occurred during daylight). This may present as separation anxiety or school avoidance.

Difficulties in concentration: the ability to learn and retain new information or to otherwise progress academically.

Substance abuse: the new onset or exacerbation of alcohol, tobacco, or other substance use may be seen in children, adolescents, and adults after a disaster.

Risk-taking behavior: increased sexual behavior or other reactive risk-taking can occur, especially among older children and adolescents.

Somatization: children with adjustment difficulties may present instead with physical symptoms suggesting a physical condition.

Developmental or social regression: children (and adults) may become less patient or tolerant of change, revert to bedwetting, or become irritable and disruptive.

Posttraumatic reactions and disorders: see Table 2.

than inquiring specifically about feelings and reactions. The adults' own reactions to the event also may diminish their ability to identify their children's needs with optimal sensitivity or reliability.[8] Finally, the parents' own difficulty adjusting to an event may, in turn, threaten children's sense of safety and security and serve as a negative model of emotional regulation.[9]

Research has shown that after a major disaster, a large proportion of children in the affected community will develop adjustment reactions, with many qualifying for a diagnosis of a mental health condition, often related to trauma, anxiety, or depression.[10] In a study conducted 6 months after the terrorist attacks of September 11, 2001, involving

a representative sample of more than 8000 students in grades 4 through 12 attending New York City public schools, 27% met criteria for 1 or more probable psychiatric disorders on the basis of self-reporting of symptoms and impairment in daily functioning. The study reported the following:

- 11% of students had PTSD;
- 8% of students had major depressive disorder;
- 12% of students had separation anxiety disorder;
- 9% of students had panic attacks; and
- 15% of students had agoraphobia (or fear of going outside or taking public transportation).

Perhaps of even greater concern, at least two-thirds of those students who self-reported mental health symptoms and impairment in daily functioning also reported that they had not sought care, even though free mental health services had been available in their schools. In addition, the vast majority (87%) of all students surveyed reported at least 1 ongoing symptom that persisted 6 months after the event, reported as follows:

- 76% of students reported often thinking about the attacks;
- 45% of students were actively trying to avoid thinking or talking about the event;
- 25% of students were experiencing difficulty concentrating;
- 24% of students were having sleep problems (including 17% with nightmares); and
- 18% of students stopped going to places or doing things that reminded them of the events of September 11.[11]

Because most children experience at least some long-term reactions to a disaster and because many children and families cannot or do not access mental health services for reasons including cost and perceived stigma, it is important to explore strategies that provide interventions and support to all children after a major disaster, rather than relying exclusively on the traditional clinical approach of triage and referral for those patients identified as needing care.

Anticipatory guidance and advice can be provided to families by pediatricians on how to identify and address the most common adjustment reactions that can be anticipated among children after a disaster (see Table 1). For example, sleep problems are common after a disaster, and children who have difficulty sleeping may develop problems with concentration, attention, learning, and academic functioning. Promoting sleep hygiene (eg, providing a consistent, quiet, and comfortable location and time for sleep that is free of noise or other distractions, preceded by a quiet and consistent bedtime ritual), may be difficult but is nonetheless important, especially when families are living in shelters or other temporary sites. Posttraumatic stress reactions are frequently observed immediately after a disaster and can be best explained to children as the way their body automatically responds after an event frightens them. Less commonly, PTSD may develop a while after the traumatic event occurred, especially among children who perceived at the time of the event that their life was in jeopardy or experienced intense fear, helplessness, or horror. Table 2 includes the diagnostic criteria for PTSD, as outlined in the *Diagnostic and Statistical Manual of Mental Disorders, Fifth Edition (DSM-5)*,[12] which include symptoms of intrusion, avoidance, negative alterations in cognitions and mood, and increased arousal that persist for at least 1 month and result in significant impairment in social, academic, or other areas of functioning.

Distress that occurs as a result of children's involvement in a disaster

TABLE 2 Symptoms of Posttraumatic Stress Disorder[24]

Exposure: The child is exposed to actual or threatened death, serious injury, or sexual violence. This may be through the child's direct experience; by witnessing the traumatic event, especially when involving a caretaker; or by the child learning that the traumatic event occurred involving a close family member or friend without any direct experience or witnessing of the event by the child.

The following symptoms must occur for more than 1 month's time:

1. Intrusion
   - The child has repeated distressing memories and/or dreams (nightmares) about the traumatic event; it is not required for children to remember the content of these distressing dreams. For some children, repetitive play activities may involve themes or aspects of the traumatic event.
   - The child may display a loss of awareness of present surroundings (dissociation) and act as if the traumatic event is reoccurring (flashbacks).
   - The child may experience intense or prolonged psychological distress and/or physiologic reactions at exposure to internal or external cues that symbolize or resemble the traumatic event.
2. Avoidance
   - The child attempts to avoid distressing memories, thoughts, feelings, activities, and/or places that remind him or her of the traumatic event.
3. Negative alterations in cognitions and mood
   - The child has problems remembering important aspects of the traumatic event.
   - The child maintains negative beliefs or expectations about oneself, others, or the world.
   - The child has thoughts about the cause or consequences of the traumatic event that lead to blame of self/others.
   - The child experiences negative emotional states, such as depression, and has trouble experiencing and expressing positive emotions.
   - The child shows a markedly diminished interest or participation in significant activities, including play.
   - The child feels distant from others, which may lead the child to become socially withdrawn and avoid people, conversations, or interpersonal situations.
4. Increased arousal and reactivity associated with the traumatic event
   - Irritable and angry outbursts (extreme temper tantrums).
   - Reckless or self-destructive behavior.
   - Hypervigilance.
   - Exaggerated startle response.
   - Problems with concentration.
   - Sleep disturbance.

often creates an additional burden for the children who may have had unresolved predisaster psychopathology or adjustment difficulties. Psychological issues that children have attempted to suppress may resurface, even if these issues are not directly related to the disaster.[10,13] As a result, unrelated events and experiences (eg, previous traumatic events or worries about the health of parents) may be the cause for what appear to be reactions to the disaster itself. This distress may be seen among adults, such as parents, as well.

In a related manner, future events and references that remind children of the losses or disturbing images, sensations, and emotions associated with the disaster event may serve as later triggers of their grief or trauma symptoms. Some examples include

anniversaries of the disaster, severe weather that reminds a child of a natural disaster, persistent signs of destruction in the community, sounds of emergency vehicles, allusions to similar events on television or in classroom lessons, or visits to health care facilities. These reminders may result in an unanticipated, acute resurgence of some of the feelings associated with the loss or crisis and catch children off guard. Parents, educators, and others who work with children should anticipate that such triggers may occur and help children anticipate and plan for how to address these feelings.

BEREAVEMENT AND SECONDARY STRESSES

Whereas the adjustment difficulties (as outlined in Table 1) that children experience after a disaster may be related to posttraumatic reactions, many will not be directly attributable to the disaster itself. Disasters may worsen preexisting problems, such as financial strain, parental depression, parenting challenges, or child behavior problems, which may have been adequately compensated or addressed in a setting of less stress.[14] Disasters often also initiate a cascade of secondary losses and stressors that may become the primary concern for a particular child or family. A child presenting with sleep problems months after a flood may be responding to marital conflict or parental distress related to financial concerns instead of solely struggling to cope with the flooding itself. After a major natural disaster, it is common to see increased unemployment or underemployment resulting in financial stress on families; a need for families to relocate resulting in changes in schools or peer groups for the children; temporary living situations that are suboptimal or causes of interpersonal conflict; or depression, substance use, or marital conflict among parents. Such an increase in marital stress, domestic violence, and parental mental health problems was demonstrated in the Gulf Coast region after Hurricane Katrina.[15,16] Child abuse has also been reported to increase after major disasters.[17] Pediatricians may see children and families dealing with such issues even if the children or adults in the family did not experience the disaster itself as traumatic but instead are reacting to secondary losses or stressors. Management of these concerns requires a different approach than trauma treatment; pediatricians need to adopt a more holistic approach to assessing adjustment and promoting coping and resiliency among children and families after a disaster. Assessments need not only to explore how children are adjusting with the disaster event itself, but also to seek information about their current life circumstances and how they are

dealing with the challenges these circumstances may pose. Given that children may withhold voicing their concerns in the presence of their parents or other family members so as not to further burden the adults who may be in distress themselves, it is important to interview the children alone with the parents' permission and child's assent when trying to assess fully their level of coping.

Given that these secondary losses and stressors may continue for even several years after a major disaster, children's adjustment difficulties may persist for a similarly extended time. Children's adjustment should not be expected before the restoration and stabilization of the home, school, and community environments and supports for children, which may not return to being fully functional for several years.

If children experience the deaths of family members or friends as a result of the disaster, bereavement may emerge as their predominant concern. In most situations, bereavement in the context of a disaster is not dissimilar from bereavement occurring in other contexts; when children have observed a violent death of a loved one, grief may be compounded by trauma reactions requiring treatment of trauma in addition to bereavement support. Children, like adults, will struggle with understanding and accepting the death and the effect it has on them and their family and the challenge of a life devoid of someone they loved.[18] Parents, teachers, and other caring adults are often reluctant to talk with children who are grieving or even to raise the topic out of a fear of causing further distress by saying the "wrong thing." Yet, the distress is caused by the reaction to the death itself, rather than any question or invitation to talk. Talking may provide some relief if not coerced. Avoiding discussion is rarely helpful and often isolates children at a time

when they are most in need of support and assistance.

Pediatricians and other pediatric health care providers can serve as a useful resource for children who have recently experienced the death of a close family member or friend by helping their caregivers understand the importance of inviting and answering their questions, providing information to help guide them in understanding and adjusting to the loss, and helping them identify strategies for coping with the associated distress. Timely information about how to involve children in the funeral or other memorialization activities, how to enlist the support of school personnel, and bereavement support services available within the community are helpful to provide, through in-person meetings, phone calls, or psychoeducational material. Practical and free resources are available for this purpose[19] (see www.aap.org/disasters/adjustment and www.achildingrief.com). A resource offering free multimedia training materials on how to support grieving children is available through the Coalition to Support Grieving Students at www.grievingstudents.org. Practical guidance on how to approach notification of children about the death of a family member or friend,[20] including within the unique context of a disaster,[21] can be found elsewhere.

RISK FACTORS FOR ADJUSTMENT DIFFICULTIES AND GUIDELINES FOR REFERRAL

In the immediate aftermath of a disaster, pediatricians need to assess both the physical and mental health of children. The primary focus is, of necessity, medical stabilization and evaluation, but a secondary mental health triage should follow shortly thereafter. Table 3 outlines the factors to be assessed during this mental health triage to identify children most in need of mental health services or other immediate attention to their mental health needs. The following factors, in particular, suggest the need for immediate mental health services: (1) dissociative symptoms, such as detachment, derealization, or depersonalization, which may present in children as appearing confused, distant, daydreaming, or aloof (such dissociation at the time of exposure has been found to be the most significant predictor of later PTSD); (2) extreme confusion or inability to concentrate or make even simple decisions; (3) evidence of extreme cognitive impairment or intrusive thoughts; (4) intense fear, anxiety, panic, helplessness, or horror; (5) depression at the time of the event[13]; (6) uncontrollable and intense grief; (7) suicidal ideation or intent; and (8)

TABLE 3 Factors Associated With an Increased Risk of Adjustment Problems After a Disaster[24]

1. Preexisting factors
   - Previous psychopathology, significant losses, attachment disturbances, limited coping skills, or other traumatic events.
   - Socioeconomic differences that result in lower levels of postdisaster resources and support.
2. Nature of disaster experience
   - Injury of the child or death or injury of those close to the child.
   - Nature and extent of exposure, including number of deaths, physical proximity to disaster, and extent of personal loss. Human-made disasters, especially terrorist attacks that have a high degree of intentionality, generally create reactions that are more prevalent and long-lasting.
   - Extent of exposure to horrific scenes (including indirectly through the media).
   - Child's perception (at the time of the event) that his or her life was in jeopardy.
3. Subsequent factors
   - Personal identification with the disaster or victims.
   - Separation of child from parents or other important caregivers as result of event.
   - Loss of property or belongings; need to relocate or other disruption in daily routine or environment.
   - Parental difficulty in coping, substance abuse, mental illness.
   - Lack of supportive family communication style.
   - Lack of community resources and support.

marked physical complaints resulting from somatization.[22] When children's caregivers are struggling themselves to cope with the event, helping the caregivers access services for themselves and/or providing a referral to a mental health provider to assist with children's coping also may be indicated.

Children's adjustment and resiliency depend on a number of factors that relate to the nature of the event itself (such as how much damage or death resulted from the event); the degree of personal effects on children or those close to them in terms of death, disability, injury, or loss of property or damage to housing; the level of exposure involving direct witnessing or viewing graphic coverage through the media or online; the degree and duration of secondary losses and stressors; the disruption caused to children's extended support system and the level of adaptation of caregivers and the degree to which they are able to create a safe and nurturing environment that promotes recovery for the children; and the nature of children's preexisting coping abilities.[23,24] Table 3 outlines the factors before, during, and after a disaster that are associated with an increased risk of difficulty adjusting after a disaster.

Separation from parents or other important caregivers is associated with increased difficulty adjusting to a disaster. Efforts to reunite children who are separated from their family by the event are a high priority.[25,26] In those situations in which children require medical treatment or observation before reunification is possible, individual volunteers can be assigned to provide consistent and ongoing support to individual children until reunification is achieved. When parents, guardians, or other family members are available, guidance by the health care team can help them serve an active and appropriate role in the evaluation and

treatment process and can help to reduce their children's distress.[3]

BASIC SUPPORTIVE SERVICES AND PSYCHOLOGICAL FIRST AID

Attention to the basic needs of individuals affected by a disaster is a top priority for the immediate response. Basic needs include food, shelter, safety, supervision, communication, and reunification with loved ones. Ensuring that these basic needs are addressed is the first step to providing emotional support.

In addition, all individuals directly affected by a disaster should be provided psychological first aid, which involves psychoeducation and supportive services to accelerate the natural healing process and promote effective coping strategies. Psychological first aid includes providing timely and accurate information to promote an understanding that will facilitate adjustment, offering appropriate (but not false) reassurance that corrects misconceptions and misperceptions that might otherwise unnecessarily increase the appraisal of risk, supplying information about likely reactions and practical strategies to facilitate coping with distress, and helping people identify supports in their family and useful resources in their community.[27] One such model for psychological first aid that is readily accessible to those outside the mental health field is Listen, Protect, and Connect.[28] Pediatricians and other pediatric health care providers should ensure that all staff in their practice setting, including front office and support staff, are familiar with psychological first aid and ready to provide such support to children and adults in the aftermath of a disaster. Given that children and families who present to health care settings are often in distress, these are useful skills that can be used on a daily basis even outside the context of a disaster. In addition, having other adults who care for children, such as staff within child care facilities and schools, also be familiar with these strategies is important to create resilient communities that are able to support children in the aftermath of a disaster.

NOTIFICATION AND MEDIA COVERAGE

Children should be informed about a disaster as soon as information becomes available. Children can sense when critical information is being withheld and when trusted adults are not being genuine; this, in turn, undermines their trust and sense of safety and compromises the ability of these adults to be later viewed as a source of support and assistance. Even very young children or those with developmental disabilities can sense the distress of trusted adults. Children also often overhear or otherwise learn information about the events, such as through the Internet or social media or from conversations with other children.

The amount of information to share with individual children may vary by the developmental level of the children or their typical coping strategies. In general, older children seek and benefit from more information. Irrespective of their age, children who generally cope by learning more and understanding more about a threat will often seek and benefit from a deeper understanding. But no matter the developmental level or usual coping style, it is best to start with simple and basic facts about the event and then take the lead from children's questions that follow about what further information or explanations will be helpful. If some time has passed since the event, children can be asked what they may have already heard or learned about the event and what questions they now have. In this way, misunderstandings and misconceptions can be identified and addressed. The goal is to help

children feel they understand what is going on enough for them to know how best to deal with the situation.

Media coverage often contains graphic images and details, evocative pictures or stories, or strong emotional content that is not helpful for children or adults. Technological advances and changes in the mass media landscape now offer a stage unlike any in history, from which disaster events can reach an enormous audience in real-time. Continuous news coverage, broadcast over the ubiquitous presence of televisions, personal computers, the Internet, and smartphones, and an increasingly sophisticated technology for live broadcasts has resulted in the unprecedented coverage of disasters in real-time and exquisite detail, allowing viewers to experience the event almost as if they were physically present. This expanded media presence has led to a broader population of children and youth with either primary or secondary exposure to an event.[8,29,30]

Parents should, therefore, limit the amount of media coverage in the immediate aftermath of a disaster for children and all members of the family, including television, radio, Internet, and social media, and remember that children often overhear and pick up on media coverage being viewed by adults. If media coverage is going to be viewed by children, parents may want to record and view it first and/ or watch along with children. In discussions, avoid graphic details and excessive information that is not helpful to understand what has happened or learn what to do to keep safe or to cope. If no further understanding is resulting from continued viewing of coverage of the event, then it is best for even adults to discontinue such viewing. Right after a disaster occurs is a good time to turn off electronic devices that are being used for entertainment and come together physically and

emotionally as a family unit to provide support to one another.

PROMOTING EFFECTIVE COPING STRATEGIES

Advocating specific coping strategies for children after a disaster can be challenging because of the interaction among a number of factors, including a child's personal characteristics, preexisting functioning, and developmental level.[10] Research on stress management has demonstrated that directly facing a problem is associated with better outcomes, and avoiding the situation or only reacting emotionally can be more problematic, but outcomes may vary depending on the nature of the stressors. Problem-focused coping may be most beneficial when stressors can be controlled by the child. Avoidant or emotion-focused coping might be more productive when stressors cannot be removed.[31] The influence of a child's caregivers is also important to consider; parents and other caring adults may be so overwhelmed themselves after a disaster that they are unable to appreciate the distress in their children. Adults often hide their own distress to protect their children or provide them false reassurance; they may intentionally or unintentionally imply that children should not be upset. In reality, if children feel worried, then they are worried. Telling them that they should not be worried is usually ineffective and undermines the potential for children to own their feelings and learn strategies to deal with them.

Although it is important for children to be encouraged to express their feelings and concerns, it is equally important that adults help foster a range of coping skills in children so that they have strategies they can use to address distress and troubling feelings. If parents can communicate some of their own distress, with an emphasis on sharing personal strategies they have used to cope effectively with that distress (that may be applicable to the children), they provide opportunities for children to learn coping strategies. For example, a parent can share that he was upset about the destruction of their home and loss of personal property and that this interfered with his sleep or caused some sadness, and then discuss how talking to another trusted adult, getting some exercise, meditating, helping others who were also affected, and so forth, helped him feel better. Pediatricians can support families by providing examples of a variety of coping strategies (eg, both problem focused and emotion focused, approach and avoidance) while modeling emotional regulation and a positive attitude. Suggesting that children contribute to a food or clothing drive for those who lost their homes or draw hopeful pictures for victims in hospitals can help children feel like they are contributing. Adolescents may wish to write positive comments in social media to encourage those who may be isolated and distressed after a disaster. Children may also benefit from the pediatrician sharing his or her own understanding of the disaster and recovery process which will help children better interpret all that is going on (eg, "The tornado created a big mess, but we are pulling together as a community," or "Living in a shelter with all the other children in the neighborhood must have been a real adventure"). Communicating with children in this manner after a disaster may help them begin to make sense of all that has occurred and increase their self-confidence because they have coped with an event that once appeared overwhelming.

Children may feel guilt or shame associated with the disaster, even when they have no objective reason to feel responsible. They may question what they did or failed to do that led to or contributed to the

impact of the disaster; they may wonder what they could have done to have improved the outcome. It is often helpful to reassure children about their lack of responsibility. When children persist in beliefs that their inadvertent comments or actions were somehow contributory (eg, a child has an argument with a parent just before the parent is killed in a car accident during a severe storm), it may be helpful to clarify that their behavior or conversation was in no way intended to cause such harm and did not do so. Although such guilt and shame may be common in the aftermath of a disaster, if left unaddressed, these painful self-incriminating emotions may cause significant distress and long-term adjustment problems. Self-blame and survivor's guilt may remain with children and can lead to long-term difficulties.[32]

Children, just as do adults, often feel powerless in the aftermath of a disaster; this may be improved if they are able to help others. It is, therefore, beneficial to help children identify practical actions they can take to aid others, whether victims of the disaster or others in need in the family or broader community.

Psychotropic medications should generally be avoided in the management of children's distress after a disaster. Children need to develop an understanding of the event and learn to express and cope with their reactions. Medication should, therefore, not be used to suppress reactions such as crying or feelings such as sadness and should not be used to blunt children's awareness of the event. Referral to or consultation with a child mental health professional with expertise in the management of childhood trauma is recommended for primary care providers when considering use of psychotropic medications for persistent or severe posttraumatic reactions.[21]

CONSULTATION TO SCHOOLS

Pediatricians can work with local schools to assist in recovery efforts for students. After a disaster, schools are likely to see negative effects on learning among their students, and staff may find it difficult to teach or manage their classes unless adequate supports are put in place immediately after the disaster and maintained until recovery has been completed. Schools can serve as an effective means to reach the broad population of children and families affected by the disaster and a cost-effective and accessible site for the delivery of basic and supportive services by professionals already familiar to the students and trusted by the families. Schools are also sites that are amenable to psychoeducation, psychological first aid, and group supportive services. Schools are particularly well suited to monitoring children's adjustment over time and can be used to provide additional mental health services or referral to community services.

Schools should have well-established guidelines for crisis response and well-trained crisis response teams.[33,34] All school staff should have basic skills in psychological first aid[28] and basic bereavement support.[18,35] Resources for training and guidance for schools responding to crisis and loss can be found at the Web site for the National Center for School Crisis and Bereavement (www.schoolcrisiscenter.org) and the Coalition to Support Grieving Students (www.grievingstudents.org).

SHORT- AND LONG-TERM INTERVENTIONS

The goal of short-term intervention is to address immediate physical needs and to keep children safe and protected from additional harm; to help children understand and begin to accept the disaster; to identify, express, validate, and cope with their feelings and reactions; to reestablish a sense of safety through routines and family connections; to start to regain a sense of mastery and control over their life; and to return to child care or school and other developmentally appropriate activities.[21,36] Children who are grieving the loss of a family member or friend may benefit from bereavement counseling or support. Those experiencing or at high-risk of developing PTSD should be offered referral to a mental health professional experienced in cognitive-behavioral therapy that addresses trauma. School-based group treatment using cognitive-behavioral treatment approaches, such as Cognitive-Behavioral Intervention for Trauma in Schools, also has been shown to be effective.[37] Children with multiple stressors and/or chronic and ongoing trauma and those with limited external supports within their family, school, and broader community are more likely to require counseling or other formal support.

In general, children are helped by returning to their routine, such as child care, school, organized activities, and sports, as soon as practical after a disaster, as long as the necessary support systems and accommodations (such as temporarily reducing or providing more time for homework assignments or tests) are in place. Expectations for children's classroom performance and behavior may need to be modified until their adjustment difficulties no longer interfere with their cognitive, emotional, and social functioning. Parents and educators may be falsely reassured, however, by a return to routine, misinterpreting that children are more resilient than they may be and are no longer in need of support or assistance once they have begun the process of recovery. Children often need ongoing support for months or longer after a major disaster, and some will require more intensive interventions. If supports and assistance are withdrawn before full recovery has occurred, some children will fail to return to their baseline level of

adjustment and coping and may show continued impairment for an extended period of time.

In the immediate aftermath of a disaster, communities often become more cohesive for a time period, with members of the community providing and receiving support that had not been expressed before the disaster. This "honeymoon phase" is often characterized by some initial improvement in coping among members of the community but is often not sustained. Some vulnerable individuals, despite an initial improvement, may be challenged without ongoing support; they may come to feel hopeless about their ability to return to their baseline functioning or doubt they will ever recover fully. Depression and suicidality, especially among adults, may therefore be seen later, such as several months after the disaster event, despite initial improvement but before substantial recovery occurs. These observations have been noted among communities affected by major disasters and represent an important vulnerability.[38,39]

In contrast, if children and adults receive sufficient and sustained support, and have the internal resources to adjust to the event, they may emerge with new skills that they can use to cope with future adversity. In this way, disasters may result in posttraumatic growth among both children and adults. Such posttraumatic growth is more likely to occur when children are provided support of sufficient intensity and duration.[24]

Schools also can provide opportunities for students to help others as they and their communities recover from the event and its aftermath. Having the opportunity to help others often assists in the adjustment and coping of the students providing such assistance. Schools also can help students identify appropriate mechanisms for memorialization and

commemoration. These activities provide a means for expressing grief and loss in a shared fashion, thereby decreasing isolation and promoting cohesion. When deaths have occurred as a result of the disaster, these means of remembrance can reaffirm the personal attachment to the individual(s) who died and reassure the bereaved that the loved one will be remembered. Any such activities should involve the active participation of children and adolescents both in the planning and implementation to ensure that they are developmentally appropriate and personally relevant for them. Simply put, a memorial planned by adults for children is most likely to be therapeutic for the adults.[18]

PROFESSIONAL SELF-CARE

Pediatricians, when they are members of the community affected by a disaster, also experience their own personal effects as well as the effects on family and friends. Despite this, they must contend with the increased needs of their patients during a time when conditions may be austere and the supports available for the practice of medicine may be significantly compromised. Physicians may find that they need to provide more direct mental health services and basic medical services while also helping families navigate the process to obtain social services. The "emotional labor" during disasters can be highly strenuous. In addition, it can be difficult to witness the distress of patients and their families (as well as that of other staff); vicarious traumatization can result from repeated exposure to the evocative stories of patients and their families. Reminding oneself that one is making a positive impact, when surrounded by enormous needs that seem beyond one's control, can be challenging. Establishment of flexible routines, monitoring oneself for negative thoughts, creating realistic professional expectations, setting healthy boundaries between personal time and professional hours, practicing daily personal stress management, making a conscious attempt to reduce compassion fatigue, and use of both professional and social supports, including counseling, will increase the likelihood that pediatricians will remain able to attend to the needs and feelings of their patients as well as their own.[6]

Pediatricians, as a group, need to acknowledge that it is acceptable to be upset when situations are particularly distressing, need to become willing to ask for and accept assistance whenever it may be helpful (as opposed to only when it is "absolutely needed"), and need to actively take steps to care for their colleagues and themselves. The American Academy of Pediatrics has identified a range of resources that pediatric health care providers can use to promote the recovery of children, families, and communities (www.aap.org/disasters/adjustment). As a professional organization, the American Academy of Pediatrics has identified professional self-care as an important priority and has focused funding, strategic planning efforts, and continuing education initiatives in this area.

Most pediatricians enter the profession because of a heartfelt desire to help children and families most in need. If adequately prepared and supported, pediatricians who are able to draw on their skills to assist children, families, and communities to recover after a disaster will find the work to be particularly rewarding, although at times exhausting. There are few other opportunities to have such a dramatic effect on the lives of children, their families, and the community.

LEAD AUTHORS

David J. Schonfeld, MD, FAAP
Thomas Demaria, PhD

DISASTER PREPAREDNESS ADVISORY COUNCIL, 2014-2015

Steven Elliot Krug, MD, FAAP, Chairperson
Sarita Chung, MD, FAAP
Daniel B. Fagbuyi, MD, FAAP
Margaret C. Fisher, MD, FAAP
Scott Needle, MD, FAAP
David J. Schonfeld, MD, FAAP

LIAISONS

John James Alexander, MD, FAAP – *US Food and Drug Administration*
Daniel Dodgen, PhD – *Office of the Assistant Secretary for Preparedness and Response*
Andrew L. Garrett, MD, MPH, FAAP – *Office of the Assistant Secretary for Preparedness and Response*
Georgina Peacock, MD, MPH, FAAP – *Centers for Disease Control and Prevention*
Sally Phillips, RN, PhD – *Department of Homeland Security, Office of Health Affairs*
Erica Radden, MD – *US Food and Drug Administration*
David Alan Siegel, MD, FAAP – *National Institute of Child Health and Human Development*

STAFF

Laura Aird, MS
Sean Diederich
Tamar Magarik Haro

COMMITTEE ON PSYCHOSOCIAL ASPECTS OF CHILD AND FAMILY HEALTH, 2014-2015

Michael W. Yogman, MD, FAAP, Chairperson
Thresia B. Gambon, MD, FAAP
Arthur Lavin, MD, FAAP
LTC Keith M. Lemmon, MD, FAAP
Gerri Mattson, MD, FAAP
Laura Joan McGuinn, MD, FAAP
Jason Richard Rafferty, MD, MPH, EdM
Lawrence Sagin Wissow, MD, MPH, FAAP

LIAISONS

Sharon Berry, PhD, LP – *Society of Pediatric Psychology*
Terry Carmichael, MSW – *National Association of Social Workers*
Edward R. Christophersen, PhD, FAAP – *Society of Pediatric Psychology*
Norah L. Johnson, PhD, RN, CPNP-BC – *National Association of Pediatric Nurse Practitioners*
Leonard Read Sulik, MD, FAAP – *American Academy of Child and Adolescent Psychiatry*

CONSULTANT

George J. Cohen, MD, FAAP

STAFF

Stephanie Domain, MS, CHES
Tamar Magarik Haro

ABBREVIATION

PTSD: posttraumatic stress disorder

REFERENCES

1. Becker-Blease KA, Turner HA, Finkelhor D. Disasters, victimization, and children's mental health. *Child Dev.* 2010;81(4):1040–1052

2. Chrisman AK, Dougherty JG. Mass trauma: disasters, terrorism, and war. *Child Adolesc Psychiatr Clin N Am.* 2014;23(2):257–279

3. American Academy of Pediatrics, Disaster Preparedness Advisory Council, Committee on Pediatric Emergency Medicine. Ensuring the health of children in disasters. In press

4. Institute of Medicine. *Preparing for the Psychological Consequences of Terrorism: A Public Health Strategy.* Washington, DC: National Academics Press; 2003

5. Hu YY, Adams RE, Boscarino JA, Laraque D. Training needs of pediatricians facing the environmental health and bioterrorism consequences of September 11th. *Mt Sinai J Med.* 2006;73(8):1156–1164

6. Madrid PA, Grant R, Reilly MJ, Redlener NB. Challenges in meeting immediate emotional needs: short-term impact of a major disaster on children's mental health: building resiliency in the aftermath of Hurricane Katrina. *Pediatrics.* 2006;117(5 pt 3):S448–S453

7. Schonfeld DJ, Gurwitch RH. Addressing disaster mental health needs of children: practical guidance for pediatric emergency health care providers. *Clin Pediatr Emerg Med.* 2009;10(3):208–215

8. Furr JM, Comer JS, Edmunds JM, Kendall PC. Disasters and youth: a meta-analytic examination of posttraumatic stress. *J Consult Clin Psychol.* 2010;78(6):765–780

9. Blaustein M, Kinniburgh KM. *Treating Traumatic Stress in Children and Adolescents: How to Foster Resilience Through Attachment, Self-Regulation, and Competency.* New York, NY: Guilford Press; 2010

10. Pfefferbaum B, Noffsinger MA, Wind LH, Allen JR. Children's coping in the context of disasters and terrorism. *J Loss Trauma.* 2014;9(1):78–97

11. Hoven CW, Duarte CS, Lucas CP, et al. Psychopathology among New York city public school children 6 months after September 11. *Arch Gen Psychiatry.* 2005;62(5):545–552

12. American Psychiatric Association. *Diagnostic and Statistical Manual of Mental Disorders, Fifth Edition (DSM-5)*. Washington, DC: American Psychiatric Association; 2013

13. Lai BS, La Greca AM, Auslander BA, Short MB. Children's symptoms of posttraumatic stress and depression after a natural disaster: comorbidity and risk factors. *J Affect Disord*. 2013;146(1):71–78

14. Scaramella LV, Sohr-Preston SL, Callahan KL, Mirabile SP. A test of the Family Stress Model on toddler-aged children's adjustment among Hurricane Katrina impacted and nonimpacted low-income families. *J Clin Child Adolesc Psychol*. 2008;37(3):530–541

15. Larrance R, Anastario M, Lawry L. Health status among internally displaced persons in Louisiana and Mississippi travel trailer parks. *Ann Emerg Med*. 2007;49(5):590–601, 601. e1–601.e12

16. Norris FH, Friedman MJ, Watson PJ. 60,000 disaster victims speak: Part II. Summary and implications of the disaster mental health research. *Psychiatry*. 2002;65(3):240–260

17. Curtis T, Miller BC, Berry EH. Changes in reports and incidence of child abuse following natural disasters. *Child Abuse Negl*. 2000;24(9):1151–1162

18. Schonfeld DJ, Quackenbush M. *The Grieving Student: A Teacher's Guide*. Baltimore, MD: Brookes Publishing; 2010

19. Schonfeld DJ, Quackenbush M. *After a Loved One Dies—How Children Grieve and How Parents and Other Adults Can Support Them*. New York, NY: New York Life Foundation; 2009

20. Schonfeld DJ. Providing support for families experiencing the death of a child. In: Kreitler S, Ben-Arush MW, Martin A, eds. *Pediatric Psycho-Oncology: Psychosocial Aspects and Clinical Interventions*. 2nd ed. West Sussex, UK: John Wiley & Sons, Ltd; 2012:223–230

21. Foltin GL, Schonfeld DJ, Shannon MW, eds. Pediatric Terrorism and Disaster Preparedness: A Resource for Pediatricians. Rockville, MD: Agency for Healthcare Research and Quality; 2006. AHRQ publication 06-0056-EF

22. Schonfeld D. Providing psychological first aid and identifying mental health needs in the aftermath of a disaster or community crisis. In: Foltin G, Tunik M, Treiber M, Cooper A, eds. Pediatric Disaster Preparedness: A Resource for Planning, Management, and Provision of Out-of-Hospital Emergency Care. New York, NY: Center for Pediatric Emergency Medicine; 2008. Available at http://cpem.med.nyu.edu/teaching-materials/pediatric-disaster-preparedness. Accessed July 27, 2015

23. Masten AS, Narayan AJ. Child development in the context of disaster, war, and terrorism: pathways of risk and resilience. *Annu Rev Psychol*. 2012;63:227–257

24. Schonfeld DJ, Gurwitch RH. Children in disasters. In: Elzouki AY, Stapleton FB, Whitley RJ, Oh W, Harfi HA, Nazer H, eds. *Textbook of Clinical Pediatrics*. 2nd ed. New York, NY: Springer-Verlag; 2012:687–698

25. Federal Emergency Management Agency. Post-disaster reunification of children: a nationwide approach. Available at: www.fema.gov/media-library-data/1384376663394-eef4a1b4269de14faff40390e4e2f2d3/Post%20Disaster%20Reunification%20of%20Children%20-%20A%20Nationwide%20Approach.pdf. Accessed July 27, 2015

26. Kimmer S, Altman B, Strauss-Riggs K. Tracking and reunification of children in disasters: a lesson and reference for health professionals. National Center for Disaster Medicine and Public Health Web site. Available at: http://ncdmph.usuhs.edu/KnowledgeLearning/2012-Learning1.htm. Accessed July 27, 2015

27. American Red Cross. *Foundations of Disaster Mental Health*. Washington, DC: American Red Cross; 2006

28. Schreiber M, Gurwitch R, Wong M. Listen, protect, connect—model & teach: psychological first aid (PFA) for students and teachers. 2006. Available at: www.ready.gov/sites/default/files/documents/files/PFA_SchoolCrisis.pdf. Accessed July 27, 2015

29. Ortiz CD, Silverman WK, Jaccard J, La Greca AM. Children's state anxiety in reaction to disaster media cues: a preliminary test of a multivariate model. *Psychol Trauma*. 2011;3(2):157–164

30. Comer JS, Furr JM, Beidas RS, Babyar HM, Kendall PC. Media use and children's perceptions of societal threat and personal vulnerability. *J Clin Child Adolesc Psychol*. 2008;37(3):622–630

31. Compas BE, Connor-Smith JK, Saltzman H, Thomsen AH, Wadsworth ME. Coping with stress during childhood and adolescence: problems, progress, and potential in theory and research. *Psychol Bull*. 2001;127(1):87–127

32. Rojas VM, Lee TN. *Childhood vs. Adults PTSD. Posttraumatic Stress Disorders in Children and Adolescents: Handbook*. New York, NY: W.W. Norton & Co Inc; 2004:237–256

33. Schonfeld DJ. *How to Prepare for and Respond to a Crisis*. 2nd ed. Alexandria, VA: Association for Supervision and Curriculum Development; 2002

34. Grant L, Schonfeld D. Emergency and disaster preparedness in schools. In: Gereige RS, Zenni EA, eds. *School Health: Policy and Practice*. 7th ed. Elk Grove Village, IL: American Academy of Pediatrics; 2015

35. Coalition to Support Grieving Students. Available at: www.grievingstudents.org. Accessed July 27, 2015

36. Schonfeld DJ. Helping children deal with terrorism. In: Osborn LM, DeWitt TG, First LR, Zenel JA, eds. *Pediatrics*. Philadelphia, PA: Elsevier Mosby; 2005:1600–1602

37. Jaycox LH, Kataoka SH, Stein BD, Langley AK, Wong M. Cognitive behavioral intervention for trauma in schools. *Journal of Applied School Psychology*. 2012;28(3):239–255

38. Lai BS, Auslander BA, Fitzpatrick SL, Podkowirow V. Disasters and depressive symptoms in children: a review. *Child Youth Care Forum*. 2014;43(4):489–504

39. van der Velden PG, Wong A, Boshuizen HC, Grievink L. Persistent mental health disturbances during the 10 years after a disaster: four-wave longitudinal comparative study. *Psychiatry Clin Neurosci*. 2013;67(2):110–118

CLINICAL REPORT Guidance for the Clinician in Rendering Pediatric Care

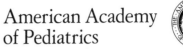

American Academy
of Pediatrics

DEDICATED TO THE HEALTH OF ALL CHILDREN™

Psychosocial Factors in Children and Youth With Special Health Care Needs and Their Families

Gerri Mattson, MD, MSPH, FAAP,[a] Dennis Z. Kuo, MD, MHS, FAAP,[b] COMMITTEE ON PSYCHOSOCIAL ASPECTS OF CHILD AND FAMILY HEALTH, COUNCIL ON CHILDREN WITH DISABILITIES

abstract

Children and youth with special health care needs (CYSHCN) and their families may experience a variety of internal (ie, emotional and behavioral) and external (ie, interpersonal, financial, housing, and educational) psychosocial factors that can influence their health and wellness. Many CYSHCN and their families are resilient and thrive. Medical home teams can partner with CYSHCN and their families to screen for, evaluate, and promote psychosocial health to increase protective factors and ameliorate risk factors. Medical home teams can promote protective psychosocial factors as part of coordinated, comprehensive chronic care for CYSHCN and their families. A team-based care approach may entail collaboration across the care spectrum, including youth, families, behavioral health providers, specialists, child care providers, schools, social services, and other community agencies. The purpose of this clinical report is to raise awareness of the impact of psychosocial factors on the health and wellness of CYSHCN and their families. This clinical report provides guidance for pediatric providers to facilitate and coordinate care that can have a positive influence on the overall health, wellness, and quality of life of CYSHCN and their families.

[a]Children and Youth Branch, Division of Public Health, North Carolina Department of Health and Human Services, Raleigh, North Carolina; and [b]Department of Pediatrics, University at Buffalo, Buffalo, New York

Drs Mattson and Kuo conceptualized, designed, drafted, reviewed, and revised the manuscript, approved the final manuscript as submitted, and agree to be accountable for all aspects of the work.

DOI: https://doi.org/10.1542/peds.2018-3171

Address correspondence to Gerri Mattson, MD, MSPH, FAAP. E-mail: gerri.mattson@dhhs.nc.gov

To cite: Mattson G, Kuo DZ, AAP COMMITTEE ON PSYCHOSOCIAL ASPECTS OF CHILD AND FAMILY HEALTH, AAP COUNCIL ON CHILDREN WITH DISABILITIES. Psychosocial Factors in Children and Youth With Special Health Care Needs and Their Families. Pediatrics. 2019;143(1):e20183171

INTRODUCTION

Children and youth with special health care needs (CYSHCN) are "those who have or are at increased risk for a chronic physical, developmental, behavioral, or emotional condition and who also require health and related services of a type or amount beyond that required for children generally."[1] This definition has been used to guide the development of family-centered, coordinated systems of care for children with special needs and families who are served by many public and private health systems, most notably by state Title V block programs administered by the federal Maternal and Child Health Bureau. This report highlights psychosocial internal (emotional or behavioral) and external (interpersonal, housing, and financial) risk and protective factors that impact growth and development, health and wellness, and quality of life for CYSHCN and their families.[2] The report offers guidance for pediatric providers to address psychosocial risk and protective factors as part of comprehensive, coordinated care within the medical home. Such care should be delivered in partnership with families, mental and behavioral health providers, child care settings, schools, social services, and other professionals and community agencies across the care spectrum. This report complements other pediatric literature in which screening and surveillance, discussion, and the management of threats to social, behavioral, emotional, and mental health in all children are addressed.[3–7]

CHANGING EPIDEMIOLOGY OF CYSHCN

According to the 2016 National Survey of Children's Health (NSCH), 19.4% of children and youth have special health care needs.[8] This is an increase from 15.1% found in the 2009–2010 National Survey of Children with Special Health Care Needs.[9] Racial and ethnic disparities are seen in prevalence, resource use, and survival rates between children who have more medically complex and less complex physical, mental health, and developmental conditions.[10–16] Studies reveal that families caring for CYSHCN experience more significant financial and caregiving demands than families of children without special health care needs.[8,9,17] Few CYSHCN (3.8%) were reported to be uninsured on the 2016 NSCH, but 29.6% of parents of CYSHCN reported inadequate insurance coverage, compared with 23.6% of parents of children without special health care needs.[8]

National surveys have shown a significant increase in the overall prevalence and severity of specific chronic conditions, including asthma, diabetes mellitus, and obesity.[11,18–22] The 2015 data from the National Health Interview Survey of the Centers for Disease Control and Prevention show a current overall asthma prevalence of 8.4% among children younger than 18 years. However, there is racial disparity, as non-Hispanic African American children have a 13.4% prevalence of asthma.[18] There have been disproportionate increases in the prevalence of obesity and severe obesity among Hispanic, non-Hispanic African American, and American Indian and/or Alaskan native children.[20,21,23] There is also a disproportionate increase in type 2 diabetes mellitus, which is believed to be related to increasing rates of obesity,[24,25] especially in African American and American Indian and/or Alaskan native children.[22–25]

The prevalence of children with medical complexity (CMC), who represent the most resource-intensive subset of CYSHCN, is also increasing. CMC typically include children with congenital, genetic, or acquired multisystem conditions who have multiple subspecialty needs as well as children with a dependence on technology for daily needs.[17,26,27] The increase in CMC is possibly related to advances in neonatal care and additional life-saving technologies.[28–30] Despite being a small subset of CYSHCN, CMC account for an increasing proportion of pediatric inpatient admissions, with hospitalization rates that doubled between 1991 and 2005.[31,32]

The overall prevalence of children with a behavioral, mental health, learning, or developmental disability as their primary chronic health condition is increasing in the United States.[6,7] Parent surveys indicate that the prevalence of attention-deficit/hyperactivity disorder (ADHD)

(currently 8.9% of children),[8] autism spectrum disorders (2.5% of children),[8] and bipolar disorders (2.2% among youth)[33] have increased over the last 2 decades.[6,7,34] ADHD has been found to be highest in the non-Hispanic multiracial group and lowest among Hispanic children. Behavioral or conduct problems are highest among non-Hispanic African American children, and autism spectrum disorders tend to be higher among non-Hispanic white children.[7] Speech disorders, ADHD, and learning disabilities are among the leading causes of limitations in play or school for children attributable to a chronic condition, and there has been a receding in importance between 1979 and 2009 in the numbers of respiratory, eye, ear, and orthopedic conditions that cause limitations for children.[35]

According to the 2016 NSCH, 42.4% of CYSHCN were reported to have an emotional, developmental, or behavioral issue.[8] Behavioral health can strongly influence health and wellness outcomes for all children and especially for CYSHCN.[36] Reviews of the literature have shown that children with chronic physical health and developmental conditions are at an increased risk for having co-occurring mental health or behavioral problems or conditions.[37,38] Internalizing problems and conditions, ranging from low self-esteem and worry to depression and anxiety, can occur in CYSHCN. CYSHCN also can experience externalizing problems and conditions, ranging from attention problems and defiant and aggressive behaviors to ADHD, conduct disorder, and oppositional defiant disorder.[38–40]

Associations of chronic illnesses with psychological and behavioral conditions, such as anxiety and depression, are well described. Such associations may be explained by biological causes, such as inflammatory processes with asthma or diabetes, and psychological causes, such as the stress of living with an adverse and potentially life-threatening condition.[36,41,42] Studies in adults reveal that comorbid mental and physical illnesses can result in more health care service needs, functional impairment, and higher medical costs compared with similar physical illnesses without the co-occurring mental health condition.[43] Fewer studies have been conducted in children, but 1 study suggests that mental health encounters may encompass a large proportion of outpatient use for some CMC.[44] A focus on psychosocial factors and wellness would appear to be an important addition to the overall chronic care model for CYSHCN.[36]

IMPACT OF PSYCHOSOCIAL FACTORS ON OVERALL HEALTH AND WELLNESS FOR CYSHCN AND THEIR FAMILIES

The biological, physical, emotional, and social environments strongly affect the capacity for children to be healthy over their life course trajectory.[45] External psychosocial factors include social determinants of health (SDH), which are defined by the Kaiser Family Foundation and World Health Organization as the "conditions in which people are born, grow, live, work and age."[46] The Centers for Disease Control and Prevention Essentials for Childhood initiative emphasizes that "[s]afe, stable, nurturing relationships and environments are essential to prevent child maltreatment…and to assure that children reach their full potential" over their lives.[47] SDH, such as housing stability and food security, have a positive influence on the health of all children and are recommended to be addressed during well-child visits.[5,46,48] Studies suggest that poor housing and neighborhood quality are associated with a greater risk for some CYSHCN experiencing a poorer quality of life.[49,50] Food insecurity may also impact CYSHCN specifically if they

have increased or specialized nutritional needs or dietary restrictions.[51]

CYSHCN have higher rates of exposure to adverse childhood experiences (ACEs) or toxic stress (eg, abuse and domestic violence).[8] According to the 2016 NSCH, 37% of CYSHCN had 2 or more ACEs, compared with 18% of children without special health care needs.[9] These ACEs are often internalized, but the negative effects may be mitigated over time by protective factors.[52–54] In addition, children with 2 or more ACEs are significantly more likely to be considered CYSHCN compared with children with no exposure to ACEs.[53] The presence of 2 or more ACEs can be linked to exacerbations of their chronic conditions, an increased risk of developing secondary conditions, poor school engagement, and even an increased risk of repeating a grade in school.[52,53] Exposure to 2 or more ACEs may be associated with smoking, using drugs, participating in earlier sexual activity, and performing violent or antisocial acts.[53,54] If CYSHCN engage in these risky behaviors, there may be an increased risk for additional short- and long-term physical and mental health problems and difficulties with following treatment recommendations as well as an increased risk for poorer health care outcomes.[50,55,56] However, studies show that CYSHCN who learn and show resilience may be able to reduce the negative effects of some ACEs. This mitigation of risk occurs especially when supports are provided for key transition points, such as starting child care, school, and work.[52,53]

Children with intellectual or developmental disabilities may be at an increased risk for physical, emotional, and sexual abuse and neglect. The reasons may include inadequate social skills, limited capacity to find help or report abuse,

lack of strategies to defend against abuse, or increased exposure to multiple caregivers and settings.[57,58] Additional challenges can occur if parents of children with disabilities lack respite, coping skills, or adequate social and community support. These stressors can put some children at risk for failing to receive needed medications or adequate medical care and can lead to abuse or neglect.[59]

Additional family stressors not considered ACEs can still negatively affect the health of some CYSHCN. These stressors include, but are not limited to, caregiver burden, poor coping skills, inadequate sleep, limited interactions with extended family and friends, reductions or loss of parental employment, and financial problems.[60–65] Family conflict, in particular, can be associated with a greater number of hospitalizations, as seen in 1 study for children with asthma.[41] Financial problems may result from multiple and costly medications, equipment, therapies or specialty appointments, and loss of income from taking time off work to care for CYSHCN.[17,66] Limited English proficiency in parents and lack of insurance are 2 stressors that may disproportionately affect the health and well-being of some immigrant families of CYSHCN.[67] Parenting stress may increase if negative perceptions of their child's illness occur, potentially leading to additional mental and physical health problems in the parents of some CYSHCN.[68] Siblings of some CYSHCN with developmental disabilities and cancer may be at risk for emotional and behavioral problems, difficulties with interpersonal relationships and functioning at school, and psychiatric conditions.[69,70] The effects on caregiver and family stress can be even greater in families with children who have higher medical complexity.[17,71]

Child care and school settings may struggle to accommodate the needs of CYSHCN, leading to increased stress, poor socialization, and poor school performance.[49,50,72–75] Some CYSHCN may lose motivation to do well in school, resulting in lower academic achievement and increased school absences.[75] Some CYSHCN may experience bullying, stereotyping, prejudice, or stigmatization from peers or others in their schools or communities. This negative experiences may lead to difficulties in school, including school avoidance.[50,76,77] Children with intellectual and developmental disabilities, seizure disorders, and other conditions affecting the central nervous system are at particular risk for school problems because of impairments in brain growth and development[78–80] with resultant effects on executive functioning skills.[38,78,80,81] Problems with attention, memory, language, and understanding social processes place some CYSHCN at an increased risk for academic failure, poor interpersonal skills, and low self-esteem.[38,78,80–82] Negative school experiences may also further exacerbate problems with adherence to medications, therapies, or other health recommendations at school.[83]

The cumulative effects of living with and managing a chronic condition may evolve further over the life span of a child.[84,85] Certain chronic physical and mental health conditions and treatments, particularly those affecting the central nervous system, may affect neurologic and cognitive function, social development, emotional regulation and awareness, and expressive and receptive communication. These effects may not be readily apparent to families, caregivers, teachers, and health care providers.[84–86] Developmental, social, and behavioral problems may be observed when age-appropriate and interpersonal competencies, abilities, and skills are not achieved.[38,78,87–90]

Escalation in levels of needed medical care can increase the development of additional mental or behavioral health problems or social concerns in children. These developments can present additional challenges in the home and in child care and school settings.[38,78,87,88,91,92]

A negative illness perception, low self-esteem, and a belief of a lack of control can increase the risk of a co-occurring mental health concern or diagnosis in some children.[93,94] Stress from unrecognized and/or untreated mental health concerns can result in increased cortisol levels, which can negatively affect physiology and metabolism and exacerbate chronic conditions, such as asthma or diabetes.[87] Unrecognized and untreated chronic complications among CYSHCN can increase the risk of developing internalizing or externalizing behavioral problems or conditions.[95,96] For example, chronic nocturnal symptoms with uncontrolled asthma or undiagnosed sleep apnea with Down syndrome can negatively affect behavioral health and quality of life.[97] Co-occurring chronic physical and mental health conditions are associated with an attempted suicide risk in excess of that predicted by the chronic mental health condition alone.[98] A focus on behavioral health and wellness as part of chronic care may help improve health outcomes for some CYSHCN and their families.[36]

SUPPORTING PSYCHOSOCIAL PROTECTIVE FACTORS FOR CYSHCN AND THEIR FAMILIES

Psychosocial protective factors can be supported at the individual, interpersonal, and community levels. Supportive and stable relationships, processes, and policies that promote resilience benefit children and can buffer against ACEs.[99–103] Developmentally appropriate and supported cognitive, language, and communication skills and abilities

may be associated with calmer temperament and higher levels of self-esteem, which can aid in coping with a chronic illness.[40,104–106] Skills for social competence have been taught by caregivers to encourage cooperation, self-control, assertion, and self-responsibility in children with mobility disorders.[99] Protective factors in some children with malignancies include comparing themselves with other children with malignancies instead of healthy peers, using positive reappraisal, spiritual or religious coping, and future-oriented thinking.[107–109]

Studies now show the importance of supporting families and communities that help CYSHCN to have positive relationships and interactions.[103] Healthy and well-functioning families may offer coping assistance for some CYSHCN.[108,110] Cohesive and connected families with stable family structures seem to be most functional.[60,110] Studies of children with autism, asthma, and diabetes suggest that instilling positive parenting beliefs helps engage parents in appropriate care.[111–114] Education of community members about a child or youth's medical condition may increase coping and resilience in some families.[110] A father's involvement in the care of a child with a chronic disease has been associated with higher treatment adherence, better psychological adjustment, and improved health for the child.[115] Higher social support for caregivers of CYSHCN has been associated with decreased psychological distress in the child and decreased risks for stress, loneliness, depression, and anxiety in caregivers.[116]

Schools can be a source of strength when there are positive parent-school partnerships and a supportive, coordinated early intervention system.[73–75] Health care providers and schools can collaborate with families on monitoring changes in health status, developing the treatment plan, and ensuring appropriate school staffing.[117,118] Schools, in partnership with families and health care providers, can play a significant role in supporting self-management of care for CYSHCN and other elements of health care transition.[119] Families, youth, providers, and school and child care staff can develop and modify an Individualized Family Service Plan, Individualized Education Program, 504 plan, or individualized health plan on the basis of medical and psychosocial needs and supports. These supports may include self-management of care and transition to adult health care systems.[117,119–122]

Fully supporting protective factors involves the development of community-based systems of care for CYSHCN that address psychosocial aspects of care.[123,124] A system of care represents a coordinated network of community-based services and supports, including the family, the medical home, child care providers, and schools. The core values include building on the strengths and needs of the youth and family. This approach has resulted in improvements in multiple domains of individual and family functioning, including the reduction of family stress and strain and increased behavioral and emotional strengths in children.[125]

ADDRESSING PSYCHOSOCIAL FACTORS IN THE MEDICAL HOME

The pediatric medical home is an ideal setting to address psychosocial factors that impact wellness and resilience for CYSHCN and their families. The medical home can conduct ongoing surveillance and screening for psychosocial factors and promote care coordination of needed services and supports.[126,127] Longitudinal, relationship-centered care may facilitate discussions about psychosocial factors, address symptoms, and increase adherence

to recommendations.[127–130] Pediatric primary care and specialty providers can promote team-based care with partners from multiple disciplines by coordinating psychosocial screening, care planning, and interventions. Additional key partners may include care managers, family navigators, social workers, psychologists, professional interpreters, and public health and social service agencies.[131] Access to comprehensive care for CYSHCN through a medical home is associated with improvements in health status, access to care, and family satisfaction. Use of a medical home approach is also associated with fewer missed school days for children, issues with child care, missed days of work, and out-of-pocket costs for families.[8,9,126,132–134]

In the 2017 *Bright Futures: Guidelines for Health Supervision of Infants, Children, and Adolescents, Fourth Edition,* the American Academy of Pediatrics (AAP) emphasizes a strength-based approach to comprehensive care and wellness for all children. The need to particularly focus on health and wellness for CYSHCN is also recognized.[5] AAP *Bright Futures* recommendations for preventive pediatric health care include developmental surveillance, general developmental screening, and screening for autism at specific ages during well-child visits.[5,135–136] Recommended surveillance and screenings are important even in the presence of an existing chronic physical or mental health condition, a developmental delay, or a disability, when appropriate.

The AAP *Bright Futures* recommendations include a psychosocial and behavioral assessment at every well-child visit that is "family centered and may include an assessment of child social emotional health, caregiver depression, and social determinants."[5,135] *Bright Futures* and the US Preventive Services Task Force recommend screening for

both postpartum depression and depression in adolescents at specified well-child visits.[5,137–139] Surveillance or screening for parental socioemotional well-being and SDH outside of the postpartum period may identify additional psychosocial risk factors for CYSHCN.[19,50,53,54,60,61,63–65] The AAP policy statement "Poverty and Child Health in the United States"[48] and an additional article about redesigning health care to address poverty[140] provide recommendations and resources for screening tools for SDH (eg, Safe Environment for Every Kid [SEEK]).

A variety of resources can help pediatric medical home providers address psychosocial risk factors using a team-based approach. These include the AAP Mental Health Initiatives Web site (https://www.aap.org/en-us/advocacy-and-policy/aap-health-initiatives/Mental-Health/Pages/Primary-Care-Tools.aspx), a tool kit called Mental Health Screening and Assessment Tools for Primary Care,[141] articles and resources from the AAP Task Force on Mental Health published in a June 2010 supplement to *Pediatrics*,[142] and a recent clinical report ("Promoting Optimal Development: Screening for Behavioral and Emotional Problems"[4]) that provides resources about specific behavioral and emotional tools and processes. The AAP Screening, Technical Assistance, and Resource Center provides a variety of resources about screening, discussion, management, and referral in primary care around child development, maternal depression, and SDH for young children (https://www.aap.org/en-us/advocacy-and-policy/aap-health-initiatives/Screening/Pages/default.aspx). These developmental, autism, and social-emotional screening tools were validated in the general population and normalized for typically developing children.[4,5,139,141,143,144] Validated quality-of-life screening questions have been used across several conditions, although more in research settings than in primary care.[145] Standardized care approaches and tools can be used to facilitate self-management that addresses psychosocial needs, adherence to treatment plans, and leverage of supportive community resources.[146,147]

Pediatric providers are encouraged to develop mental health competencies for direct patient care and for coordination with community resources.[3] Pediatric providers can use evidence-based techniques (eg, motivational interviewing) to address mental health concerns and social determinants identified with screening in the medical home setting. Such approaches may be used by providers while waiting for further evaluation of the child and even while a child is receiving treatment by a mental health provider.[3,130] Interventions may include counseling about family-focused physical activity guidelines, good nutrition, and improved sleep routines.[36,131] Common elements among psychosocial interventions include the use of motivational interviewing strategies to communicate hope, empathy, and loyalty; use of plain language; asking permission to ask questions or share information; and partnering with families.[130] Such elements have been found to be effective in building alliances, increasing disclosure, and facilitating discussions about psychosocial strengths and concerns.[129,130] Pediatric providers on the care team may not serve as the primary provider to deliver mental health counseling and interventions, but they can support integrated interdisciplinary efforts and partnerships.[36] A team-based approach may include the use of designated staff for wellness promotion, collocation of services (eg, social workers

and psychologists), or referrals to community services for mental health assessment, counseling, and interventions.[131]

Behavioral health integration has been described as a useful "approach and model of delivering care that comprehensively addresses the primary care, behavioral health, specialty care, and social support needs of children and youth with behavioral health issues in a manner that is continuous and family-centered."[148] Behavioral health integration can aid the medical home as needs occur from infancy through adolescence and into young adulthood.[149] Practices with collocated behavioral health providers or real-time access to short-term mental health support have seen improved timely evaluations of child and family functioning, increased referrals for more specialized evaluations, and improved access to direct behavioral health services for CYSHCN.[3,150] Mindfulness and relaxation training may also be effective with stress and can be taught to parents and children.[151] However, not all practices have collocated or integrated behavioral health providers; therefore, pediatric providers are encouraged, as mentioned earlier, to develop some mental health competencies for use in primary care to enhance their delivery of direct patient care and coordination with community resources.[3] Formal care coordinators, as part of the medical home team, can assist with identifying and strengthening protective relationships to help support and monitor strategies and interventions with child care providers, schools, home health agencies, behavioral health providers, social service workers, and a variety of other professionals.[152] Care coordinators can be employed by the practice or another entity and can help facilitate management and referral

and follow-up related to community resources.[3,140,152]

These community relationships can help increase awareness, communication, and transparency of the care directed by the medical home.[152] The medical home, in partnership with care coordinators and community partners, may promote planned transition from pediatric to adult health care that addresses psychosocial risk and protective factors. Planned transition includes structured assessments and planning (beginning in early adolescence) addressing SDH as well as guardianship and other legal issues. The goal is to minimize breaks in continuous care and lessen parental concern, particularly for chronic conditions accompanied by cognitive impairment.[119]

Implementation of the medical home model entails a quality improvement approach and practice transformation activities. Such activities may include a patient registry, care tracking, team-based care, and special care protocols. Strategies could include a previsit process that may include routine psychosocial screening, scheduling additional time during appointments, and identifying a team member and/or care coordinator. Additional efforts include electronic health record integration and workflow changes to incorporate screening, discussion, referrals, and follow-up as part of a comprehensive, integrated plan of care. Such a plan of care includes patient- and family-identified psychosocial goals and priorities.[48,124,153]

Individual provider and practice challenges to the medical home include time, training, and lack of knowledge about available resources.[4,154] Community and system barriers include inadequate payments, a shortage of pediatric psychiatrists and developmental-behavioral pediatricians,[155] limited community mental health resources, and limited services and abilities in communities to address SDH (eg, housing).[48,149] Flexible population-based payment models and the use of payment incentives could help to encourage increased management of psychosocial health and well-being as part of care for chronic conditions and could help to increase the use of more screening tools.[48,153]

ADDITIONAL STRATEGIES TO SUPPORT SYSTEMS ADDRESSING PSYCHOSOCIAL FACTORS

Pediatricians represent only 1 stakeholder interested in the comprehensive system of care for CYSHCN and their families. Title V Maternal and Child Health programs, health plans, insurers, state Medicaid and Children's Health Insurance Program agencies, children's hospitals, health services researchers, families, and consumers developed national standards for a system of care for CYSHCN in 2014 and then updated these standards in 2017.[124]

Recommendations for pediatric medical home teams include developing processes and protocols in collaboration with other community agencies (eg, Part C early intervention and home health) and professionals. These agencies may also perform psychosocial screenings and refer CYSHCN for further assessment of concerns. Collaboration could allow the medical home team to reduce duplication of efforts and ensure referred services regardless of who conducted the screening. Service linkage, timely communication, and appropriate data sharing can be used to promote an integrated plan of care that includes psychosocial goals and priorities from CSYHCN and their families.[124] The resource titled *Managing Chronic Health Needs in Child Care and Schools*[72] and the AAP policy statement on the role of school nurses and the medical home[117] offer collaborative strategies to support social-emotional health, which influences health, school attendance, and academic performance.[117,118]

Pediatric medical home providers and parents can learn about and be linked to several home- and community-based services and supports to help assess and address psychosocial needs for CYSHCN and their families. Respite care, palliative care, and hospice care and home-based services are examples of these services.[124] Parents may be supported through home visiting and parenting support programs regardless of whether they are specific for CYSHCN.[156–158] One parenting program, called the Positive Parenting Program or Triple P, offers a series of parenting modules called Stepping Stones, which was developed specifically for use with parents of children with developmental disabilities. Stepping Stones modules address self-efficacy, self-sufficiency, self-management, personal agency, and problem solving with parents of children with developmental disabilities. However, not all states offer Triple P Stepping Stones modules, and some states that do offer it have limited access to these modules.[159,160] Parent-to-parent support groups may help some families of CYSHCN share a social identity, experience personal growth, and learn coping strategies.[161]

Several programs serve as clearinghouses about services and supports for families. One example is the early childhood coordinated referral and system building programs called Help Me Grow (www.helpmegrownational.org/). Help Me Grow is now available in 26 states to help connect providers and families to developmental screening and services.[140] The Community Services Locator (https://www.ncemch.org/knowledge/community.php) is another clearinghouse of information that provides Web sites and phone numbers that can be used to assist with accessing national, state, and local resources for child care, early childhood education, special education services, family support, financial support, health and wellness, and parenting programs.[140] A third example is the United Way 211 line (http://www.211.org/pages/about), which is a telephone and Internet-based resource that is available 24 hours a day, 7 days a week, throughout most of the United States.[140] The 211 line can provide information about a wide variety of resources in multiple languages about housing, food pantries, and utilities in addition to child care, early education, and many other services to address SDH.[140]

RECOMMENDATIONS

Health and wellness for CYSHCN are particularly sensitive to psychosocial risk and protective factors. Pediatric providers, particularly from the primary care–based medical home, are in the position to screen for, manage, and coordinate longitudinal care in which psychosocial factors of health among CYSHCN and their families are addressed. The following suggestions are offered to pediatricians involved in caring for CYSHCN:

1. Follow *Bright Futures* recommendations and guidance for CYSHCN and their families. Recommendations include the promotion of health and wellness as well as timely assessments of child social-emotional health, parental and/or caregiver depression, and SDH.

2. Use practice transformation strategies, such as quality improvement, patient registries, and previsit planning, to promote psychosocial screening and assessment, referrals, and follow-up among CYSHCN and their families. A good resource is the AAP Practice Transformation site (https://www.aap.org/en-us/

professional-resources/practice-Transformation/Pages/practice-transformation.aspx).

3. Use team-based care strategies, care protocols, and dedicated care coordinators (if available) to recognize psychosocial protective factors and ameliorate risk factors. This strategy may involve collocation, consultation, comanagement, and/or integration with behavioral health specialists as part of medical home and specialty care teams.

4. Consider strategies for working with child care and school staff to monitor progress, reduce absences, and improve learning experiences and academic performance for CYSHCN.

5. Advocate for flexible payment redesign with Medicaid and other insurers. Payment redesign may better support wellness and chronic care management for CYSHCN and their families. Flexible payment redesign may include payments for mental health treatment, care coordination, and collocation or comanagement with behavioral health and other specialists or disciplines.

6. Promote evidence-based interventions and strategies in the medical home and subspecialty settings to support psychosocial development of CYSHCN, parenting competencies, and family resilience.

7. Advocate for research on adaptions of existing psychosocial screening tools and interventions for CYSHCN.

8. Advocate for community-based resources and strategies to address SDH and the reduction of disparities for CYSHCN and their families.

9. Pediatric providers and state AAP chapters can partner with Title V Maternal and Child Health CYSHCN programs in supporting implementation of the Association of Maternal and Child Health Program's Standards for Systems of Care for CYSHCN. These standards include increasing access for CYSHCN to quality medical homes, ease of use of community services, and transitioning across the life span.

LEAD AUTHORS

Gerri Mattson, MD, MSPH, FAAP
Dennis Z. Kuo, MD, MHS, FAAP

COMMITTEE ON PSYCHOSOCIAL ASPECTS OF CHILD AND FAMILY HEALTH, 2017–2018

Michael Yogman, MD, FAAP, Chairperson
Rebecca Baum, MD, FAAP
Thresia B. Gambon, MD, FAAP
Arthur Lavin, MD, FAAP
Gerri Mattson, MD, FAAP
Raul Montiel Esparza, MD
Arwa A. Nasir, MBBS, MSc, MPH, FAAP
Lawrence Sagin Wissow, MD, MPH, FAAP

LIAISONS

Amy Starin, PhD – *National Association of Social Workers*
Edward Christophersen, PhD, FAAP – *Society of Pediatric Psychology*
Sharon Berry, PhD, LP – *Society of Pediatric Psychology*
Norah L. Johnson, PhD, RN, CPNP-PC – *National Association of Pediatric Nurse Practitioners*
Abigail B. Schlesinger, MD – *American Academy of Child and Adolescent Psychiatry*
Aaron Pikcilingis – *Family Partnerships Network*

STAFF

Karen Smith
Tamar Magarik Haro

COUNCIL ON CHILDREN WITH DISABILITIES EXECUTIVE COMMITTEE, 2017–2018

Dennis Z. Kuo, MD, MHS, FAAP, Chairperson
Susan Apkon, MD, FAAP
Timothy J. Brei, MD, FAAP
Lynn F. Davidson, MD, FAAP
Beth Ellen Davis, MD, MPH, FAAP
Kathryn A. Ellerbeck, MD, FAAP
Susan L. Hyman, MD, FAAP
Mary O'Connor Leppert, MD, FAAP
Garey H. Noritz, MD, FAAP
Christopher J. Stille, MD, MPH, FAAP
Larry Yin, MD, MSPH, FAAP

FORMER COUNCIL ON CHILDREN WITH DISABILITIES EXECUTIVE COMMITTEE MEMBERS

Amy J. Houtrow, MD, PhD, MPH, FAAP
Kenneth W. Norwood Jr, MD, FAAP, Immediate Past Chairperson

LIAISONS

Peter J. Smith, MD, MA, FAAP – *Section on Developmental and Behavioral Pediatrics*
Edwin Simpser, MD, FAAP – *Section on Home Care*
Georgina Peacock, MD, MPH, FAAP – *Centers for Disease Control and Prevention*
Marie Mann, MD, MPH, FAAP – *Maternal and Child Health Bureau*
Cara Coleman, JD, MPH – *Family Voices*

STAFF

Alexandra Kuznetsov, RD

ABBREVIATIONS

AAP: American Academy of Pediatrics
ACE: adverse childhood experience
ADHD: attention-deficit/hyperactivity disorder
CMC: children with medical complexity
CYSHCN: children and youth with special health care needs
NSCH: National Survey of Children's Health
SDH: social determinants of health

PEDIATRICS (ISSN Numbers: Print, 0031-4005; Online, 1098-4275).

Copyright © 2019 by the American Academy of Pediatrics

FINANCIAL DISCLOSURE: The authors have indicated they have no financial relationships relevant to this article to disclose.

FUNDING: No external funding.

POTENTIAL CONFLICT OF INTEREST: The authors have indicated they have no potential conflicts of interest to disclose.

REFERENCES

1. McPherson M, Arango P, Fox H, et al. A new definition of children with special health care needs. *Pediatrics.* 1998;102(1 pt 1):137–140

2. Fee RJ, Hinton VJ. Resilience in children diagnosed with a chronic neuromuscular disorder. *J Dev Behav Pediatr.* 2011;32(9):644–650

3. Committee on Psychosocial Aspects of Child and Family Health; Task Force on Mental Health. Policy statement—the future of pediatrics: mental health competencies for pediatric primary care. *Pediatrics.* 2009;124(1):410–421

4. Weitzman C, Wegner L; Section on Developmental and Behavioral Pediatrics; Committee on Psychosocial Aspects of Child and Family Health; Council on Early Childhood; Society for Developmental and Behavioral Pediatrics; American Academy of Pediatrics. Promoting optimal development: screening for behavioral and emotional problems [published correction appears in *Pediatrics.* 2015;135(5):946]. *Pediatrics.* 2015;135(2):384–395

5. Hagan JF, Shaw JS, Duncan PM, eds. *Bright Futures: Guidelines for Health Supervision of Infants, Children, and Adolescents.* 4th ed. Elk Grove Village, IL: American Academy of Pediatrics; 2017

6. Boyle CA, Boulet S, Schieve LA, et al. Trends in the prevalence of developmental disabilities in US children, 1997-2008. *Pediatrics.* 2011;127(6):1034–1042

7. Perou R, Bitsko RH, Blumberg SJ, et al; Centers for Disease Control and Prevention (CDC). Mental health surveillance among children—United States, 2005-2011. *MMWR Suppl.* 2013;62(2):1–35

8. Child and Adolescent Health Measurement Initiative; Data Resource Center for Child and Adolescent Health. 2016 National Survey of Children's Health (NSCH) data query. Available at: http://childhealthdata.org/browse/survey/results?q=4562&r. Accessed March 5, 2018

9. US Department of Health and Human Services; Health Resources and Services Administration; Maternal and Child Health Bureau. *The National Survey of Children With Special Health Care Needs Chartbook 2009–2010.* Rockville, MD: US Department of Health and Human Services; 2013

10. Berry JG, Bloom S, Foley S, Palfrey JS. Health inequity in children and youth with chronic health conditions. *Pediatrics.* 2010;126(suppl 3):S111–S119

11. Akinbami LJ, Moorman JE, Garbe PL, Sondik EJ. Status of childhood asthma in the United States, 1980-2007. *Pediatrics.* 2009;123(suppl 3):S131–S145

12. Wu YW, Croen LA, Shah SJ, Newman TB, Najjar DV. Cerebral palsy in a term population: risk factors and neuroimaging findings. *Pediatrics.* 2006;118(2):690–697

13. Lipton R, Good G, Mikhailov T, Freels S, Donoghue E. Ethnic differences in mortality from insulin-dependent diabetes mellitus among people less than 25 years of age. *Pediatrics.* 1999;103(5 pt 1):952–956

14. Centers for Disease Control and Prevention (CDC). Racial disparities in median age at death of persons with Down syndrome—United States, 1968-1997. *MMWR Morb Mortal Wkly Rep.* 2001;50(22):463–465

15. Boneva RS, Botto LD, Moore CA, Yang Q, Correa A, Erickson JD. Mortality associated with congenital heart defects in the United States: trends and racial disparities, 1979-1997. *Circulation.* 2001;103(19):2376–2381

16. Linabery AM, Ross JA. Childhood and adolescent cancer survival in the US by race and ethnicity for the diagnostic period 1975-1999. *Cancer.* 2008;113(9):2575–2596

17. Kuo DZ, Cohen E, Agrawal R, Berry JG, Casey PH. A national profile of caregiver challenges among more medically complex children with special health care needs. *Arch Pediatr Adolesc Med.* 2011;165(11):1020–1026

18. Centers for Disease Control and Prevention. Most recent asthma data. Available at: https://www.cdc.gov/asthma/most_recent_data.htm. Accessed April 3, 2017

19. Perrin JM, Bloom SR, Gortmaker SL. The increase of childhood chronic conditions in the United States. *JAMA.* 2007;297(24):2755–2759

20. Kelly AS, Barlow SE, Rao G, et al; American Heart Association; Atherosclerosis, Hypertension, and Obesity in the Young Committee of the Council on Cardiovascular Disease in the Young; Council on Nutrition, Physical Activity and Metabolism; Council on Clinical Cardiology. Severe obesity in children and adolescents: identification, associated health risks, and treatment approaches: a scientific statement from the American Heart Association. *Circulation.* 2013;128(15):1689–1712

21. Skinner AC, Skelton JA. Prevalence and trends in obesity and severe obesity among children in the United States, 1999-2012. *JAMA Pediatr.* 2014;168(6):561–566

22. Dabelea D, Mayer-Davis EJ, Saydah S, et al; SEARCH for Diabetes in Youth Study. Prevalence of type 1 and type 2 diabetes among children and adolescents from 2001 to 2009. *JAMA.* 2014;311(17):1778–1786

23. Adams AK, Quinn RA, Prince RJ. Low recognition of childhood overweight and disease risk among Native-American caregivers. *Obes Res.* 2005;13(1):146–152

24. Reinehr T. Type 2 diabetes mellitus in children and adolescents. *World J Diabetes.* 2013;4(6):270–281

25. Goran MI, Ball GD, Cruz ML. Obesity and risk of type 2 diabetes and cardiovascular disease in children and adolescents. *J Clin Endocrinol Metab.* 2003;88(4):1417–1427

26. Cohen E, Kuo DZ, Agrawal R, et al. Children with medical complexity: an emerging population for clinical and research initiatives. *Pediatrics.* 2011;127(3):529–538

27. Berry JG, Hall M, Neff J, et al. Children with medical complexity and Medicaid: spending and cost savings. *Health Aff (Millwood).* 2014;33(12):2199–2206

28. van der Lee JH, Mokkink LB, Grootenhuis MA, Heymans HS, Offringa M. Definitions and measurement of chronic health conditions in

childhood: a systematic review. *JAMA.* 2007;297(24):2741–2751

29. Stiller C. Epidemiology of cancer in adolescents. *Med Pediatr Oncol.* 2002;39(3):149–155

30. van der Veen WJ. The small epidemiologic transition: further decrease in infant mortality due to medical intervention during pregnancy and childbirth, yet no decrease in childhood disabilities [in Dutch]. *Ned Tijdschr Geneeskd.* 2003;147(9):378–381

31. Simon TD, Berry J, Feudtner C, et al. Children with complex chronic conditions in inpatient hospital settings in the United States. *Pediatrics.* 2010;126(4):647–655

32. Burns KH, Casey PH, Lyle RE, Bird TM, Fussell JJ, Robbins JM. Increasing prevalence of medically complex children in US hospitals. *Pediatrics.* 2010;126(4):638–646

33. Merikangas KR, Cui L, Kattan G, Carlson GA, Youngstrom EA, Angst J. Mania with and without depression in a community sample of US adolescents. *Arch Gen Psychiatry.* 2012;69(9):943–951

34. Visser SN, Danielson ML, Bitsko RH, et al. Trends in the parent-report of health care provider-diagnosed and medicated attention-deficit/hyperactivity disorder: United States, 2003-2011. *J Am Acad Child Adolesc Psychiatry.* 2014;53(1):34–46.e2

35. Halfon N, Houtrow A, Larson K, Newacheck PW. The changing landscape of disability in childhood. *Future Child.* 2012;22(1):13–42

36. Boat TF, Filigno S, Amin RS. Wellness for families of children with chronic health disorders. *JAMA Pediatr.* 2017;171(9):825–826

37. Hysing M, Elgen I, Gillberg C, Lie SA, Lundervold AJ. Chronic physical illness and mental health in children. Results from a large-scale population study. *J Child Psychol Psychiatry.* 2007;48(8):785–792

38. Pinquart M, Shen Y. Behavior problems in children and adolescents with chronic physical illness: a meta-analysis. *J Pediatr Psychol.* 2011;36(9):1003–1016

39. Inkelas M, Raghavan R, Larson K, Kuo AA, Ortega AN. Unmet mental health need and access to services for children with special health care needs and their families. *Ambul Pediatr.* 2007;7(6):431–438

40. Theunissen SC, Rieffe C, Netten AP, et al. Self-esteem in hearing-impaired children: the influence of communication, education, and audiological characteristics. *PLoS One.* 2014;9(4):e94521

41. Goodwin RD, Bandiera FC, Steinberg D, Ortega AN, Feldman JM. Asthma and mental health among youth: etiology, current knowledge and future directions. *Expert Rev Respir Med.* 2012;6(4):397–406

42. Hood KK, Beavers DP, Yi-Frazier J, et al. Psychosocial burden and glycemic control during the first 6 years of diabetes: results from the SEARCH for Diabetes in Youth study. *J Adolesc Health.* 2014;55(4):498–504

43. Melek S, Norris D. *Chronic Conditions and Comorbid Psychological Disorders.* Seattle, WA: Milliman; 2008

44. Kuo DZ, Melguizo-Castro M, Goudie A, Nick TG, Robbins JM, Casey PH. Variation in child health care utilization by medical complexity. *Matern Child Health J.* 2015;19(1):40–48

45. Fine A, Kotelchuck M, Adess N, Pies C. *Policy Brief. A New Agenda for MCH Policy and Programs: Integrating a Life Course Perspective.* Martinez, CA: Contra Costa Health Services; 2009

46. Heiman HJ, Artigo S. *Beyond Health Care: The Role of Social Determinants in Promoting Health and Health Equity.* San Francisco, CA: Kaiser Family Foundation; 2015. Available at: https://www.issuelab.org/resources/22899/22899.pdf. Accessed October 24, 2018

47. Centers for Disease Control and Prevention, National Center for Injury Prevention and Control, Division of Violence Prevention. Essentials for childhood: steps to create safe, stable, nurturing relationships and environments. Available at: https://www.cdc.gov/violenceprevention/pdf/essentials_for_childhood_framework.pdf. Accessed November 4, 2017

48. Council on Community Pediatrics. Poverty and child health in the United States. *Pediatrics.* 2016;137(4):e20160339

49. Coutinho MT, McQuaid EL, Koinis-Mitchell D. Contextual and cultural risks and their association with family asthma management in urban children. *J Child Health Care.* 2013;17(2):138–152

50. Atkinson M, Rees D, Davis L. Disability and economic disadvantage: facing the facts. *Arch Dis Child.* 2015;100(4):305–307

51. Rose-Jacobs R, Fiore JG, de Cuba SE, et al. Children with special health care needs, supplemental security income, and food insecurity. *J Dev Behav Pediatr.* 2016;37(2):140–147

52. Bethell CD, Newacheck PW, Fine A, et al. Optimizing health and health care systems for children with special health care needs using the life course perspective. *Matern Child Health J.* 2014;18(2):467–477

53. Bethell CD, Newacheck P, Hawes E, Halfon N. Adverse childhood experiences: assessing the impact on health and school engagement and the mitigating role of resilience. *Health Aff (Millwood).* 2014;33(12):2106–2115

54. Anda RF, Felitti VJ, Bremner JD, et al. The enduring effects of abuse and related adverse experiences in childhood. A convergence of evidence from neurobiology and epidemiology. *Eur Arch Psychiatry Clin Neurosci.* 2006;256(3):174–186

55. Bonnie RJ, Stratton K, Kwan LY, eds; Committee on the Public Health Implications of Raising the Minimum Age for Purchasing Tobacco Products; Board on Population Health and Public Health Practice; Institute of Medicine. *Public Health Implications of Raising the Minimum Age of Legal Access to Tobacco Products.* Washington, DC: National Academies Press; 2015

56. Weitzman ER, Ziemnik RE, Huang Q, Levy S. Alcohol and marijuana use and treatment nonadherence among medically vulnerable youth. *Pediatrics.* 2015;136(3):450–457

57. Murphy NA, Elias ER. Sexuality of children and adolescents with developmental disabilities. *Pediatrics.* 2006;118(1):398–403

58. Martinello E. Reviewing risks factors of individuals with intellectual disabilities as perpetrators of sexually abusive behaviors. *Sex Disabil.* 2015;33(2):269–278

59. Hibbard RA, Desch LW; American Academy of Pediatrics Committee on Child Abuse and Neglect; American Academy of Pediatrics Council on Children With Disabilities. Maltreatment of children with disabilities. *Pediatrics.* 2007;119(5):1018–1025

60. Churchill SS, Villareale NL, Monaghan TA, Sharp VL, Kieckhefer GM. Parents of children with special health care needs who have better coping skills have fewer depressive symptoms. *Matern Child Health J.* 2010;14(1):47–57

61. Hatzmann J, Peek N, Heymans H, Maurice-Stam H, Grootenhuis M. Consequences of caring for a child with a chronic disease: employment and leisure time of parents. *J Child Health Care.* 2014;18(4):346–357

62. Meltzer LJ, Booster GD. Sleep disturbance in caregivers of children with respiratory and atopic disease. *J Pediatr Psychol.* 2016;41(6):643–650

63. Siden H, Steele R. Charting the territory: children and families living with progressive life-threatening conditions [published correction appears in *Paediatr Child Health.* 2015;20(8):466–467]. *Paediatr Child Health.* 2015;20(3):139–144

64. Fedele DA, Grant DM, Wolfe-Christensen C, Mullins LL, Ryan JL. An examination of the factor structure of parenting capacity measures in chronic illness populations. *J Pediatr Psychol.* 2010;35(10):1083–1092

65. Cidav Z, Marcus SC, Mandell DS. Implications of childhood autism for parental employment and earnings. *Pediatrics.* 2012;129(4):617–623

66. Romley JA, Shah AK, Chung PJ, Elliott MN, Vestal KD, Schuster MA. Family-provided health care for children with special health care needs. *Pediatrics.* 2017;139(1):e20161287

67. Singh GK, Yu SM, Kogan MD. Health, chronic conditions, and behavioral risk disparities among U.S. immigrant children and adolescents. *Public Health Rep.* 2013;128(6):463–479

68. Cousino MK, Hazen RA. Parenting stress among caregivers of children with chronic illness: a systematic review. *J Pediatr Psychol.* 2013;38(8):809–828

69. Goudie A, Havercamp S, Jamieson B, Sahr T. Assessing functional impairment in siblings living with children with disability. *Pediatrics.* 2013;132(2). Available at: www.pediatrics.org/cgi/content/full/132/2/e476

70. Houtzager BA, Oort FJ, Hoekstra-Weebers JE, Caron HN, Grootenhuis MA, Last BF. Coping and family functioning predict longitudinal psychological adaptation of siblings of childhood cancer patients. *J Pediatr Psychol.* 2004;29(8):591–605

71. Rehm RS. Nursing's contribution to research about parenting children with complex chronic conditions: an integrative review, 2002 to 2012. *Nurs Outlook.* 2013;61(5):266–290

72. Donoghue EA, Kraft CA, eds. *Managing Chronic Health Needs in Child Care and Schools.* Elk Grove Village, IL: American Academy of Pediatrics; 2010

73. Murdock KK, Robinson EM, Adams SK, Berz J, Rollock MJ. Family-school connections and internalizing problems among children living with asthma in urban, low-income neighborhoods. *J Child Health Care.* 2009;13(3):275–294

74. O'Connor M, Howell-Meurs S, Kvalsvig A, Goldfeld S. Understanding the impact of special health care needs on early school functioning: a conceptual model. *Child Care Health Dev.* 2015;41(1):15–22

75. Forrest CB, Bevans KB, Riley AW, Crespo R, Louis TA. School outcomes of children with special health care needs. *Pediatrics.* 2011;128(2):303–312

76. Vranda MN, Mothi SN. Psychosocial issues of children infected with HIV/AIDS. *Indian J Psychol Med.* 2013;35(1):19–22

77. Van Cleave J, Davis MM. Bullying and peer victimization among children with special health care needs. *Pediatrics.* 2006;118(4). Available at: www.pediatrics.org/cgi/content/full/118/4/e1212

78. Pinquart M, Teubert D. Academic, physical, and social functioning of children and adolescents with chronic physical illness: a meta-analysis. *J Pediatr Psychol.* 2012;37(4):376–389

79. Leitner Y. The co-occurrence of autism and attention deficit hyperactivity disorder in children - what do we know? *Front Hum Neurosci.* 2014;8:268

80. Liogier d'Ardhuy X, Edgin JO, Bouis C, et al. Assessment of cognitive scales to examine memory, executive function and language in individuals with Down syndrome: implications of a 6-month observational study. *Front Behav Neurosci.* 2015;9:300

81. Schott N, Holfelder B. Relationship between motor skill competency and executive function in children with Down's syndrome. *J Intellect Disabil Res.* 2015;59(9):860–872

82. Hajek CA, Yeates KO, Anderson V, et al. Cognitive outcomes following arterial ischemic stroke in infants and children. *J Child Neurol.* 2014;29(7):887–894

83. Gidman W, Cowley J, Mullarkey C, Gibson L. Barriers to medication adherence in adolescents within a school environment [abstract]. *Arch Dis Child.* 2011;96(suppl 1):A64

84. Berg AT. Epilepsy, cognition, and behavior: the clinical picture. *Epilepsia.* 2011;52(suppl 1):7–12

85. Packer RJ, Gurney JG, Punyko JA, et al. Long-term neurologic and neurosensory sequelae in adult survivors of a childhood brain tumor: childhood cancer survivor study. *J Clin Oncol.* 2003;21(17):3255–3261

86. Reiter-Purtill J, Vannatta K, Gerhardt CA, Correll J, Noll RB. A controlled longitudinal study of the social functioning of children who completed treatment of cancer. *J Pediatr Hematol Oncol.* 2003;25(6):467–473

87. Cottrell D. Prevention and treatment of psychiatric disorders in children with chronic physical illness. *Arch Dis Child.* 2015;100(4):303–304

88. Hocking MC, McCurdy M, Turner E, et al. Social competence in pediatric brain tumor survivors: application of a model from social neuroscience and

developmental psychology. *Pediatr Blood Cancer*. 2015;62(3):375–384

89. Walterfang M, Bonnot O, Mocellin R, Velakoulis D. The neuropsychiatry of inborn errors of metabolism. *J Inherit Metab Dis*. 2013;36(4):687–702

90. Rantanen K, Eriksson K, Nieminen P. Social competence in children with epilepsy--a review. *Epilepsy Behav*. 2012;24(3):295–303

91. Ingerski LM, Modi AC, Hood KK, et al. Health-related quality of life across pediatric chronic conditions. *J Pediatr*. 2010;156(4):639–644

92. Kirk S, Glendinning C. Developing services to support parents caring for a technology-dependent child at home. *Child Care Health Dev*. 2004;30(3):209–218; discussion 219

93. Zeltner NA, Huemer M, Baumgartner MR, Landolt MA. Quality of life, psychological adjustment, and adaptive functioning of patients with intoxication-type inborn errors of metabolism - a systematic review. *Orphanet J Rare Dis*. 2014;9:159

94. Rizou I, De Gucht V, Papavasiliou A, Maes S. Illness perceptions determine psychological distress and quality of life in youngsters with epilepsy. *Epilepsy Behav*. 2015;46:144–150

95. May ME, Kennedy CH. Health and problem behavior among people with intellectual disabilities. *Behav Anal Pract*. 2010;3(2):4–12

96. Sivertsen B, Hysing M, Elgen I, Stormark KM, Lundervold AJ. Chronicity of sleep problems in children with chronic illness: a longitudinal population-based study. *Child Adolesc Psychiatry Ment Health*. 2009;3(1):22

97. Boergers J, Koinis-Mitchell D. Sleep and culture in children with medical conditions. *J Pediatr Psychol*. 2010;35(9):915–926

98. Barnes AJ, Eisenberg ME, Resnick MD. Suicide and self-injury among children and youth with chronic health conditions. *Pediatrics*. 2010;125(5):889–895

99. Alriksson-Schmidt AI, Wallander J, Biasini F. Quality of life and resilience in adolescents with a mobility disability. *J Pediatr Psychol*. 2007;32(3):370–379

100. McLeroy KR, Bibeau D, Steckler A, Glanz K. An ecological perspective on health promotion programs. *Health Educ Q*. 1988;15(4):351–377

101. Barros L, Gaspar de Matos M, Batista-Foguet JM. Chronic diseases, social context and adolescent health. *Revista Brasileira de Terapias Cognitivas*. 2008;4(1):123–141

102. Rutter M. Psychosocial resilience and protective mechanisms. *Am J Orthopsychiatry*. 1987;57(3):316–331

103. Sege R, Bethell C, Linkenbach J, Jones JA, Klika B, Pecora PJ. *Balancing Adverse Childhood Experiences With HOPE: New Insights Into the Role of Positive Experience on Child and Family Development*. Boston, MA: The Medical Foundation; 2017. Available at: www.cssp.org. Accessed November 4, 2017

104. Blackman JA, Conaway MR. Developmental, emotional and behavioral co-morbidities across the chronic health condition spectrum. *J Pediatr Rehabil Med*. 2013;6(2):63–71

105. Hintermair M. Self-esteem and satisfaction with life of deaf and hard-of-hearing people—a resource-oriented approach to identity work. *J Deaf Stud Deaf Educ*. 2008;13(2):278–300

106. Pinquart M. Self-esteem of children and adolescents with chronic illness: a meta-analysis. *Child Care Health Dev*. 2013;39(2):153–161

107. Harter S. *The Construction of the Self: A Developmental Perspective*. New York, NY: The Guilford Press; 1999

108. Hildenbrand AK, Alderfer MA, Deatrick JA, Marsac ML. A mixed methods assessment of coping with pediatric cancer. *J Psychosoc Oncol*. 2014;32(1):37–58

109. Sansom-Daly UM, Wakefield CE. Distress and adjustment among adolescents and young adults with cancer: an empirical and conceptual review. *Transl Pediatr*. 2013;2(4):167–197

110. Hall HR, Neely-Barnes SL, Graff JC, Krcek TE, Roberts RJ, Hankins JS. Parental stress in families of children with a genetic disorder/disability and the resiliency model of family stress, adjustment, and adaptation. *Issues Compr Pediatr Nurs*. 2012;35(1):24–44

111. Bekhet AK, Johnson NL, Zauszniewski JA. Effects on resilience of caregivers of persons with autism spectrum disorder: the role of positive cognitions. *J Am Psychiatr Nurses Assoc*. 2012;18(6):337–344

112. Johnson N, Frenn M, Feetham S, Simpson P. Autism spectrum disorder: parenting stress, family functioning and health-related quality of life. *Fam Syst Health*. 2011;29(3):232–252

113. Idalski Carcone A, Ellis DA, Weisz A, Naar-King S. Social support for diabetes illness management: supporting adolescents and caregivers. *J Dev Behav Pediatr*. 2011;32(8):581–590

114. Ellis DA, King P, Naar-King S, Lam P, Cunningham PB, Secord E. Effects of family treatment on parenting beliefs among caregivers of youth with poorly controlled asthma. *J Dev Behav Pediatr*. 2014;35(8):486–493

115. Wysocki T, Gavin L. Psychometric properties of a new measure of fathers' involvement in the management of pediatric chronic diseases. *J Pediatr Psychol*. 2004;29(3):231–240

116. Morelli SA, Lee IA, Arnn ME, Zaki J. Emotional and instrumental support provision interact to predict well-being. *Emotion*. 2015;15(4):484–493

117. Council on School Health. Role of the school nurse in providing school health services. *Pediatrics*. 2016;137(6):e20160852

118. Perrin JM, Anderson LE, Van Cleave J. The rise in chronic conditions among infants, children, and youth can be met with continued health system innovations. *Health Aff (Millwood)*. 2014;33(12):2099–2105

119. Cooley WC, Sagerman PJ; American Academy of Pediatrics; American Academy of Family Physicians; American College of Physicians; Transitions Clinical Report Authoring Group. Supporting the health care transition from adolescence to adulthood in the medical home. *Pediatrics*. 2011;128(1):182–200

120. Lipkin PH, Okamoto J; Council on Children With Disabilities; Council on School Health. The individuals with disabilities education act (IDEA) for

children with special educational needs. *Pediatrics*. 2015;136(6). Available at: www.pediatrics.org/cgi/content/full/136/6/e1650

121. Adams RC, Tapia C; Council on Children With Disabilities. Early intervention, IDEA part C services, and the medical home: collaboration for best practice and best outcomes. *Pediatrics*. 2013;132(4). Available at: www.pediatrics.org/cgi/content/full/132/4/e1073

122. Cartwright JD; American Academy of Pediatrics Council on Children With Disabilities. Provision of educationally related services for children and adolescents with chronic diseases and disabling conditions. *Pediatrics*. 2007;119(6):1218–1223

123. Stroul BA, Blau GM, Friedman RM. *Updating the System of Care Concept and Philosophy*. Washington, DC: National Technical Assistance Center for Children's Mental Health, Georgetown University Center for Child and Human Development; 2010. Available at: https://gucchdtacenter.georgetown.edu/resources/Call%20Docs/2010Calls/SOC_Brief2010.pdf. Accessed March 7, 2018

124. Association of Maternal and Child Health Programs; Lucile Packard Foundation for Children's Health. *Standards for Systems of Care for Children and Youth With Special Health Care Needs Version 2.0*. Washington, DC: Association of Maternal and Child Health Programs;2017 . Available at: http://www.amchp.org/programsandtopics/CYSHCN/Documents/Standards for Systems of Care for Children and Youth with Special Health Care Needs Version 2.0.pdf. Accessed September 15, 2017

125. Texas System of Care. A better future for Texas children: the impact of system of care. Available at: www.txsystemofcare.org/wp-content/uploads/2013/02/TXSOC_outcomes.pdf. Accessed March 7, 2018

126. Turchi RM, Berhane Z, Bethell C, Pomponio A, Antonelli R, Minkovitz CS. Care coordination for CSHCN: associations with family-provider relations and family/child outcomes. *Pediatrics*. 2009;124(suppl 4):S428–S434

127. Little P, Everitt H, Williamson I, et al. Observational study of effect of patient centredness and positive approach on outcomes of general practice consultations. *BMJ*. 2001;323(7318):908–911

128. Thom DH, Kravitz RL, Bell RA, Krupat E, Azari R. Patient trust in the physician: relationship to patient requests. *Fam Pract*. 2002;19(5):476–483

129. Wissow LS, Larson SM, Roter D, et al; SAFE Home Project. Longitudinal care improves disclosure of psychosocial information. *Arch Pediatr Adolesc Med*. 2003;157(5):419–424

130. Wissow L, Anthony B, Brown J, et al. A common factors approach to improving the mental health capacity of pediatric primary care. *Adm Policy Ment Health*. 2008;35(4):305–318

131. Katkin JP, Kressly SJ, Edwards AR, et al; Task Force on Pediatric Practice Change. Guiding principles for team-based pediatric care. *Pediatrics*. 2017;140(2):e20171489

132. Kuhlthau KA, Bloom S, Van Cleave J, et al. Evidence for family-centered care for children with special health care needs: a systematic review. *Acad Pediatr*. 2011;11(2):136–143

133. Cooley WC, McAllister JW, Sherrieb K, Kuhlthau K. Improved outcomes associated with medical home implementation in pediatric primary care. *Pediatrics*. 2009;124(1):358–364

134. Arauz Boudreau AD, Van Cleave JM, Gnanasekaran SK, Kurowski DS, Kuhlthau KA. The medical home: relationships with family functioning for children with and without special health care needs. *Acad Pediatr*. 2012;12(5):391–398

135. Committee on Practice and Ambulatory Medicine; Bright Futures Periodicity Schedule Workgroup. 2017 recommendations for preventive pediatric health care. *Pediatrics*. 2017;139(4):e20170254

136. Myers SM, Johnson CP; American Academy of Pediatrics Council on Children With Disabilities. Management of children with autism spectrum disorders. *Pediatrics*. 2007;120(5):1162–1182

137. Earls MF; Committee on Psychosocial Aspects of Child and Family Health; American Academy of Pediatrics. Incorporating recognition and management of perinatal and postpartum depression into pediatric practice. *Pediatrics*. 2010;126(5):1032–1039

138. O'Connor E, Rossom RC, Henninger M, Groom HC, Burda BU. Primary care screening for and treatment of depression in pregnant and postpartum women: evidence report and systematic review for the US Preventive Services Task Force. *JAMA*. 2016;315(4):388–406

139. Forman-Hoffman V, McClure E, McKeeman J, et al. Screening for major depressive disorder in children and adolescents: a systematic review for the U.S. Preventive Services Task Force. *Ann Intern Med*. 2016;164(5):342–349

140. Fierman AH, Beck AF, Chung EK, et al. Redesigning health care practices to address childhood poverty. *Acad Pediatr*. 2016;16(suppl 3):S136–S146

141. American Academy of Pediatrics. Mental health screening and assessment tools for primary care. In: *Addressing Mental Health Concerns in Primary Care: A Clinician's Toolkit*. Elk Grove Village, IL: American Academy of Pediatrics; 2012

142. Foy JM, Perrin J; American Academy of Pediatrics Task Force on Mental Health. Enhancing pediatric mental health care: strategies for preparing a community. *Pediatrics*. 2010;125(suppl 3):S75–S86

143. Council on Children With Disabilities; Section on Developmental Behavioral Pediatrics; Bright Futures Steering Committee; Medical Home Initiatives for Children With Special Needs Project Advisory Committee. Identifying infants and young children with developmental disorders in the medical home: an algorithm for developmental surveillance and screening [published correction appears in *Pediatrics*. 2006;118(4):1808–1809]. *Pediatrics*. 2006;118(1):405–420

144. Johnson CP, Myers SM; American Academy of Pediatrics Council on Children With Disabilities. Identification and evaluation of children with autism spectrum disorders. *Pediatrics*. 2007;120(5):1183–1215

145. Varni JW, Limbers CA, Burwinkle TM. Impaired health-related quality of life in children and adolescents with chronic conditions: a comparative analysis of 10 disease clusters and 33 disease categories/severities utilizing the PedsQL 4.0 Generic Core Scales. *Health Qual Life Outcomes*. 2007;5:43

146. Modi AC, Pai AL, Hommel KA, et al. Pediatric self-management: a framework for research, practice, and policy. *Pediatrics*. 2012;129(2). Available at: www.pediatrics.org/cgi/content/full/129/2/e473

147. Lozano P, Houtrow A. Supporting self-management in children and adolescents with complex chronic conditions. *Pediatrics*. 2018;141(suppl 3):S233–S241

148. Substance Abuse and Mental Health Services Administration and Health Resources and Services Administration Center for Integrated Health Solutions. *Integrating Behavioral Health and Primary Care for Children and Youth: Concepts and Strategies*. Washington, DC: Substance Abuse and Mental Health Services Administration and Health Resources and Services Administration Center for Integrated Health Solutions; 2013. Available at: https://static1.squarespace.com/static/545cdfcce4b0a64725b9f65a/t/553e7ef4e4b09e24c5c935db/1430159092492/13_June_CIHS_Integrated_Care_System_for_Children_final.pdf. Accessed November 11, 2017

149. Tyler ET, Hulkower RL, Kaminski JW. Behavioral health integration in pediatric primary care: considerations and opportunities for policymakers, planners, and providers. 2017.

Available at: https://www.milbank.org/wp-content/uploads/2017/03/MMF_BHI_REPORT_FINAL.pdf. Accessed November 11, 2017

150. Kuehn BM. Pediatrician-psychiatrist partnerships expand access to mental health care. *JAMA*. 2011;306(14):1531–1533

151. Fjorback LO, Arendt M, Ørnbøl E, Fink P, Walach H. Mindfulness-based stress reduction and mindfulness-based cognitive therapy: a systematic review of randomized controlled trials. *Acta Psychiatr Scand*. 2011;124(2):102–119

152. Council on Children With Disabilities; Medical Home Implementation Project Advisory Committee. Patient- and family-centered care coordination: a framework for integrating care for children and youth across multiple systems. *Pediatrics*. 2014;133(5). Available at: www.pediatrics.org/cgi/content/full/133/5/e1451

153. Landon BE. Structuring payments to patient-centered medical homes. *JAMA*. 2014;312(16):1633–1634

154. Hochstein M, Sareen H, Olson L, O'Connor K, Inkelas M, Halfon N. *Periodic Survey #46. A Comparison of Barriers to the Provision of Developmental Assessments and Psychosocial Screenings During Pediatric Health Supervision*. Elk Grove Village, IL: American Academy of Pediatrics; 2001. Available at: https://www.aap.org/en-us/professional-resources/Research/Pages/PS46_AcomparisonofBarrierstotheProvisionofDevelopmentalAssessmentsandpsychosocialscreeningsduringpediatrichealthsupervision.aspx. Accessed March 7, 2018

155. Bridgemohan C, Bauer NS, Nielsen BA, et al. A workforce survey on developmental-behavioral pediatrics. *Pediatrics*. 2018;141(3):e20172164

156. Tschudy MM, Toomey SL, Cheng TL. Merging systems: integrating home visitation and the family-centered medical home. *Pediatrics*. 2013;132(suppl 2):S74–S81

157. Jones K, Daley D, Hutchings J, Bywater T, Eames C. Efficacy of the Incredible Years Basic parent training programme as an early intervention for children with conduct problems and ADHD. *Child Care Health Dev*. 2007;33(6):749–756

158. Sanders MR, Turner KM, Markie-Dadds C. The development and dissemination of the Triple P-Positive Parenting Program: a multilevel, evidence-based system of parenting and family support. *Prev Sci*. 2002;3(3):173–189

159. Mazzucchelli TG, Sanders MR. *Stepping Stones Triple P: A Population Approach to the Promotion of Competent Parenting of Children With Disability*. Queensland, Australia: University of Queensland; 2012

160. Tellegen C. *Outcomes From a Randomised Controlled Trial Evaluating a Brief Parenting Intervention With Parents of Children With an Autism Spectrum Disorder*. Queensland, Australia: University of Queensland; 2012

161. Shilling V, Morris C, Thompson-Coon J, Ukoumunne O, Rogers M, Logan S. Peer support for parents of children with chronic disabling conditions: a systematic review of quantitative and qualitative studies. *Dev Med Child Neurol*. 2013;55(7):602–609

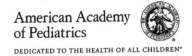

American Academy
of Pediatrics
DEDICATED TO THE HEALTH OF ALL CHILDREN®

Guidance for the Clinician in
Rendering Pediatric Care

CLINICAL REPORT

Psychosocial Support for Youth Living With HIV

abstract

Jaime Martinez, MD, FAAP, Rana Chakraborty, MD, FAAP,
and the COMMITTEE ON PEDIATRIC AIDS

This clinical report provides guidance for the pediatrician in addressing the psychosocial needs of adolescents and young adults living with HIV, which can improve linkage to care and adherence to life-saving antiretroviral (ARV) therapy. Recent national case surveillance data for youth (defined here as adolescents and young adults 13 to 24 years of age) revealed that the burden of HIV/AIDS fell most heavily and disproportionately on African American youth, particularly males having sex with males. To effectively increase linkage to care and sustain adherence to therapy, interventions should address the immediate drivers of ARV compliance and also address factors that provide broader social and structural support for HIV-infected adolescents and young adults. Interventions should address psychosocial development, including lack of future orientation, inadequate educational attainment and limited health literacy, failure to focus on the long-term consequences of near-term risk behaviors, and coping ability. Associated challenges are closely linked to the structural environment. Individual case management is essential to linkage to and retention in care, ARV adherence, and management of associated comorbidities. Integrating these skills into pediatric and adolescent HIV practice in a medical home setting is critical, given the alarming increase in new HIV infections in youth in the United States. *Pediatrics* 2014;133:558–562

KEY WORDS
HIV, pediatrics, youth, psychosocial support, antiretroviral therapy

ABBREVIATIONS
ARV—antiretroviral
cART—combination antiretroviral therapy
LGBT—lesbian, gay, bisexual, and transgender

www.pediatrics.org/cgi/doi/10.1542/peds.2013-4061

doi:10.1542/peds.2013-4061

All clinical reports from the American Academy of Pediatrics automatically expire 5 years after publication unless reaffirmed, revised, or retired at or before that time.

PEDIATRICS (ISSN Numbers: Print, 0031-4005; Online, 1098-4275).

BACKGROUND

The US government released a National Strategy for HIV/AIDS in 2010, in which 3 common goals were stated: (1) to reduce the number of individuals who become HIV infected; (2) to increase access to care and improve health outcomes in HIV-infected individuals; and (3) to reduce HIV-related health disparities.[1] These goals reflect significant progress in treatment of HIV infection with effective combination antiretroviral therapy (cART). This approach requires an ever-vigilant approach to long-term antiretroviral (ARV) adherence ($\geq$95%) for optimal virologic suppression and to offset the emergence of drug-resistant HIV so that future treatment options remain viable. Unfortunately many HIV-positive youth are not consistently linked into or retained in care. Youth who miss clinic appointments are more likely to develop life-threatening opportunistic infections. Poor adherence to cART is also associated with increased secondary HIV transmission.[2]

Epidemiology

HIV-infected youth consist of 2 distinct populations: those who acquired HIV infection perinatally and those infected horizontally either by transfusion of blood products or by risk behaviors, including sexual activity and intravenous drug use. As of 2010, there were an estimated 10 797 perinatally HIV-infected people in the United States and dependent areas, and 76% of those affected were ≥13 years of age at the time of the analysis.[3] Recent surveillance data from 2009 and 2010 reveal that youth account for 26% of all new HIV infections in the United States. Nearly 75% and 46% of the 12 200 new HIV infections in youth were attributable to males having sex with males and African American adolescents and young adults, respectively.[4] Stigma, discrimination,[5] infrequent condom use, alcohol and drug use, and having sex with older partners[6] contributed to an even higher risk for acquiring HIV infection, disproportionately affecting minority youth residing in the south and the northeastern United States. An estimated 60% of individuals were unaware of their underlying HIV infection.[7]

Challenges to ARV Adherence Among HIV-Infected Youth in the United States

Poor adherence to ARV therapy has been documented for both perinatally and horizontally HIV-infected youth. Many children infected with HIV perinatally have survived into their second or third decade of life with cART. However, during adolescence a number of psychological and social factors influence decision-making and create challenges for effective ARV adherence. A retrospective multicenter study of adolescents who acquired HIV perinatally reported that adolescents and young adults had the highest risk for resistance to available ARVs secondary to poor drug adherence.[8,9] Similar findings among adolescents and young adults who acquired HIV horizontally are reported, with as few as 24% in 1 study achieving virologic suppression at 3 years after initiation of cART.[10] Such observations reinforce the need to design, implement, and evaluate strategies to increase and sustain adherence to therapy in this group. Interventions must factor the adolescents' stage of development, education level, health literacy and coping ability, and structural environment.[11] Factors that have been implicated in poor levels of adherence and ARV efficacy include poverty, inadequate food access,[12,13] unstable housing,[8] limited educational attainment, lack of stable employment, substance abuse, denial, stigma, homophobia, and discrimination.[14]

HIV Disclosure to Perinatally HIV-Infected Youth

As perinatally HIV-infected children approach adolescence, disclosure of their serostatus becomes essential for personal health maintenance and secondary HIV prevention. The first longitudinal study to examine the impact of disclosure of HIV status on health-related quality of life outcomes documented a median age at disclosure of 11 years. There were no significant changes over time in general health perception, psychological status, physical functioning, social/role functioning, or health care use domains. There was also no significant difference between time trends in quality of life scores before and after disclosure of HIV status, suggesting that diagnostic disclosure to children should not be delayed for fear of a negative impact on quality of life.[15] Disclosure prior to sexual activity is also a public health issue affecting secondary HIV transmission.

Stigma and Disclosure in Horizontally HIV-Infected Youth

Horizontally HIV-infected youth have historically experienced rejection, violence, and discrimination following disclosure of their HIV status. These experiences reflect prevalent societal stigma toward individuals who have acquired HIV through perceived risk behavior. The detrimental effect of HIV stigma on youth is often reported as more significant than the disease itself[9] and negatively impacts ARV adherence. In one study, individuals who have HIV who reported high levels of HIV stigma were 3 times more likely to report problems with adherence.[8] In contrast, when youth reported high levels of satisfaction with health care providers, this ameliorated the negative impact of stigma on adherence to treatment.[16]

Children and Youth Who Are in Foster Care or Homeless

Children who have HIV infection are often placed in foster care. Provision of medical services, including hospitalization, can be initially complicated by limited acquisition and communication of medical information. Eliminating barriers to sharing confidential information between medical providers, mental health case managers, and the foster care agency can improve care of the child or adolescent living with HIV.[17] Institutional confidentiality and privacy policies guiding the care of HIV-infected youth should be developed.[18] Samples of confidentiality policies can be found in *Bright Futures*.[19] A complete medical history may be unavailable at the initial visit, and physicians must be prepared to document the circumstances surrounding the unavailability of previous medical records and provide service with limited knowledge of the youth's family, past medical or ARV history, or immunization status.[20]

Studies indicate that youth aging out of foster care at 18 years of age and those who are lesbian, gay, bisexual, and transgender (LGBT) are especially susceptible to homelessness.[21] The former, particularly minority youth, have limited experience in independent living and lack the financial and social supports required to become independent.[22,23] Many are at increased risk for sexual victimization, school dropout, substance abuse, and mental health comorbidities. Homeless adolescents and young adults frequently engage in prostitution in exchange for money, food, or shelter. The literature estimates that nightly in the United States, homeless youth can number between 1.6 and 2 million, including those living in shelters, on the streets, or in other temporary accommodations. Significantly, LGBT youth account for 20% to 40% of all homeless youth in the United States[24–26] and are 6 to 12 times more likely to become HIV infected than other youth.[27] Homeless youth are 7 times as likely to die from AIDS and 16 times as likely to have HIV infection diagnosed as the general youth population.[26] These youth experience high rates of trauma and abuse before and during their experience of homelessness. Violence is reported in many forms, including physical (50%–82%), sexual (26%–39%), and family abuse (50%).[28]

Acceptance of an HIV Diagnosis and Self-Disclosure to Others

Studies have revealed that youth who have chronic and/or terminal illness experience similar difficulty adjusting to their diagnosis, predominantly with medical management.[29–32] However, HIV-infected youth have the unique difficulty of also living with stigma, which can interfere with their ability to adjust and cope.[33,34] Significant stressors include acceptance of their diagnosis and rejection by others following disclosure.[35] Many fail to keep their medical appointments and present much later with opportunistic infections.

Schooling

Graduating from school is a major milestone for all youth. Youth living with HIV infection are most concerned about disclosure to peers causing HIV stigmatization and adversely impacting social functioning. Youth living with HIV infection report changing grades after being given their diagnosis, with some ultimately dropping out of school. Like many youth who have chronic disease, HIV-infected youth in school have the added stress of skipping classes for medical appointments, which can negatively affect their grades.[35]

THE RESPONSE TO IDENTIFIED PSYCHOSOCIAL NEEDS

1. Youth-Friendly Services

HIV Disclosure, Confidentiality, and Stigma

(a) Confidentiality and privacy policies should be implemented. Given that homophobia, discrimination, and violence often affect HIV-positive LGBT adolescents and young adults, better outcomes are reported in health care settings where there are confidentiality and privacy policies that are discussed during enrollment and at subsequent clinic visits.[18,36,37] Standard forms for and policies on confidentiality as well as policies on privacy for youth are available and can be modified as state or local jurisdictions legally permit.[38]

(b) HIV stigma should be addressed within a developmentally appropriate unit offering comprehensive medical services like a medical home,[16] with patients engaged in trusting relationships with health care providers and being kept well informed of the status of their illness.[16,39]

Denial and Coping With the Diagnosis of HIV Infection

(c) Services should address how youth can cope with their HIV diagnosis. Infrastructure in the medical home that promotes coping through family, peer groups, and spiritual groups as well as professional involvement can improve adherence to clinic appointments and ARV therapy.[16]

Case Management and Multidisciplinary Care in the Medical Home

(d) The sole provision of medical treatment is not sufficient to engage and retain HIV-infected youth in care. Service models that include consideration of gender, race and ethnicity, developmental stage, mental health, family composition, peer reference groups and relationships, economic resources, sexuality, and sexual behaviors are more likely to improve outcomes.[40]

(e) Effective medical treatment should be inclusive of flexible scheduling and a multidisciplinary team approach that includes aggressive case management and care coordination.[41,42]

(f) Patients should be assigned to a physician-led medical home team that can regularly provide all of the medical services and continuity of care.[41]

(g) Medical care services should facilitate prompt access to mental health services.

(h) Regular multidisciplinary team meetings should be scheduled to include all providers involved in the patient's care.

2. Structural Program Elements

(a) Addressing barriers to health care use may assist youth in improving disease self-management. Perceived needs in 1 study of 107 HIV-infected youth included access to mental health services (45%), alcohol and drug treatment (14%), transportation to health care settings (40%), and housing (47%). Youth who expressed these needs were unable or unwilling to "focus on accessing" HIV comprehensive health care.[41,43]

(b) Youth buddies are peer advocates who conduct peer-to-peer counseling. When youth buddies are used as part of the comprehensive medical services team, they can be effective in engaging and retaining youth in care.[41]

3. Social Media

Health Insurance Portability and Accountability Act-compliant secure messaging through the Internet, mobile phones, and social media can be used for improving appointment and medication adherence. Almost all adolescents and young adults have used the Internet and mobile phones in their daily lives.[44] Ninety-five percent of youth report using the Internet and are avid users of social media, with 90% of 13- to 17-year-olds reporting its use, 80% reporting a current profile on a social network site, and 22% having a Twitter account.[45–50]

4. Advocacy

Pediatricians should advocate for resources that are necessary to provide optimal care for HIV-infected adolescents and young adults to include social support, rehabilitation, education, and access to basic necessities, including stable housing, without which the best medical care may prove ineffective. Pediatricians can advocate at the community and legislative/public policy levels (http://www.aap.org/en-us/advocacy-and-policy/Pages/Advocacy-and-Policy.aspx).

LEAD AUTHORS

Jaime Martinez, MD, FAAP
Rana Chakraborty, MD, FAAP

COMMITTEE ON PEDIATRIC AIDS, 2012–2013

Rana Chakraborty, MD, FAAP, Chairperson
Grace M. Aldrovandi, MD, FAAP
Ellen Gould Chadwick, MD, FAAP
Ellen Rae Cooper, MD, FAAP
Athena Kourtis, MD, FAAP
Jaime Martinez, MD, FAAP
Elizabeth Montgomery Collins, MD, FAAP

LIAISONS

Kenneth L. Dominguez, MD, MPH – *Centers for Disease Control and Prevention*
Lynne M. Mofenson, MD, FAAP – *National Institute of Child Health and Human Development*

CONSULTANT

Gordon E. Schutze, MD, FAAP

STAFF

Anjie Emanuel, MPH

REFERENCES

1. The White House Office of National AIDS Policy. *National HIV/AIDS Strategy for the United States*. Washington, DC: The White House Office of National AIDS Policy; 2010. Available at: http://aids.gov/federal-resources/national-hiv-aids-strategy/nhas.pdf. Accessed September 10, 2013

2. Cohen MS, Chen YQ, McCauley M, et al. Prevention of HIV-1 infection with early antiretroviral therapy. *N Engl J Med*. 2011;365(6):493–505

3. Centers for Disease Control and Prevention. Diagnoses of HIV infection in the United States and dependent areas, 2011. HIV Surveillance Report. 2011;23. Available at: http://www.cdc.gov/hiv/library/reports/surveillance/2011/surveillance_Report_vol_23.html. Accessed September 10, 2013

4. Centers for Disease Control and Prevention. Vital signs: HIV infection, testing, and risk behaviors among youths—United States. *MMWR Morb Mortal Wkly Rep*. 2012;61(47):971–976

5. Wong CF, Weiss G, Ayala G, Kipke MD. Harassment, discrimination, violence, and illicit drug use among young men who have sex with men. *AIDS Educ Prev*. 2010;22(4):286–298

6. Hurt CB, Matthews DD, Calabria MS, et al. Sex with older partners is associated with primary HIV infection among men who have sex with men in North Carolina. *J Acquir Immune Defic Syndr*. 2010;54(2):185–190

7. Centers for Disease Control and Prevention. Monitoring selected national HIV prevention and care objectives by using HIV surveillance data—United States and six U.S. dependent areas—2010. HIV Surveillance Supplemental Report. 2012;17(3 Pt A). Available at: http://www.cdc.gov/hiv/library/reports/surveillance/2010/surveillance_Report_vol_18_no_2.html. Accessed September 10, 2013

8. Martinez J, Bell D, Camacho R, et al. Adherence to antiviral drug regimens in HIV-infected adolescent patients engaged in care in a comprehensive adolescent and young adult clinic. *J Natl Med Assoc*. 2000;92(2):55–61

9. Hosek SG, Harper GW, Domanico R. Predictors of medication adherence among HIV-infected youth. *Psychol Health Med*. 2005;10(2):166–179

10. Flynn PM, Rudy BJ, Lindsey JC, et al. Long-term observation of adolescents initiating HAART therapy: three-year follow-up. *AIDS Res Hum Retroviruses*. 2007;23(10):1208–1214

11. Garcia C. Conceptualization and measurement of coping during adolescence: a review of the literature. *J Nurs Scholarsh*. 2010;42(2):166–185

12. Chandrasekhar A, Gupta A. Nutrition and disease progression pre-highly active antiretroviral therapy (HAART) and post-HAART: can good nutrition delay time to HAART and affect response to HAART? *Am J Clin Nutr*. 2011;94(6):1703S–1715S

13. Raiten DJ. Nutrition and pharmacology: general principles and implications for HIV. *Am J Clin Nutr*. 2011;94(6):1697S–1702S

14. Koenig LJ, Bachanas PJ. Adherence to medications for HIV: teens say, "Too many, too big, too often. In: Lyon ME, D'Angelo LJ, eds. *Teenagers, HIV, and AIDS*. Westport, CT: Praeger; 2006:45–66

15. Butler AM, Williams PL, Howland LC, Storm D, Hutton N, Seage GR III. Pediatric AIDS Clinical Trials Group 219C Study Team. Impact of disclosure of HIV infection on health-related quality of life among children and adolescents with HIV infection. *Pediatrics*. 2009;123(3):935–943

16. Martinez J, Harper G, Carleton RA, et al; Adolescent Medicine Trials Network. The impact of stigma on medication adherence among HIV-positive adolescent and young adult females and the moderating effects of coping and satisfaction with health care. *AIDS Patient Care STDS.* 2012;26(2):108–115

17. American Academy of Pediatrics, Committee on Pediatric AIDS. Identification and care of HIV-exposed and HIV-infected infants, children, and adolescents in foster care. *Pediatrics.* 2000;106(1 Pt 1):149–153. Reaffirmed June 2011

18. American Academy of Pediatrics, Committee on Adolescence. Achieving quality health services for adolescents. *Pediatrics.* 2008;121(6):1263–1270

19. American Academy of Pediatrics, Bright Futures Steering Committee. Bright Futures Adolescent Supplemental Questionnaire 15 to 17 Year Visits. Available at: http://brightfutures.aap.org/pdfs/Other%203/D.Adol.SQ.Patient.15-17yr.pdf. Accessed September 10, 2013

20. [No authors listed.]. Special considerations for the health supervision of children and youth in foster care. *Paediatr Child Health (Oxford).* 2008;13(2):129–133

21. Edidin JP, Ganim Z, Hunter SJ, Karnik NS. The mental and physical health of homeless youth: a literature review. *Child Psychiatry Hum Dev.* 2012;43(3):354–375

22. Hyde J. From home to the street: understanding young people's transitions into homelessness. *J Adolesc.* 2005;28(2):171–183

23. Fowler PJ, Toro PA, Miles BW. Pathways to and from homelessness and associated psychosocial outcomes among adolescents leaving the foster care system. *Am J Public Health.* 2009;99(8):1453–1458

24. National Alliance to End Homelessness. *Youth Homelessness Series, Brief No. 1: Fundamental Issues to Prevent and End Youth Homelessness.* Washington, DC: National Alliance to End Homelessness; 2006

25. Rew L, Taylor-Seehafer M, Thomas NY, Yockey RD. Correlates of resilience in homeless adolescents. *J Nurs Scholarsh.* 2001;33(1):33–40

26. Ray N. *Lesbian, Gay, Bisexual and Transgender Youth: An Epidemic of Homelessness.* New York, NY: National Gay and Lesbian Task Force Policy Institute and the National Coalition for the Homeless; 2006

27. Rotheram-Borus MJ, Song J, Gwadz M, Lee M, Van Rossem R, Koopman C. Reductions in HIV risk among runaway youth. *Prev Sci.* 2003;4(3):173–187

28. Ferguson KM. Exploring family environment characteristics and multiple abuse experiences among homeless youth. *J Interpers Violence.* 2009;24(11):1875–1891

29. Gavaghan MP, Roach JE. Ego identity development of adolescents with cancer. *J Pediatr Psychol.* 1987;12(2):203–213

30. Lavigne J, Faier-Routman J. Psychological adjustment to pediatric physical disorders: a meta-analytic review. *J Pediatr Psychol.* 1992;17(2):133–157

31. Sayer AG, Hauser ST, Jacobson AM, Willett JB, Cole CF. Developmental influences on adolescent health. In: Wallander JL, Siegel LJ, eds. *Adolescent Health Problems.* New York, NY: Guilford Press; 1995:22–51

32. Wallander JL, Thompson RJ. Psychosocial adjustment of children with chronic physical conditions. In: Roberts MD, ed. *Handbook of Pediatric Psychology,* 2nd ed. New York, NY: Guilford Press; 1995:124–142

33. Brown LK, Lourie KJ, Pao M. Children and adolescents living with HIV and AIDS: a review. *J Child Psychol Psychiatry.* 2000;41(1):81–96

34. Rao D, Ketwaletswe TC, Hosek SG, Martinez J, Rodriguez F. Stigma and social barriers to medication adherence with urban youth living with HIV. *AIDS Care.* 2007;19(1):28–33

35. Hosek SG, Harper GW, Lemos D, Martinez J; Adolescent Medicine Trials Network for HIV/AIDS Interventions. An ecological model of stressors experienced by youth newly diagnosed with HIV. *J HIV AIDS Prev Child Youth.* 2008;9(2):192–218

36. AIDS Alliance for Children. *Youth and Families. Finding HIV-Positive Youth And Bringing Them Into Care.* Washington, DC: AIDS Alliance for Children, Youth and Families; 2005

37. Stanford PD, Monte DA, Briggs FM, et al. Recruitment and retention of adolescent participants in HIV research: findings from the REACH (Reaching for Excellence in Adolescent Care and Health) Project. *J Adolesc Health.* 2003;32(3):192–203

38. American Academy of Pediatrics, Bright Futures Steering Committee. Introduction to the Bright Futures Visits. Available at: http://brightfutures.aap.org/pdfs/Guidelines_PDF/12-Introduction_to_the_Bright_Futures_Visits.pdf. Accessed September 10, 2013

39. Urowitz S, Deber R. How consumerist do people want to be? Preferred role in decision-making of individuals with HIV/AIDS. *Health Policy.* 2008;3(3):e168–e182

40. Johnson RL, Martinez J, Botwinick G, et al. Introduction: what youth need: adapting HIV care models to meet the lifestyles and special needs of adolescents and young adults. *J Adolesc Health.* 2003;33(suppl):4–9

41. Johnson RL, Botwinick G, Sell RL, et al. The utilization of treatment and case management services by HIV infected youth. *J Adolesc Health.* 2003;33(suppl):31–38

42. Martinez J, Hosek SG, Carleton RA. Screening and assessing violence and mental health disorders in a cohort of inner city HIV positive youth between 1998–2006. *AIDS Patient Care STDS.* 2009;23(6):469–475

43. Martinez J, Bell D, Dodds S, et al. Transitioning youth into care (linking identified HIV infected youth at outreach sites in the community to hospital based clinics and or community based health centers). *J Adolesc Health.* 2003;33(suppl):23–30

44. Allison A, Bauermeister JA, Bull S, et al. The intersection of youth, technology, and new media with sexual health: moving the research agenda forward. *J Adolesc Health.* 2012;51(3):207–212

45. Lenhart A, Madden M, Smith A, et al. *Teens, Kindness and Cruelty on Social Network Sites: How American Teens Navigate the New World of "Digital Citizenship.".* Washington, DC: Pew Research Center's Internet and American Life Project; 2011

46. Media CS. Social Media, Social Life: How Teens View Their Digital Lives. A Common Sense Media Research Study. June 26, 2012. Available at: http://www.commonsensemedia.org/research/social-media-social-life. Accessed September 10, 2013

47. Lenhart A, Madden M, McGill AR, Smith A. *Teens and Social Media: The Use of Social Media Gains a Greater Foothold in Teen Life as They Embrace the Conversational Nature of Interactive Online Media.* Washington, DC: Pew Internet and American Life Project; 2007

48. Malesky LA Jr. Predatory online behavior: modus operandi of convicted sex offenders in identifying potential victims and contacting minors over the internet. *J Child Sex Abuse.* 2007;16(2):23–32

49. Smith-Rohrberg D, Mezger J, Walton M, et al. Impact of enhanced services on virologic outcomes in a directly administered antiretroviral therapy trial for HIV-infected drug users. *J Acquir Immune Defic Syndr.* 2006;43(suppl):S48–S53

50. Purnel M, Santos K, Balthazar C. Using technology to retain young MSM in an open label pre-exposure prophylaxis study [abstr WEPE271]. Paper presented at: 19th International AIDS Conference; July 22–27, 2012; Washington, DC

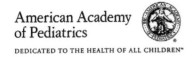

Guidance for the Clinician in
Rendering Pediatric Care

CLINICAL REPORT

Supporting the Family After the Death of a Child

abstract

The death of a child can have a devastating effect on the family. The pediatrician has an important role to play in supporting the parents and any siblings still in his or her practice after such a death. Pediatricians may be poorly prepared to provide this support. Also, because of the pain of confronting the grief of family members, they may be reluctant to become involved. This statement gives guidelines to help the pediatrician provide such support. It describes the grief reactions that can be expected in family members after the death of a child. Ways of supporting family members are suggested, and other helpful resources in the community are described. The goal of this guidance is to prevent outcomes that may impair the health and development of affected parents and children. *Pediatrics* 2012;130:1164—1169

Esther Wender, MD, and THE COMMITTEE ON PSYCHOSOCIAL ASPECTS OF CHILD AND FAMILY HEALTH

KEY WORDS
child death, family support, grief, pediatrician, parents, siblings

This document is copyrighted and is property of the American Academy of Pediatrics and its Board of Directors. All authors have filed conflict of interest statements with the American Academy of Pediatrics. Any conflicts have been resolved through a process approved by the Board of Directors. The American Academy of Pediatrics has neither solicited nor accepted any commercial involvement in the development of the content of this publication.

The guidance in this report does not indicate an exclusive course of treatment or serve as a standard of medical care. Variations, taking into account individual circumstances, may be appropriate.

www.pediatrics.org/cgi/doi/10.1542/peds.2012-2772

doi:10.1542/peds.2012-2772

All clinical reports from the American Academy of Pediatrics automatically expire 5 years after publication unless reaffirmed, revised, or retired at or before that time.

PEDIATRICS (ISSN Numbers: Print, 0031-4005; Online, 1098-4275).

INTRODUCTION

The death of an infant, child, or adolescent, from any cause, has a devastating effect on the family. For parents, the loss of a child defies the natural order. In our era, parents do not expect to bury their children. The death of a child or adolescent also often means there is a sibling or siblings who experience their own significant loss. The pediatrician is in a position to help family members cope, both with the immediate loss and then the ongoing effect of the child's death. Because of the general good health of children in our society, pediatricians are often unfamiliar with how to deal with the death of a child, however. Or they may feel that addressing this event is too emotionally painful. This report identifies the most important issues to be considered and suggests ways the pediatrician can and should help.

PARENTAL GRIEF

The death of a child of any age is extremely painful for parents. Parents have an obligation and a strong emotional need to protect their children from harm. Most parents experience a profound sense of guilt when harm comes to their child, even if through no fault of their own. Parents invest much of their hopes and wishes for the future in their children. All of these factors lead to a devastating grief that is much longer lasting than most people realize.[1] The depth of parental grief often shocks and surprises others. It is common for grieving parents to be unable to function for varying times after their child's death. They may spend days in bed, away from work, and unable to carry out household tasks. It is common for parents to have great difficulty eating and sleeping. The thought that life is not worth living is frequent, as are thoughts that one might be "going crazy."

ISSUES RELATED TO THE CIRCUMSTANCES OF THE DEATH

Death as the Result of Chronic Illness or Disability

When a child or adolescent's death results from chronic illness or disability, it is likely that the pediatrician has been involved in the patient's care and may have a long-standing relationship with the family. Although the family may have anticipated the death, the grief will still likely be profound. Even when the child has had severe disability or has suffered, the parents' sense of grief and loss is not usually diminished. When there has been a long-standing relationship with the family surrounding the child's illness or disability, the family also may suffer from the loss of the relationship with the pediatrician. Under these circumstances, the pediatrician's continuing involvement with the family may be especially important.

Sudden, Unexpected Death

Injuries are the single most common reason for death in children and adolescents. In adolescents, suicide and homicide are also a common cause of death. Pediatricians may not immediately be aware of the death in such circumstances. If there is a brief period of survival after the event, the pediatrician may be involved; however, these deaths often occur in the emergency department. If this situation is the case, the emergency physician should inform the pediatrician of the death, including the details of the last hours of care.[2,3] If not actually witnessed by the parents, these details will often be what haunts the

parents' thoughts in the months after the death. Pediatricians may hear about the death of a child or adolescent who was one of their patients from the news or from their office staff or other parents in their practice. Although the pediatrician was not involved at the time of the death, if there has been a relationship with the family and if there are surviving siblings who are still patients in the practice, the pediatrician has an important role in supporting the family.

Infant Death

In the case of infant death, many physicians fail to appreciate the intense attachment to the fetus and infant and the extent to which parents and other family members invest in that infant's imagined future. The grief at this loss is intense, and the surviving siblings also may be deeply affected. The physician should recognize the depth of these feelings and be prepared to provide the kind of support outlined in this statement.

Helpful Responses and Those That Hurt

The most helpful response after a child or adolescent death is to provide an opportunity to meet with the parents, face to face, and to just listen, responding in ways that encourage the parents to talk. Frequently, in the context of an unexpected death, physicians fail to respond at all. This failure to respond may contribute to the family's pain. Many physicians find the thought of losing a child so terrible that they avoid contact with the grieving parents rather than confront their own fears. Others find it difficult to be with parents who are crying or showing their grief in other ways. Physicians often hold the mistaken belief that talking about the death will be harmful because such talk will reawaken and prolong the parents'

grief.[4] Quite the contrary, grieving parents report that acknowledging their grief is important, and they seldom forget the pain of a friend, family member, or physician who fails to make contact after such a loss.[5] If pediatricians have a relationship with a family, they should always contact the parents when they learn of the death of a child in that family, including the pediatrician who hears about the death from the news or from others in the community. Such contact should be more than attendance at a viewing or a funeral. At such formal times of grieving, personal contact is not possible, and parents are usually in shock and unable to ask the questions that may be on their minds. The most helpful response is a face-to-face visit.[6] The purpose of such an encounter is to acknowledge the death and allow the parents to talk. The pediatrician might say, simply, "I'm so sorry to hear about _____'s death. What a terrible loss for you and your family." Attempts to alleviate the grief by providing advice are usually ineffective and may be hurtful. Expressions of religious interpretation may or may not be appropriate and should be tailored to what the pediatrician knows of the family's beliefs. Comments made to parents of children with disabilities, such as "he/she is better off now," are often perceived as diminishing the value of the child. Some parents, however, may voice this thought themselves.

Duration of Grieving

Many people are surprised at how long parents may grieve the loss of a child. The period of a year of grieving is acknowledged by many religions and cultural practices, but commonly, parents experience significant grief for much longer. Parents frequently report waves of grief that include reliving the traumatic details of the injury or visions of the person suffering the final stages of a fatal illness.

Anniversaries of the death and important dates, such as the child's birthday, bring recurring waves of grief, often for several years. Family events, such as graduations, marriages, and births, reawaken grief. These events are reminders of the hopes and dreams shattered by the child's death. Eventually, and the period of time varies greatly, parents describe a gradual pattern of change. They no longer relive the experiences at the time of death, and they are able to remember common and happy events in the child's life with less pain and even with pleasure. This change is, however, usually measured in years. Parents frequently report that their greatest fear is that the child will be forgotten, so failing to mention or talk about the child who has died confirms these fears.

Helping During Prolonged Grief

Every parent grieves in his or her own way, and the pediatrician should not expect a prescribed timetable of grieving. Parents find it painful to hear a statement such as, "You should get over it and get on with your life." Yet such statements are frequently made. Self-help support groups, such as The Compassionate Friends and Bereaved Parents USA (see Resources section), are specifically designed for parents whose children have died and provide some of the best help for this prolonged grieving process.[7] These peer-led support groups provide an atmosphere in which it is possible to talk about the loss without the pressure to "get over it." Also, most parents are comforted by an environment in which others have been through a similar experience and in which they meet those who have survived this devastating loss. Descriptive studies confirm that many parents resolve their grief by talking about their loss in an accepting environment.[4] Family members who are discouraged from expressing their grief

may find it more difficult to get past the most painful part of their grieving and function effectively. Pediatricians are encouraged to learn about the support groups in their community and how they function. They can then refer parents who might benefit from such groups (see Resources).

Special Circumstances

The death of a child, no matter what the cause, is devastating. But there are some circumstances that make this loss particularly difficult. When the death occurs by suicide or through the child's use of alcohol or drugs, the guilt experienced by parents can be particularly strong. Homicide or injuries that are caused by negligence, such as by drunk driving, produce intense anger. The grief also may be especially intense if the parent's actions may have contributed to the death, such as in situations in which supervision was lacking or if the parent was driving when an injury occurred. Parents in these circumstances may require special help through counseling or therapy. If the cause of a child's death might be filicide, special circumstances beyond the scope of this statement must be addressed.

Complicated Grief, Medication, and Grief Counseling

In this report, the term "complicated grief" refers to the situation when grief is so intense and/or prolonged that the pediatrician believes that professional mental health evaluation or treatment is required. It is difficult to specify either the symptoms or the circumstances when this point is reached, but a few general guidelines can be given. Complicated grief occurs most frequently when the parent is already experiencing a psychiatric problem, or the parent may have had a psychiatric disorder in the past. Most obviously, when a parent is already experiencing

depression, the death of his or her child is likely to exacerbate that problem. Other psychiatric disorders also may worsen with such a death. Another situation that is known to result in a more serious grief reaction is the death of a child when the parent-child relationship has been a troubled one[8]; however, grief (including intense and prolonged grief, as described previously) is a normal reaction to the loss of a child. In most situations, medication is not needed and can be counterproductive. If, however, the pediatrician judges the grief to be especially intense and debilitating, medication may be needed, and a referral to a mental health specialist should be considered.

Grief counseling is available and/or provided under a variety of circumstances. In situations of injury death in which a number of people have been killed, such as in an airplane crash, grief counselors may provide help in the immediate aftermath. Also, in most communities and at most hospitals, grief counseling groups meet, usually for a prescribed period of time, typically lasting from 6 to 8 weeks. Such groups usually are not designed just for parents who have lost children. Although these groups are helpful to many parents, they do not address the long-term issues mentioned previously. Grief counselors can be especially helpful when they are trained to recognize the complicated grief described previously and can make appropriate referrals.

SIBLINGS

Siblings in a family in which an infant, child, or adolescent has died are sometimes called "the forgotten mourners."[9] This phrase acknowledges that the grief of siblings is often neglected because parents are the focus of grieving within the family. The pediatrician is in a unique position to provide support to siblings who are in their practice, both at the time of death of their brother or sister and in the context of the sibling's ongoing health care. What follows are suggestions on how to provide this type of care.

Initially, particularly in the case of sudden, unexpected death, the problem may be that parents may not be able to provide ongoing support to their surviving children in the midst of their own grief. For very young siblings for whom the need for parental support is great, this problem may be acute. Members of the extended family may be in the position to help once the need is identified. When not available, however, other social services may need to be recruited to provide support. Older siblings often experience an ongoing lack of emotional support and feel abandoned by their grieving parents. The pediatrician may be in the best position to assess these issues and identify other resources if needed.

The way siblings respond to the death of a brother or a sister of any age varies depending on the developmental age of the sibling, and this response changes as the sibling matures. The reactions to death in the family and the changes that occur during development are discussed elsewhere in the pediatric literature[10]; however, there are special issues associated with sibling loss that are less well known and are reviewed here.

Survivor Guilt

Survivor guilt in siblings is common, especially in situations of unexpected death. Guilty feelings may be especially strong in siblings who have experienced intense sibling rivalry. Before the death, the sibling may have had negative feelings about the deceased, or there may have been harsh words spoken during angry arguments. The sibling may have harbored thoughts wishing that harm would come to his or her brother or sister. These thoughts and words may haunt the surviving sibling. Such thoughts and memories may be emotionally crippling unless talked about in counseling or dealt with in therapy.

Overprotection

Parents commonly fear that their surviving child or children will also die. These fears may lead to serious overprotection of surviving siblings, such as restricting age-appropriate activities. Behavior problems in these siblings may stem from the need to break free from stifling overprotection. Pediatricians should be sensitive to this possibility and should counsel parents under such circumstances.

Idealization and the Replacement Child

Parents and other family members frequently idealize the deceased child. Parents often create shrines to memorialize the child, which may reinforce this idealization. Siblings, especially younger ones, may be jealous and resent this picture of the idealized child. The surviving sibling may feel he or she cannot live up to that ideal and may respond with rebellious behavior. Parents also may come to view a surviving sibling, particularly a younger one, as a replacement for the child who died.[11] In this situation, the family member projects on to the surviving sibling his or her hopes and wishes for the child who died. The sibling may sense the parents' feelings and rebel against these wishes and hopes, especially if they are unrealistic. If pediatricians recognize these dynamics, they can be discussed with the parents, and suggestions can be made to address the sibling's feelings.[12] A referral for therapy may be needed if the problem persists.

Assuming the Parental Role

It is especially common for older siblings to assume a parental role when parents are absorbed with their own grief. Although this reaction may be adaptive in the early months of the parents' grief journey, it may become maladaptive as the sibling matures. The pediatrician should look for this situation and help the parent and surviving sibling to relinquish this distortion of family roles.

General Issues of Sibling Grief

One's siblings play a special role in a child's growth and development. Siblings share family secrets, and no one else in a child's life may share that experience. Siblings also have a special role to play in protecting each other in the wider environment of school and playground. Surviving siblings may experience a profound sadness at the loss of this special relationship and may find it helpful to talk about this aspect of their loss.

Providing Sibling Support

If a surviving sibling is in the pediatrician's practice, the clinician should find a way to follow that sibling's emotional development and intervene when problems are detected. One suggestion is to place a picture of the deceased child in the sibling's chart as a reminder whenever that sibling is seen in ongoing health care. A helpful approach is to raise the issue of the brother's or sister's death at well-child visits. The surviving sibling's feelings and thoughts will change with time. The pediatrician should be aware that siblings may refuse to talk about their deceased brother or sister at first. The pediatrician should honor this resistance but be persistent in raising the issue, because this reaction often changes over time.

Some self-help support groups provide support for siblings who are old enough to benefit from talking to other young people who have suffered a similar loss. Support for siblings may also be provided by schools, religious organizations, and groups such as scouts or other organizations. Knowledge of these and other such services in one's community allows the pediatrician to tap other sources of support (see Resources).

SUMMARY

The death of an infant, child, or adolescent is a devastating experience for the family. The pediatrician is in a special position to help families through their grief experience. The ultimate goal of such support is the prevention of problems that may result from such trauma. The following are suggestions for pediatricians regarding this support.

1. Expect that grief after the loss of a child is intense and long lasting.

2. Recognize that failing to acknowledge the death of an infant, child, or adolescent who was a patient can contribute to the family's pain. A telephone call or a face-to-face visit with the parent(s) of a patient who has died is encouraged.

3. Follow up with and provide guidance to surviving siblings who are still patients. Providing guidance to siblings requires recognition of the special issues experienced by grieving siblings.

4. Understand that the duration of grieving within a family after the loss of a child is longer than many expect and is usually measured in years.

5. Recognize the power of self-help support groups in helping parents get through the prolonged grief after their child's death. Be aware of the presence of such groups in the community and make referrals when indicated.

6. Be aware that when the death of a child or adolescent is by suicide, through the use of alcohol or drugs, or through homicide, the grief is especially intense and is accompanied by intense guilt and/or anger. Consider referral for counseling or therapy in these cases.

7. Be aware that complicated grief is more likely when the parent has a preexisting psychiatric problem or when there was a troubled parent-child relationship before death. In such cases, referral to a mental health specialist may be indicated. Most intense and prolonged grief is normal, however, and the use of medication is usually not helpful.

RESOURCES

The Compassionate Friends

A national self-help support organization with >600 local chapters. Many local chapters have special groups for siblings. National office telephone number (toll free): 877-969-0010; Web site: www.compassionatefriends.org.

SHARE

Support for those touched by the death of an infant through miscarriage, stillbirth, or newborn death. Web site: www.nationalshare.org.

BEREAVED PARENTS OF THE USA (BP/USA)

Provides support, care, and compassion for bereaved parents, siblings, and grandparents. Web site: www.bereavedparentsusa.org.

SURVIVORS OF SUICIDE (SOS)

Support for those who have lost a loved one to suicide. Web site: www.survivorsofsuicide.com.

LEAD AUTHOR

Esther H. Wender, MD

COMMITTEE ON PSYCHOSOCIAL ASPECTS OF CHILD AND FAMILY HEALTH, 2011–2012

Benjamin S. Siegel, MD, Chairperson
Mary I. Dobbins, MD
Andrew S. Garner, MD, PhD
Laura J. McGuinn, MD
John Pascoe, MD, MPH
David L. Wood, MD, MPH
Michael W. Yogman, MD

LIAISONS

Ronald T. Brown, PhD — *Society of Pediatric Psychology*
Terry Carmichael, MSW — *National Association of Social Workers*
Mary Jo Kupst, PhD — *Society of Pediatric Psychology*
D. Richard Martini, MD — *American Academy of Child and Adolescent Psychiatry*
Mary Sheppard, MS, RN, PNP, BC — *National Association of Pediatric Nurse Practitioners*

LIAISONS

George J. Cohen, MD

STAFF

Karen S. Smith
Tamar Mangarik Haro

REFERENCES

1. Finkbeiner A. *After the Death of a Child: Living with Loss Through the Years.* Baltimore, MD: Johns Hopkins University Press; 1996

2. American Academy of Pediatrics Committee on Pediatric Emergency Medicine, American College of Emergency Physicians Pediatric Emergency Medicine Committee. Death of a child in the emergency department: Joint statement by the American Academy of Pediatrics and the American College of Emergency Physicians. *Pediatrics.* 2002;110(4): 839–840 (under revision as of January 2012)

3. Knapp J, Mulligan-Smith D; American Academy of Pediatrics Committee on Pediatric Emergency Medicine. Death of a child in the emergency department. *Pediatrics.* 2005;115(5):1432–1437

4. Taneja GS, Brenner RA, Klinger R, Trumble AC, Qian C, Klebanoff M. Participation of next of kin in research following sudden, unexpected death of a child. *Arch*

Pediatr Adolesc Med. 2007;161(5):453–456

5. Macdonald ME, Liben S, Carnevale FA, et al. Parental perspectives on hospital staff members' acts of kindness and commemoration after a child's death. *Pediatrics.* 2005;116(4):884–890

6. Wessel MA. The primary pediatrician's role when a death occurs in a family in one's practice. *Pediatr Rev.* 2003;24(6):183–185

7. Picton C, Cooper BK, Close D, Tobin J. Bereavement support groups: timing of participation and reasons for joining. *Omega.* 2001;43(3):247–258

8. Hendrickson KC. Morbidity, mortality, and parental grief: a review of the literature on the relationship between the death of a child and the subsequent health of parents. *Palliat Support Care.* 2009;7(1):109–119

9. Brent DA. A death in the family: the pediatrician's role. *Pediatrics.* 1983;72(5):645–651

10. American Academy of Pediatrics. Committee on Psychosocial Aspects of Child and Family Health. The pediatrician and childhood bereavement. *Pediatrics.* 2000;105(2):445–447

11. Cain AC, Cain BS. On replacing a child. *J Am Acad Child Psychiatry.* 1964;3(July):443–456

12. Horsley G, Horsley H. *Teen Grief Relief: Parenting with Understanding, Support and Guidance.* Highland City, FL: Rainbow Books; 2007

CLINICAL REPORT   Guidance for the Clinician in Rendering Pediatric Care

American Academy
of Pediatrics

DEDICATED TO THE HEALTH OF ALL CHILDREN™

Supporting the Grieving Child and Family

David J. Schonfeld, MD, FAAP, Thomas Demaria, PhD, COMMITTEE ON PSYCHOSOCIAL ASPECTS OF CHILD AND FAMILY HEALTH, DISASTER PREPAREDNESS ADVISORY COUNCIL

abstract

The death of someone close to a child often has a profound and lifelong effect on the child and results in a range of both short- and long-term reactions. Pediatricians, within a patient-centered medical home, are in an excellent position to provide anticipatory guidance to caregivers and to offer assistance and support to children and families who are grieving. This clinical report offers practical suggestions on how to talk with grieving children to help them better understand what has happened and its implications and to address any misinformation, misinterpretations, or misconceptions. An understanding of guilt, shame, and other common reactions, as well an appreciation of the role of secondary losses and the unique challenges facing children in communities characterized by chronic trauma and cumulative loss, will help the pediatrician to address factors that may impair grieving and children's adjustment and to identify complicated mourning and situations when professional counseling is indicated. Advice on how to support children's participation in funerals and other memorial services and to anticipate and address grief triggers and anniversary reactions is provided so that pediatricians are in a better position to advise caregivers and to offer consultation to schools, early education and child care facilities, and other child congregate care sites. Pediatricians often enter their profession out of a profound desire to minimize the suffering of children and may find it personally challenging when they find themselves in situations in which they are asked to bear witness to the distress of children who are acutely grieving. The importance of professional preparation and self-care is therefore emphasized, and resources are recommended.

Clinical reports from the American Academy of Pediatrics benefit from expertise and resources of liaisons and internal (AAP) and external reviewers. However, clinical reports from the American Academy of Pediatrics may not reflect the views of the liaisons or the organizations or government agencies that they represent.

The guidance in this report does not indicate an exclusive course of treatment or serve as a standard of medical care. Variations, taking into account individual circumstances, may be appropriate.

All clinical reports from the American Academy of Pediatrics automatically expire 5 years after publication unless reaffirmed, revised, or retired at or before that time.

DOI: 10.1542/peds.2016-2147

Accepted for publication Jun 27, 2016

PEDIATRICS (ISSN Numbers: Print, 0031-4005; Online, 1098-4275).

Copyright © 2016 by the American Academy of Pediatrics

FINANCIAL DISCLOSURE: The authors have indicated they do not have a financial relationship relevant to this article to disclose.

FUNDING: No external funding.

POTENTIAL CONFLICT OF INTEREST: The authors have indicated they have no potential conflicts of interest to disclose.

To cite: Schonfeld DJ, Demaria T, AAP COMMITTEE ON PSYCHOSOCIAL ASPECTS OF CHILD AND FAMILY HEALTH, DISASTER PREPAREDNESS ADVISORY COUNCIL. Supporting the Grieving Child and Family. Pediatrics. 2016;138(3):e20162147

INTRODUCTION

At some point in their childhood, the vast majority of children will experience the death of a close family member or friend[1,2]; approximately 1 in 20 children in the United States experiences the death of a parent by the age of 16.[3] Despite the high prevalence of bereavement among children, many pediatricians are uncomfortable talking with and supporting grieving children.[4]

Bereavement is a normative experience that is universal in nature, but this does not minimize the impact of a loss. The death of someone close to a child often has a profound and lifelong effect on the child and may result in a range of both short- and long-term reactions. Pediatricians, within a patient-centered medical home, are in an excellent position to provide anticipatory guidance to caregivers before, during, and after a loss and can provide assistance and support in a number of areas, including the following:

- exploring and confirming that children understand what has occurred and what death means;

- helping to identify reactions such as guilt, fear, worry, or depressive symptoms that suggest the need for further discussion or services;

- providing reassurance to children who become concerned about their own health or those of family members;

- offering support to grieving children and their families to minimize their distress and accelerate their adjustment;

- informing families about local resources that can provide additional assistance; and

- offering advice on funeral attendance of children.

Pediatricians also can play an important role in supporting parents and other caregivers after the death of a child, even in the absence of surviving siblings.[4–6] In addition, children may experience grief in response to a range of other losses, such as separation from parents because of deployment, incarceration, or divorce, which may be helped by similar caring strategies.

This clinical report is a revision of an earlier clinical report that

introduced some of the key issues that pediatricians should consider in providing support to grieving children.[7] Guidance is available elsewhere regarding how to support families faced with the impending or recent death of their child,[4,8] including practical advice on how to approach notification of parents about the death of their child in a hospital setting[8,9] or in the unique context of a disaster.[10] Because traumatic events often involve loss, complementary information on providing psychosocial support in the aftermath of a crisis can be found in a recent clinical report,[11] which may be particularly relevant to pediatricians providing care in emergency departments and intensive care settings.

IDENTIFYING CHILDREN'S LOSS EXPERIENCES

In a busy pediatric practice, it is likely that a pediatrician interacts with a child who is grieving a death virtually every week, if not every day. But many children who are grieving show few outward signs during an office visit. From an early age, children learn that questions or discussion about death make many adults uncomfortable; they learn not to talk about death in public. In the context of a recent death, children may also be reluctant to further burden grieving family members with their own concerns.

Children's questions about the impact of a personal loss can be quite poignant and/or frame the experience in concrete and direct terms that underscore the immediacy and reality of the loss to adults (eg, "If Mommy died, does that mean that she won't be here even for my birthday? How can I live the rest of my life without her?"). Adolescents who are in a better position to appreciate the secondary losses and other implications of a significant loss may raise concerns

that surviving adults may not have yet appreciated (eg, "I don't know if I ever will feel comfortable having my own children when I grow up, without Mom there to help me."). When children ask such questions or make similar comments, surviving family members may become tearful and/or obviously upset. Children may misinterpret these expressions of grief triggered by their questions as evidence that the questions themselves were hurtful or inappropriate. They subsequently may remain silent and grieve alone, without support. In addition, when children lose a parent or other close family member, they are often fearful that others they count on for support may also die and leave them all alone. Children may find it particularly unsettling to observe their surviving caregivers struggling and often respond to their surviving parent(s) demonstrations of grief by offering support or assistance (eg, "Don't worry Daddy, I can help do many of the things Mommy used to do; we are going to be okay."), rather than asking for help themselves, which may convince surviving caregiver(s) that the child is coping and has no need for assistance. For this reason, it is important for pediatricians to offer to speak with children privately after a family death to identify their understanding, concerns, and reactions without children feeling that they need to protect surviving caregivers.

Caregivers who are struggling with their own personal grief may be particularly reluctant, or even unable, to recognize or accept their children's grief. The reality is that many children in this situation are grieving alone, postponing expressing their grief until a time when it feels safer, or seeking support elsewhere, such as at school or after-school programs where they can talk about their feelings and concerns with adults who have personal distance from the loss.

Young children, in particular, may not yet understand the implications the death may have for them or their family. Children and their families may wish to seek advice but view death as a normative experience that does not warrant professional assistance and may not realize that their pediatrician may be interested in helping and able to assist them. During an incidental pediatric office visit, children may be reluctant to raise the topic because they worry that they will start crying or otherwise embarrass themselves. They may be afraid to start a discussion in the pediatric office or at school because they worry that once they start to cry, they will be unable to compose themselves by the end of an office visit or a conversation at school. Children may also express their grief indirectly through their behavior or attempt to address their feelings through play. Grief is, in many ways, a private experience. Older children, especially, may elect to keep their feelings and concerns to themselves unless caring adults invite and facilitate discussion. These are among the many reasons why pediatricians may be unaware of a death involving a close family member or friend of one of their patients.

Pediatricians can increase the likelihood that children and families will bring significant losses to their attention by directly informing families, often during the initial visit and periodically thereafter, that they are interested in hearing about major changes in the lives of patients and their families, such as deaths of family members or friends, financial or marital concerns of the family, planned or recent moves, traumatic events in the local community or neighborhood, or problems or concerns at school or with peer relationships. At subsequent visits, pediatricians can ask whether any major changes or potential stressors at home, at school, or within the community have occurred or are anticipated.[12] Practices that respond to these needs as they arise in families, by inviting conversations, expressing concern, and offering information and referral, create an atmosphere in which families are more likely to disclose their occurrence and actively seek assistance and support.

INITIATING THE CONVERSATION

Pediatricians and other caring adults often worry that asking children about the recent death of someone close to them may upset them. In the immediate aftermath of a major loss, the loss is almost always on survivors' minds. Although a question about the death may lead to an expression of sadness, it is the death itself, and not the question, that is the cause of the distress. Inviting children to express their feelings allows them to express their sadness; it does not cause it. In contrast, avoiding the subject may create more problems. Children may interpret the silence as evidence that adults are unaware of their loss, feel that their loss is trivial and unworthy of comment, are disinterested in their grief, are unwilling or unable to assist, or view the child as unable to cope even with support. Instead, the following steps can be used to initiate the conversation[13]:

- Express your concern. It is okay to be tearful or simply to let them know you feel sorry someone they care about has died.

- Be genuine; children can tell when adults are authentic. Do not tell the child you will miss her grandfather if you have never met him; instead, let the child know that you appreciate that he was important to her and you feel sorry she had to experience such a loss.

- Listen and observe; talk less. Simply being present while the child is expressing grief and tolerating the unpleasant affect can be very helpful.

- Invite discussion using open-ended questions such as "How are you doing since your mother died?" or "How is your family coping?"

- Limit the sharing of your personal experiences. Keep the focus on the child's loss and feelings.

- Offer practical advice, such as suggestions about how to answer questions that might be posed by peers or how to talk with teachers about learning challenges.

- Offer appropriate reassurance. Do not minimize children's concerns but let them know that over time you do expect that they will become better able to cope with their distress.

- Communicate your availability to provide support over time. Do not require children or families to reach out to you for such support, but rather, make the effort to schedule follow-up appointments and reach out by phone or e-mail periodically.

Adults are often worried that they will say the wrong thing and make matters worse. In the context of talking with a patient who has recently experienced a death, caregivers may wish to consider the following suggestions[13]:

- Although well intentioned, attempts to "cheer up" individuals who are grieving are usually neither effective nor appreciated. Anything that begins with "at least" should be reconsidered (eg, "at least he isn't in pain anymore," "at least you have another brother"). Such comments may minimize professionals' discomfort in being with a child who is grieving but do not help children express and cope with their feelings.

- Do not instruct children to hide their emotions (eg, "You need to be strong; you are the man of the house now that your father has died.").

- Avoid communicating that you know how they feel (eg, "I know exactly what you are going through."). Instead, ask them to share their feelings.

- Do not tell them how they ought to feel ("You must feel angry.").

- Avoid comparisons with your own experiences. When adults share their own experiences in the context of recent loss, it shifts the focus away from the child. If your loss is perceived by the child as less important, the comparison can be insulting (eg, "I know what you are going through after the death of your father. My cat died this week."). If your experience appears worse (eg, "I understand your grandfather died. When I was your age, both my mother and father died in a car accident."), the child may feel compelled to comfort you and be reluctant to ask for help.

The use of expressive techniques, such as picture drawing or engaging children in an activity while talking with them, may be helpful in some situations in which children appear reluctant to address the topic in direct conversation. Pediatricians can also provide written information to families about how to support grieving children (eg, *After a Loved One Dies: How Children Grieve and How Parents and Other Adults Can Support Them*, which is freely available and can be accessed through the coping and adjustment Web page of the American Academy of Pediatrics at https://www.aap.org/en-us/advocacy-and-policy/aap-health-initiatives/Children-and-Disasters/Pages/Promoting-Adjustment-and-Helping-Children-Cope.aspx).[14] Books written specifically for younger children that help them develop a better understanding of death or that help children and adolescents cope and adjust with a

personal loss (eg, Guiding Your Child Through Grief is one such resource for older children[15]) can be found through recommendations of a children's librarian or at bookstores. Pediatricians can identify a few books to recommend and, ideally, may even choose to stock their offices with a couple of copies to lend to families.

CHILDREN'S DEVELOPMENTAL UNDERSTANDING OF DEATH

Before the development of object permanence, something out of view is felt to be literally "out of mind." Therefore, it is unlikely that infants in their first 6 months of life can truly grieve. But as children develop object permanence during the second half of the first year of life, they begin to acquire the ability to appreciate the possibility of true loss. It is therefore not coincidental that peek-a-boo emerges during this time period as a game played by children in all cultures, wherein the child shows heightened concern at separation and joy at reunion, as if "playing" with the idea of loss. Infants and toddlers play this game repeatedly as they try to understand and deal with the potentiality of loss. It has been suggested that peek-a-boo is one of many games that children play that might allude to loss or death. In fact, "peek-a-boo" is translated literally from Old English as "alive-or-dead." Parents who worry that it is too early to raise the topic of death with their preschool- or even school-aged children likely do not realize that they began communicating with their children about loss at an early age.

Research has shown that there are 4 concepts that children come to understand that help them make sense of, and ultimately cope with, death: irreversibility, finality (nonfunctionality), causality, and universality (inevitability).[14–19] On average, most children will develop an understanding of these concepts, outlined in Table 1, by 5

to 7 years of age. Personal loss or a terminal illness before this age has been associated with a precocious understanding of these concepts[19]; education has been shown to accelerate children's understanding as well.[20] The death of a pet in early childhood can be used as an opportunity to help young children both understand death and learn to express and cope with loss.

Understanding the concepts of death can be viewed as a necessary precondition, but not necessarily sufficient, for acceptance and adjustment. Children at a very young age can understand that death is irreversible; indeed, even toddlers come to learn "all-gone." But accepting that someone about whom you care deeply will never return is difficult even for adults. Pediatricians can counsel parents to help children understand these concepts and assess children's comprehension directly through simple questions. Parents can be encouraged to be patient with children's repetitive questions after a loss, which may occur over an extended period of time. For young children, such questions may reflect attempts to develop a more complete understanding over time as cognitive development progresses.

Misinformation or misconceptions can impair children's adjustment to loss. Literal misinterpretations are common among young children. For example, children may become resistant to attending a wake after being told that their parent's body will be placed in the casket; adults often assume this is because of a fear of dead bodies. But some children, when told that the "body" is placed in 1 location, may conclude that the head is placed elsewhere; their reluctance to attend the wake may be attributable to a fear of viewing their parent decapitated. It is best not to assume the reasons for children's worries or hesitation but instead ask what they are thinking about. Young

TABLE 1 Component Death Concepts and Implications of Incomplete Understanding for Adjustment to Loss

Irreversibility: death is a permanent phenomenon from which there is no recovery or return
• Example of incomplete understanding: the child expects the deceased to return, as if from a trip
• Implication of incomplete understanding: failure to comprehend this concept prevents the child from detaching personal ties to the deceased, a necessary first step in successful mourning

Finality (nonfunctionality): death is a state in which all life functions cease completely
• Example of incomplete understanding: the child worries about a buried relative being cold or in pain; the child wishes to bury food with the deceased
• Implication of incomplete understanding: may lead to preoccupation with physical suffering of the deceased and impair readjustment

Inevitability (universality): death is a natural phenomenon that no living being can escape indefinitely
• Example of incomplete understanding: the child views significant individuals (ie, self, parents) as immortal
• Implication of incomplete understanding: if the child does not view death as inevitable, he/she is likely to view death as punishment (either for actions or thoughts of the deceased or the child), leading to excessive guilt and shame

Causality: the child develops a realistic understanding of the causes of death
• Example of incomplete understanding: the child who relies on magical thinking is apt to assume responsibility for the death of a loved one by assuming that bad thoughts or unrelated actions were causative
• Implication of incomplete understanding: tends to lead to excessive guilt that is difficult for the child to resolve

Reprinted with permission from Schonfeld D. Crisis intervention for bereavement support: a model of intervention in the children's school. *Clin Pediatr (Phila)*. 1989;28(1):29.

children also may have difficulty understanding why families would choose to cremate a loved one after death. Providing developmentally appropriate explanations for parents and other caregivers to use to address common questions can be helpful and reassuring (eg, explaining to preschool-aged children that once people die, their body stops working permanently and they no longer are able to move, think, or feel pain, which is why it is okay to cremate the body, or use high temperatures to turn the body into ashes).

To minimize misinterpretations, it is best to avoid euphemisms; especially with younger children, it is important to use the word "dead" or "died." For example, a young child told that a family member is in eternal sleep may become afraid of going to sleep himself. Religious explanations can be shared with children of any age according to the wishes of their caregivers. But because religious concepts tend to be abstract and therefore more likely to be misunderstood by young children, it is important to also share with children factual information based on the physical reality. For example, a young child told only that a brother died "because he was such a good baby God wanted him back at his side" may begin to fear attending church (if this is viewed as "God's

home") and misbehave whenever brought to religious services.

Children with intellectual disabilities will generally benefit from explanations geared toward their level of cognitive functioning, followed by questions to assess the degree of comprehension and to probe for any misunderstandings. Children with neurodevelopmental disorders, such as autism spectrum disorder, may benefit from practical suggestions about communicating their feelings and needs, as well as additional support to promote coping. Children unable to communicate verbally may show their grief through nonspecific signs or behaviors, such as weight loss or head banging. To provide support after a death, parents and other caregivers can draw on the strategies and approaches that have worked with their children in the past to provide comfort when faced with other stressors and to explain challenging concepts.

ADOLESCENTS

Adolescents may have a mature conceptual understanding of death, but they still experience challenges adjusting to the death of a close family member or friend.[21] Although they are capable of rational thinking, adolescents, like adults, nonetheless benefit from additional explanation

and discussion in addition to emotional support. Although they often turn to peers for support and assistance in many situations, after the death of a close family member or friend, they can benefit from the additional physical and emotional presence of adults. Unfortunately, many adolescents receive limited explanation or support after a death. Often, surviving caregivers rely on them to take on more adult responsibilities, such as contributing to the care of younger siblings and performing more chores within the home, and may count on them to serve the role of a confidante and source of emotional support for the caregivers themselves. Pediatricians may be able to assist in such cases by encouraging adult caregivers to identify their own support, such as through faith-based organizations, community-based support groups, or professional counseling.

Juniors or seniors in high school are at a point in their development when they may be particularly vulnerable to difficulties in coping with the death of a close family member or friend. This is a time of heightened academic demands, and the common short-term negative effect on academic productivity may be compounded by the high level of academic scrutiny characteristic of applying to college. Completing high school and leaving family to pursue their own education or career is a challenging transition for adolescents and often involves stress and ambivalence. A recent death can exacerbate academic and personal challenges. Youth anticipating leaving home for school or career may feel guilty about leaving other family members who are grieving or worry that they will have difficulty coping when separated from their family, friends, and familiar supports. These young people may arrive in college to face peers who are unaware of their loss, unfamiliar with how best to provide them with support, and focused on pursuits and activities that seem incongruous with their grief. The food, people, and settings that normally provide them solace and comfort may be lacking at a time when they are most needed. Pediatricians can support these adolescents by staying connected with them during the transition and helping them and their families identify supports and resources at college and in their family's community.[13]

GUILT AND SHAME

Because of the egocentrism and magical thinking that are characteristic of young children's understanding of causality, children will often assume that there was something they did, did not do, or should have done that would have prevented the death of someone close to them and develop guilt over a death. Even older children, and indeed adults, often feel guilty when there is no logical, objective reason for them to feel responsible for a death. People may assume some responsibility because it helps them believe that, by taking actions they failed to take before, they can prevent the future deaths of others about whom they care deeply and feel more in control. For example, if a child assumes that the reason his father died was because he attended

a friend's party rather than staying home to monitor his father, he can reassure himself that his mother will be okay as long as he never leaves the home at night again. The alternative to this kind of thinking is accepting that we have limited influence over tragic events, but that reality leaves many feeling helpless. It is frightening to realize someone else we care about could die at any time, no matter what we do. But assuming fault for a death in this manner does not prevent future loss, and the resulting guilt contributes to further distress. In situations in which children's actions clearly contributed to the cause of death (eg, a child who accidentally discharges a firearm that results in the death of someone) or when children persist in feeling responsible (whether such guilt is logical), pediatricians should consider referral for counseling. In the context of ongoing support, children can be helped to either dismiss illogical guilt or come to forgive themselves for unintended actions they believe have contributed in some way to the death.

Children are also more likely to feel guilty about a death when the preexisting relationship with the deceased was ambivalent or conflicted. The relationship between adolescents and their parents often has some element of such ambivalence or conflict as the adolescent strives for independence, and conflict is more likely to be present if the deceased had a chronic mental or physical illness or problem with substance abuse or had been abusive, neglectful, or absent (eg, incarcerated or deployed). Guilt of other family members may also lead to difficulties: for example, it can distort the relationships between parents and surviving children after the death of a sibling.[22]

It is helpful for pediatricians to approach children who have lost a loved one to presume that guilt may be present, even when there is no

logical reason for it. Pediatricians can explain that they know there is nothing that the child did, failed to do, or could have done to change the outcome but wonder if the child ever believes that he or she somehow contributed to the death as many children do in similar situations. They can explain that feeling bad does not mean you did anything bad and feeling guilty does not mean you are guilty. When pediatricians help children express their guilt associated with a death, it allows children to begin to challenge their faulty assumptions about personal responsibility and promotes a refocusing on the child's feelings about the loss.

Children also may experience guilt over surviving after a sibling died or feeling relief after a death that followed a lengthy illness. In the setting of a protracted illness, family members and friends often experience anticipatory grieving. They can imagine the death and experience graduated feelings of loss, but when it becomes overwhelming they can reassure themselves that their loved one is still alive. Anticipating the death allows them to accomplish some of the "work" of grief before the death actually occurs. But this is a painful process, and at some point, many individuals in this situation will wish for the death to occur. Although they may couch this in terms of hoping for the person who is dying to be able to end his or her suffering, the death would also end some of their own emotional suffering as they anticipate the death of a loved one and free them of their responsibility to focus much of their time and efforts on the needs of the person who is critically ill. This situation can result in further guilt and complicate the grieving process.[8]

When children assume that the cause of the death was the result of the actions, inactions, or thoughts of the person who died, they may feel ashamed of the person who died and/or the death and reluctant to talk with others about their loss. Shame is also likely to complicate bereavement when the death is somehow stigmatized, such as death from suicide or resulting from criminal activity or substance abuse. This shame further isolates grieving children from the support and assistance of concerned peers and adults.

Suicide is often complicated by both guilt and shame among survivors. As a result, discussion about the cause of death is often limited, and children may struggle to understand the cause or circumstances of the death. Open communication helps prevent suicide from becoming a "family secret," which may further disrupt the grieving process. If the explanations are too simplistic, concerns may be increased. For example, if children are told only, "Your uncle killed himself because he was very, very sad," they will likely notice that extended family members and friends, who are overwhelmed with grief, may look "very, very sad" and worry that they, too, will kill themselves. A preferable explanation might aim to convey that suicide is usually the result of underlying depression or other mental health problems; it may also be related to alcohol or other substance abuse. It is important to emphasize that suicide is not generally a logical "choice" made by someone who is thinking clearly and able to consider a range of solutions to problems. In addition, children should be encouraged to communicate when they are distressed or feeling depressed, informed about where they can go for advice and assistance, and instructed not to keep in confidence when peers or others communicate to them that they are considering self-harm.[23] Sample scripts and language for discussing suicide with children at different developmental levels, prepared by the National Center for School Crisis and Bereavement,

can be used by schools to respond to a death by suicide of a student or member of the school staff (freely available at www.schoolcrisiscenter. org).

SECONDARY AND CUMULATIVE LOSSES

Although children generally show a remarkable resiliency and ability to adjust to the death of someone close to them, nonetheless, they do not "get over" a death in 6 months or a year. Rather, they spend the rest of their life accommodating the absence. In fact, many find the second year more difficult than the first. The first year after the death is filled with many anticipated challenges: the first holiday or birthday without a loved one or the first father-daughter dance after the father's death. Expectations typically are reduced (ie, the child expects to feel sad at the first special holiday without a loved one), and multiple supports are usually in place. But when these special occasions are still not joyful in the second year, children may wonder if they will ever be able to experience joy again. Unfortunately, by this point in time, the support they may have received from extended family, teachers, coaches, and others at school and in the community has probably already ended. However, the sense of loss is persistent, and without proper support it may be perceived as overwhelming. Maintaining support for children and families is important well beyond the initial period of grief.

When children experience a death of someone close to them, they lose not only the person who died (ie, the primary loss) but also everything that person had contributed or would have contributed to their life (ie, secondary losses). Common secondary losses include the following:

- change in lifestyle (eg, altered financial status of the family after the death of a parent);

- relocation resulting in a change in school and peer group;

- less interaction with friends or relatives of the person who died (eg, friends of a child's sister no longer visit after the sister dies);

- loss of shared memories;

- decreased special attention (eg, a child may no longer value participating in sports activities without his parent there to cheer for him);

- decreased availability of the surviving parent (who may need to work more hours or who becomes less available emotionally because of depression); and

- a decreased sense of safety and trust in the world.

Relationships that seemed incidental may take on new meaning after they are no longer available. For example, after the death of his sister, a younger brother may now miss the advice and guidance provided by his sister's boyfriend, who no longer visits. Other losses may not become apparent until years later. A 5-year-old girl experiencing the death of her grandmother who was her primary caregiver may not realize until many years later that she has lost her grandmother's advice and support as she faces puberty or her first date, or on the first night her newborn infant cries inconsolably. At each new milestone, the loss of someone for whom we care deeply is redefined and grief is revisited.

When children experience a death at a young age, they may also not fully understand the death or its implications. Each new developmental stage, as cognitive development advances and experience widens, may prompt a resurfacing of their grief and be accompanied by questions that permit the child to come to a more mature understanding of the death and its implications.

Subsequent losses and stressors also add to the challenge of adaptation. Children who have experienced traumatic events or significant losses in the context of sufficient support and internal capacity to cope may experience posttraumatic growth and emerge with increased resiliency and new skills to cope with future adversity. These children may shift their life goals to align more with public service; place a higher priority on family, friends, spirituality, and helping others; or become more empathic.[11,24] But in communities that are characterized by high rates of violence, poverty, and frequent deaths of peers and young family members, such supports are generally not present or are insufficient to meet the heightened need. Children in such environments do not somehow "get used to death" or become desensitized. Rather, these losses make them progressively more vulnerable to future stresses and loss. Children in these circumstances often come to appreciate that adults in their communities are unable to provide for their safety and are unwilling or unable to provide support and learn not to seek assistance from these adults because they know it is unlikely to be offered. One reason children and adolescents in these environments may instead turn to peers (and gangs) is to seek such support, which may contribute to high-risk behaviors that jeopardize their safety. They may engage in risky behaviors out of fear for their own mortality and the need to challenge these fears by engaging in the same behaviors they know to be dangerous. Only by surviving these risks can children and adolescents reassure themselves that they are safe, at least for the moment. In this context, it becomes critical that adults in our society take responsibility for ensuring that the environment is safe for children and adolescents, especially in communities characterized by violence, poverty, and frequent loss,

and that we provide them with the support and assistance they need to cope with loss and crisis.

GRIEF TRIGGERS AND ANNIVERSARY REACTIONS

Grief triggers evoke sudden reminders of the person who died that can cause powerful emotional responses in children who are grieving. Although they are most common in the first few months after the death, they may happen months or years later, although the strength of the emotions generally lessens with time. Some triggers, such as a Mother's Day activity in class or a father-daughter dance at school, are easier to identify, but grief triggers can be ubiquitous and often difficult to anticipate. A child may pass by a stranger wearing the same perfume as her aunt or hear a song that her grandfather used to sing and be reminded of the loss. Parents can work with teachers to both minimize likely triggers in school settings and create a "safety" plan wherein students know they can leave the classroom if necessary. If children know that they can leave if they need to, they are less likely to feel overwhelmed or afraid they will cry in class. As a result, they will rarely need to exit and are more able to remain within the classroom and engaged in the classwork.[13]

Anniversaries of the death, birthdays of the deceased, holidays, special events, and major transitions (eg, changing schools, graduating high school, moving homes) are also times when a loved one's absence will be acutely felt. Pediatricians can help the family find ways to meaningfully honor these events. The medical home is uniquely well suited to provide ongoing periodic bereavement support. Pediatricians should invite children and their families to reach out for assistance and advice as children adjust to the loss over time. However, many

individuals who are grieving may not anticipate the challenges posed by anniversaries or events or may feel uncomfortable imposing on the physician for advice for what they believe to be a normative and universal experience. Pediatricians can, instead, schedule follow-up appointments to coincide with such timed events (eg, just before the start of a new school year; just before the first-year anniversary of the death), when modest changes in the timing make it practical, or can call, write, or e-mail a patient/family periodically to check in and let the child and family know of their continued availability and interest. Pediatricians interested in providing significant direct bereavement support for children and families within their practice can explore coding by time for counseling and coordination of care to maximize reimbursement for these services. When the pediatrician lets the family know he or she is still concerned and available, it increases the chances that the child or family will seek advice and assistance when needed.

FUNERAL ATTENDANCE

Children, like adults, often benefit from participating in funerals, wakes, and other memorial or commemorative activities after the death of a close family member or friend. It provides them with an opportunity to grieve in the presence of family and friends while receiving their support and, as appropriate to the family, solace from their spiritual beliefs. Parents and other caregivers sometimes exclude children from funerals and wakes for fear that the experience may be upsetting or because they, themselves, are grieving and unsure whether they can provide appropriate support. Children who are excluded from memorial or funeral services often resent not being able to participate in a meaningful activity involving someone they care deeply about and may wonder what is so terrible that is being done to the loved one that it is not suitable for them to view. What they imagine is likely to be far worse than the reality.

It is best to invite children to participate in wakes, funerals, or memorial services, to the extent they wish. Begin by providing basic information in simple terms about what children can expect from the experience. For example, include information about whether there will be an open casket and anticipated cultural and religious rituals (eg, guests may be invited to place some dirt on the coffin at the gravesite), as well as how people may be expected to behave (eg, some people may be crying and very upset; humorous stories and memories may be shared). Ask children what additional information they would like and what questions they might have. Children should not be forced or coerced to participate in particular rituals or to attend the funeral or wake. If older children who had a very close relationship with the deceased (eg, teenagers whose parent has died) indicate they do not want to attend the funeral, it is helpful to explore the reason for their not wishing to attend and ask them to describe what accommodations might be made in the plans to meet their needs (eg, they prefer not to attend the wake but will attend the funeral service). But, as with all true invitations, the decision is ultimately left to the child. Families can work with children to identify alternate ways for them to recognize the death, such as a private visit to the funeral home once the casket has been closed or a visit to the gravesite after the burial. All children can be invited to make meaningful but developmentally appropriate decisions about the service of an immediate family member; they may be permitted to select a flower arrangement or a picture of the parent to be displayed at the wake.

It can be helpful to assign an adult whom the child knows well but who is not personally grieving (eg, a teacher, babysitter, or relative who is close to the child but less familiar with the deceased) to accompany and monitor the child throughout the services. If the child is fidgeting or appears distressed, the adult can suggest they go for a walk and inquire about how the child is coping with the experience. If the child prefers to stand outside of the room and hand out prayer cards, that level of participation can be accommodated without disrupting the experience for other grieving family members (ie, the child would be less able to stay outside of the room if being watched by the mother who feels it important to stand by her husband's coffin throughout the wake). Older children and adolescents may wish to invite a close friend to sit with them during the service or assist with greeting guests as they approach the room. Suggestions on how to address the needs of children related to commemoration and memorialization involving a crisis, especially in a school setting, can be found elsewhere.[11,13]

CULTURAL SENSITIVITY

Different cultures have a range of traditional practices and rituals as well as expectations around how members of their culture typically mourn the death of a family member or close friend. Although it is helpful for pediatricians to know something about these cultural differences, it is important to remember that the fundamental experience of grief is universal.

Knowledge of the common practices of a particular culture may not accurately predict how a family or individual from that culture will behave. Many families have mixed backgrounds and/or have been exposed to different cultures through their communities or schools. Parents sometimes have different beliefs or practices from their children. Families or individuals may choose to follow practices of a different culture if they seem to align better with their current preferences. Assumptions about how someone ought to mourn in a particular culture may result in a stereotype that could cloud our perceptions and make us miss opportunities to be helpful. Pediatricians should therefore ask families what they feel would be most helpful for their family or for individuals within the family.

The best approach is to be present, authentic, and honest. Approach children and their families with an open mind and heart and be guided by what you see, hear, and feel. The following are questions that may assist in this process:

- "Can you tell me how your family and your culture recognize and cope with the death of a family member?"

- "How does this fit with your own preferences at this time?"

- "Can you help me understand how I can best be of help to you and your family?"

WORKING WITH SCHOOLS

Children typically experience at least temporary academic challenges after the death of a close friend or family member. The effect the loss has on learning may first appear weeks or even months later. Some children may even respond to a death by overachieving in school. Children with learning problems that predated the loss may experience a marked worsening.

In general, it is best for the family to anticipate at least brief difficulties in learning and concentration and to establish a proactive relationship with the school to coordinate supports at school with those within the home. If schools wait for academic failure to become apparent, then school becomes a source of additional distress rather than a potential support. Instead, academic expectations should be modified as needed and supports put into place in anticipation of a possible need.

Caregivers and educators can work together to identify the level of academic work that feels appropriate and achievable at a particular point of time in the recovery process after a major loss. Some modifications that may be considered include the following:

- adapting assignments (eg, allow a student to prepare a written presentation if he feels uncomfortable with an oral presentation; substitute smaller projects for a large project that may feel overwhelming in scope);

- changing the focus or timing of a lesson (eg, excuse the student from a lesson on substance abuse if her sister recently died of a drug overdose or consider postponing it to later in the semester);

- reducing and coordinating homework and extracurricular activities so that the student is able to meet expectations for what is being required; or

- modifying or excusing the student from tests or placing more weight on grades achieved before the death.

The goal is to maintain reasonable expectations while providing the support and accommodations so that the student can achieve at that level and be prepared for successful advancement to the next grade level.[13]

Pediatricians can help provide training to schools about how best to support grieving students and provide consultation after a death has occurred involving a member of the school community.[11,13,25-27]

The Coalition to Support Grieving Students was formed to develop a set of resources broadly approved by 10 of the leading professional organizations of school professionals to guide educators and other school personnel in supporting and caring for their grieving students. The resources are available at no charge to the public at www.grievingstudents.org. The video-training modules feature expert commentary, school professionals who share their observations and advice, and bereaved children and family members who offer their own perspective on living with loss. Handouts and reference materials oriented for classroom educators, principals/administrators, and student support personnel that summarize the training videos, as well as a range of additional resources, can be downloaded from the Web site. Although developed for use by educators, the materials are applicable for the professional development of pediatric health care providers as well. Many are also appropriate for other sites where child congregate care is provided, including early learning centers, preschools, and in-home day care settings. Those caring for children younger than school age similarly benefit from the support and training that can be provided by pediatricians.

COMPLICATED MOURNING AND INDICATIONS FOR REFERRAL

In the immediate aftermath of a death, the reactions of children and adults can be quite extreme and varied. It is best to avoid the tendency to judge or try to categorize such acute reactions as either "normal" or "abnormal." If children or adults appear to be at risk of harming themselves or others, action should be immediately taken to preserve safety. Pediatricians should be aware of community resources for bereavement support. These resources may include the following:

- bereavement support groups and camps (a listing of national and regional services and resources for grieving children can be found at http://www.newyorklife.com/nyl/v/index.jsp?contentId=143564&vgnextoid=755540bf8c442310VgnVCM100000ac841cacRCRD);

- school-based programs and services;

- counselors who are interested and qualified in counseling children who are grieving; and

- other mental health professionals trained to counsel grieving children who are also experiencing depression, anxiety, or trauma symptoms.

As noted previously, adults in the family may benefit from their own support so that they do not depend unduly on their children for emotional support and so they are better able to discern and address the needs of their grieving children.

Grief from the death of a close family member or friend can dominate children's lives in the immediate aftermath of the loss, causing disinterest in engaging in previously enjoyed activities, compromising peer relationships, interfering with the ability to concentrate and learn, causing regressive or risk-taking behavior, or creating a challenge to healthy social and emotional development. But with time and adequate support, grieving children learn that their lives in the absence of the deceased, although permanently altered, nonetheless can be meaningful and increasingly characterized by moments of satisfaction and joy. Children who instead experience complicated mourning may fail to show such adjustment over time.[28] They may experience difficulty with daily functioning at school or at home that persists months after the death. They may become preoccupied with thoughts about the deceased or develop nonadaptive behaviors, such as tobacco, alcohol, or other substance use; promiscuous sexual behavior; or delinquent or other risky behaviors. Referral for counseling is particularly important in this context. More immediate or urgent referral is indicated if children show deep or sustained sadness or depression, especially if they are perceived to be at risk of suicidal behavior.

PROFESSIONAL PREPARATION AND SELF-CARE

Pediatricians often enter the profession because of a desire to help children grow, develop, and be healthy and happy. Understandably, pediatricians can find it difficult to witness children's distress as they grieve the death of someone about whom they care deeply. Many pediatricians have received limited training about how to support grieving children. It is difficult to believe you are helping people when they remain in such distress. You want to help people feel "better," but when they freely express their sorrow in the immediate aftermath of a death, it is difficult to know that you are helping them ultimately adjust and cope. Following up with children and their families over time and actively inquiring about how they are continuing to adjust will help the pediatrician support and observe the course of recovery and understand his or her role in that process. Professional preparation and education are helpful; resources are available on various professional Web sites (eg, the American Academy of Pediatrics at www. aap.org/disasters/adjustment; the Coalition to Support Grieving Students at www.grievingstudents. org; or the National Center for School Crisis and Bereavement at www. schoolcrisiscenter.org). Pediatricians can also seek out and request professional development training through professional meetings, through grand rounds, from other

continuing medical education venues, and via retreats and psychosocial rounds in hospital settings.

Children's grief may also trigger reminders of loss and other reactions in pediatricians. It may remind adults of their own losses or raise thoughts or concerns about the well-being of those they love. Children's grief is often unfiltered and pure; their questions are direct and poignant. It is difficult to witness a child's grief and not feel an effect personally. In fact, not being affected should not even be an expectation or a goal. Nonetheless, pediatricians should monitor their reactions and feelings and limit their support to what they feel ready and able to provide to any particular family at that point in time. If the family is in need of additional supportive services, the pediatrician can seek the assistance of a professional colleague in the office or through referral to someone in the community.

It is important for pediatricians to examine and understand their personal feelings about death to be effective in providing support to children who have experienced a personal loss or who are faced with their own impending death. Often, this understanding will involve an awareness of the effects of deaths of patients on pediatricians' professional and personal lives. The culture in medicine needs to acknowledge that it is understandable to feel upset when bearing witness to something that is upsetting. As professionals, pediatricians should offer support to our colleagues and seek out and accept support for ourselves.

Pediatricians who do provide support to grieving children and families often have a meaningful and lasting impact. A relatively modest effort to provide compassion and support can have a dramatic effect. It can help reduce the amount of time grieving children feel confused, isolated, and overwhelmed. Pediatricians will not

be able to take away the pain and sorrow (and should not see that as their goal), but they can significantly reduce the suffering and minimize the negative effects of loss on children's lives and developmental courses.

LEAD AUTHORS

David J. Schonfeld, MD, FAAP
Thomas Demaria, PhD

CONTRIBUTING AUTHOR

Sharon Berry, PhD, LP, ABPP

COMMITTEE ON PSYCHOSOCIAL ASPECTS OF CHILD AND FAMILY HEALTH, 2015–2016

Michael Yogman, MD, FAAP, Chairperson
Nerissa S. Bauer, MD, MPH, FAAP
Thresia Gambon, MD, FAAP
Arthur Lavin, MD, FAAP
Keith Lemmon, MD, FAAP
Gerri Mattson, MD, FAAP
Jason Rafferty, MD, MPH, EdM
Lawrence Wissow, MD, MPH, FAAP

LIAISONS

Sharon Berry, PhD, LP, ABPP — *Society of Pediatric Psychology*
Terry Carmichael, MSW — *National Association of Social Workers*
Edward R. Christopherson, PhD, FAAP (hon) — *Society of Pediatric Psychology*
Norah Johnson, PhD, RN, CPNP — *National Association of Pediatric Nurse Practitioners*
L. Read Sulik, MD — *American Academy of Child and Adolescent Psychiatry*

CONSULTANT

George Cohen, MD, FAAP

STAFF

Stephanie Domain, MS

DISASTER PREPAREDNESS ADVISORY COUNCIL

Steven E. Krug, MD, FAAP, Chairperson
Sarita Chung, MD, FAAP, Member
Daniel B. Fagbuyi, MD, FAAP, Member
Margaret C. Fisher, MD, FAAP, Member
Scott M. Needle, MD, FAAP, Member
David J. Schonfeld, MD, FAAP, Member

LIAISONS

John James Alexander, MD, FAAP — *US Food and Drug Administration*
Daniel Dodgen, PhD — *Office of the Assistant Secretary for Preparedness and Response*
Eric J. Dziuban, MD, DTM, CPH, FAAP — *Centers for Disease Control and Prevention*

Andrew L. Garrett, MD, MPH, FAAP – *Office of the Assistant Secretary for Preparedness and Response*

Ingrid Hope, RN, MSN – *Department of Homeland Security Office of Health Affairs*

Georgina Peacock, MD, MPH, FAAP – *Centers for Disease Control and Prevention*

Erica Radden, MD – *US Food and Drug Administration*

David Alan Siegel, MD, FAAP – *National Institute of Child Health and Human Development*

STAFF

Laura Aird, MS

Sean Diederich

Tamar Magarik Haro

REFERENCES

1. Ewalt P, Perkins L. The real experience of death among adolescents: an empirical study. *Soc Casework.* 1979;60(99):547–551

2. Hoven CW, Duarte CS, Lucas CP, et al. Psychopathology among New York city public school children 6 months after September 11. *Arch Gen Psychiatry.* 2005;62(5):545–552

3. Mahon MM. Children's concept of death and sibling death from trauma. *J Pediatr Nurs.* 1993;8(5):335–344

4. Wender E; Committee on Psychosocial Aspects of Child And Family Health. Supporting the family after the death of a child. *Pediatrics.* 2012;130(6):1164–1169

5. Meert KL, Eggly S, Kavanaugh K, et al. Meaning making during parent-physician bereavement meetings after a child's death. *Health Psychol.* 2015;34(4):453–461

6. Section on Hospice and Palliative Medicine; Committee on Hospital Care. Pediatric palliative care and hospice care commitments, guidelines, and recommendations. *Pediatrics.* 2013;132(5):966–972

7. American Academy of Pediatrics Committee on Psychosocial Aspects of Child and Family Health. The pediatrician and childhood bereavement. *Pediatrics.* 2000;105(2):445–447. Reaffirmed March 2013

8. Schonfeld D. Providing support for families experiencing the death of a child. In: Kreitler S, Ben-Arush MW, Martin A, eds. *Pediatric Psycho-oncology: Psychosocial Aspects and Clinical Interventions.* 2nd ed. West Sussex, United Kingdom: John Wiley & Sons Ltd; 2012:223–230

9. Leash R. *Death Notification: A Practical Guide to the Process.* Hinesburg, VT: Upper Access; 1994

10. Foltin GL, Schonfeld DJ, Shannon MW, eds. *Pediatric Terrorism and Disaster Preparedness: A Resource for Pediatricians.* Rockville, MD: Agency for Healthcare Research and Quality; 2006. AHRQ publication 06-0056-EF

11. Schonfeld D, Demaria T; Disaster Preparedness Advisory Council; Committee on Psychosocial Aspects of Child and Family Health. Providing psychosocial support to children and families in the aftermath of disaster and crisis: a guide for pediatricians. *Pediatrics.* 2015;136(4):e1120–e1130

12. Hagan JF, Shaw JS, Duncan PM, eds. *Bright Futures: Guidelines for Health Supervision of Infants, Children, and Adolescents.* 3rd ed. Elk Grove Village, IL: American Academy of Pediatrics; 2008

13. Schonfeld D, Quackenbush M. *The Grieving Student: A Teacher's Guide.* Baltimore, MD: Brookes Publishing; 2010

14. Schonfeld D, Quackenbush M. *After a Loved One Dies—How Children Grieve and How Parents and Other Adults Can Support Them.* New York, NY: New York Life Foundation; 2009

15. Emswiler M, Emswiler J. *Guiding Your Child Through Grief.* New York, NY: Bantam Books; 2000

16. Panagiotaki G, Nobes G, Ashraf A, Aubby H. British and Pakistani children's understanding of death: cultural and developmental influences. *Br J Dev Psychol.* 2015;33(1):31–44

17. Schonfeld DJ. Talking with children about death. *J Pediatr Health Care.* 1993;7(6):269–274

18. Schonfeld D. Death during childhood. In: Augustyn M, Zuckerman B, Caronna E, eds. *The Zuckerman Parker Handbook of Developmental and Behavioral Pediatrics for Primary Care.* 3rd ed. Philadelphia, PA: Lippincott Williams & Wilkins; 2011:441–445

19. Speece MW, Brent SB. Children's understanding of death: a review of three components of a death concept. *Child Dev.* 1984;55(5):1671–1686

20. Schonfeld DJ, Kappelman M. The impact of school-based education on the young child's understanding of death. *J Dev Behav Pediatr.* 1990;11(5):247–252

21. Stikkelbroek Y, Bodden DH, Reitz E, Vollebergh WA, van Baar AL. Mental health of adolescents before and after the death of a parent or sibling. *Eur Child Adolesc Psychiatry.* 2016;25(1):49–59

22. Krell R, Rabkin L. The effects of sibling death on the surviving child: a family perspective. *Fam Process.* 1979;18(4):471–477

23. Shain B; Committee on Adolescence. Suicide and suicide attempts in adolescents. *Pediatrics.* 2016;138(1):e20161420

24. Schonfeld D, Gurwitch R. Children in disasters. In: Elzouki AY, Stapleton FB, Whitley RJ, Oh W, Harfi HA, Nazer H, eds. *Textbook of Clinical Pediatrics.* 2nd ed. New York, NY: Springer; 2011:687–698

25. Schonfeld DJ. Crisis intervention for bereavement support: a model of intervention in the children's school. *Clin Pediatr (Phila).* 1989;28(1):27–33

26. Schonfeld D, Lichtenstein R, Kline M, Speese-Linehan D. *How to Respond to and Prepare for a Crisis.* 2nd ed. Alexandria, VA: Association for Supervision and Curriculum Development; 2002

27. Schonfeld D; US Department of Education. Coping with the death of a student or staff member. *ERCMExpress.* 2007;3(2):1–12

28. Rando T. *Treatment of Complicated Mourning.* Champaign, IL: Research Press; 1993

SECTION 8
Mental Health Competencies

POLICY STATEMENT Organizational Principles to Guide and Define the Child Health
Care System and/or Improve the Health of all Children

American Academy
of Pediatrics

DEDICATED TO THE HEALTH OF ALL CHILDREN™

Mental Health Competencies for Pediatric Practice

Jane Meschan Foy, MD, FAAP,[a] Cori M. Green, MD, MS, FAAP,[b] Marian F. Earls, MD, MTS, FAAP,[c] COMMITTEE ON PSYCHOSOCIAL ASPECTS OF CHILD AND FAMILY HEALTH, MENTAL HEALTH LEADERSHIP WORK GROUP

abstract

Pediatricians have unique opportunities and an increasing sense of responsibility to promote healthy social-emotional development of children and to prevent and address their mental health and substance use conditions. In this report, the American Academy of Pediatrics updates its 2009 policy statement, which proposed competencies for providing mental health care to children in primary care settings and recommended steps toward achieving them. This 2019 policy statement affirms the 2009 statement and expands competencies in response to science and policy that have emerged since: the impact of adverse childhood experiences and social determinants on mental health, trauma-informed practice, and team-based care. Importantly, it also recognizes ways in which the competencies are pertinent to pediatric subspecialty practice. Proposed mental health competencies include foundational communication skills, capacity to incorporate mental health content and tools into health promotion and primary and secondary preventive care, skills in the psychosocial assessment and care of children with mental health conditions, knowledge and skills of evidence-based psychosocial therapy and psychopharmacologic therapy, skills to function as a team member and comanager with mental health specialists, and commitment to embrace mental health practice as integral to pediatric care. Achievement of these competencies will necessarily be incremental, requiring partnership with fellow advocates, system changes, new payment mechanisms, practice enhancements, and decision support for pediatricians in their expanded scope of practice.

[a]Department of Pediatrics, School of Medicine, Wake Forest University, Winston-Salem, North Carolina; [b]Department of Pediatrics, Weill Cornell Medicine, Cornell University, New York, New York; and [c]Community Care of North Carolina, School of Medicine, University of North Carolina at Chapel Hill, Chapel Hill, North Carolina

Policy statements from the American Academy of Pediatrics benefit from expertise and resources of liaisons and internal (AAP) and external reviewers. However, policy statements from the American Academy of Pediatrics may not reflect the views of the liaisons or the organizations or government agencies that they represent.

Drs Foy, Green, and Earls contributed to the drafting and revising of this manuscript; and all authors approved the final manuscript as submitted.

The guidance in this statement does not indicate an exclusive course of treatment or serve as a standard of medical care. Variations, taking into account individual circumstances, may be appropriate.

All policy statements from the American Academy of Pediatrics automatically expire 5 years after publication unless reaffirmed, revised, or retired at or before that time.

To cite: Foy JM, Green CM, Earls MF , AAP COMMITTEE ON PSYCHOSOCIAL ASPECTS OF CHILD AND FAMILY HEALTH, MENTAL HEALTH LEADERSHIP WORK GROUP. Mental Health Competencies for Pediatric Practice. *Pediatrics.* 2019; 144(5):e20192757

INTRODUCTION

A total of 13% to 20% of US children and adolescents experience a mental* disorder in a given year.[1] According to the seminal Great Smoky Mountain Study, which has managed a cohort of rural US youth since 1992, 19% of youth manifested impaired mental functioning without meeting the criteria for diagnosis as a mental disorder (ie, subthreshold symptoms).[2] The authors of this study have since shown that adults who had a childhood mental disorder have 6 times the odds of at least 1 adverse adult outcome in the domain of health, legal, financial, or social functioning compared with adults without childhood disorders, even after controlling for childhood psychosocial hardships. Adults who had impaired functioning and subthreshold psychiatric symptoms during childhood—termed "problems" in this statement—have 3 times the odds of adverse outcomes as adults.[3] These findings underscore the importance to adult health of both mental health disorders and mental health problems during childhood.

The prevalence of mental health disorders and problems (collectively termed "conditions" in this statement) in children and adolescents is increasing and, alarmingly, suicide rates are now the second leading cause of death in young people from 10 to 24 years of age.[4–6] Furthermore, nearly 6 million children were considered disabled in 2010–2011, an increase of more than 15% from a decade earlier; among these children, reported disability related to physical illnesses decreased by 11.8%, whereas disability related to neurodevelopmental and mental health conditions increased by 20.9%.[5] Although the highest rates of reported neurodevelopmental and mental health disabilities were seen in children living in poverty, the greatest increase in prevalence of reported neurodevelopmental and mental health disabilities occurred, unexpectedly, among children living in socially advantaged households (income ≥400% of the federal poverty level).[5]

Comorbid mental health conditions often complicate chronic physical conditions, decreasing the quality of life for affected children and increasing the cost of their care.[7–12] Because of stigma, shortages of mental health specialists, administrative barriers in health insurance plans, cost, and other barriers to mental health specialty care, an estimated 75% of children with mental health disorders go untreated.[13–16] Primary care physicians are the sole physician managers of care for an estimated 4 in 10 US children with attention-deficit/hyperactivity disorder (ADHD) and one-third with mental disorders overall.[17]

In 2009, the American Academy of Pediatrics (AAP) issued a policy statement, "The Future of Pediatrics: Mental Health Competencies for Pediatric Primary Care," proposing competencies—skills, knowledge, and attitudes—requisite to providing mental health care of children in primary care settings and recommending steps toward achieving them.[18] In the policy, the AAP documented the many forces driving the need for enhancements in pediatric mental health practice.

Updates to the Previous Statement

In the years since publication of the original policy statement on mental health competencies, increases in childhood mental health morbidity and mortality and a number of other developments have added to the urgency of enhancing pediatric mental health practice. A federal parity law has required that insurers cover mental health and physical health conditions equivalently.[19,20] Researchers have shown that early positive and adverse environmental influences—caregivers' protective and nurturing relationships with the child, social determinants of health, traumatic experiences (ecology), and genetic influences (biology)—interact to affect learning capacities, adaptive behaviors, lifelong physical and mental health, and adult productivity, and pediatricians have a role to play in addressing chronic stress and adverse early childhood experiences.[21–24] Transformative

changes in the health care delivery system—payment for value, system- and practice-level integration of mental health and medical services, crossdiscipline accountability for outcomes, and the increasing importance of the family- and patient-centered medical home—all have the potential to influence mental health care delivery.[25–27] Furthermore, improving training and competence in mental health care for future pediatricians—pediatric subspecialists as well as primary care pediatricians—has become a national priority of the American Board of Pediatrics[28,29] and the Association of Pediatric Program Directors.[30]

In this statement, we (1) discuss the unique aspects of the pediatrician's role in mental health care; (2) articulate competencies needed by the pediatrician to promote healthy social-emotional development, identify risks and emerging symptoms, prevent or mitigate impairment from mental health symptoms, and address the mental health and substance use conditions prevalent among children and adolescents in the United States; and (3) recommend achievable next steps toward enhancing mental health practice to support pediatricians in providing mental health care. The accompanying technical report, "Achieving the Pediatric Mental Health Competencies," is focused on strategies to train future pediatricians and prepare practices for achieving the competencies.[31]

Uniqueness of the Pediatrician's Role in Mental Health Care

Traditional concepts of mental health care as well as mental health payment systems build on the assumption that treatment must follow the diagnosis of a disorder. However, this diagnostic approach does not take into account the many opportunities afforded pediatricians, both in general and subspecialty practice, to promote mental health and to offer primary and secondary prevention. Nor do these traditional concepts address the issue that many children have impaired functioning although they do not meet the diagnostic criteria for a specific mental disorder. Consequently, pediatric mental health competencies differ in some important respects from competencies of mental health professionals. The unique role of pediatricians in mental health care stems from the "primary care advantage," which is a developmental mind-set, and their role at the front lines of children's health care.[32] Primary care pediatricians typically see their patients longitudinally, giving them the opportunity to develop a trusting and empowering therapeutic relationship with patients and their families; to promote social-emotional health with every contact, whether for routine health supervision, acute care, or care of a child's chronic medical or developmental condition; to prevent mental health problems through education and anticipatory guidance; and to intervene in a timely way if and when risks, concerns, or symptoms emerge. Recognizing the longitudinal and close relationships that many pediatric subspecialists have with patients and families, the authors of this statement have expanded the concept of primary care advantage to the "pediatric advantage."

Pediatric subspecialists, like pediatric primary care clinicians, need basic mental health competencies. Children and adolescents with somatic manifestations of mental health problems often present to pediatric medical subspecialists or surgical specialists for evaluation of their symptoms; awareness of mental health etiologies has the potential to prevent costly and traumatic workups and expedite referral for necessary mental health services.[33] Children and adolescents with chronic medical conditions have a higher prevalence of mental health problems than do their peers without those conditions; and unrecognized mental health problems, particularly anxiety and depression, often drive excessive use of medical services in children with a chronic illness and impede adherence to their medical treatment.[34] Furthermore, children and adolescents with serious and life-threatening medical and surgical conditions often experience trauma, such as painful medical procedures, disfigurement, separation from loved ones during hospitalizations, and their own and their loved ones' fears about prognosis.[35] For these reasons, mental health competencies involving clinical assessment, screening, early intervention, referral, and comanagement are relevant to pediatric subspecialists who care for children with chronic conditions. Subspecialists have the additional responsibility of coordinating any mental health services they provide with patients' primary care clinicians to prevent duplication of effort, connect children and families to accessible local resources, and reach agreement on respective roles in monitoring patients' mental health care.

Integration of Mental Health Care Into Pediatric Workflow

The AAP Task Force on Mental Health (2004–2010) spoke to the importance of enhancing pediatricians' mental health practice while recognizing that incorporating mental health care into a busy pediatric practice can be a daunting prospect. The task force offered an algorithm, the "Primary Care Approach to Mental Health Care," depicting a process by which mental health services can be woven into practice flow, and tied each step in the algorithm to *Current Procedural Terminology* coding guidance that can potentially support those mental health–related activities in a fee-for-service environment.[32] The AAP Mental Health Leadership Work Group (2011–present) recently updated this to the "Algorithm: A Process for Integrating Mental Health Care Into Pediatric Practice" (see Fig 1). The AAP has a number of resources to assist with coding for mental health care.

The pediatric process for identifying and managing mental health problems is similar to the iterative process of caring for a child with fever and no focal findings: the clinician's initial assessment of the febrile child's severity of illness determines if there is a serious problem that urgently requires further diagnostic evaluation and treatment; if not, the clinician advises the family on symptomatic care and watchful waiting and advises the family to return for further assessment if symptoms persist or worsen. Similarly, a mental health concern of the patient, family, or child care and/or school personnel (or scheduling of a routine health supervision visit [algorithm step 1]) triggers a preliminary psychosocial assessment (algorithm step 2). This initial assessment can be expedited by use of previsit collection of data and screening tools (electronic or paper and pencil), which the clinician can review in advance of the visit, followed by a brief interview and observations to explore findings (both positive and negative) and the opportunity to highlight the child's and family's strengths, an important element of supportive, family-centered care. Finding a problem that is not simply a normal behavioral variation (algorithm step 3) necessitates triage for a psychiatric and/or social emergency and, if indicated, immediate care in the subspecialty or social service system (algorithm steps 9 and 10). In making these determinations, it is important to understand the family context, namely, the added risks conferred by adverse social determinants of health, which may exacerbate the problem and precipitate an emergency.

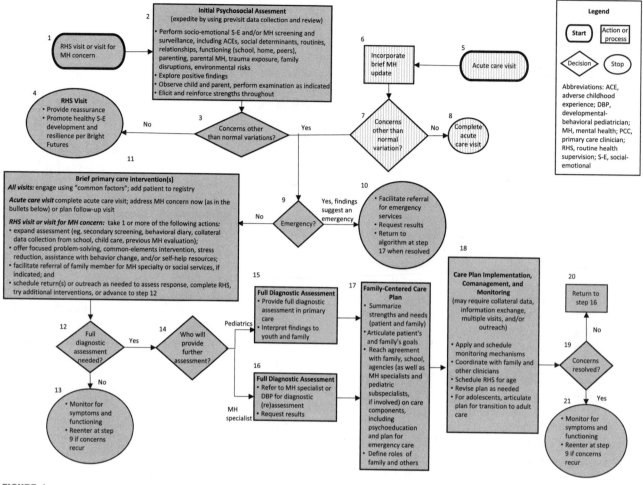

FIGURE 1

Mental health (MH) care in pediatric practice. ACE, adverse childhood experience; RHS, routine health supervision; S-E, social-emotional.

Intervention will need to include supports to address social determinants.

If an identified problem is not an emergency, the clinician can undertake 1 or more brief interventions, as time allows, during the current visit or at follow-up visit(s) (algorithm step 11). These interventions may include iteratively expanding the assessment, for example, by using secondary screening tools, gathering information from school personnel or child care providers, or having the family create a diary of problem behaviors and their triggers. Brief interventions may also include referral of a family member for assistance in addressing his or her own social or mental health problems that may be contributing to the child's difficulties. In addition, brief interventions may include evidence-informed techniques to address the child's symptoms, as described in the section immediately below.

When indicated by findings of the assessment and/or by failure to respond to brief therapeutic interventions, a full diagnostic assessment can be performed, either by the pediatrician (algorithm step 15) at a follow-up visit or through referral to a specialist (algorithm step 16), followed by the steps of care planning and implementation, comanagement, and monitoring the child's progress (algorithm steps 17 and 18).

Brief Interventions: Addressing Mental Health Symptoms in the Context of a Busy Pediatric Practice

Although disorder-specific, standardized psychosocial treatments have been a valuable advance in the mental health field generally, their real-world application to the care of children and adolescents has been limited by the fact that many young people are "diagnostically heterogeneous"; that is, they manifest symptoms of multiple disorders or problems, and their manifestations are variably triggered by events and by their social environment. These limitations led researchers in the field of psychotherapy to develop and successfully apply "transdiagnostic" approaches to the care of children and adolescents, addressing multiple disorders and problems by using a single protocol and allowing for more flexibility in selecting and sequencing interventions.[36]

A number of transdiagnostic approaches are proving to be adaptable for use as brief interventions in pediatric settings. The goals of brief therapeutic interventions for children and adolescents with emerging symptoms of mild to moderate severity are to improve the patient's functioning, reduce distress in the patient and parents, and potentially prevent a later disorder. For children and adolescents identified as needing mental health and/or developmental-behavioral specialty involvement, goals of brief interventions are to help overcome barriers to their accessing care, to ameliorate symptoms and distress while awaiting completion of the referral, and to monitor the patient's functioning and well-being while awaiting higher levels of care. Brevity of these interventions, ideally no more than 10 to 15 minutes per session, mitigates disruption to practice flow. Although formal evaluation of these adaptations is in its early stages, authors of studies suggest that they can be readily learned by pediatric clinicians and are beneficial to the child and family.[37] Table 1 is used to excerpt several of these adaptations from a summary by Wissow et al.[37]

All of these approaches feature prominently in the pediatric mental health competencies; 2 require further explanation.

"Common-factors" communication skills, so named because they are components of effective interventions common to diverse therapies across multiple diagnoses, are foundational among the proposed pediatric mental health competencies. These communication techniques include clinician interpersonal skills that help to build a therapeutic alliance—the felt bond between the clinician and patient and/or family, a powerful factor in facilitating emotional and psychological healing—which, in turn, increases the patient and/or family's optimism, feelings of well-being, and willingness to work toward improved health. Other common-factors techniques target feelings of anger, ambivalence, and hopelessness, family conflicts, and barriers to behavior change and help seeking. Still other techniques keep the discussion focused, practical, and organized. These techniques come from family therapy, cognitive therapy, motivational interviewing, family engagement, family-focused pediatrics, and solution-focused therapy.[38] They have been proven useful and effective in addressing mental health symptoms in pediatrics across the age spectrum and can be readily acquired by experienced clinicians.[39] Importantly, when time is short, the clinician can also use them to bring a visit to a supportive close while committing his or her loyalty and further assistance to the patient and family—that is, reinforcing the therapeutic alliance, even as he or she accommodates to the rapid pace of the practice.

See Table 2 for the HELP mnemonic, developed by the AAP Task Force on Mental Health to summarize components of the common-factors approach.

"Common-elements" approaches can also be used as brief interventions. They differ from common factors in that instead of applying to a range of diagnoses that are not causally related, common elements are semispecific components of psychosocial therapies that apply to a group of related conditions.[40–43] In this approach, the clinician caring for a patient who manifests a cluster of causally related symptoms—for example, fearfulness and avoidant behaviors—draws interventions from evidence-based psychosocial therapies for a related set of disorders—in this example, anxiety disorders. Thus, as a first-line intervention to help an anxious child, the pediatrician coaches the parent to provide gradual exposure to feared activities or objects and to model brave behavior—common elements in a number of effective psychosocial treatments for anxiety disorders. Such interventions can be definitive or a means to reduce distress and ameliorate symptoms while a child is awaiting mental health specialty assessment and/or care. Table 3 is used to summarize promising common-elements approaches applicable to common pediatric primary care problems.

TABLE 1 Promising Adaptations of Mental Health Treatment for Primary Care

Pediatric Settings	Parallels in Mental Health Services
Emphasis on patient-centered care and joint decision-making building trust and activation	Common-factors psychotherapeutic processes promoting engagement, optimism, alliance
Initial treatment often presumptive or relatively nonspecific	Stepped-care models with increasing specificity of diagnosis and intensity of treatment
Treatment based on brief counseling focused on patient-identified problems	"Common elements"
Links with community services, advice addressing family and social determinants	Peer and/or family navigators

Adapted from Wissow LS, van Ginneken N, Chandna J, Rahman A. Integrating children's mental health into primary care. *Pediatr Clin North Am.* 2016; 63(1):101.

TABLE 2 Common-Factors Approach: HELP Build a Therapeutic Alliance

H = Hope

    Hope facilitates coping. Increase the family's hopefulness by describing your realistic expectations for improvement and reinforcing the strengths and assets you see in the child and family. Encourage concrete steps toward whatever is achievable.

E = Empathy

    Communicate empathy by listening attentively, acknowledging struggles and distress, and sharing happiness experienced by the child and family.

L^2 = Language, Loyalty

    Use the child or family's own language (not a clinical label) to reflect your understanding of the problem as they see it and to give the child and family an opportunity to correct any misperceptions.

    Communicate loyalty to the family by expressing your support and your commitment to help now and in the future.

P^3 = Permission, Partnership, Plan

    Ask the family's permission for you to ask more in-depth and potentially sensitive questions or make suggestions for further evaluation or management.

    Partner with the child and family to identify any barriers or resistance to addressing the problem, find strategies to bypass or overcome barriers, and find agreement on achievable steps (or simply an achievable first step) aligned with the family's motivation. The more difficult the problem, the more important is the promise of partnership.

    On the basis of the child's and family's preferences and sense of urgency, establish a plan (or incremental first step) through which the child and family will take some action(s), work toward greater readiness to take action, or monitor the problem and follow-up with you. (The plan might include, eg, keeping a diary of symptoms and triggers, gathering information from other sources such as the child's school, making lifestyle changes, applying parenting strategies or self-management techniques, reviewing educational resources about the problem or condition, initiating specific treatment, seeking referral for further assessment or treatment, or returning for further family discussion.)

Adapted from Foy JM; American Academy of Pediatrics, Task Force on Mental Health. Enhancing pediatric mental health care: algorithms for primary care. *Pediatrics.* 2010;125(suppl 3): S110.

Certain evidence-based complementary and integrative medicine approaches may also lend themselves to brief interventions: for example, relaxation and other self-regulation therapies reveal promise in assisting children to manage stress and build their resilience to trauma and social adversities.[43] Other brief interventions include coaching parents in managing a particular behavior (eg, "time-out" for disruptive behavior[44]) or, more broadly, strategies to reduce stress in the household and to foster a sense of closeness and emotional security, for example, reading together,[45] sharing outdoor time,[46] or parent-child "special time"—a regularly scheduled period as brief as 5 to 10 minutes set aside for a one-on-one, interactive activity of the child's choice.[47] Self-help resources may also be useful (eg, online depression management).[48]

Encouragement of healthy habits, such as sufficient sleep (critically important to children's mental health and resilience as well as their parents'), family meals, active play, time and content limits on media exposure, and prosocial activities with peers can be used as "universal" brief interventions across an array of presenting problems as well as a means to promote mental wellness and resilience.[49]

For a more detailed summary of psychosocial interventions and the evidence supporting them, see PracticeWise Evidence-Based Child and Adolescent Psychosocial Interventions at www.aap.org/mentalhealth. Psychosocial interventions that have been studied in primary care are listed in Common Elements of Evidence-Based Practice Amenable to Primary Care: Indications and Sources at www.aap.

org/mentalhealth. With training, pediatricians can achieve competence in applying brief interventions such as these in primary care or, potentially, subspecialty settings.[37,50–52]

MENTAL HEALTH COMPETENCIES

The Accreditation Council for Graduate Medical Education has organized competencies into 6 domains: patient care, medical knowledge, interpersonal and communication skills, practice-based learning and improvement, professionalism, and systems-based practice.[53] We have used this framework to develop a detailed outline of pediatric mental health competencies for use by pediatric educators; this outline is available at www.aap.org/mentalhealth. Competencies most salient to this statement are listed in Tables 4 and 5.

TABLE 3 Most Frequently Appearing Common Elements in Evidence-Based Practices, Grouped by Common Presenting Problems in Pediatric Primary Care

Presenting Problem Area	Most Common Elements of Related Evidence-Based Practices
Anxiety	Graded exposure, modeling
ADHD and oppositional problems	Tangible rewards, praise for child and parent, help with monitoring, time-out, effective commands and limit setting, response cost
Low mood	Cognitive and/or coping methods, problem-solving strategies, activity scheduling, behavioral rehearsal, social skills building

Adapted from Wissow LS, van Ginneken N, Chandna J, Rahman A. Integrating children's mental health into primary care. *Pediatr Clin North Am.* 2016; 63(1):103.

Clinical Skills

All pediatricians need skills to promote mental health, efficiently perform psychosocial assessments, and provide primary and secondary preventive services (eg, anticipatory guidance, screening). They need to be able to triage for psychiatric emergencies (eg, suicidal or homicidal intent, psychotic thoughts) and social emergencies (eg, child abuse or neglect, domestic violence, other imminent threats to safety). Pediatricians need to be able to establish a therapeutic alliance with the patient and family and take initial action on any identified mental health and social concerns, as described above. All pediatricians also need to know how to organize the care of patients who require mental health specialty referral or consultation, facilitate transfer of trust to mental health specialists, and coordinate their patients' mental health care with other clinicians, reaching previous agreement on respective roles, such as who will prescribe and monitor medications and how communication will take place. The care team might include any of the individuals listed in Table 6, on- or off-site. For a discussion of collaborative care models that integrate services of mental health and pediatric professionals, see the accompanying technical report.[31]

The clinical role of the pediatrician will depend on the patient's condition and level of impairment, interventions and supports needed, patient and family priorities and preferences, pediatrician's self-perception of efficacy and capacity, and accessibility of community services.

TABLE 4 Core Pediatric Mental Health Competencies: Clinical Skills

Pediatricians providing care to children and adolescents can maximize the patient's and family's health, agency, sense of safety, respect, and partnership by developing competence in performing the following activities:

Promotion and primary prevention
  Promote healthy emotional development by providing anticipatory guidance on healthy lifestyles and stress management
  Routinely gather an age-appropriate psychosocial history, applying appropriate tools to assist with data gathering

Secondary prevention
  Identify and evaluate risk factors to healthy emotional development and emerging symptoms that could cause impairment or suggest future mental health problems, applying appropriate tools to assist with screening and refer to community resources when appropriate (ie, parenting programs)

Assessment
  Recognize mental health emergencies such as suicide risk, severe functional impairment, and complex mental health symptoms that require urgent mental health specialty care
  Analyze and interpret results from mental health screening, history, physical examination, and observations to determine what brief interventions may be useful and whether a full diagnostic assessment is needed
  Diagnose school-aged children and adolescents with the following disorders: ADHD, common anxiety disorders (separation anxiety disorder, social phobia, generalized anxiety disorder), depression, and substance use

Treatment
  Apply fundamental (common factors, motivational interviewing) communications skills to engage youth and families and overcome barriers to their help seeking for identified social and mental health problems
  Apply common-factors skills and common elements of evidence-based psychosocial treatments to initiate the care of the following:
    Children and youth with medical and developmental conditions who manifest comorbid mental health symptoms
    Depressed mothers and their children
    Infants and young children manifesting difficulties with communication and/or attachment or other signs and symptoms of emotional distress (eg, problematic sleep, eating behaviors)
    Children and adolescents presenting with the following:
      Anxious or avoidant behaviors
      Exposure to trauma or loss
      Impulsivity and inattention, with or without hyperactivity
      Low mood or withdrawn behaviors
      Disruptive or aggressive behaviors
      Substance use
      Learning difficulties
  When a higher level of care is needed for symptoms listed above, integrate patient and/or family strengths, needs, and preferences, the clinician's own skills, and available resources into development of a care plan for children and adolescents with mental health problem(s), alone, with the practice care team, or in collaboration with mental health specialists
  Demonstrate proficiency in selecting, prescribing, and monitoring (for response and adverse effects) ADHD medications and selective serotonin reuptake inhibitors that have a safety and efficacy profile appropriate to use in pediatric care
  Develop a contingency or crisis plan for a child or adolescent
  Develop a safety plan with patients and parents for children and adolescents who are suicidal and/or depressed
  Apply strategies to actively monitor adverse and positive effects of nonpharmacologic and pharmacologic therapy
  Facilitate a family's and patient's engagement with and transfer of trust (ie, "warm handoff") to a mental health professional
  Demonstrate an accurate understanding of privacy regulations
  Refer, collaborate, comanage, and participate as a team member in coordinating mental health care with specialists and in transitioning adolescents with mental health needs to adult primary care and mental health specialty providers

TABLE 5 Core Pediatric Mental Health Competencies: Practice Enhancements

Pediatricians providing care to children and adolescents can improve the quality of their practice's (and network's) mental health services by developing competence in performing the following activities

Establish collaborative and consultative relationships—within the practice, virtually, or off-site—and define respective roles in assessment, treatment, coordination of care, exchange of information, and family support

Build a practice team culture around a shared commitment to embrace mental health care as integral to pediatric practice and an understanding of the impact of trauma on child well-being

Establish systems within the practice (and network) to support mental health services; elements may include the following:

Preparation of office staff and professionals to create an environment of respect, agency, confidentiality, safety, and trauma-informed care;

Preparation of office staff and professionals to identify and manage patients with suicide risk and other mental health emergencies;

Electronic health record prompts and culturally and/or linguistically appropriate educational materials to facilitate offering anticipatory guidance and to educate youth and families on mental health and substance use topics and resources;

Routines for gathering the patient's and family's psychosocial history, conducting psychosocial and/or behavioral assessment;

Registries, evidence-based protocols, and monitoring and/or tracking mechanisms for patients with positive psychosocial screen results, adverse childhood experiences and social determinants of health, behavioral risks, and mental health problems;

Directory of mental health and substance use disorder referral sources, school-based resources, and parenting and family support resources in the region;

Mechanisms for coordinating the care provided by all collaborating providers through standardized communication; and

Tools for facilitating coding and billing specific to mental health.

Systematically analyze the practice by using quality improvement methods with the goal of mental health practice improvement

---

Disorders such as maladaptive aggression[54,55] and bipolar disorder[56] may require medications for which pediatricians will need specialized training or consultation from physician mental health specialists to prescribe (eg, antipsychotics, lithium). Comanagement—formally defined as "collaborative and coordinated care that is conceptualized, planned, delivered, and evaluated by 2 or more health care providers"[57]—is a successful approach for complex mental conditions in children and adolescents. Both general pediatricians and pediatric subspecialists will benefit from these collaborative skills. These skills also enable pediatricians to help adolescents with mental health conditions and their families transition the adolescent's care to adult primary and mental health specialty care at the appropriate time, as pediatricians do other patients with special health care needs.

Misperceptions about privacy regulations (eg, the Health Insurance Portability and Accountability Act of 1996,[58] federal statutes and regulations regarding substance abuse treatment [42 US Code § 290dd–2; 42 Code of Federal Regulations 2.11],[59] and state-specific regulations) often impede collaboration by limiting communication among clinicians who are providing services. In most instances, pediatricians are, in fact, allowed to exchange information with other clinicians involved in a patient's care, even without the patient or guardian's consent. Pediatricians need an accurate understanding of privacy regulations to ensure that all clinicians involved in the mutual care of a patient share information in an appropriate and timely way (see https://www.aap.org/en-us/advocacy-and-policy/aap-health-initiatives/Mental-Health/Pages/HIPAA-Privacy-Rule-and-Provider-to-Provider-Communication.aspx).

Other necessary clinical skills are specific to the age, presenting problem of the patient, and type of therapy required, as described in the following sections.

Infants and Preschool-aged Children

For infants and preschool-aged children, the signs and symptoms of emotional distress may be varied and nonspecific and may manifest themselves in the child, in the parent, or in their relationship. When consistently outside the range of normal development, these young children and families typically require specialized diagnostic assessment (based on the *Diagnostic Classification of Mental Health and Developmental*

TABLE 6 Potential Mental Health Care Team Members

Patient and family

One or more PCC

Any other pediatric team member who has forged a bond of trust with the family (eg, nurse, front desk staff, medical assistant)

Mental health medical consultant (eg, child psychiatrist, developmental-behavioral pediatrician, adolescent specialist, pediatric neurologist), directly involved or consulting with PCC by phone or telemedicine link

Psychologist, social worker, advanced practice nurse, substance use counselor, early intervention specialist, or other licensed specialist(s) trained in the relevant evidence-based psychosocial therapy

School-based professionals (eg, guidance counselor, social worker, school nurse, school psychologist)

Representative of involved social service agency

Medical subspecialist(s) or surgical specialist

Parent educator

Peer navigator

Care manager

PCC, primary care clinician.

Disorders of Infancy and Early Childhood[60]), intensive parenting interventions, and treatment by developmental-behavioral specialists or mental health specialists with expertise in early childhood. Consequently, pediatric mental health competencies for the care of this age group involve overcoming any barriers to referral, guiding the family in nurturing and stimulating the child, counseling on parenting and behavioral management techniques, referring for diagnostic assessment and dyadic (attachment-focused) therapy as indicated, and comanaging care. When social risk factors are identified (eg, maternal depression, poverty, food insecurity), the pediatrician's role is to connect the family to needed resources.

School-aged Children and Adolescents

The AAP Task Force on Mental Health identified common manifestations of mental health problems in school-aged children and adolescents as depression (low mood), anxious and avoidant behaviors, impulsivity and inattention (with or without hyperactivity), disruptive behavior and aggression, substance use, and learning difficulty and developed guidance to assist pediatric clinicians in addressing these problems.[61] Recognizing that 75% of children who need mental health services do not receive them, the AAP went on to publish a number of additional educational resources on these topics, specifically for pediatricians.[62–64] Additional tools are available online at www.aap.org/mentalhealth. Children and adolescents who have experienced trauma may manifest any combination of these symptoms.[65,66] Children and adolescents with an underlying mental condition may present with somatic symptoms (eg, headache, abdominal pain, chest pain, limb pain, fatigue) or eating abnormalities.[67,68] Furthermore, children and adolescents may experience impaired functioning at home, at school, or

with peers, even in the absence of symptoms that reach the threshold for a diagnosis.[2,69,70]

Once a pediatrician has identified a child or adolescent with 1 or more of these manifestations of a possible mental health condition (collectively termed "mental health concerns" in this statement, indicating that they are undifferentiated as to disorder, problem, or normal variation), the pediatrician needs skills to differentiate normal variations from problems from disorders and to diagnose, at a minimum, conditions for which evidence-based primary care assessment and treatment guidance exists—currently ADHD,[71] depression,[72,73] and substance use.[74] Pediatricians also need knowledge and skills to diagnose anxiety disorders, which are among the most common disorders of childhood, often accompany and adversely affect the care of chronic medical conditions, and when associated with no more than mild to moderate impairment, are often amenable to pediatric treatment.[66] A number of disorder-specific rating scales and functional assessment tools are applicable to use in pediatrics, both to assist in diagnosis and to monitor the response to interventions; these have been described and referenced in the document "Mental Health Tools for Pediatrics" at www.aap.org/mentalhealth.

Although the diagnostic assessment of children presenting with aggressive behaviors often requires mental health specialty involvement, pediatricians can use a stepwise approach to begin the assessment and offer guidance in selecting psychosocial interventions in the community for further diagnosis and treatment, as outlined in the guideline, "Treatment of Maladaptive Aggression in Youth (T-MAY)," available at www.ahrq.gov/sites/default/files/wysiwyg/chain/practice-tools/tmay-final.pdf.

Pharmacologic and Psychosocial Therapies

Many pharmacologic and psychosocial therapies have been proven effective in treating children with mental health disorders. Pharmacologic therapies may be more familiar to pediatricians than psychosocial therapies; however, psychosocial therapies, either alone or in combination with pharmacologic therapies, may be more effective in some circumstances. For example, American Academy of Child and Adolescent Psychiatry guidelines recommend at least 2 trials of psychosocial treatment before starting medication in young children up to 5 years of age.[75] Studies involving children and adolescents in several specific age groups have revealed the advantage of combined psychosocial and medication treatment over either type of therapy alone for ADHD in 7- to 9-year-old children,[76] common anxiety disorders in 7- to 9-year-old children,[77] and depression in 12- to 17-year-old children,[78] and benefits of combined therapy likely go well beyond these age groups. Furthermore, many children with mild or subthreshold anxiety or depression are likely to benefit from psychosocial therapy, mind-body approaches, and self-help resources without medication.[48,66,79] Although pediatricians may feel pressured to prescribe only medication in these and other situations because it is generally more accessible and/or expedient,[80] knowledge of these other approaches is necessary to offer children these choices. If needed community services are not available, pediatricians can use common-elements approaches in the pediatric office and advocate for evidence-based therapies to be offered by the mental health community.

Certain disorders (ADHD, common anxiety disorders, depression), if associated with no more than moderate impairment, are amenable to primary care medication management because there are indicated medications with a well-established safety profile (eg, a variety of ADHD medications and certain selective serotonin reuptake inhibitors).[81] Ideally, pediatric subspecialists would also be knowledgeable about these medications, their adverse effects, and their interactions with medications prescribed in their subspecialty practice. Necessary clinical skills are summarized in Table 4.

Practice Enhancements

Effective mental health care requires the support of office and network systems. Competencies requisite to establishing and sustaining these systems are outlined in Table 5.

PROGRESS TO DATE

Despite many efforts to enhance the competence of pediatric residents and practicing pediatricians (see accompanying technical report "Achieving the Pediatric Mental Health Competencies"[31]), change in mental health practice during the last decade has been modest, as measured by the AAP's periodic surveys of members. National data reveal that in 2013, only 57% of pediatricians were consistently treating ADHD and less than a quarter were treating any other disorder.[82] Although fewer barriers were reported in 2013 than in 2004, most pediatricians surveyed in 2013 reported that they had inadequate training in treating child mental health problems, a lack of confidence to counsel children, and limited time for these problems.[83]

In the accompanying technical report, we address the barriers of training and confidence.[31] The barrier of limited time for mental health care may one day become an artifact of volume-based care and the payment systems that have incentivized it. Value-based payment, expanded clinical care teams, and integration of

mental health care into pediatric settings may provide new incentives and opportunities for mental health practice, improve quality of care, and result in improved outcomes for both physical and mental health conditions. In the interim, the AAP recognizes that although the proposed competencies are necessary to meet the needs of children, pediatricians will necessarily achieve them through incremental steps that rely on improved third-party payment for their mental health services and access to expertise in mental health coding and billing to support the time required for mental health practice.

RECOMMENDATIONS

The recommendations that follow build on the 2009 policy statement[18] and assumptions drawn from review of available literature; the recognized, well-documented, and growing mental health needs of the pediatric population; expert opinion of the authoring bodies; and review and feedback by additional relevant AAP entities. There are striking geographic variations in access to pediatric mental health services from state to state and within states, from urban to rural areas.[84] By engaging in the kind of partnerships described in the first point below, pediatricians can prioritize their action steps and implement them, incrementally, in accordance with their community's needs. With the pediatric advantage in mind, the AAP recommends that pediatricians engage in the following:

partner with families, youth, and other child advocates; mental health, adolescent, and developmental specialists; teachers; early childhood educators; health and human service agency leaders; local and state chapters of mental health specialty organizations; and/or AAP chapter and national leaders with the goal of improving the organizational and financial base of mental health care, depending on

the needs of a particular community or practice; this might include such strategies as:

advocating with insurers and payers for appropriate payment to pediatricians and mental health specialists for their mental health services (see the Chapter Action Kit in Resources);

using appropriate coding and billing practices to support mental health services in a fee-for-service payment environment (see Chapter Action Kit in Resources);

participating in development of models of value-based and bundled payment for integrated mental health care (see the AAP Practice Transformation Web site in Resources); and/or

identifying gaps in key mental health services in their communities and advocating to address deficiencies (see Chapter Action Kit in Resources);

pursue quality improvement and maintenance of certification activities that enhance their mental health practice, prioritizing suicide prevention (see Quality Improvement and/or Maintenance of Certification in Resources);

explore collaborative care models of practice, such as integration of a mental health specialist as a member of the medical home team, consultation with a child psychiatrist or developmental-behavioral pediatrician, or telemedicine technologies that both enhance patients' access to mental health specialty care and grow the competence and confidence of involved pediatricians (see AAP Mental Health Web site in Resources);

build relationships with mental health specialists (including school-based providers) with whom they can collaborate in enhancing their mental health knowledge and skills, in identifying and providing emergency care to children and adolescents at risk for suicide, and in comanaging children with primary mental health conditions and physical conditions with mental health comorbidities (see Chapter Action Kit in Resources);

pursue educational strategies (eg, participation in a child psychiatry consultation network, collaborative office rounds, learning collaborative, miniature fellowship, AAP chapter, or health system network initiative) suited to their own learning style and skill level for incrementally achieving the mental health competencies outlined in Tables 4 and 5 (see accompanying technical report for in-depth discussion of educational strategies);

advocate for innovations in medical school education, residency and fellowship training, and continuing medical education activities to increase the knowledge base and skill level of future pediatricians in accordance with the mental health competencies outlined in Tables 4 and 5; and

promote and participate in research on the delivery of mental health services in pediatric primary care and subspecialty settings.

In the accompanying technical report,[31] we highlight successful educational initiatives and suggest promising strategies for achieving the mental health competencies through innovations in the training of medical students, pediatric residents, fellows, preceptors, and practicing pediatricians and through support in making practice enhancements.

CONCLUSIONS

The AAP recognizes pediatricians' unique opportunities to promote children's healthy socioemotional development, strengthen children's resilience to the many stressors that face them and their families, and recognize and address the mental health needs that emerge during childhood and adolescence. These opportunities flow from the pediatric advantage, which includes longitudinal, trusting, and empowering relationships with patients and their families and the nonstigmatizing, family friendliness of pediatric practices. Fully realizing this advantage will depend on pediatricians developing or honing their mental health knowledge and skills and enhancing their mental health practice. To that end, this statement outlines mental health competencies for pediatricians, incorporating evidence-based clinical approaches that are feasible within pediatrics, supported by collaborative relationships with mental health specialists, developmental-behavioral pediatricians, and others at both the community and practice levels.

Enhancements in pediatric mental health practice will also depend on system changes, new methods of financing, access to reliable sources of information about existing evidence and new science, decision support, and innovative educational methods (discussed in the accompanying technical report[31]). For this reason, attainment of the competencies proposed in this statement will, for most pediatricians, be achieved incrementally over time. Gains are likely to be substantial, including the improved well-being of children, adolescents, and families and enhanced satisfaction of pediatricians who care for them.

RESOURCES

AAP Clinical Tools and/or Tool Kits

AAP clinical tools and/or tool kits include the following:

Addressing Mental Health Concerns in Primary Care: A Clinician's Toolkit;

Health Insurance Portability and Accountability Act of 1996 Privacy Rule and Provider to Provider Communication;

Mental Health Initiatives Chapter Action Kit; and

AAP Coding Fact Sheets (AAP log-on required).

AAP Policies

AAP policies include the following:

ADHD: Clinical Practice Guideline for the Diagnosis, Evaluation, and Treatment of Attention-Deficit/ Hyperactivity Disorder in Children and Adolescents (November 2011);

Guidelines for Adolescent Depression in Primary Care (GLAD-PC): Part I. Practice Preparation, Identification, Assessment, and Initial Management (endorsed by the AAP March 2018);

Guidelines for Adolescent Depression in Primary Care (GLAD-PC): Part II. Treatment and Ongoing Management (endorsed by the AAP March 2018);

Policy Statement: Incorporating Recognition and Management of Perinatal and Postpartum Depression Into Pediatric Practice (January 2019);

Technical Report: Incorporating Recognition and Management of Perinatal and Postpartum Depression Into Pediatric Practice (January 2019);

Policy Statement: Early Childhood Adversity, Toxic Stress, and the Role of the Pediatrician: Translating Developmental Science Into Lifelong Health (January 2012; reaffirmed July 2016);

Technical Report: The Lifelong Effects of Early Childhood Adversity and Toxic Stress (January 2012; reaffirmed July 2016);

Clinical Report: Mind-Body Therapies in Children and Youth (September 2016);

The Prenatal Visit (July 2018);

Clinical Report: Promoting Optimal Development: Screening for

Behavioral and Emotional Problems (February 2015);

Policy Statement: Substance Use Screening, Brief Intervention, and Referral to Treatment (July 2016); and

Clinical Report: Substance Use Screening, Brief Intervention, and Referral to Treatment (July 2016).

Quality Improvement and/or Maintenance of Certification

Quality improvement and/or Maintenance of Certification resources include the following:

Education in Quality Improvement for Pediatric Practice: Bright Futures - Middle Childhood and Adolescence;

Education in Quality Improvement for Pediatric Practice: Substance Use - Screening, Brief Intervention, Referral to Treatment; and

American Board of Pediatrics Quality Improvement Web site.

AAP Publications

AAP publications include the following:

AAP Developmental Behavioral Pediatrics, Second Edition;

Mental Health Care of Children and Adolescents: A Guide for Primary Care Clinicians;

Promoting Mental Health in Children and Adolescents: Primary Care Practice and Advocacy;

Pediatric Psychopharmacology for Primary Care;

Quick Reference Guide to Coding Pediatric Mental Health Services 2019; and

Thinking Developmentally.

AAP Reports

AAP reports include the following:

Improving Mental Health Services in Primary Care: A Call to Action for the Payer Community (AAP log-on required); and

Reducing Administrative and Financial Barriers.

Web Sites

Web site resources include the following:

AAP Mental Health Web site;

AAP Practice Transformation Web site;

National Center for Medical Home Implementation;

The Resilience Project; and

Screening Technical Assistance and Resource Center.

Lead Authors

Jane Meschan Foy, MD, FAAP

Cori M. Green, MD, MS, FAAP

Marian F. Earls, MD, MTS, FAAP

Committee on Psychosocial Aspects of Child and Family Health, 2018–2019

Arthur Lavin, MD, FAAP, Chairperson

George LaMonte Askew, MD, FAAP

Rebecca Baum, MD, FAAP

Evelyn Berger-Jenkins, MD, FAAP

Thresia B. Gambon, MD, FAAP

Arwa Abdulhaq Nasir, MBBS, MSc, MPH, FAAP

Lawrence Sagin Wissow, MD, MPH, FAAP

Former Committee on Psychosocial Aspects of Child and Family Health Members

Michael Yogman, MD, FAAP, Former Chairperson

Gerri Mattson, MD, FAAP

Jason Richard Rafferty, MD, MPH, EdM, FAAP

Liaisons

Sharon Berry, PhD, ABPP, LP – *Society of Pediatric Psychology*

Edward R. Christophersen, PhD, FAAP – *Society of Pediatric Psychology*

Norah L. Johnson, PhD, RN, CPNP-BC – *National Association of Pediatric Nurse Practitioners*

Abigail Boden Schlesinger, MD – *American Academy of Child and Adolescent Psychiatry*

Rachel Shana Segal, MD – *Section on Pediatric Trainees*

Amy Starin, PhD – *National Association of Social Workers*

Mental Health Leadership Work Group, 2017–2018

Marian F. Earls, MD, MTS, FAAP, Chairperson

Cori M. Green, MD, MS, FAAP

Alain Joffe, MD, MPH, FAAP

Staff

Linda Paul, MPH

ABBREVIATIONS

AAP: American Academy of Pediatrics

ADHD: attention-deficit/hyperactivity disorder

---

*The term "mental" throughout this statement is intended to encompass "behavioral," "psychiatric," "psychological," "emotional," and "substance use" as well as family context and community-related concerns. Accordingly, factors affecting mental health include precipitants such as child abuse and neglect, separation or divorce of parents, domestic violence, parental or family mental health issues, natural disasters, school crises, military deployment of children's loved ones, incarceration of a loved one, and the grief and loss accompanying any of these issues or the illness or death of family members. Mental also is intended to encompass somatic manifestations of psychosocial issues, such as eating disorders and gastrointestinal symptoms. This use of the term is not to suggest that the full range or severity of all mental health conditions and concerns falls within the scope of pediatric practice but, rather, that children and adolescents may suffer from the full range and severity of mental health conditions and psychosocial stressors. As such, children with mental health needs, similar to children with special

physical and developmental needs, are children for whom pediatricians provide care in the medical home and in subspecialty practice.

DOI: https://doi.org/10.1542/peds.2019-2757

Address correspondence to Jane Meschan Foy, MD, FAAP. E-mail: foy.jane@gmail.com

PEDIATRICS (ISSN Numbers: Print, 0031-4005; Online, 1098-4275).

FINANCIAL DISCLOSURE: The authors have indicated they have no financial relationships relevant to this article to disclose.

FUNDING: No external funding.

POTENTIAL CONFLICT OF INTEREST: The authors have indicated they have no potential conflicts of interest to disclose.

REFERENCES

1. Perou R, Bitsko RH, Blumberg SJ, et al; Centers for Disease Control and Prevention (CDC). Mental health surveillance among children—United States, 2005-2011. *MMWR Suppl.* 2013; 62(2):1–35

2. Burns BJ, Costello EJ, Angold A, et al. Children's mental health service use across service sectors. *Health Aff (Millwood).* 1995;14(3):147–159

3. Copeland WE, Wolke D, Shanahan L, Costello EJ. Adult functional outcomes of common childhood psychiatric problems: a prospective, longitudinal study. *JAMA Psychiatry.* 2015;72(9): 892–899

4. Slomski A. Chronic mental health issues in children now loom larger than physical problems. *JAMA.* 2012;308(3): 223–225

5. Houtrow AJ, Larson K, Olson LM, Newacheck PW, Halfon N. Changing trends of childhood disability, 2001-2011. *Pediatrics.* 2014;134(3):530–538

6. Heron M. Deaths: Leading causes for 2016. National Vital Statistics Reports; Vol 67. *No 6.* Hyattsville, MD: National Center for Health Statistics. 2018. Available at: https://www.cdc.gov/nchs/data/nvsr/nvsr67/nvsr67_06.pdf. Accessed September 22, 2019

7. Suryavanshi MS, Yang Y. Clinical and economic burden of mental disorders among children with chronic physical conditions, United States, 2008-2013. *Prev Chronic Dis.* 2016;13:E71

8. Barlow JH, Ellard DR. The psychosocial well-being of children with chronic disease, their parents and siblings: an overview of the research evidence base. *Child Care Health Dev.* 2006;32(1):19–31

9. Perrin JM, Gnanasekaran S, Delahaye J. Psychological aspects of chronic health conditions. *Pediatr Rev.* 2012;33(3): 99–109

10. Hood KK, Beavers DP, Yi-Frazier J, et al. Psychosocial burden and glycemic control during the first 6 years of diabetes: results from the SEARCH for Diabetes in Youth study. *J Adolesc Health.* 2014;55(4):498–504

11. Shomaker LB, Tanofsky-Kraff M, Stern EA, et al. Longitudinal study of depressive symptoms and progression of insulin resistance in youth at risk for adult obesity. *Diabetes Care.* 2011; 34(11):2458–2463

12. Roy-Byrne PP, Davidson KW, Kessler RC, et al. Anxiety disorders and comorbid medical illness. *Gen Hosp Psychiatry.* 2008;30(3):208–225

13. American Academy of Child and Adolescent Psychiatry, Committee on Health Care Access and Economics Task Force on Mental Health. Improving mental health services in primary care: reducing administrative and financial barriers to access and collaboration. *Pediatrics.* 2009;123(4):1248–1251

14. Merikangas KR, He JP, Brody D, et al. Prevalence and treatment of mental disorders among US children in the 2001-2004 NHANES. *Pediatrics.* 2010; 125(1):75–81

15. Merikangas KR, He JP, Burstein M, et al. Service utilization for lifetime mental disorders in U.S. adolescents: results of the National Comorbidity Survey-Adolescent Supplement (NCS-A). *J Am Acad Child Adolesc Psychiatry.* 2011; 50(1):32–45

16. Whitney DG, Peterson MD. US national and state-level prevalence of mental health disorders and disparities of mental health care use in children. *JAMA Pediatr.* 2019;173(4):389–391

17. Anderson LE, Chen ML, Perrin JM, Van Cleave J. Outpatient visits and medication prescribing for US children with mental health conditions. *Pediatrics.* 2015;136(5). Available at: www.pediatrics.org/cgi/content/full/136/5/e1178

18. Committee on Psychosocial Aspects of Child and Family Health and Task Force on Mental Health. Policy statement--The future of pediatrics: mental health competencies for pediatric primary care. *Pediatrics.* 2009;124(1):410–421

19. Centers for Medicare & Medicaid Services (CMS), HHS. Medicaid and Children's Health Insurance Programs; Mental Health Parity and Addiction Equity Act of 2008; the application of mental health parity requirements to coverage offered by Medicaid managed care organizations, the Children's Health Insurance Program (CHIP), and alternative benefit plans. Final rule. *Fed Regist.* 2016;81(61):18389–18445

20. Cauchi R, Hanson K; National Conference of State Legislators. Mental health benefits: state laws mandating or regulating. 2015. Available at: www.ncsl.org/research/health/mental-health-benefits-state-mandates.aspx. Accessed September 8, 2017

21. Garner AS, Shonkoff JP; Committee on Psychosocial Aspects of Child and

Family Health; Committee on Early Childhood, Adoption, and Dependent Care; Section on Developmental and Behavioral Pediatrics. Early childhood adversity, toxic stress, and the role of the pediatrician: translating developmental science into lifelong health. *Pediatrics*. 2012;129(1). Available at: www.pediatrics.org/cgi/content/full/129/1/e224

22. Shonkoff JP, Garner AS; Committee on Psychosocial Aspects of Child and Family Health; Committee on Early Childhood, Adoption, and Dependent Care; Section on Developmental and Behavioral Pediatrics. The lifelong effects of early childhood adversity and toxic stress. *Pediatrics*. 2012;129(1). Available at: www.pediatrics.org/cgi/content/full/129/1/e232

23. McLaughlin KA, Greif Green J, Gruber MJ, et al. Childhood adversities and first onset of psychiatric disorders in a national sample of US adolescents. *Arch Gen Psychiatry*. 2012;69(11): 1151–1160

24. Levine ME, Cole SW, Weir DR, Crimmins EM. Childhood and later life stressors and increased inflammatory gene expression at older ages. *Soc Sci Med*. 2015;130:16–22

25. Council on Children with Disabilities and Medical Home Implementation Project Advisory Committee. Patient- and family-centered care coordination: a framework for integrating care for children and youth across multiple systems. *Pediatrics*. 2014;133(5). Available at: www.pediatrics.org/cgi/content/full/133/5/e1451

26. Croghan TW, Brown JD. *Integrating Mental Health Treatment Into the Patient Centered Medical Home*. Rockville, MD: Agency for Healthcare Research and Quality; 2010

27. Internal Revenue Service, Department of the Treasury; Employee Benefits Security Administration, Department of Labor; Centers for Medicare & Medicaid Services, Department of Health and Human Services. Final rules under the Paul Wellstone and Pete Domenici Mental Health Parity and Addiction Equity Act of 2008; technical amendment to external review for multi-state plan program. Final rules. *Fed Regist*. 2013;78(219):68239–68296

28. Leslie L; American Board of Pediatrics. Finding allies to address children's mental and behavioral needs. 2016. Available at: https://blog.abp.org/blog/finding-allies-address-childrens-mental-and-behavioral-needs. Accessed September 12, 2017

29. McMillan JA, Land M Jr, Leslie LK. Pediatric residency education and the behavioral and mental health crisis: a call to action. *Pediatrics*. 2017;139(1): e20162141

30. McMillan JA, Land ML Jr, Rodday AM, et al. Report of a joint Association of Pediatric Program Directors-American Board of Pediatrics workshop: Preparing Future Pediatricians for the Mental Health Crisis. *J Pediatr*. 2018; 201:285–291

31. Green CM, Foy JM, Earls MF; American Academy of Pediatrics, Committee on Psychosocial Aspects of Child and Family Health; Mental Health Leadership Work Group. Technical report: achieving the pediatric mental health competencies. *Pediatrics*. 2019;144(5): e20192758

32. Foy JM; American Academy of Pediatrics, Task Force on Mental Health. Enhancing pediatric mental health care: report from the American Academy of Pediatrics Task Force on Mental Health. Introduction. *Pediatrics*. 2010;125(suppl 3):S69–S74

33. Samsel C, Ribeiro M, Ibeziako P, DeMaso DR. Integrated behavioral health care in pediatric subspecialty clinics. *Child Adolesc Psychiatr Clin N Am*. 2017;26(4): 785–794

34. Bernal P. Hidden morbidity in pediatric primary care. *Pediatr Ann*. 2003;32(6): 413–418–422

35. Janssen JS. Medical trauma. Available at: https://www.socialworktoday.com/news/enews_0416_1.shtml. Accessed November 3, 2018

36. Marchette LK, Weisz JR. Practitioner Review: empirical evolution of youth psychotherapy toward transdiagnostic approaches. *J Child Psychol Psychiatry*. 2017;58(9):970–984

37. Wissow LS, van Ginneken N, Chandna J, Rahman A. Integrating children's mental health into primary care. *Pediatr Clin North Am*. 2016;63(1):97–113

38. Wissow L, Anthony B, Brown J, et al. A common factors approach to improving the mental health capacity of pediatric primary care. *Adm Policy Ment Health*. 2008;35(4):305–318

39. Wissow LS, Gadomski A, Roter D, et al. Improving child and parent mental health in primary care: a cluster-randomized trial of communication skills training. *Pediatrics*. 2008;121(2): 266–275

40. Chorpita BF, Daleiden EL, Weisz JR. Identifying and selecting the common elements of evidence based interventions: a distillation and matching model. *Ment Health Serv Res*. 2005;7(1):5–20

41. Chorpita BF, Daleiden EL, Park AL, et al. Child STEPs in California: a cluster randomized effectiveness trial comparing modular treatment with community implemented treatment for youth with anxiety, depression, conduct problems, or traumatic stress. *J Consult Clin Psychol*. 2017;85(1):13–25

42. Tynan WD, Baum R. *Adapting Psychosocial Interventions to Primary Care. Mental Health Care of Children and Adolescents: A Guide for Primary Care Clinicians*. Itasca, IL: American Academy of Pediatrics; 2018

43. Kemper KJ, Vora S, Walls R; Task Force on Complementary and Alternative Medicine; Provisional Section on Complementary, Holistic, and Integrative Medicine. American Academy of Pediatrics. The use of complementary and alternative medicine in pediatrics. *Pediatrics*. 2008; 122(6):1374–1386. Reaffirmed January 2013

44. Sanders MR, Bor W, Morawska A. Maintenance of treatment gains: a comparison of enhanced, standard, and self-directed Triple P-Positive Parenting Program. *J Abnorm Child Psychol*. 2007;35(6):983–998

45. High PC, Klass P; Council on Early Childhood. Literacy promotion: an essential component of primary care pediatric practice. *Pediatrics*. 2014; 134(2):404–409

46. Yogman M, Garner A, Hutchinson J, Hirsh-Pasek K, Golinkoff RM; Committee on Psychosocial Aspects of Child and Family Health; Council on Communications and Media. The power

of play: a pediatric role in enhancing development in young children. *Pediatrics*. 2018;142(3):e20182058

47. Howard BJ. Guidelines for Special Time. In: Jellinek M, Patel BP, Froehle MC, eds. *Bright Futures in Practice: Mental Health—Volume II. Tool Kit*. Arlington, VA: National Center for Education in Maternal and Child Health; 2002

48. van Straten A, Cuijpers P, Smits N. Effectiveness of a Web-based self-help intervention for symptoms of depression, anxiety, and stress: randomized controlled trial. *J Med Internet Res*. 2008;10(1):e7

49. Foy JM, ed. *Promoting Mental Health in Children and Adolescents: Primary Care Practice and Advocacy*. Itasca, IL: American Academy of Pediatrics; 2018

50. Weersing VR, Brent DA, Rozenman MS, et al. Brief behavioral therapy for pediatric anxiety and depression in primary care: a randomized clinical trial. *JAMA Psychiatry*. 2017;74(6): 571–578

51. Walkup JT, Mathews T, Green CM. Transdiagnostic behavioral therapies in pediatric primary care: looking ahead. *JAMA Psychiatry*. 2017;74(6):557–558

52. Leslie LK, Mehus CJ, Hawkins JD, et al. Primary health care: potential home for family-focused preventive interventions. *Am J Prev Med*. 2016;51(4 suppl 2): S106–S118

53. Accreditation Council on Graduate Medical Education. ACGME core competencies. Available at: https://www.ecfmg.org/echo/acgme-core-competencies.html. Accessed March 9, 2018

54. Knapp P, Chait A, Pappadopulos E, Crystal S, Jensen PS; T-MAY Steering Group. Treatment of maladaptive aggression in youth: CERT guidelines I. Engagement, assessment, and management. *Pediatrics*. 2012;129(6). Available at: www.pediatrics.org/cgi/content/full/129/6/e1562

55. Scotto Rosato N, Correll CU, Pappadopulos E, Chait A, Crystal S, Jensen PS; Treatment of Maladaptive Aggressive in Youth Steering Committee. Treatment of maladaptive aggression in youth: CERT guidelines II. Treatments and ongoing management. *Pediatrics*. 2012;129(6). Available at:

www.pediatrics.org/cgi/content/full/129/6/e1577

56. Shain BN; Committee on Adolescence. Collaborative role of the pediatrician in the diagnosis and management of bipolar disorder in adolescents. *Pediatrics*. 2012;130(6). Available at: www.pediatrics.org/cgi/content/full/130/6/e1725

57. Stille CJ. Communication, comanagement, and collaborative care for children and youth with special healthcare needs. *Pediatr Ann*. 2009; 38(9):498–504

58. American Academy of Pediatrics. Mental health initiatives: HIPAA privacy rule and provider to provider communication. Available at: https://www.aap.org/en-us/advocacy-and-policy/aap-health-initiatives/Mental-Health/Pages/HIPAA-Privacy-Rule-and-Provider-to-Provider-Communication.aspx. Accessed March 9, 2018

59. Office of the Federal Register. Confidentiality of substance use disorder patient records. Available at: https://www.federalregister.gov/documents/2017/01/18/2017-00719/confidentiality-of-substance-use-disorder-patient-records. Accessed March 9, 2018

60. Zero to Three. *DC:0-5 Diagnostic Classification of Mental Health and Developmental Disorders of Infancy and Early Childhood*. Washington, DC: Zero to Three; 1994. Available at: https://www.zerotothree.org/our-work/dc-0-5. Accessed November 1, 2017

61. American Academy of Pediatrics. *Addressing Mental Health Concerns in Primary Care: A Clinician's Toolkit*. Elk Grove Village, IL: American Academy of Pediatrics; 2010

62. Adam H, Foy J. *Signs and Symptoms in Pediatrics*. Elk Grove Village, IL: American Academy of Pediatrics; 2015

63. McInerny TK, Adam HM, Campbell DE, eds, et al. *Textbook of Pediatric Care*, 2nd ed. Elk Grove Village, IL: American Academy of Pediatrics; 2016

64. American Academy of Pediatrics. Pediatric care online. Available at: https://pediatriccare.solutions.aap.org/Pediatric-Care.aspx. Accessed November 3, 2018

65. Knapp P. The Iterative Mental Health Assessment. In: Foy JM, ed. *Mental Health Care of Children and Adolescents: A Guide for Primary Care Clinicians*, vol. Vol 1. Itasca, IL: American Academy of Pediatrics; 2010:pp 173–226

66. Wissow LS. Anxiety and Trauma-Related Distress. In: Foy JM, ed. *Mental Health Care of Children and Adolescents: A Guide for Primary Care Clinicians*, vol. Vol 1. Itasca, IL: American Academy of Pediatrics; 2018:pp 433–456

67. Baum R, Campo J. Medically Unexplained Symptoms. In: Foy JM, ed. *Mental Health Care of Children and Adolescents: A Guide for Primary Care Clinicians*, vol. Vol 1. Itasca, IL: American Academy of Pediatrics; 2018:pp 649–659

68. Schneider M, Fisher M. Eating Abnormalities. In: Foy JM, ed. *Mental Health Care of Children and Adolescents: A Guide for Primary Care Clinicians*, vol. Vol 1. Itasca, IL: American Academy of Pediatrics; 2018:pp 477–506

69. Angold A, Costello EJ, Farmer EM, Burns BJ, Erkanli A. Impaired but undiagnosed. *J Am Acad Child Adolesc Psychiatry*. 1999;38(2):129–137

70. Lewinsohn PM, Shankman SA, Gau JM, Klein DN. The prevalence and co-morbidity of subthreshold psychiatric conditions. *Psychol Med*. 2004;34(4): 613–622

71. Wolraich M, Brown L, Brown RT, et al; Subcommittee on Attention-Deficit/Hyperactivity Disorder; Steering Committee on Quality Improvement and Management. ADHD: clinical practice guideline for the diagnosis, evaluation, and treatment of attention-deficit/hyperactivity disorder in children and adolescents. *Pediatrics*. 2011;128(5): 1007–1022

72. Zuckerbrot RA, Cheung A, Jensen PS, Stein REK, Laraque D; GLAD-PC Steering Group. Guidelines for Adolescent Depression in Primary Care (GLAD-PC): part I. practice preparation, identification, assessment, and initial management. *Pediatrics*. 2018;141(3): e20174081

73. Cheung AH, Zuckerbrot RA, Jensen PS, Laraque D, Stein REK; GLAD-PC STEERING GROUP. Guidelines for Adolescent Depression in Primary Care (GLAD-PC): part II. Treatment and ongoing

management. *Pediatrics*. 2018;141(3): e20174082

74. Levy SJ, Williams JF; Committee on Substance Use and Prevention. Substance use screening, brief intervention, and referral to treatment. *Pediatrics*. 2016;138(1):e20161211

75. Gleason MM, Egger HL, Emslie GJ, et al. Psychopharmacological treatment for very young children: contexts and guidelines. *J Am Acad Child Adolesc Psychiatry*. 2007;46(12):1532–1572

76. The MTA Cooperative Group. Multimodal Treatment Study of Children with ADHD. A 14-month randomized clinical trial of treatment strategies for attention-deficit/hyperactivity disorder. *Arch Gen Psychiatry*. 1999;56(12):1073–1086

77. Walkup JT, Albano AM, Piacentini J, et al. Cognitive behavioral therapy, sertraline, or a combination in childhood anxiety. *N Engl J Med*. 2008;359(26):2753–2766

78. March J, Silva S, Petrycki S, et al; Treatment for Adolescents With Depression Study (TADS) Team. Fluoxetine, cognitive-behavioral therapy, and their combination for adolescents with depression: Treatment for Adolescents With Depression Study (TADS) randomized controlled trial. *JAMA*. 2004;292(7):807–820

79. Wissow LS. Low Mood. In: Foy JM, ed. *Mental Health Care of Children and Adolescents: A Guide for Primary Care Clinicians*, vol. Vol 1. Itasca, IL: American Academy of Pediatrics; 2018:pp 617–636

80. Smith BL. Inappropriate prescribing. *Monit Psychol*. 2012;43(6):36

81. Riddle MA, ed. *Pediatric Psychopharmacology for Primary Care*. Elk Grove Village, IL: American Academy of Pediatrics; 2015

82. Stein RE, Storfer-Isser A, Kerker BD, et al. Beyond ADHD: how well are we doing? *Acad Pediatr*. 2016;16(2):115–121

83. Horwitz SM, Storfer-Isser A, Kerker BD, et al. Barriers to the identification and management of psychosocial problems: changes from 2004 to 2013. *Acad Pediatr*. 2015;15(6):613–620

84. Hudson CG. Disparities in the geography of mental health: implications for social work. *Soc Work*. 2012;57(2):107–119

TECHNICAL REPORT

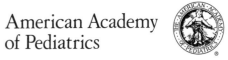

American Academy of Pediatrics

DEDICATED TO THE HEALTH OF ALL CHILDREN™

Achieving the Pediatric Mental Health Competencies

Cori M. Green, MD, MS, FAAP,[a] Jane Meschan Foy, MD, FAAP,[b] Marian F. Earls, MD, FAAP,[c] COMMITTEE ON PSYCHOSOCIAL ASPECTS OF CHILD AND FAMILY HEALTH, MENTAL HEALTH LEADERSHIP WORK GROUP

abstract

Mental health disorders affect 1 in 5 children; however, the majority of affected children do not receive appropriate services, leading to adverse adult outcomes. To meet the needs of children, pediatricians need to take on a larger role in addressing mental health problems. The accompanying policy statement, "Mental Health Competencies for Pediatric Practice," articulates mental health competencies pediatricians could achieve to improve the mental health care of children; yet, the majority of pediatricians do not feel prepared to do so. In this technical report, we summarize current initiatives and resources that exist for trainees and practicing pediatricians across the training continuum. We also identify gaps in mental health clinical experience and training and suggest areas in which education can be strengthened. With this report, we aim to stimulate efforts to address gaps by summarizing educational strategies that have been applied and could be applied to undergraduate medical education, residency and fellowship training, continuing medical education, maintenance of certification, and practice quality improvement activities to achieve the pediatric mental health competencies. In this report, we also articulate the research questions important to the future of pediatric mental health training and practice.

[a]Department of Pediatrics, Weill Cornell Medicine, Cornell University and New York–Presbyterian Hospital, New York, New York; [b]Department of Pediatrics, School of Medicine, Wake Forest University, Winston-Salem, North Carolina; and [c]Community Care of North Carolina, School of Medicine, University of North Carolina at Chapel Hill, Chapel Hill, North Carolina

All authors contributed to the drafting and revising of this manuscript and approved the final manuscript as submitted.

Technical reports from the American Academy of Pediatrics benefit from expertise and resources of liaisons and internal (AAP) and external reviewers. However, technical reports from the American Academy of Pediatrics may not reflect the views of the liaisons or the organizations or government agencies that they represent.

The guidance in this report does not indicate an exclusive course of treatment or serve as a standard of medical care. Variations, taking into account individual circumstances, may be appropriate.

All technical reports from the American Academy of Pediatrics automatically expire 5 years after publication unless reaffirmed, revised, or retired at or before that time.

DOI: https://doi.org/10.1542/peds.2019-2758

Address correspondence to Cori M. Green, MD, MS, FAAP. E-mail: cmg9004@med.cornell.edu

PEDIATRICS (ISSN Numbers: Print, 0031-4005; Online, 1098-4275).

To cite: Green CM, Foy JM, Earls MF, AAP COMMITTEE ON PSYCHOSOCIAL ASPECTS OF CHILD AND FAMILY HEALTH, MENTAL HEALTH LEADERSHIP WORK GROUP. Achieving the Pediatric Mental Health Competencies. Pediatrics. 2019; 144(5):e20192758

INTRODUCTION

Mental health disorders have surpassed physical conditions as the most common reasons children have impairments and limitations.[1] Mental health disorders affect 1 in 5 children; however, a shortage of mental health specialists, stigma, cost, and other barriers prevent the majority of affected children from receiving appropriate services.[2–4] Pediatricians have unique opportunities and a growing sense of responsibility to promote healthy social-emotional development of children and to prevent and address their mental health and substance use problems. In 2009, the American Academy of Pediatrics (AAP) published a policy statement proposing mental health competencies for pediatric primary care and recommended steps toward achieving them.[5] The policy statement

"Mental Health Competencies for Pediatric Practice,"[6] accompanying this technical report, affirms and, importantly, provides updates to incorporate new science on early brain development, to articulate the pediatrician's role in addressing social determinants of health and trauma, and to consider mental health practice in subspecialty, as well as primary care, settings.

Currently, the majority of pediatricians do not feel prepared to achieve these mental health competencies.[7,8] Furthermore, more than half of pediatric program directors (PDs) surveyed in 2011 were unaware of the 2009 competencies, making it unlikely that training programs have enhanced their curriculum to prepare future pediatricians to achieve them.[9] With this technical report, we aim to stimulate efforts to address these gaps by summarizing educational strategies that have been applied and could be applied to undergraduate medical education, residency and fellowship training, continuing medical education (CME), maintenance of certification, and quality improvement activities to achieve the pediatric mental health competencies proposed in the accompanying policy statement. This report also articulates research questions important to the future of pediatric mental health training and practice.

HISTORY

Deficiencies in mental health training have been recognized for more than 4 decades, and in the 1980s, the AAP first called for improved education of pediatricians in the care of children with psychosocial and mental health problems.[10,11] Pediatric trainees and graduates since the 1980s report feeling less prepared to care for these children than they do children with other pediatric conditions.[12,13] Surveys over 3 decades have

documented little change in their reported preparedness, despite the considerable efforts described below.[14–16]

In 1997, the Accreditation Council for Graduate Medical Education (ACGME) mandated that all pediatric residency programs include a 4-week developmental-behavioral pediatrics (DBP) rotation.[17] Completion of all 4 weeks of this rotation has had a positive effect on pediatricians' self-reported competence, practices, and willingness to accept responsibility for providing mental health care.[18,19] However, change in mental health practice has been modest, as measured by the AAP's periodic surveys of members, and mental health training is still not emphasized during residency and is considered to be suboptimal per PDs.[8,9,20,21] Advances in science have continued to demonstrate the interplay between the environment—particularly the child's social environment—and both physical and mental health; the pervasiveness of environmental influence makes it evident that mental health training needs to expand beyond a single rotation. Well-meaning efforts to address deficiencies in mental competencies by requiring DBP rotations and/or offering clinical rotations in psychiatry may have the unintended consequence of implying that mental health is primarily the domain of DBP subspecialists or child psychiatrists.[22] Ideally, mental health content and practice experiences would be integrated throughout the pediatric curriculum, during both inpatient and outpatient experiences, conveying the message that mental health competencies are integral to all aspects of pediatric practice.

AAP RESPONSES

In response to the needs of practicing pediatricians, the AAP Task Force on Mental Health (2004–2010) published a supplement to

Pediatrics[23] describing the rationale for enhancing pediatric mental health care, offering community-level and practice-level strategies to support enhanced pediatric mental health care, and presenting algorithms for integrating mental health care into the flow of primary care pediatric practice. The task force also published *Addressing Mental Health Concerns in Primary Care: A Clinician's Toolkit*,[24] providing an array of pragmatic tools to assess a practice's capacity for providing mental health care, to build capacity when needed, and to operationalize the process laid out in the supplement. Also, within this toolkit, symptom "cluster" guidance offered a pragmatic clinical approach to addressing the common symptom constellations faced in pediatrics: anxiety, low mood, disruptive behavior and aggression, inattention and impulsivity, substance use, learning difficulty, and social-emotional symptoms in young children. This guidance has subsequently been incorporated into several publications of the AAP: *Signs and Symptoms in Pediatrics*,[25] *Textbook of Pediatric Care, Second Edition*,[26] *Pediatric Care Online*,[27] and *Mental Health Care of Children and Adolescents: A Guide for Primary Care Clinicians*.[28] The AAP has also published or endorsed clinical guidelines, reports, or statements guiding the assessment and management of attention-deficit/hyperactivity disorder (ADHD),[29] depression,[30,31] maladaptive aggression,[32,33] early social-emotional problems,[34] early childhood trauma and toxic stress,[35] and substance use.[36]

The AAP Mental Health Leadership Work Group (2011 to present), in collaboration with other AAP groups, has offered additional resources: a set of videos on using motivational interviewing (MI) to address mental health problems, e-mail notification about new publications relevant to pediatric mental health, Webinars, a curriculum and course for continuity clinic preceptors (see below), and a Web site with mental health resources.[37,38] Unfortunately, dissemination and evaluation of these approaches remain a challenge, and the mental health toolkit and other materials created to help pediatricians integrate mental health into their practice have not reached the majority of pediatricians.[39,40]

RESPONSES OF ACCREDITING BODIES

Improving training and competence in mental health care for future pediatricians—subspecialists as well as primary care pediatricians—has increasingly received national attention and is now a priority of the American Board of Pediatrics (ABP).[41,42] In 2013, the ACGME and ABP created the "Pediatric Milestones Project" to assess incremental achievement of pediatric competencies across the career span, from novice to expert.[43] Seventeen entrustable professional activities (EPAs)—professional units of work that define a specialty—were developed for general pediatrics.[44,45] A number of EPAs have implications for mental health care, and one—number 9—specifically states that the general pediatrician should be able to "assess and manage patients with common behavior/mental health problems."[45] This EPA lists the following functions expected of the pediatrician: (1) identify and manage common behavioral/mental health issues, (2) refer and/or comanage patients with appropriate specialist(s), (3) know mental health resources available in one's community, (4) know team member roles and/or monitor care, and (5) provide developmentally and culturally sensitive care. This EPA reinforces many of the mental health competencies from the 2009 AAP statement[5] and the accompanying policy statement "Mental Health Competencies for Pediatric Practice."

Pediatric medical subspecialty practices are at times the de facto medical home for children with chronic conditions who are at a higher risk than their peers for mental health problems.[46,47] However, subspecialists often focus on their organ system, and studies have revealed that subspecialists are not routinely inquiring about psychosocial and mental health problems in children with chronic medical conditions or referring them for mental health care.[48,49] Promisingly, the majority of PDs agree that all trainees, regardless of future career plans, need to be competent in identifying, referring, and comanaging children with mental health problems. However, only half of PDs believe trainees going into a subspecialty should be responsible for mental health treatment.[42]

PURPOSE OF THIS REPORT

With this report, we identify gaps in mental health clinical experience and education across the training continuum and describe innovative strategies created and/or tested to improve pediatricians' ability to care for children with mental health problems. As reflected in the material below, efforts to date have been focused mainly on pediatric residency training programs and CME efforts.

PROMISING APPROACHES ACROSS THE EDUCATIONAL CONTINUUM

Undergraduate Medical Education

Currently, the Liaison Committee on Medical Education includes communication skills as 1 of the 9 mandated areas of content.[50] Although there are no specifications as to which skills should be taught and how, medical school curricula offer opportunities to enhance physician-patient communication and professionalism. The first step in addressing any mental health concern is to engage the family and build a therapeutic relationship by using

communication skills such as MI and a "common-factors" approach, which builds on MI (see Discussion in accompanying policy statement[6]). These skills (eg, building hope, providing empathy, partnering with families, rolling with resistance, managing conflict) are necessary in all aspects of patient care and should be emphasized and taught throughout the continuum of medical education, starting with medical school.

It is essential that medical students choosing pediatrics be aware of and be prepared for their role in caring for pediatric mental health problems. The Council on Medical Student Education in Pediatrics does include pediatric behavior in its third-year competencies and objectives.[51] However, whether this is emphasized and whether preceptors model the provision of care to children with mental health problems during pediatric rotations is unknown. These questions should be addressed in further study.

Graduate Medical Education

As of 2013, 68% of practicing pediatricians reported receiving no training in MI during residency training, and more than half reported receiving no training in other interviewing techniques.[19] Until medical schools consistently provide this training, residency programs will need to provide it and ensure trainees' competence in these skills, and regardless of when it is introduced, preceptors will need to model and reinforce evidence-based communication skills.[21,42] Unfortunately, only 20% of PDs currently report that their residents receive optimal training in common-factors communication skills.[21]

It is promising that most residents believe they are responsible for identifying and referring children with mental health problems, yet few believe they are responsible for treating them.[52] In the unified theory of health behavior change, intention is what is most predictive of behavior,[53] yet for trainees and practicing pediatricians, perceived responsibility does not always lead to practicing in a way that is consistent with that perception.[18,54] This discrepancy between intent and practice is likely the result of a learning environment that does not provide the teaching and support needed to practice the requisite skills.[54,55] Trainees request experiential learning opportunities to care for children with mental health problems.[55] This request aligns with principles of andragogy (ie, to build self-efficacy, the clinical learning environment must provide opportunities to learn and practice skills guided by knowledgeable clinicians who can role model and demonstrate these skills).[56]

In response, educational interventions have included not only curriculum development but also a variety of instructional methods: role plays,[38] videos,[57,58] standardized patients (SPs),[59,60] and training alongside mental health professionals and trainees.[52,61,62] Successful interventions have used multimodal approaches, allowing trainees to gain knowledge and practice skills. Specifically, Fallucco et al[59] demonstrated that interns who received instruction using both didactics and SP trainings had increased knowledge and confidence in assessing for suicide compared with trainees who received only the lecture, those who received only the SP training, or controls who did not receive either of these experiences. Jee et al[60] had similar results combining case-based didactics with the use of SPs, leading to increased confidence among trainees in use of anxiety screening tools and later practices in performing a warm handoff (ie, an in-person, facilitated transfer of care from the trainee to another provider).

Additional examples highlight important caveats. One institution

created a multimodal instructional approach using role plays, cases, and SPs on screening for substance use, brief intervention, and referral to treatment, which increased trainees' knowledge and confidence in the screening technique; however, these gains declined over time.[63] Another institution successfully implemented a multimodal curriculum for addressing substance use using screening, brief intervention, and referral to treatment while also creating an assessment tool to measure performance. Residents improved in patient-centered discussions and identifying motives and plans when practicing skills with SPs.[64] At another institution, the combination of computer modules and SPs to teach how to assess and diagnose depression improved trainees' interpersonal skills, diagnostic skills, and confidence in treatment of depression; however, gaps in history taking and assessment for comorbidities remained.[65] These findings reinforce the need for ongoing assessment of trainees' skills and, importantly, their practice of skills to supplement curricular efforts.

As an attempt to stimulate mental health training nationally, the AAP created a curriculum and training for pediatric continuity clinic preceptors and trainees in the common-factors approach.[38] This curriculum was created with various teaching modalities, including videos and role plays, with flexibility in implementation so that it can be adapted regardless of program characteristics. A faculty guide was included as an attempt to provide guidance for preceptors who may not have learned these concepts already. The curriculum has been disseminated by the AAP online and at national meetings as an attempt to train preceptors to deliver the modules. However, this curriculum has yet to be evaluated, and the

majority of PDs are not familiar with the contents of the AAP curriculum.[40]

Trainees have stated that the most effective way they will learn to provide mental health care is for their own pediatric preceptors to model the mental health practices,[55] yet many pediatricians, including continuity preceptors, do not feel competent to serve as role models for mental health practice.[8,20,55] As an attempt to fill this gap, more than half of residency continuity clinics have an on-site developmental-behavioral pediatrician, social worker, child psychiatrist, psychologist, or other mental health specialist.[21,42] Although the role of these mental health specialists is not clear and likely varies between sites, PDs and residents trained in clinics with enhanced mental health services do report increased confidence and competence in systems-based practice and in coordinating and collaborating with mental health specialists.[9,52,61,62]

One study revealed that residents training on-site with mental health professionals were more likely to identify and refer patients with ADHD and reported that having the support of an on-site professional made them more comfortable to delve into their patients' problems.[52] However, as stated in the accompanying policy statement, pediatricians should be able to manage common mental health problems themselves, and having an on-site mental health provider has not been shown to increase trainees' practice of treating mental health problems. It is necessary to clarify the role of on-site mental health professionals as teachers rather than simply referral sources; their purpose is to increase the knowledge and skills of trainees and preceptors rather than offer them a way to avoid caring for mental health issues that are within pediatricians' scope of practice. Further study is needed to delineate how an on-site mental health professional can best impact practices because there are currently no financial structures to support them as preceptors without direct patient care responsibilities.

Study of successful integrated models has underscored the importance of preparing behavioral health providers to work within a primary care culture —for example, accommodating interruptions for consultation, participating in interdisciplinary meetings for peer-to-peer problem solving, and allowing unscheduled time for collaboration with other team members on unanticipated behavioral health issues.[66] Educational resources, including well-developed competencies, are available to guide mental health/ substance use professionals in serving as primary care team members, comanagers, or consultants.[67] Some psychiatry residency programs and a number of other mental health professional programs have started training licensed mental health trainees in integrated programs (ie, programs that combine mental health and primary care services in a single site).[68,69] One innovative program providing interdisciplinary training is the "buddy system," in which pediatric and mental health trainees were paired to teach skills in integration and collaboration; its premise is that interdisciplinary team meetings help clinicians from different backgrounds to develop and understand each other's work and services.[70] Impacts of this program are currently unknown, but it will likely lead to improved skills in collaboration between primary care pediatricians and mental health specialists. In 1 pediatric residency program, having pediatric and mental health trainees see patients in the same clinic has improved collaboration skills.[71]

The ACGME requires 6 months of individualized learning for pediatric residents; because subspecialty-bound residents are likely to focus on their future subspecialty during this time, this requirement may result in their receiving less training in caring for mental health problems.[72] Currently, the ACGME guidelines for subspecialty training in pediatrics do specify communication and interpersonal skills that are expected of all fellows, regardless of specialty, including working and collaborating as a team member, but there is no mention of providing fully integrated care that would include addressing psychosocial and mental health concerns.[73] Many pediatric subspecialty clinics incorporate a mental health professional as a team member, and there is likely some crossfertilization of the fellows and subspecialists who participate in these models; however, the mental health professional typically has a clinical rather than an educational role and is often stretched thin with inpatient duties.[49] Additional research is needed to address how best to prepare future specialists to integrate mental health care into their practice.

The need to improve pediatric graduates' training in mental health has been established, and the initiatives discussed above reveal promise. However, at this point, evaluation of educational interventions has mainly been limited to self-reported confidence, competence, and practices.[18,19,52] More assessment tools to measure competence are needed to evaluate the impact of educational innovations.[42] It will also be important to study actual practices and patient outcomes related to educational interventions.

Education of Experienced Clinicians

Educational efforts have successfully reached experienced pediatricians, building on skills they have developed over years of working with children and families. For instance, Wissow et al[74] have demonstrated that experienced primary care clinicians (PCCs) can acquire common-factors skills (described in the accompanying policy statement and above) and that the skills are helpful across a range of mental health conditions.[75,76] Children treated by PCCs trained in the common-factors techniques have shown modest but significant improvement in mental health functioning, and their parents have shown reduction in distress compared with children treated by clinicians who did not receive this training.[75,76]

Practicing pediatricians often feel that treating mental health problems is outside their scope of practice and often report that they do not have time to effectively implement psychosocial interventions.[8,18] Brief interventions that pediatricians can learn readily and implement in a short time period may offer a solution. See the accompanying policy statement for a full discussion.[6] Research will be necessary to develop and hone strategies for training residents and fellows in these approaches.

Several groups of mental health educators have successfully developed comprehensive training and CME programs to prepare mental health specialists and primary care professionals for their respective roles in collaborative practice.[77–79] The AAP is collecting information about such trainings on its Mental Health Initiatives Web site (https://www.aap.org/en-us/advocacy-and-policy/aap-health-initiatives/Mental-Health/Pages/Collaborative-Projects.aspx). The following are several examples:

The Resource for Advancing Children's Health Institute offers a 3-day mini-fellowship for primary care physicians using active learning methods to teach how to improve skills in recognition, diagnosis, and treatment of children with mental health disorders. This is followed by 6 months of biweekly case conferences. This program has changed physicians' practice patterns, as measured by an increase in the quality of referrals and a decrease in emergency department referrals, both of which can lead to decreased health care costs.[80] In New York, Project Training and Education for the Advancement of Children's Health uses the Resource for Advancing Children's Health mini-fellowship to train primary care physicians and offers a telepsychiatry consult line for support in diagnosis and management and to help find appropriate referrals. This program has trained more than 600 primary care physicians and consulted on over 8000 children and adolescents using telepsychiatry. Trained physicians felt more confident in addressing mental health problems with their patients and were motivated by the supportive and positive interactions with mental health specialists.[77,81]

In Massachusetts, a regional network of child psychiatrists offering real-time telephone consultation and referral to PCCs in Massachusetts enhanced the capacity of PCCs to care for children with diagnostic comorbidity, complicated ADHD, anxiety, and depression.[82–85] The Massachusetts Child Psychiatry Access Program has the resources to provide consultation and care coordination to 95% of the state's children, and in 2013, it had already served more than 10 500 children.[86] This program has been well received by pediatricians and now has expanded to offer support for mothers with depression.[87] At least 27 states have such consultation networks.[88] Congress authorized Pediatric Mental Health Care Access grants (§10002) that are modeled after the Massachusetts Child Psychiatry Access Program to support the development of new or improvement of existing pediatric

mental health care telehealth access programs.[89]

Clinicians may also work toward enhancing mental health competence in maintenance of certification by using such quality improvement programs as Education in Quality Improvement for Pediatric Practice, AAP chapter-led quality improvement learning collaboratives, and development of relevant pay-for-performance and quality indicators for health plans. A growing number of educational resources developed by the AAP, the ABP, the American Academy of Family Physicians, the National Association of Pediatric Nurse Practitioners, the American Psychiatric Association, the National Association of Social Workers, the American Academy of Child and Adolescent Psychiatry, and the American Psychological Association are available on each organization's Web site.

Even when practicing pediatricians acquire the knowledge and skills needed to integrate mental health into primary care, time and other practice barriers (culture, processes) may impede intentions from becoming practices. Building Mental Wellness was a state initiative developed by the Ohio Chapter of the AAP as a way to engage practices and primary care physicians in integrating mental health.[90] This initiative successfully taught physicians skills in prevention, identification, and management of mental health problems using online educational sessions. Importantly, this program also addressed organizational climate, culture, and care processes. Study of uptake of this program revealed that practice organization and culture were associated with the uptake of interventions, suggesting that education alone will not transform pediatricians' practices, but focus on office processes, culture, and climate is needed as well.[91]

The American Medical Association has suggested 10 steps to improve office culture including first diagnosing team culture by using measurement tools and brainstorming improvements and creating processes to improve teamwork and communication to change a practice's culture.[92] As discussed in the policy statement, thinking of a mental health concern (eg, inattention and impulsivity) similarly to fever may help clarify processes: an initial visit to assess severity and offer symptomatic care (antipyretic for fever or brief common-elements intervention such as helping parents apply effective behavioral management techniques for inattention and impulsivity), follow-up visits and further assessment possibly using objective measures if symptoms persist (a complete blood cell count for fever or a rating scale such as the Vanderbilt to assess for ADHD), targeted treatment if a diagnosis is made (antibiotics for a pneumonia or stimulants and behavioral therapy for ADHD), and referral if first-line treatment fails and/or severity worsens (the emergency department for respiratory distress or mental health specialist for complicated ADHD).

The AAP mental health toolkit, as mentioned previously, offers tools to support mental health processes in practices. Other tools have been developed and studied, such as a brief intervention for anxiety using an anxiety action plan.[93] Study of this tool, which is comparable to an asthma action plan, has shown it to be feasibly implemented into primary care and helpful in reducing children's symptoms. Maternal depression screening was successfully implemented into practice in North Carolina by Community Care of North Carolina through a guided Maintenance of Certification Part 4 activity that reached over 100 PCCs (www.

communitycarenc.org). Outreach by regional quality improvement coordinators in 14 regions across the state and "1-pagers" for practices resulted in high rates of implementation of perinatal depression screening (87% at all 1-month well visits, as of quarter 4, 2018). Technical assistance to practices included use of the screening tool, support resources for mothers, evidence-based dyadic therapies, referral, and follow-up. Similar progress has been seen with adolescent depression screening. Lastly, approaching mental health concerns through a stepwise approach as described through the AAP algorithm (see accompanying policy statement) can make it more feasible to implement in busy practices.

Expansion of the medical home team to include a mental health provider is financially feasible in some payment environments and clinically beneficial to patients and families.[94–97] In addition, it offers PCCs the benefit of crossdisciplinary learning through experiences such as collaborative care planning, clinical problem solving, and comanagement of patients with mental health morbidities and comorbidities.[98–100] These integrated models of care in which a licensed mental health specialist is on-site in a primary care practice have shown promise in improving access to mental health care for patients, improving patient functioning and productivity, and improving patient and provider satisfaction.[94,100–103] The majority of mental health care is provided during well-child visits and spans the continuum from promotion, to screening, to initiation of medications.[28] However, simply placing a mental health specialist on-site in pediatric practices may not necessarily enhance pediatricians' own mental health skills or practice; the roles of both the mental health specialist and pediatrician(s) must be well thought out and clear to avoid

inappropriate referral to the on-site mental health specialist of patients ideally managed by the PCC.[104] In addition, there are barriers to sustaining integrated models of care in fee-for-service plans because productivity of the mental health professional is variable.[102,105] As mentioned in the accompanying policy statement, systems changes are needed for pediatricians to achieve the proposed mental health competencies.

For some subspecialties, guidelines have specified inclusion of a mental health professional as a team member. For example, the International Society for Pediatric and Adolescent Diabetes "Clinical Practice Consensus Guidelines 2014" for care of children and adolescents with type 1 diabetes mellitus state "Resources should be made available to include professionals with expertise in the mental health and behavioral health of children and adolescents within the interdisciplinary diabetes health care team. These mental health specialists should include psychologists, social workers, and psychiatrists."[106] A recent supplement to *Pediatric Blood and Cancer* outlined 15 evidence-based standards for the psychosocial care of children with hematologic and oncologic conditions and their families, including 1 on integrating a mental health team member.[107] Even when such standards exist, however, there is no assurance that an integrated model can be implemented or sustained in a given clinical setting.[108] Additional research is needed to assess whether these models of care better integrate mental health into the care of children with chronic physical conditions.

PROMISING DIRECTIONS

Achieving the proposed competencies will require new educational approaches and evaluation of their

effectiveness, as well as significant enhancement in the interest and competence of pediatric faculty members who serve as teachers and role models. On the basis of experiences described above and the opinion of experts, the following strategies seem most promising and are offered here for the consideration of pediatric educators:

- prioritize training in common-factors communication skills for all pediatric faculty and for learners at all levels;
- incorporate the mental health competencies into curricular objectives, as described in the ABP EPA number 9, "assess and manage patients with common behavior/mental health problems,"[45] in accordance with the level of training;
- incorporate the promotion of healthy social-emotional development into the residency curriculum, including reinforcing strengths in the child and family and identifying risks to healthy social-emotional development and emerging symptoms to prevent or mitigate impairment from future mental health symptoms;
- prepare medical educators and preceptors to model, teach, and assess mental health competencies;
- consider including mental health specialists and/or developmental specialists as copreceptors and team members in teaching clinics (both general pediatric and subspecialty), inpatient rounds, and other clinical teaching settings, taking care to ensure that learners participate in mental health care, not just refer to specialists;
- consider incorporating trainees in psychology, social work, child psychiatry, DBP, and other specialties as team members in continuity and subspecialty clinics;
- consider addition of clinical experience(s) in child psychiatry to pediatric residency programs,

either as a block rotation or, preferably, a longitudinal experience;

- monitor their learners' success in achieving the mental health competencies and ensure ongoing opportunities to practice skills; and

- participate in and/or support research to answer such questions as:

- ○ What do medical students know about the role pediatricians play and will play in caring for children with mental health problems?

- ○ How much exposure is there during the pediatric clerkship to mental health promotion, primary and secondary prevention, and care of pediatric mental health problems?

- ○ What are the best educational strategies to change attitudes and encourage the pediatric community that mental health care is within their scope of practice?

- ○ What are the most effective ways to teach foundational communication skills to inexperienced as well as experienced clinicians?

- ○ How can common elements of evidence-based psychosocial treatments be most effectively adapted for pediatric practice? What impact do they have? How can they be incorporated into residency training and CME?

- ○ Which competencies are most relevant to subspecialty pediatric practice and therefore necessary to residency and/or fellowship training?

- ○ How can achievement of competence in providing mental health care be assessed within the context of residency and fellowship training?

- ○ How can practicing subspecialists be engaged in enhancing their mental health practice and improving coordination with PCCs and mental health specialists

around the mental health needs of their patients?

- ○ Which collaborative models are most effective with respect to outcomes for children? Which are most effective for enhancing pediatricians' competence?

- ○ How can pediatricians not currently able or motivated to enhance their mental health competence or practice best be engaged?

- ○ Will better preparing pediatricians to care for mental health problems in their practice improve the mental health care of children and reduce the societal burden of untreated mental health problems?

CONCLUSIONS

Attainment of the mental health competencies proposed in the accompanying AAP policy statement will require innovative educational methods and research as described in this report. Significant enhancement in pediatric faculty competence, medical education, pediatric residency and fellowship training, and practicing pediatricians' own educational efforts will also be needed, along with effective assessment methods to document learners' progress toward achieving the competencies. These changes will continue to require investments by the AAP and its partner organizations, pediatric educators, and pediatricians working at both the community and practice levels.

AAP RESOURCES

Clinical Tools and/or Tool Kits

AAP clinical tools and/or tool kits include the following:

Addressing Mental Health Concerns in Primary Care: A Clinician's Toolkit;

Common Elements;

Hope, Empathy, Loyalty, Language, Permission, Partnership, Plan ("HELP") mnemonic;

Mental Health Algorithm; and

Mental Health Symptom Cluster Guidance.

Education, Training Materials, and/or Videos

AAP education, training materials, and/or videos include the following:

Mental Health Residency Curriculum; and

Implementing Mental Health Priorities in Practice video series.

PUBLICATIONS AND/OR BOOKS

AAP publications and/or books include the following:

Developmental Behavioral Pediatrics;

Mental Health Care of Children and Adolescents: A Guide for Primary Care Clinicians; and

Pediatric Psychopharmacology for Primary Care.

Reports

AAP reports include the report "Reducing Administrative and Financial Barriers."

Web Site

Web site resources include the AAP mental health Web site.

LEAD AUTHORS

Cori M. Green, MD, MS, FAAP

Jane Meschan Foy, MD, FAAP

Marian F. Earls, MD, FAAP

COMMITTEE ON PSYCHOSOCIAL ASPECTS OF CHILD AND FAMILY HEALTH, 2018–2019

Arthur Lavin, MD, FAAP, Chairperson

George LaMonte Askew, MD, FAAP

Rebecca Baum, MD, FAAP

Evelyn Berger-Jenkins, MD, FAAP

Thresia B. Gambon, MD, FAAP

Arwa Abdulhaq Nasir, MBBS, MSc, MPH, FAAP

Lawrence Sagin Wissow, MD, MPH, FAAP

FORMER COMMITTEE ON PSYCHOSOCIAL ASPECTS OF CHILD AND FAMILY HEALTH MEMBERS

Michael Yogman, MD, FAAP, Former Chairperson

Gerri Mattson, MD, FAAP

Jason Richard Rafferty, MD, MPH, EdM, FAAP

LIAISONS

Sharon Berry, PhD, ABPP, LP – *Society of Pediatric Psychology*

Edward R. Christophersen, PhD, FAAP – *Society of Pediatric Psychology*

Norah L. Johnson, PhD, RN, CPNP-BC – *National Association of Pediatric Nurse Practitioners*

Abigail Boden Schlesinger, MD – *American Academy of Child and Adolescent Psychiatry*

Rachel Shana Segal, MD – *Section on Pediatric Trainees*

Amy Starin, PhD – *National Association of Social Workers*

MENTAL HEALTH LEADERSHIP WORK GROUP, 2017–2018

Marian F. Earls, MD, FAAP, Chairperson

Cori M. Green, MD, MS, FAAP

Alain Joffe, MD, MPH, FAAP

STAFF

Linda Paul, MPH

ABBREVIATIONS

AAP: American Academy of Pediatrics
ABP: American Board of Pediatrics
ACGME: Accreditation Council for Graduate Medical Education
ADHD: attention-deficit/hyperactivity disorder
CME: continuing medical education
DBP: developmental-behavioral pediatrics
EPA: entrustable professional activity
MI: motivational interviewing
PCC: primary care clinician
PD: program director
SP: standardized patient

FINANCIAL DISCLOSURE: The authors have indicated they have no financial relationships relevant to this article to disclose.

FUNDING: No external funding.

POTENTIAL CONFLICT OF INTEREST: The authors have indicated they have no potential conflicts of interest to disclose.

REFERENCES

1. Halfon N, Houtrow A, Larson K, Newacheck PW. The changing landscape of disability in childhood. *Future Child.* 2012;22(1):13–42

2. American Academy of Child and Adolescent Psychiatry, Committee on Health Care Access and Economics Task Force on Mental Health. Improving mental health services in primary care: reducing administrative and financial barriers to access and collaboration. *Pediatrics.* 2009;123(4): 1248–1251

3. Merikangas KR, He JP, Brody D, et al. Prevalence and treatment of mental disorders among US children in the 2001-2004 NHANES. *Pediatrics.* 2010; 125(1):75–81

4. Merikangas KR, He JP, Burstein M, et al. Service utilization for lifetime mental disorders in U.S. adolescents: results of the National Comorbidity Survey-Adolescent Supplement (NCS-

A). *J Am Acad Child Adolesc Psychiatry.* 2011;50(1):32–45

5. Committee on Psychosocial Aspects of Child and Family Health; Task Force on Mental Health. Policy statement—the future of pediatrics: mental health competencies for pediatric primary care. *Pediatrics.* 2009;124(1):410–421

6. Foy JM, Green CM, Earls MF; Committee on Psychosocial Aspects of Child and Family Health; Mental Health Leadership Work Group. Mental health competencies for pediatric practice. *Pediatrics.* 2019;144(5):e20192757

7. Fox HB, McManus MA, Klein JD, et al. Adolescent medicine training in pediatric residency programs. *Pediatrics.* 2010;125(1):165–172

8. Horwitz SM, Storfer-Isser A, Kerker BD, et al. Barriers to the identification and management of psychosocial problems: changes from 2004 to 2013. *Acad Pediatr.* 2015;15(6):613–620

9. Green C, Hampton E, Ward MJ, Shao H, Bostwick S. The current and ideal state of mental health training: pediatric program director perspectives. *Acad Pediatr.* 2014;14(5): 526–532

10. Haggerty RJ. The changing role of the pediatrician in child health care. *Am J Dis Child.* 1974;127(4):545–549

11. Green M, Brazelton TB, Friedman DB, et al; American Academy of Pediatrics Committee on Psychosocial Aspects of Child and Family Health. Pediatrics and the psychosocial aspects of child and family health. *Pediatrics.* 1982;70(1): 126–127

12. Burns BJ, Scott JE, Burke JD Jr, Kessler LG. Mental health training of primary care residents: a review of recent literature (1974-1981). *Gen Hosp Psychiatry.* 1983;5(3):157–169

13. Dworkin PH, Shonkoff JP, Leviton A, Levine MD. Training in developmental

pediatrics. How practitioners perceive the gap. *Am J Dis Child*. 1979;133(7):709–712

14. Freed GL, Dunham KM, Switalski KE, Jones MD Jr, McGuinness GA; Research Advisory Committee of the American Board of Pediatrics. Recently trained general pediatricians: perspectives on residency training and scope of practice. *Pediatrics*. 2009;123(suppl 1):S38–S43

15. Camp BW, Gitterman B, Headley R, Ball V. Pediatric residency as preparation for primary care practice. *Arch Pediatr Adolesc Med*. 1997;151(1):78–83

16. Rosenberg AA, Kamin C, Glicken AD, Jones MD Jr. Training gaps for pediatric residents planning a career in primary care: a qualitative and quantitative study. *J Grad Med Educ*. 2011;3(3):309–314

17. Coury DL, Berger SP, Stancin T, Tanner JL. Curricular guidelines for residency training in developmental-behavioral pediatrics. *J Dev Behav Pediatr*. 1999;20(suppl 2):S1–S38

18. Horwitz SM, Caspary G, Storfer-Isser A, et al. Is developmental and behavioral pediatrics training related to perceived responsibility for treating mental health problems? *Acad Pediatr*. 2010;10(4):252–259

19. Stein RE, Storfer-Isser A, Kerker BD, et al. Does length of developmental behavioral pediatrics training matter? *Acad Pediatr*. 2017;17(1):61–67

20. Stein RE, Storfer-Isser A, Kerker BD, et al. Beyond ADHD: how well are we doing? *Acad Pediatr*. 2016;16(2):115–121

21. Shahidullah JD, Kettlewell PW, Palejwala MH, et al. Behavioral health training in pediatric residency programs: a national survey of training directors. *J Dev Behav Pediatr*. 2018;39(4):292–302

22. Stein RE. Are we on the right track? Examining the role of developmental behavioral pediatrics. *Pediatrics*. 2015;135(4):589–591

23. Foy JM; American Academy of Pediatrics Task Force on Mental Health. Enhancing pediatric mental health care: algorithms for primary care. *Pediatrics*. 2010;125(suppl 3):S109–S125

24. American Academy of Pediatrics. *Addressing Mental Health Concerns in Primary Care: A Clinician's Toolkit*. Elk Grove Village, IL: American Academy of Pediatrics; 2010

25. Adam H, Foy J. *Signs and Symptoms in Pediatrics*. Elk Grove Village, IL: American Academy of Pediatrics; 2015

26. McInerny TK, Adam HM, Campbell DE, eds, et al. *Textbook of Pediatric Care*, 2nd ed. Elk Grove Village, IL: American Academy of Pediatrics; 2016

27. American Academy of Pediatrics. Pediatric care online. Available at: https://pediatriccare.solutions.aap.org/Pediatric-Care.aspx. Accessed November 3, 2018

28. Foy JM. *Mental Health Care of Children and Adolescents: A Guide for Primary Care Clinicians*. Itasca, IL: American Academy of Pediatrics; 2018

29. Wolraich ML, Hagan JF Jr., Allan C, et al; Subcommittee on Children and Adolescents With Attention-Deficit/Hyperactive Disorder. Clinical practice guideline for the diagnosis, evaluation, and treatment of attention-deficit/hyperactivity disorder in children and adolescents. *Pediatrics*. 2019;144(4):e20192528

30. Zuckerbrot RA, Cheung A, Jensen PS, Stein REK, Laraque D; GLAD-PC Steering Group. Guidelines for Adolescent Depression in Primary Care (GLAD-PC): part I. Practice preparation, identification, assessment, and initial management. *Pediatrics*. 2018;141(3):e20174081

31. Cheung AH, Zuckerbrot RA, Jensen PS, Laraque D, Stein REK; GLAD-PC Steering Group. Guidelines for Adolescent Depression in Primary Care (GLAD-PC): part II. Treatment and ongoing management. *Pediatrics*. 2018;141(3):e20174082

32. Knapp P, Chait A, Pappadopulos E, Crystal S, Jensen PS; T-MAY Steering Group. Treatment of maladaptive aggression in youth: CERT guidelines I. Engagement, assessment, and management. *Pediatrics*. 2012;129(6). Available at: www.pediatrics.org/cgi/content/full/129/6/e1562

33. Scotto Rosato N, Correll CU, Pappadopulos E, et al; Treatment of Maladaptive Aggressive in Youth Steering Committee. Treatment of maladaptive aggression in youth: CERT guidelines II. Treatments and ongoing management. *Pediatrics*. 2012;129(6). Available at: www.pediatrics.org/cgi/content/full/129/6/e1577

34. Gleason MM, Goldson E, Yogman MW; Council on Early Childhood; Committee on Psychosocial Aspects of Child and Family Health; Section on Developmental and Behavioral Pediatrics. Addressing early childhood emotional and behavioral problems. *Pediatrics*. 2016;138(6):e20163025

35. Garner AS, Shonkoff JP; Committee on Psychosocial Aspects of Child and Family Health; Committee on Early Childhood, Adoption, and Dependent Care; Section on Developmental and Behavioral Pediatrics. Early childhood adversity, toxic stress, and the role of the pediatrician: translating developmental science into lifelong health. *Pediatrics*. 2012;129(1). Available at: www.pediatrics.org/cgi/content/full/129/1/e224

36. Levy SJ, Williams JF; Committee on Substance Use and Prevention. Substance use screening, brief intervention, and referral to treatment. *Pediatrics*. 2016;138(1):e20161211

37. American Academy of Pediatrics. Mental health initiatives: implementing mental health priorities in practice. Available at: https://www.aap.org/en-us/advocacy-and-policy/aap-health-initiatives/Mental-Health/Pages/implementing_mental_health_priorities_in_practice.aspx. Accessed May 17, 2019

38. American Academy of Pediatrics. Mental health initiatives: residency curriculum. Available at: https://www.aap.org/en-us/advocacy-and-policy/aap-health-initiatives/Mental-Health/Pages/Residency-Curriculum.aspx. Accessed May 17, 2019

39. Garner AS, Storfer-Isser A, Szilagyi M, et al. Promoting early brain and child development: perceived barriers and the utilization of resources to address them. *Acad Pediatr*. 2017;17(7):697–705

40. Green C. Mental health initiatives. In: Association of Pediatric Program Directors 2017 Annual Spring Meeting Pre-Meeting Workshop: The Behavioral/Mental Health Crisis: Preparing Future Pediatricians to Meet the Challenge: April 5, 2017; Anaheim, CA. Available at:

https://www.appd.org/home/pdf/ABP_APPD_Training_Behavioral_Mental_Health.pdf. Accessed September 27, 2019

41. McMillan JA, Land M Jr, Leslie LK. Pediatric residency education and the behavioral and mental health crisis: a call to action. *Pediatrics.* 2017;139(1): e20162141

42. McMillan JA, Land ML Jr, Rodday AM, et al. Report of a joint association of pediatric program directors-American Board of Pediatrics workshop: preparing future pediatricians for the mental health crisis. *J Pediatr.* 2018; 201:285–291

43. Hicks PJ, Englander R, Schumacher DJ, et al. Pediatrics milestone project: next steps toward meaningful outcomes assessment. *J Grad Med Educ.* 2010; 2(4):577–584

44. Ten Cate O, Chen HC, Hoff RG, et al. Curriculum development for the workplace using Entrustable Professional Activities (EPAs): AMEE guide No. 99. *Med Teach.* 2015;37(11): 983–1002

45. American Board of Pediatrics. Entrustable professional activities for general pediatrics. 2016. Available at: https://www.abp.org/entrustable-professional-activities-epas. Accessed May 23, 2019

46. Boat TF, Land ML Jr, Leslie LK. Health care workforce development to enhance mental and behavioral health of children and youths. *JAMA Pediatr.* 2017;171(11):1031–1032

47. Perrin JM, Gnanasekaran S, Delahaye J. Psychological aspects of chronic health conditions. *Pediatr Rev.* 2012;33(3): 99–109

48. Green C, Stein REK, Storfer-Isser A, et al. Do subspecialists ask about and refer families with psychosocial concerns? A comparison with general pediatricians. *Matern Child Health J.* 2019;23(1):61–71

49. Samsel C, Ribeiro M, Ibeziako P, DeMaso DR. Integrated behavioral health care in pediatric subspecialty clinics. *Child Adolesc Psychiatr Clin N Am.* 2017;26(4): 785–794

50. Liaison Committee on Education. *Functions and Structure of a Medical School: Standards for Accreditation of Medical Education Programs Leading to the MD Degree.* Washington, DC: Association of American Medical Colleges and American Medical Association; 2018

51. Council on Medical Student Education in Pediatrics. Curricular competencies and objectives. 2017. Available at: https://www.comsep.org/curriculum-competencies-and-objectives/ Accessed September 27, 2019

52. Ragunanthan B, Frosch EJ, Solomon BS. On-site mental health professionals and pediatric residents in continuity clinic. *Clin Pediatr (Phila).* 2017;56(13): 1219–1226

53. Guilamo-Ramos V, Jaccard J, Dittus P, Collins S. Parent-adolescent communication about sexual intercourse: an analysis of maternal reluctance to communicate. *Health Psychol.* 2008;27(6):760–769

54. Green C. How can we use education to improve the mental health of today's children? In: Association of Pediatric Program Directors 2017 Annual Spring Meeting Pre-Meeting Workshop: The Behavioral/Mental Health Crisis: Preparing Future Pediatricians to Meet the Challenge: April 5, 2017; Anaheim, CA. Available at: https://www.appd.org/home/pdf/ABP_APPD_Training_Behavioral_Mental_Health.pdf. Accessed September 27, 2019

55. Hampton E, Richardson JE, Bostwick S, Ward MJ, Green C. The current and ideal state of mental health training: pediatric resident perspectives. *Teach Learn Med.* 2015;27(2):147–154

56. Kaufman DM. Applying educational theory in practice. *BMJ.* 2003;326(7382): 213–216

57. Bauer NS, Sullivan PD, Hus AM, Downs SM. Promoting mental health competency in residency training. *Patient Educ Couns.* 2011;85(3): e260–e264

58. Kutner L, Olson CK, Schlozman S, et al. Training pediatric residents and pediatricians about adolescent mental health problems: a proof-of-concept pilot for a proposed national curriculum. *Acad Psychiatry.* 2008;32(5): 429–437

59. Fallucco EM, Hanson MD, Glowinski AL. Teaching pediatric residents to assess adolescent suicide risk with a standardized patient module. *Pediatrics.* 2010;125(5):953–959

60. Jee SH, Baldwin C, Dadiz R, Jones M, Alpert-Gillis L. Integrated mental health training for pediatric and psychology trainees using standardized patient encounters. *Acad Pediatr.* 2018;18(1): 119–121

61. Garfunkel LC, Pisani AR, leRoux P, Siegel DM. Educating residents in behavioral health care and collaboration: comparison of conventional and integrated training models. *Acad Med.* 2011;86(2):174–179

62. Bunik M, Talmi A, Stafford B, et al. Integrating mental health services in primary care continuity clinics: a national CORNET study. *Acad Pediatr.* 2013;13(6):551–557

63. Schram P, Harris SK, Van Hook S, et al. Implementing adolescent Screening, Brief Intervention, and Referral to Treatment (SBIRT) education in a pediatric residency curriculum. *Subst Abus.* 2015;36(3):332–338

64. Ryan S, Pantalon MV, Camenga D, Martel S, D'Onofrio G. Evaluation of a pediatric resident skills-based screening, brief intervention and referral to treatment (SBIRT) curriculum for substance use. *J Adolesc Health.* 2018;63(3):327–334

65. Lewy C, Sells CW, Gilhooly J, McKelvey R. Adolescent depression: evaluating pediatric residents' knowledge, confidence, and interpersonal skills using standardized patients. *Acad Psychiatry.* 2009;33(5):389–393

66. Cohen DJ, Davis MM, Hall JD, Gilchrist EC, Miller BF. *A Guidebook of Professional Practices for Behavioral Health and Primary Care Integration: Observations From Exemplary Sites.* Rockville, MD: Agency for Healthcare Research and Quality; 2015

67. Miller BF, Gilchrist EC, Ross KM, Wong SL, Blount A, Peek CJ. Core competencies for behavioral health providers working in primary care. 2016. Available at: http://farleyhealthpolicycenter.org/wp-content/uploads/2016/02/Core-Competencies-for-Behavioral-Health-Providers-Working-in-Primary-Care.pdf. Accessed May 17, 2019

68. Burkey MD, Kaye DL, Frosch E. Training in integrated mental health-primary care models: a national survey of child psychiatry program directors. *Acad Psychiatry*. 2014;38(4):485–488

69. Zomorodi M, de Saxe Zerden L, Alexander L, Nance-Floyd B; Healthcare PROMISE team. Engaging students in the development of an interprofessional population health management course. *Nurse Educ*. 2017; 42(1):5–7

70. Moran M. Innovative 'buddy system' teaches collaboration. *Psychiatr News*. 2014;49(9). Available at: https://psychnews.psychiatryonline.org/doi/10.1176/appi.pn.2014.5a15/. Accessed May 17, 2019

71. Pisani AR, leRoux P, Siegel DM. Educating residents in behavioral health care and collaboration: integrated clinical training of pediatric residents and psychology fellows. *Acad Med*. 2011;86(2):166–173

72. Accreditation Council on Graduate Medical Education. ACGME core competencies. Available at: https://www.ecfmg.org/echo/acgme-core-competencies.html. Accessed March 9, 2018

73. Accreditation Council on Graduate Medical Education. ACGME program requirements for graduate medical education in the subspecialties of pediatrics. 2016. Available at: https://www.acgme.org/Portals/0/PFAssets/ProgramRequirements/CPRFellowship2019.pdf Accessed September 27, 2019

74. Wissow LS, Gadomski A, Roter D, et al. Improving child and parent mental health in primary care: a cluster-randomized trial of communication skills training. *Pediatrics*. 2008;121(2):266–275

75. Wissow LS, Brown JD, Krupnick J. Therapeutic alliance in pediatric primary care: preliminary evidence for a relationship with physician communication style and mothers' satisfaction. *J Dev Behav Pediatr*. 2010; 31(2):83–91

76. Wissow L, Anthony B, Brown J, et al. A common factors approach to improving the mental health capacity of pediatric primary care. *Adm Policy Ment Health*. 2008;35(4):305–318

77. Gadomski AM, Wissow LS, Palinkas L, et al. Encouraging and sustaining integration of child mental health into primary care: interviews with primary care providers participating in Project TEACH (CAPES and CAP PC) in NY. *Gen Hosp Psychiatry*. 2014;36(6):555–562

78. Integrated Primary Care. The portal to information and tools for the integration of behavioral health and primary care. Available at: https://sites.google.com/view/integratedprimarycare2/training. Accessed September 27, 2019

79. The Resource for Advancing Children's Health Institute. Child and adolescent training institute in evidence-based psychotherapies (CATIE). Available at: www.thereachinstitute.org/services/for-healthcare-organizations/staff-training/child-adolescent-training-in-evidence-based-psychotherapies-catie-1. Accessed March 26, 2019

80. McCaffrey ESN, Chang S, Farrelly G, Rahman A, Cawthorpe D. Mental health literacy in primary care: Canadian Research and Education for the Advancement of Child Health (CanREACH). *Evid Based Med*. 2017; 22(4):123–131

81. Kaye DL, Fornari V, Scharf M, et al. Description of a multi-university education and collaborative care child psychiatry access program: New York State's CAP PC. *Gen Hosp Psychiatry*. 2017;48:32–36

82. Dvir Y, Wenz-Gross M, Jeffers-Terry M, Metz WP. An assessment of satisfaction with ambulatory child psychiatry consultation services to primary care providers by parents of children with emotional and behavioral needs: the Massachusetts Child Psychiatry Access Project University of Massachusetts parent satisfaction study. *Front Psychiatry*. 2012;3:7

83. Massachusetts Child Psychiatry Access Project. Available at: www.mcpap.org. Accessed March 26, 2019

84. Sarvet B, Gold J, Bostic JQ, et al. Improving access to mental health care for children: the Massachusetts Child Psychiatry Access Project. *Pediatrics*. 2010;126(6):1191–1200

85. Van Cleave J, Le TT, Perrin JM. Point-of-care child psychiatry expertise: the Massachusetts Child Psychiatry Access Project. *Pediatrics*. 2015;135(5):834–841

86. Straus JH, Sarvet B. Behavioral health care for children: the Massachusetts Child Psychiatry Access Project. *Health Aff (Millwood)*. 2014;33(12):2153–2161

87. Byatt N, Biebel K, Moore Simas TA, et al. Improving perinatal depression care: the Massachusetts Child Psychiatry Access Project for Moms. *Gen Hosp Psychiatry*. 2016;40:12–17

88. National Network of Child Psychiatry Access Programs. Available at: http://web.jhu.edu/pedmentalhealth/nncpap_members.html. Accessed September 27, 2019

89. Health Resources and Services Administration. Pediatric Mental Health Care Access Program. Available at: https://www.hrsa.gov/grants/fundingopportunities/default.aspx?id=f1fe7b69-4d80-4a92-a3e8-aecee0fbbdee. Accessed March 26, 2019

90. American Academy of Pediatrics Ohio Chapter. Building mental wellness. Available at: http://ohioaap.org/projects/building-mental-wellness/. Accessed March 26, 2019

91. King MA, Wissow LS, Baum RA. The role of organizational context in the implementation of a statewide initiative to integrate mental health services into pediatric primary care. *Health Care Manage Rev*. 2018;43(3):206–217

92. Association Medical Association. Team culture: strengthen team cohesion and engagement. 2015. Available at: https://edhub.ama-assn.org/steps-forward/module/2702515. Accessed March 26, 2019

93. Ginsburg GS, Drake K, Winegrad H, Fothergill K, Wissow L. An open trial of the Anxiety Action Plan (*AxAP*): a brief pediatrician-delivered intervention for anxious youth. *Child Youth Care Forum*. 2016;45(1):19–32

94. Asarnow JR, Rozenman M, Wiblin J, Zeltzer L. Integrated medical-behavioral care compared with usual primary care for child and adolescent behavioral health: a meta-analysis. *JAMA Pediatr*. 2015;169(10):929–937

95. Richardson LP, McCarty CA, Radovic A, Suleiman AB. Research in the integration of behavioral health for adolescents and young adults in

primary care settings: a systematic review. *J Adolesc Health.* 2017;60(3): 261–269

96. Kaplan-Sanoff M, Talmi A, Augustyn M. Infusing mental health services into primary care for very young children and their families. *Zero Three.* 2012; 33(2):73–77

97. Talmi A, Fazio E. Commentary: promoting health and well-being in pediatric primary care settings: using health and behavior codes at routine well-child visits. *J Pediatr Psychol.* 2012; 37(5):496–502

98. Greene CA, Ford JD, Ward-Zimmerman B, Honigfeld L, Pidano AE. Strengthening the coordination of pediatric mental health and medical care: piloting a collaborative model for freestanding practices. *Child Youth Care Forum.* 2016;45(5):729–744

99. Pidano AE, Marcaly KH, Ihde KM, Kurowski EC, Whitcomb JM. Connecticut's enhanced care clinic initiative: early returns from pediatric-behavioral health partnerships. *Fam Syst Health.* 2011;29(2):138–143

100. Talmi A, Muther EF, Margolis K, et al. The scope of behavioral health integration in a pediatric primary care setting. *J Pediatr Psychol.* 2016;41(10): 1120–1132

101. Blount A, ed. *Integrated Primary Care: The Future of Medical and Mental Health Collaboration.* New York, NY: W. W. Norton and Company, Inc; 1998

102. Kolko DJ, Perrin E. The integration of behavioral health interventions in children's health care: services, science, and suggestions. *J Clin Child Adolesc Psychol.* 2014;43(2):216–228

103. Williams J, Shore SE, Foy JM. Co-location of mental health professionals in primary care settings: three North Carolina models. *Clin Pediatr (Phila).* 2006;45(6):537–543

104. Horwitz S, Storfer-Isser A, Kerker BD, et al. Do on-site mental health professionals change pediatricians' responses to children's mental health problems? *Acad Pediatr.* 2016;16(7): 676–683

105. Ader J, Stille CJ, Keller D, et al. The medical home and integrated behavioral health: advancing the policy agenda. *Pediatrics.* 2015;135(5):909–917

106. Delamater AM, de Wit M, McDarby V, Malik J, Acerini CL; International Society for Pediatric and Adolescent Diabetes. ISPAD Clinical Practice Consensus Guidelines 2014. Psychological care of children and adolescents with type 1 diabetes. *Pediatr Diabetes.* 2014; 15(suppl 20):232–244

107. Wiener L, Kazak AE, Noll RB, Patenaude AF, Kupst MJ. Standards for the psychosocial care of children with cancer and their families: an introduction to the special issue. *Pediatr Blood Cancer.* 2015;62(suppl 5): S419–S424

108. Freeman DS, Hudgins C, Hornberger J. Legislative and policy developments and imperatives for advancing the Primary Care Behavioral Health (PCBH) model. *J Clin Psychol Med Settings.* 2018;25(2):210–223

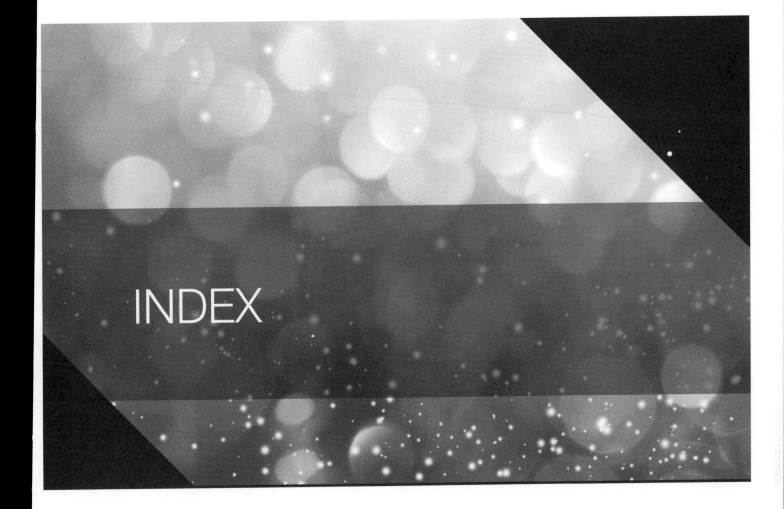

Page numbers followed by *f* indicate a figure.
Page numbers followed by *t* indicate a table.